Updates on Neonatal Chronic Lung Disease

Updates on Neonatal Chronic Lung Disease

Edited by

SUHAS G. KALLAPUR, MD
Professor of Pediatrics
Chief, Divisions of Neonatology and Developmental Biology
David Geffen School of Medicine at UCLA
UCLA Mattel Children's Hospital
Los Angeles, California

GLORIA S. PRYHUBER, MD
Professor
Pediatrics and Environmental Medicine
University of Rochester Medical Center
New York, United States

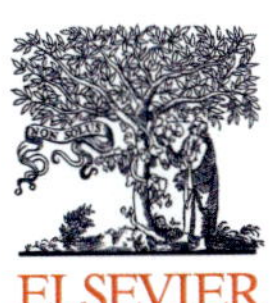

ELSEVIER

Updates on Neonatal Chronic Lung Disease ISBN: 978-0-323-68353-1

Publisher: Patrick Manley
Acquisition Editor: Kerry Holland
Editorial Project Manager: Sara Pianavilla
Production Project Manager: Sreejith Viswanathan
Cover Designer: Alan Studholme

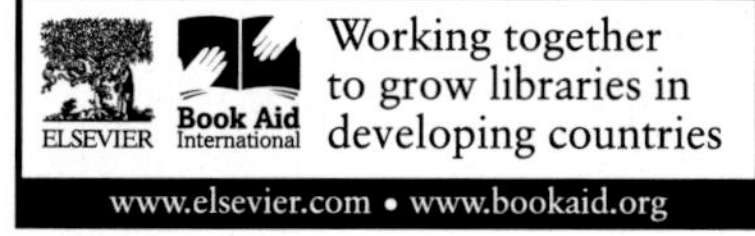

List of Contributors

Steven H. Abman, MD
Section of Pulmonary Medicine and Pediatric Heart Lung Center
Department of Pediatrics
University of Colorado School of Medicine
Aurora, CO, United States

Professor
Pediatrics
University of Colorado Health Sciences Center
Aurora, CO, United States

Director
Pediatric Heart Lung Center
The Children's Hospital
Aurora, CO, United States

Namasivayam Ambalavanan, MBBS, MD
Division of Neonatology
Department of Pediatrics
University of Alabama at Birmingham
Birmingham, AL, United States

Maryanne E. Ardini-Poleske
Senior Study Director
Biostatistics and Epidemiology Unit
RTI International

Judy L. Aschner, MD
Department of Pediatrics
Joseph M Sanzari Children's Hospital at Hackensack University Medical Center
Hackensack Meridian School of Medicine
Hackensack, NJ, United States

Albert Einstein College of Medicine
Bronx, NY, United States

John E. Baatz, PhD
Professor
Department of Pediatrics
Medical University of South Carolina
Charleston, SC, United States

Christopher D. Baker, MD
Section of Pulmonary Medicine and Pediatric Heart Lung Center
Department of Pediatrics
University of Colorado School of Medicine
Aurora, CO, United States

Elizabeth K. Baker, MBBS (Hons)
Research Fellow
Newborn Research Centre
The Royal Women's Hospital
Melbourne, VIC, Australia

Department of Obstetrics and Gynaecology
The University of Melbourne
Melbourne, VIC, Australia

Vineet Bhandari, MBBS, MD, DM
Section of Neonatal-Perinatal Medicine
Department of Pediatrics
Drexel University College of Medicine
Philadelphia, PA, United States

Douglas Bush, MD
Division of Pediatric Pulmonology
Mount Sinai Kravis Children's Hospital
Icahn School of Medicine at Mount Sinai
New York, NY, United States

Jeanie L.Y. Cheong, MD
Neonatal Paediatrician,Clinical Sciences
Murdoch Children's Research Institute
Melbourne, VIC, Australia

Neonatal Services
The Royal Women's Hospital
Melbourne, VIC, Australia

Department of Obstetrics and Gynaecology
The University of Melbourne
Melbourne, VIC, Australia

Marianne C. Chiafery, DNP, MS, PNP-C
Associate Professor of Clinical Nursing
University of Rochester School of Nursing
Rochester, NY United States

Joseph M. Collaco, MD, PhD
Associate Professor of Pediatrics
Johns Hopkins University School of Medicine
Baltimore, MD, United States

Carl T. D'Angio, MD
Professor
Pediatrics and Medical Humanities & Bioethics
University of Rochester School of Medicine and Dentistry
Rochester, NY, United States

Attending Neonatologist
Golisano Children's Hospital
University of Rochester Medical Center
Rochester, NY, United States

Peter G. Davis, MD
Professor/Director of Neonatal Medicine
The Royal Women's Hospital
Melbourne, VIC, Australia

The Department of Obstetrics and Gynaecology
University of Melbourne
Melbourne, VIC, Australia

Gail H. Deutsch, MD
Department of Laboratories
Seattle Children's Hospital
Seattle, WA, United States

Professor
Department of Pathology
University of Washington School of Medicine and Seattle Children's Hospital
Seattle, WA, United States

Kalsang Dolma, MD
Division of Neonatology
Department of Pediatrics
University of Alabama at Birmingham
Birmingham, AL, United States

Lex W. Doyle, MD
Professor of Neonatal Paediatrics
Department of Obstetrics and Gynaecology and Department of Paediatrics
The University of Melbourne
Melbourne, VIC, Australia

Research Office
The Royal Women's Hospital
Melbourne, VIC, Australia

Clinical Sciences
Murdoch Children's Research Institute
Melbourne, VIC, Australia

Andrew M. Dylag, MD
Division of Neonatology
Department of Pediatrics
University of Rochester School of Medicine and Dentistry
Rochester, NY, United States

Osayame A. Ekhaguere, MBBS, MPH
Department of Pediatrics
Section of Neonatal-Perinatal Medicine
Indiana University
Indianapolis, IN, United States

Stavros Garantziotis, MD
Division of Intramural Research
National Institute of Environmental Health Sciences
Research Triangle Park
Durham, NC, United States

William W. Hay, Jr., MD
Professor
Pediatrics
University of Colorado School of Medicine
Aurora, CO, United States

Nara S. Higano, PhD
Research Associate
Cincinnati Children's Hospital
Cincinnati, OH, United States

John Ibrahim, MD
Department of Pediatrics
Division of Newborn Medicine
University of Pittsburgh
Pittsburgh, PA, United States

Erik A. Jensen, MD, MSCE
Assistant Professor, Pediatrics
University of Pennsylvania
Attending Neonatologist
Division of Neonatology and Department of Pediatrics
The Children's Hospital of Philadelphia
Philadelphia, PA, United States

Martin Keszler, MD
Professor of Pediatrics
Director of Respiratory Services
Pediatrics, Associate Director of NICU
Women and Infants Hospital
Alpert Medical School of Brown University
Providence, RI, United States

Haresh Kirpalani, BM, MSc
Professor Neonatology
Department of Pediatrics
Division of Neonatology
The Children's Hospital of Philadelphia
Philadelphia, PA, United States

Emeritus Professor
Clinical Epidemiology
McMaster University
Hamilton, ON, Canada

K. Lim Kua, MD
Department of Pediatrics
Section of Neonatal-Perinatal Medicine
Indiana University
Indianapolis, IN, United States

Satyan Lakshminrusimha, MBBS, MD, FAAP
Professor and Chair
Pediatrics UC Davis
Sacramento, CA, United States

Charitharth Vivek Lal, MD
Division of Neonatology
Department of Pediatrics
University of Alabama at Birmingham
Birmingham, AL, United States

Sean Leary, BS
Section of Neonatal-Perinatal Medicine
Department of Pediatrics
Drexel University College of Medicine
Philadelphia, PA

Susan K. Lynch, MD
The Comprehensive Center for Bronchopulmonary Dysplasia
Nationwide Children's Hospital, and the Department of Pediatrics
The Ohio State University College of Medicine
Columbus, OH, United States

Daniel T. Malleske, MD
The Comprehensive Center for Bronchopulmonary Dysplasia
Nationwide Children's Hospital, and the Department of Pediatrics
The Ohio State University College of Medicine
Columbus, OH, United States

Erica W. Mandell, MD
Section of Neonatology and Pediatric Heart Lung Center
Department of Pediatrics
University of Colorado School of Medicine
Aurora, CO, United States

Thomas J. Mariani, PhD
Professor of Pediatrics (Neonatology)
Biomedical Genetics and Environmental Medicine
Vice Chair for Research
Department of Pediatrics
Director
Pediatric Molecular and Personalized Medicine Program
University of Rochester
Rochester, NY, United States

Richard J. Martin, MD
Division of Neonatology
Department of Pediatrics
Rainbow Babies & Children's Hospital
Case Western Reserve University School of Medicine
Cleveland, OH, United States

Cindy T. McEvoy, MD, MCR
Department of Pediatrics and Obstetrics
Gynecology
Oregon Health & Science University
Portland, OR, United States

Sharon A. McGrath-Morrow, MD, MBA
Professor of Pediatrics
Johns Hopkins University School of Medicine
Baltimore, MD, United States

Robin McKinney, MD
Assistant Professor of Pediatrics
Pediatric Critical Care Medicine
The Warren Alpert Medical School of Brown University
Providence, RI, United States

Ravi S. Misra, PhD
Research Assistant Professor
University of Rochester-Golisano Children's Hospital
Department of Pediatrics-Neonatology
Rochester, NY, United States

Leif D. Nelin, MD
Dean W Jeffers Chair in Neonatology
Nationwide Children's Hospital
Professor and Chief
Neonatology
The Ohio State University
Columbus, OH, United States

Ekta U. Patel, DO
Department of Pediatrics
Medical University of South Carolina
Charleston, SC, United States

Gloria S. Pryhuber, MD
Professor
Pediatrics and Environmental Medicine
University of Rochester Medical Center
New York, United States

Colby L. Day Richardson, MD
Assistant Professor
Department of Pediatrics
University of Florida Health
Jacksonville, FL, United States

Rita M. Ryan
Professor
Case Western Reserve University
Rainbow Babies & Children's Hospital
Cleveland, OH, United States

Rashmin C. Savani, MBChB
Center for Pulmonary & Vascular Biology and Division of Neonatal-Perinatal Medicine
Professor and William Buchanan Chair
Department of Pediatrics
University of Texas Southwestern Medical Center
Dallas, TX, United States

Kristin Scheible, MD
Associate Professor
Department of Pediatrics/Division of Neonatology
University of Rochester
Rochester, NY, United States

Barbara Schmidt, MD, MSc
Department of Health Research Methods, Evidence, and Impact
McMaster University
Hamilton, ON, Canada

Professor Emeritus
Division of Neonatology and Department of Pediatrics
The Children's Hospital of Philadelphia and The University of Pennsylvania
Philadelphia, PA, United States

Edward G. Shepherd, MD
Section Chief
Neonatology
Nationwide Children's Hospital
Associate Professor
The Ohio State University
Columbus, OH, United States

Lannae Strueby, MSc, MD, FRCPC
Neonatologist
Division of Neonatal-Perinatal Medicine
Department of Pediatrics
University of Saskatchewan
Saskatoon, SK, Canada

Bernard Thébaud, MD, PhD, FRCPC
Division of Neonatology
Department of Pediatrics
Children's Hospital of Eastern Ontario Research Institute
Ottawa, ON, Canada

Sinclair Centre for Regenerative Medicine
Ottawa Hospital Research Institute
Ottawa, ON, Canada

Department of Cellular and Molecular Medicine
University of Ottawa
Ottawa, ON, Canada

Payam Vali, MD
Assistant Professor
Pediatrics University of California Davis
Sacramento, CA, United States

Jason C. Woods, PhD
Director
Center for Pulmonary Imaging Research
Co-director
Cincinnati BPD Center
Professor
Pulmonary Medicine and Radiology
Cincinnati Children's Hospital Medical Center
Professor of Pediatrics
University of Cincinnati School of Medicine
Cincinnati, OH, United States

Contents

CHAPTER 1

Bronchopulmonary Dysplasia, the Chronic Lung Disease of Premature Infants

COLBY L. DAY RICHARDSON, MD • EKTA U. PATEL, DO • JOHN E. BAATZ, PHD • RITA M. RYAN

The progression from an embryo to a fully developed human is a complex process involving an intricate interplay of genes, growth factors, hormones, and tissues, as well as maternal/placental environment. Disruptions on a cellular level at any stage have the potential to cause benign variations, devastating structural or developmental insults, or death. Additionally, a more ***global disruption*** occurs when, for either fetal or maternal reasons, an infant is born prematurely, and development must continue *ex utero*. Years of laboratory research and clinical experience have provided us with some understanding of lung development, as well as standards of clinical care and treatments designed to gently support respiratory effort and create an *ex utero* environment that is conducive to normal lung development. However, despite our best efforts, chronic lung disease of prematurity, or bronchopulmonary dysplasia (BPD), continues to exist. Rather, very little progress has been made in significantly reducing the occurrence of BPD.

But what is prematurity-associated lung disease? As we are taught throughout medical training: children are not simply small adults. Similarly, lung disease of prematurity is not the same disease as adult chronic lung disease simply occurring in infants. In order to understand the pathophysiology of this unique disease process, it is imperative to have an understanding of the basic physiology of normal lung development and normal lung vasculature development in the fetus.

REVIEW OF LUNG DEVELOPMENT

One of the most astounding properties of biologic evolution is the ability to understand the overarching goals of development in terms of desired final function. For example, when studying the physiologic development of the lungs, it is best to start with a summary of the ultimate purpose and function of the lungs: gas exchange. In order to function in gas exchange, there must be a conduit of air into the organism, a conduit of air out of the organism, and an intermediary location where air can interact with the bloodstream to deposit oxygen and obtain carbon dioxide. Furthermore, the accessible bloodstream must have a way to then connect systemically in order to ferry the oxygen around the body and return with carbon dioxide. Human development achieves these goals remarkably well if allowed to progress as planned and over the appropriate gestational length of time.

The respiratory tract begins as a budding from the primitive foregut as early as 3 weeks following conception. Development of the respiratory tract is a long process, continuing throughout gestation and into childhood and adolescence. Over the course of a normal 40-week gestation, the fetal respiratory tract undergoes several stages of development: the embryonic stage, the pseudoglandular stage, the canalicular stage, the saccular stage, and the alveolar stage (Fig. 1.1). These stages of respiratory tract development are not scientifically discrete and, therefore, have some overlap in weeks of gestation, but serve to describe distinct stages of development that must occur for the eventual evolution of a functional and architecturally sound gas exchange unit. The *embryonic stage* of development encompasses weeks three through seven of human gestation and is concerned mainly with the development of the larger, proximal respiratory tract, including the main right and left bronchi and the subsequent branching of the bronchioles. The *pseudoglandular stage* occurs between weeks five and seventeen of gestation during which bronchiole branching is completed and

Updates on Neonatal Chronic Lung Disease. https://doi.org/10.1016/B978-0-323-68353-1.00001-4

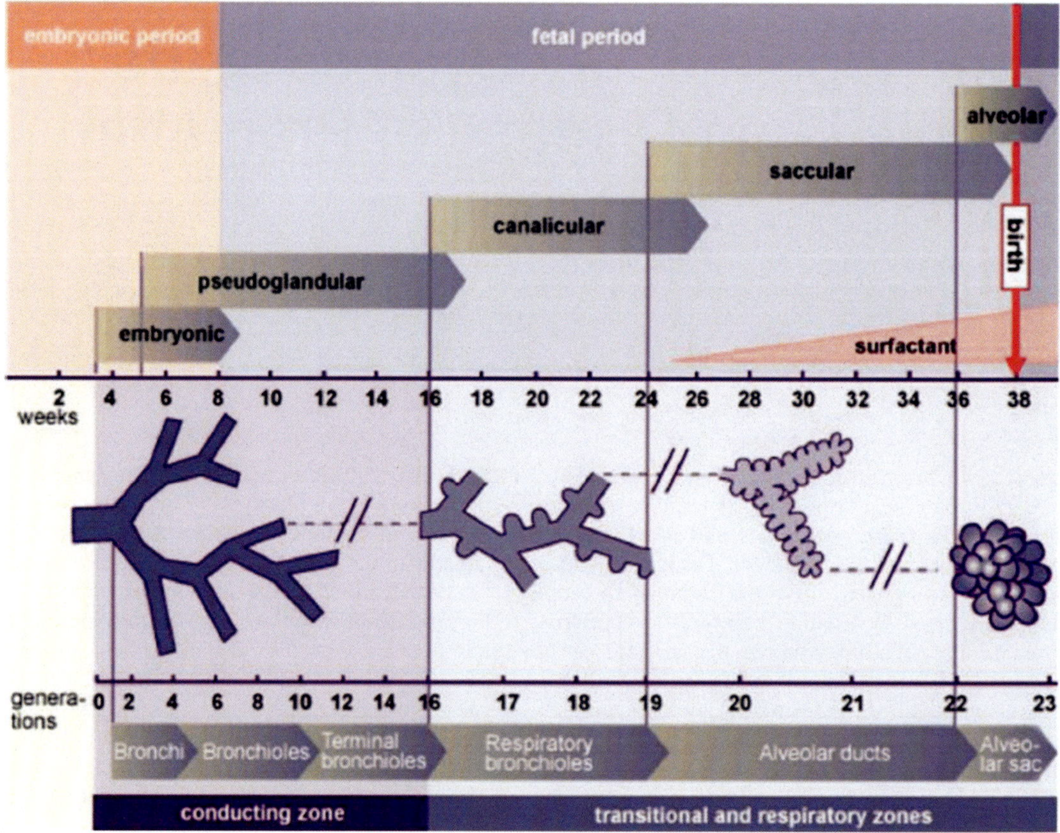

FIG. 1.1 Stages of lung development. (Permission for reprint granted from www.embyrology.ch.)

primitive acini have formed distally. The embryonic and pseudoglandular stages create the conduit in and out of the lungs for air mentioned above, and these stages lay the groundwork for the development of the actual gas exchange unit.

The *canalicular stage*, occurring during weeks 16 through 26 of gestation, represents the earliest stage of lung development during which preterm birth may result in a viable infant (toward the later weeks of this stage). As such, this stage of lung development represents the earliest and most primitive version of functional gas exchange in the lungs, at the alveolar-capillary interface. To achieve gas exchange, there is differentiation of lung epithelial cells, rudimentary production of surfactant (although less than when the lung is fully developed), expansion of the vascular capillary bed, and thinning of mesenchyme. By the end of the canalicular stage, the architectural structure for the larger airways and the gas exchange unit has been created, and it is left to the saccular and alveolar stages of lung development to fine-tune the process to make it energy efficient.

The *saccular stage* of lung development occurs from weeks 24 through 38 of gestation and features development of improved surface area and decreased diffusion distance for gas exchange, as well as cellular differentiation for the creation of surfactant-producing cells. The final stage, *the alveolar stage*, starts at 36 weeks gestation and continues for years thereafter, with maturation of the alveoli.[1,2]

REVIEW OF LUNG VASCULATURE DEVELOPMENT

Lung vasculature develops in conjunction with the respiratory tree, beginning at the earliest embryonic stages, through complex interactions with surrounding mesenchyme. Initially, a vascular bed develops. Subsequently, connections are made between this vascular bed and the developing pulmonary arteries and pulmonary veins. Lung vasculature development is absolutely essential; without development of the pulmonary vasculature, there will be no branching morphogenesis or lung development.[3] During gestation, it is not enough for the vasculature to simply develop in relative physical proximity to the burgeoning airways; there is a critical need for the developing pulmonary capillary network to be as closely approximated to the alveoli as possible to aid in the diffusion of gases. Even if the pulmonary capillary bed is sufficiently developed, if it is not close enough to the distal airspaces, there will be dysfunctional gas exchange.

While *in utero*, the majority of fetal blood flow (90%) is shunted away from the lungs via either the foramen ovale or the ductus arteriosus, shunting blood from the right side of the heart to the left without passing through the pulmonary vascular bed. However, once the placental connection is severed *ex utero*, the infant is dependent upon oxygenation via pulmonary gas exchange, and the fetal circulation must transition to the neonatal circulation. In some infants, with persistent pulmonary hypertension of the newborn (PPHN), this transition does not occur properly and the newborn continues to have high pulmonary vascular tone leading to an impaired ability to oxygenate, and, in severe cases, an inability to exchange carbon dioxide efficiently. In other infants, with alveolar capillary dysplasia, the blood vessels are not close enough to the alveoli, and the infants have lethally impaired gas exchange.

BRONCHOPULMONARY DYSPLASIA

The most common lung development–related disruption is preterm birth itself and the resultant development of bronchopulmonary dysplasia (BPD), or chronic lung disease of prematurity. As medical technology and other treatments have advanced, the gestational age at which infants are considered viable has changed dramatically, and, as a result, the potential population of preterm infants at risk for the development of BPD has increased, as less mature infants become more likely to survive. With the limits of viability at approximately 22–23 weeks gestation, these extremely preterm infants are born in the midst of the canalicular stage of lung development, at which time the basics of lung structure and the rudimentary gas exchange unit are just being created. Despite undeniable advances in promoting the survival of preterm and extremely preterm infants, there has not been an improvement in rates of BPD. While exogenous surfactant may be helpful in replacing endogenous surfactant function until the body generates its own, surfactant deficiency is not the only developmental abnormality of the premature lung. In a review of 20 years of data, Stoll et al. found an increase in survival, especially in extremely preterm infants, as well as a significant increase in survival without significant morbidities in infants born at 25–28 weeks gestation.[4] For the most part, individual morbidities appeared to be stable or mildly improved over the 20-year period, including necrotizing enterocolitis, severe intracranial hemorrhage and periventricular leukomalacia, late-onset sepsis, and severe retinopathy of prematurity. However, BPD was the only morbidity that actually showed an increase in incidence, making this disease process a definite priority for the development of more effective preventative strategies and treatments.[4]

One of the continued issues with studying BPD is the problem of nomenclature and definition. Currently, BPD is defined by its treatment rather than its unique pathophysiology, likely due to the complex interplay of multiple factors in the development of BPD. To understand the progression of our understanding of BPD, it is important to review the history behind its definition.[5]

HISTORY OF BRONCHOPULMONARY DYSPLASIA

In 1967, the term bronchopulmonary dysplasia was coined by Dr. Northway (a radiologist) and colleagues at Stanford following a retrospective study of infants with respiratory distress syndrome (RDS, called hyaline membrane disease then, and reflecting primary surfactant deficiency) who received "intensive therapy," defined as requiring at least 24 hours of artificial ventilation and high oxygen (80%–100% FiO_2).[6] At the time of Northway's study, hyaline membrane disease or RDS had been discussed for approximately a decade, but the subsequent chronic lung disease stage post RDS in premature infants had not been clearly characterized. Through the evaluation of radiographs and autopsy specimens, Northway characterized BPD as a staged healing process with Stage I lasting two to three days and representing an acute phase of RDS. Radiographically, infants in Stage I had granular opacities, air bronchograms, and widespread atelectasis. Stage II was described as lasting four to ten days and was called the "period of regeneration" with complete opacification of the bilateral lung fields on X-ray of the sickest infants in this stage. The third stage was considered a period of transition to chronic disease and defined as lasting 10 to 20 days. Radiographs included in Northway's study are consistent with what is now referred to as cystic BPD. In the final stage, Stage IV (>1 month), the infants had progressed to chronic disease with continued cystic areas of lucency on X-ray. Northway's study also included histologic examination of lungs obtained during autopsy on those infants who died. Histologically, the progression from stages I through IV included initial hyaline membranes and atelectasis progressing to necrosis, edema, smooth muscle hypertrophy, increased collagen deposition, and metaplasia.[6] This landmark paper from the 1960s included discussions of potential contributors to the development of BPD in at-risk infants, including positive pressure ventilation and oxygen toxicity. Remarkably, these continue to be considered major factors in the development of chronic lung disease and remain targets for improved therapies.

DEFINITIONS OF BRONCHOPULMONARY DYSPLASIA

In medicine, it is necessary to create definitions for diagnoses for multiple reasons. First, without a defined diagnosis, appropriate treatment plans and follow-up regimens cannot be performed and scheduled. Second, a lack of diagnosis results in an inability to communicate as a team regarding medical treatments and plans. Third, diagnoses allow for more global communication among medical centers to share data, perform research, and ultimately create standards of care that are evidence-based. This third reason also highlights the need for diagnostic definitions to be specific and detailed, otherwise it would be difficult to characterize the effectiveness and reproducibility of treatments and to monitor their safety. One limitation of this necessity is the fact that disease processes can change over time, whether due to changing patient populations, changing environmental factors, or changing therapies. This creates the need to periodically reevaluate the pathology being grouped under a certain diagnosis and determine whether the diagnosis definition requires modification, or whether new diagnoses must be created. The evolution of BPD as a diagnosis is a prime example of the need for periodic reevaluation of clinical disease definitions.

Since Northway's study defined Stage IV as the chronic disease portion of BPD, occurring at greater than 1 month of age, the main diagnostic criterion for BPD became the requirement of oxygen at 28 days of age. In 1988, Shennan et al. published a study of over 600 infants with birthweights less than 1500 g, after following the subjects for 2 years.[7] The authors had the goal of determining diagnosis criteria for BPD that would be more accurate than the requirement of oxygen at 28 days in predicting long-term pulmonary outcomes. They found an oxygen requirement at 36 weeks postmenstrual age (PMA) had a significant increase in predictive value for abnormal pulmonary function in the first 2 years of life, whereas the traditional criteria of oxygen at 28 days of life had poor predictive value for ultimate abnormal pulmonary function in infants whose birthweights were <1500 g and at lower gestational ages. In an effort to ensure that infants with risk for developing BPD were not missed, a broad definition was used for abnormal pulmonary function, including death, oxygen requirement at 40 weeks PMA, respiratory tract surgery, 2 + hospital admissions for respiratory disease, wheezing requiring medication, chest X-ray changes, or clinical respiratory symptoms along with poor growth, poor tone, or neurodevelopmental disability. (Table1.1)[7]

In 1999, Dr. Alan Jobe presented the concept of "new BPD".[8] In this report, it was suggested that progress in neonatal treatment modalities both antenatally and postnatally resulted in a new form of BPD, often occurring in infants with supposedly "milder" lung disease early in their NICU stay with a more pronounced appearance of alveolar simplification.[8] Although fibrosis still occurs in babies who die with BPD, the "new BPD" concept brought to our attention the alveolar simplification and "growth arrest" seen with our most immature survivors.[9] This idea that the pathophysiology of BPD was changing without a concomitant change in the diagnostic definition was addressed at the National Institutes of Health (NIH) National Heart, Lung and Blood Institute (NHLBI)-sponsored workshop in 2000, during which a new graded BPD definition was proposed,[9] referred to in this chapter as the 2000 NHLBI workshop definition. In this new BPD definition, infants are separated based on gestational age of <32 weeks versus gestational age ≥32 weeks and then assessed at a designated time point to be divided into mild, moderate, or severe BPD based on the level of respiratory support required. Of note, to progress to the staged BPD characterizations, the infant must have required oxygen therapy for at least 28 days cumulative, but the remainder of the mild, moderate, and severe classifications is based upon respiratory support required at 36 weeks PMA. Hence, the "2000 NHLBI workshop definition" encompasses both the original findings from Northway in 1967 by including the requirement of at least 28 days of supplemental oxygen exposure, but also uses the evidence that continued need for respiratory support at a later PMA correlates better with future lung disease suggested by the Shennan definition. Infants are characterized as "mild" BPD if at 36 weeks PMA they are breathing room air. Infants are diagnosed with

TABLE 1.1
Summary of bronchopulmonary dysplasia Definition Nomenclature.

Study (Year)	Description	Definition	Comments
Northway et al. (1967)	"Bronchopulmonary dysplasia (BPD)" coined	Four stages comprising acute RDS, regeneration, transition to chronic disease, and chronic disease (at >1 month of age/28 days of life). Chronic stage with cyanosis, oxygen requirement, CXR changes.	• Authors note that BPD follows acute RDS and its development appears to be impacted by oxygen exposure.
Shennan et al. (1988)	BPD	Requirement of oxygen therapy at 36 weeks PMA.	• Large follow-up study of 2-year-old children with history of BW < 1500 g. Outcome utilized was abnormal pulmonary findings at 2 years of age. • Recognized that 28 days was simply a marker of prematurity and made this change due to extremely preterm infants having increased survival.
Jobe et al. (2001) NIH NHLBI workshop on bronchopulmonary dysplasia, June 2000 "NHLBI 2000 workshop definition"	Severity-based BPD, 2000 NHLBI workshop definition	Infants requiring 28 days of supplemental oxygen are then evaluated at 36 weeks PMA for respiratory support required, resulting in categorization as mild, moderate, or severe BPD.	• First to recognize that grading severity of BPD was important. • The exact timeline at which infants are evaluated for respiratory support needs is slightly varied whether infant was <32 weeks GA or ≥32 weeks GA. • Complicated definition
Walsh et al. (2003)	Physiologic BPD	Standardized room air challenge added at 36 weeks PMA for those infants in moderate BPD group based on NHLBI 2000 definition.	• Recognized that the rate of BPD was dependent on saturation target.
Ryan et al. (2006)	2000 NHLBI workshop definition + physiologic BPD	Nomenclature suggestion only: Combination of the NHLBI 2000 severity-based BPD definition combined with the physiologic BPD definition proposed by Walsh et al.	• First to suggest using the term "grade" formally (so that the generic term "BPD" could be used by clinicians as needed) rather than the more subjective "mild, moderate, severe" descriptions

Continued

TABLE 1.1
Summary of bronchopulmonary dysplasia Definition Nomenclature.—cont'd

Study (Year)	Description	Definition	Comments
Higgins et al. (2018) "NICHD 2018 definition"	Graded BPD	Grades I through IIIA.	• Improved inclusion of nontraditional BPD phenotypes and early deaths likely due to BPD before 36 weeks. • Addressed newer respiratory support modalities and support with 21% oxygen.

"moderate" BPD if they require less than 30% FiO_2, and with "severe" BPD if they require greater than or equal to 30% FiO_2 and/or they require positive pressure (defined as positive pressure ventilation or nasal continuous positive airway pressure) at 36 weeks PMA.[9] Of note, this definition does not specifically address those infants who are on nasal cannula at 21%–100% FiO_2, nor does it address "effective" FiO_2, or consider infants requiring ventilation for nonlung reasons. Walsh and colleagues tackled the concern that different saturation target thresholds by various practitioners and/or institutions would result in varying levels of BPD from one place to another.[10] They introduced the concept of the "physiologic" definition of BPD, by adding a physiologic "test" for BPD to the new graded BPD diagnosis created at the 2000 NHLBI workshop. The physiologic test consisted of a stepwise room air challenge in infants included in the moderate BPD group at 36 weeks PMA. If these infants successfully maintained saturations of greater than or equal to 88% for 60 minutes on room air following the stepwise wean of FiO_2, they were given a diagnosis of "No BPD". If, however, their saturations fell to less than 88% in the 60 minutes period, they were given the BPD diagnosis. The group reported a strong correlation between this physiologic, real-time test at 36 weeks PMA and subsequent discharge home on oxygen.[10] The Shennan definition of BPD was compared with the 2000 NHLBI workshop definition in a paper by Pomar and colleagues in 2018 as well.[11] The investigators in this paper performed a retrospective study of approximately 250 infants with gestational age at birth <30 weeks and determined that the 2000 NHLBI workshop definition of BPD was more likely to identify infants with BPD, with 71% of infants classified with BPD by the NHLBI workshop definition, whereas only 39% were classified with BPD by the Shennan definition.[11]

Dr. Ryan articulated some of the frustrations practicing neonatologists encounter in using these definitions clinically in her 2006 Journal of Perinatology editorial.[12] In this editorial, Dr. Ryan recommends the combination of the 2000 NHLBI workshop definition with the physiologic definition proposed by Walsh, creating a truly graded definition of BPD (Grade 1 through 3) with further designation of "P" (Grade 1P through 3P) indicating that infants have had a formal assessment of their physiologic need for support at 36 weeks PMA.[12] A recent Canadian study proposed utilizing the need for respiratory support at 40 weeks PMA as a preferred time point to predict future lung disease; however, many infants have been discharged home prior to 40 weeks PMA, making this a less useful definition.[13] A group of investigators were again brought together by the NIH National Institute of Child Health and Human Development (NICHD)[14] and have addressed some of the glaring deficiencies to create a definition that will cover the current therapies used, including deaths before 36 weeks PMA from what seems to be evolving BPD. This last point is critical for testing potentially harmful therapies in preterm infants earlier in their NICU course, before an "official" BPD diagnosis is made. Finally, over the last decade, the role of pulmonary vascular disease (PVD) of prematurity has also become a main concern in relation to the definition of the pathophysiology of BPD[5]; we discuss this in more detail below. We certainly have known for some time that the vasculature is markedly abnormal in babies who die with BPD, as documented in human samples in the landmark paper by Bhatt and colleagues from the University of Rochester and followed up by important contributions by Abman and Thebaud.[3,15,16]

Another difficulty with the past and current definitions of BPD is that they do not allow for early identification of infants who will go on to have severe chronic lung disease of prematurity, thereby limiting clinicians' abilities to target the most at-risk infants for preventative therapies. Many of us can identify evolving BPD clinically but because of the prescriptive diagnosis at 36 weeks' PMA, we do not have a good name for this disease process prior to 36 weeks, which, of course, does not magically appear at 36 0/7 weeks. We continue to suggest that "BPD" be a discretionary clinical term nomenclature,[12] while the "official" "Grade I, II, or III" BPD nomenclature as in the NICHD new workshop definition be used for final discharge diagnoses/classification. We must have a way to categorize infants at discharge for purposes of communicating with our pediatric pulmonology and primary care colleagues, as well as have more precise outcomes for clinical research analysis.(Table 1.2)

PROP COHORT—A LARGE PROSPECTIVELY FOLLOWED-UP COHORT OF INFANTS WITH BPD (NICU AND POST DISCHARGE)

The Prematurity and Respiratory Outcomes Program (PROP) is an NHLBI and NICHD jointly funded mechanism to support single-center grants to identify and examine possible biomarkers of neonatal chronic lung disease. Additionally, it created a large ($n = 835$), current (enrolled after 2012), observational cohort for studies of common interest including the current definition and identification of infants with BPD, respiratory support patterns in the NICU, types of respiratory medications these infants receive while in the NICU within the first year post discharge, and how these babies' lungs perform at 1 year on pulmonary function testing. Many of the findings from this large multicenter study are still in progress. Several of the papers currently available, such as Maitre et al. and Pryhuber et al., focus on the need for the cohort and a review of definitions for BPD, originating with the 1967 Northway paper.[17,18] Poindexter et al. applies three BPD definitions to the PROP cohort: the Shennan definition, the 2000 NHLBI workshop definition, and the Walsh "physiologic" definition after room air challenge.[19] The PROP investigators further modified the Shennan definition to assign infants discharged home before 36 weeks PMA without respiratory support to the "no BPD" category (at the time of the Shennan study, infants were not regularly discharged home prior to 36 weeks PMA and the definition was determined at exactly 36 0/7 weeks). The 2000 NHLBI workshop definition was also modified to omit the requirement of a cumulative 28 oxygen days due to difficulty in obtaining these data and it not being particularly clinician-friendly. This modification resulted in infants who were previously characterized as "mild BPD", now characterized as "no BPD." This study highlights several shortcomings of our standard definitions of BPD; most notably, the inability to characterize newer respiratory support modalities, such as those on high flow nasal cannula but low FiO_2 support and those on low flow nasal cannula with 100% FiO_2 support. Additionally, current definitions have an excessive chance of missing assignment of diagnosis as indicated by the need to modify the definitions for this study and assign the baby as "BPD-unclassified."[19] This prompted those at the 2018 NICHD Workshop for BPD to develop yet another definition of BPD, but one that is more clinician-friendly and practical. (Table 1.3)[14]

POST NICU DISCHARGE RESPIRATORY DISEASE OR RESPIRATORY DISEASE DURING INFANCY

Post-prematurity respiratory disease, or "PRD", was identified by Keller and colleagues using clinical parameters over the first year post discharge (e.g., hospitalizations

TABLE 1.2
Challenges With BPD Nomenclature.

- Changing ventilation modalities
- Changing patient population
- Difficulties with true clinical and physiologic correlation
- Variations in clinical practice impacting diagnosis
- Weighing need for including severity versus simplicity of a simple "yes/no" diagnosis
- Need for early identification and prevention
- Need for correlation with longer-term respiratory morbidity
- Identifying the ideal assessment point and including those infants who die with evolving BPD prior to the assessment point
- Incorporating that BPD is more than one phenotype
- Incorporating pulmonary vascular disease in definition

for a respiratory problem, home respiratory support, pulmonary symptoms, and prescribed respiratory medications).[20] When correlating PRD with various NICU and maternal factors, the investigators were able to show that a diagnosis of BPD is, in fact, a predictor of more lung dysfunction over the first-year post discharge. However, it is not as strong of a predictor as many neonatologists or pediatricians would assume, and the study demonstrated that non-BPD babies can also have future lung disease, and, in particular, these babies can require respiratory medications in the first year even when no BPD diagnosis was made.[20] Ideally, a new definition will be more useful for predicting longer-term pulmonary outcomes so that a formal BPD diagnosis can be a better-performing surrogate to be used when new therapies become available. There may be some refinements of BPD status at a later corrected gestational age (CGA), as PROP investigators continue to utilize this data set. PROP will produce the largest set of infants with 1-year CGA pulmonary function tests correlated to the NICU course. Additionally, the large number of studies being performed on the PROP cohort may help elucidate the complexities of the development of BPD, possibly generating new therapeutic options for those infants diagnosed with BPD, and, most importantly, it may establish new methods of identifying those infants most at risk for BPD. Data presented in preliminary format at the 2016 NICHD BPD Workshop (published in 2018) showed that the most commonly used respiratory medication in the NICU is caffeine, with multiple medications reviewed including surfactant, inhaled nitric oxide (iNO), caffeine, postnatal steroids, and diuretics [Greenberg JM and Ryan RM, personal communication]. After discharge, over the first year post discharge, the use of diuretics decreases significantly, while inhaled medications (both albuterol and inhaled steroids) increase over the first year in these former preterm infants <29 weeks' gestation at birth.[21] Remarkably, at any given time in the first year, 67%–75% of these infants born before 29 weeks' gestation are on no respiratory medication. For any individual infant, approximately half will receive at least one respiratory medication over the first year post discharge; less mature infants are more at risk. One recent PROP study evaluated the effects of diuretics in extremely preterm infants and demonstrated no improvement in respiratory support requirements with the use of diuretics.[22] However, another recent study demonstrated widespread use of diuretics in these premature neonates [Greenberg JM and Ryan RM, personal communication]. Considering that diuretics are widely used in NICUs

TABLE 1.3
NICHD 2018 Definition of BPD.

NICHD BPD definition* is applied at 36 weeks PMA to those babies with GA <32 weeks†			
	FiO2 requirement at 36 weeks PMA		
Invasive mechanical ventilation		21	>21
Non-invasive high flow respiratory support (NIPPV, NCPAP, NC ≥3LPM)	21	22-29	≥30
Non-invasive 'low flow' respiratory support (NC 1 - <3LPM, hood O_2)	22-29	≥30	
Non-invasive 'low flow' respiratory support (NC <1LPM)	22-70	>70	

**Higgins RD, Jobe AH, Koso-Thomas M, et al. Bronchopulmonary Dysplasia: Executive Summary of a Workshop. J Pediatr. 06 2018;197:300-308.*
†Prior to 36 weeks PMA, clinicians may use ungraded terminology of BPD during the evolving BPD time period

yellow, Grade I; blue, Grade II; red, Grade III

NICHD, National Institute of Child Health and Human Development; BPD, bronchopulmonary dysplasia; PMA, postmenstrual age; GA, gestational age; NCPAP, nasal continuous positive airway pressure; NIPPV, nasal intermittent positive pressure ventilation; NC, nasal cannula; LPM, liters per minute across the country, a rigorous study evaluating the efficacy is needed with a critical discussion on an accepted end point. Clement Ren et al. studied the PROP cohort with regard to tidal breathing measurements using respiratory inductance plethysmography.[23] Finally, a subset of patients from the PROP cohort have been studied using pulmonary function testing at 1 year of age and we hope to have more information from these data shortly [Davis SD and Voynow JA, personal communication].

ETIOLOGY AND PATHOGENESIS OF BRONCHOPULMONARY DYSPLASIA

Although histopathology and other aspects of pathogenesis are discussed in detail in other chapters within this book, here we will briefly review the etiology to provide a context for the definition(s). It is widely accepted that BPD most certainly has a multifactorial etiology, making it impossible to have a single event after premature delivery that can be used as a branch point to predict definite BPD versus no BPD. Antenatal contributors to BPD that have been proposed include genetic predisposition, maternal smoking, maternal hypertension, maternal infection, in utero and *ex utero* inflammation, and intrauterine growth restriction, among others.[14,24] Postnatally, proposed contributors include oxygen toxicity, inflammation (e.g., necrotizing enterocolitis) and postnatal infection, mechanical ventilation, and extrauterine growth restriction/malnutrition, among others.[6,25] Utilizing the PROP data set, Ryan et al. reexamined the association between race and BPD and demonstrated that black infants have less BPD, despite being born at an overall earlier gestation and receiving less antenatal steroids than white infants.[26] However, despite having a lower incidence of BPD, black infants are more likely to have PRD at 1 year CGA.[26] This finding raises the question of whether this racial discrepancy for predisposition to BPD is determined by genetics, or a difference in environmental exposures, or a combination of factors. Few studies have demonstrated that preterm black infants have lower pulmonary function indices (notably forced expiratory flow rates, and forced exhaled volumes) when tested during early infancy, provocatively suggesting racial differences in pulmonary development.[27–30] However, as with most complex medical diagnoses, the most likely answer is that a combination of factors contributes to differing rates of BPD between black and white infants.

The PROP cohort has not been studied yet to examine predisposing factors for BPD (other than race) and we will have to await the analysis from this recent large cohort data set. However, several enticing biomarker studies from the cohort have come to light. Scheible et al. evaluated more than 150 infants ranging from 23 to 42 weeks gestational age and found that decreased serum T-cell expression of CD31 at time of NICU discharge is significantly associated with increased risk of PRD at 1 year of life.[31] This was particularly useful in the extremely low gestational age newborns (ELGAN) group evaluated, since, in this discrete group, gestational age alone was not found to be very predictive of PRD at 1 year of life. Misra et al. found that both proinflammatory CD4+ T-cells and T regulatory cell numbers were altered in chorioamnionitis-exposed BPD infants, further implicating immune dysregulation in the development of BPD and identifying areas ripe for study with the ultimate goal of elucidating biomarkers for this chronic disease of prematurity.[32] Benjamin et al. have focused on the expression of RAGE (receptor for advanced glycation end products) in various forms of lung disease, and noted in their 2018 PROP study that preterm infants with severe BPD have decreased RAGE levels in the first week of life, making this a potential biomarker for long-term respiratory disease.[33] A very detailed review of potential biomarkers currently being studied, including biomarkers from infant blood, urine, and bronchoalveolar lavage fluid, as well as biomarkers from maternal blood, and potential genetic biomarkers was created by Rivera and colleagues.[34] While biomarkers may become the diagnostic gold standard for BPD prediction, investigators are still struggling to find a single (or multiple) sensitive, disease-specific, easily obtainable, and financially feasible biomarker(s) for BPD.

PULMONARY VASCULAR DISEASE

Pulmonary vascular complications in BPD are discussed in greater detail in the chapter by Abman et al. As the population of surviving extremely preterm infants continues to grow, our investigation into the "growth arrest" of the lung increases and other comorbidities have begun to emerge. We know that the lungs grow best in the hypoxic environment that occurs *in utero*, and that part of the detrimental effect of high oxygen exposure is due to impairment of vascular development.[35] These vascular changes disrupt the alveolar-capillary interface leading to impaired gas exchange which increases the need for prolonged oxygen requirements and mechanical ventilation. Prolonged mechanical ventilation and protracted oxygen supplementation, along with extreme prematurity, oligohydramnios, intrauterine growth restriction, and maternal preeclampsia and hypertension, have all been implicated as risk factors for pulmonary hypertension (PHTN) in the context of BPD (BPD-PHTN).[36]

Although the spectrum of PHTN varies in infants with BPD, the mortality rate is high with only 50% survival at 2 years after a diagnosis of severe PHTN.[37] The identification of PHTN in infants with BPD requires a high index of suspicion as clinical signs and symptoms of PHTN may overlap with signs of respiratory problems. Although cardiac catheterization is the gold standard for diagnosing PHTN, it is not practical as a screening modality within this fragile population and noninvasive measures such as echocardiogram (ECHO) need further refinement. As BPD-PHTN has evolved rapidly as an important clinical presentation in the NICU, training in targeted neonatal ECHO (tnECHO) should begin to incorporate right heart evaluation so neonatologists can better manage these infants minute to minute. It is critical that the ECHO be performed by cardiologists or neonatologists with experience in this population, who can assess for the presence of pulmonary vein stenosis (PVS). An infant with PVS can be inappropriately diagnosed with "pulmonary hypertension" due to elevated RV pressures prompting the neonatology team to treat with vasodilators which can worsen the respiratory symptoms.

Management of PHTN in infants with BPD first involves improving the underlying lung disease. Periods of hypoxia should be avoided (because of the vasoconstriction effect on the pulmonary vasculature which will then chronically stress the right ventricle); therefore oxygen saturations should be targeted to ≥95% when there is proven PHTN.[38] Other factors that can contribute should be identified, including evaluations for chronic reflux or aspiration, anatomical or dynamic airway abnormalities, lung edema, and others so that appropriate treatment can eliminate further lung injury.[39] When those efforts fail to improve these infants, pharmacological therapies may be beneficial; however, the optimal therapy is controversial given the lack of randomized trials. iNO therapy has been used anecdotally in BPD-PHTN; usually it is used in acute clinical scenarios, perhaps while waiting for other medications to achieve effectiveness and while addressing other primary respiratory issues. In these patients, the vasoreactivity testing during cardiac catheterization may help to further guide optimal dosing of iNO therapy, but there is limited evidence to support this course of treatment for any extended period in the former premature infant population.

Sildenafil citrate is another medication that can be used to reduce pulmonary artery pressures.[40] Long-term studies have shown that chronic sildenafil treatment for BPD-PHTN infants is safe and effective[41]; therefore, in 2014 the FDA issued a statement stating that sildenafil may be acceptable in cases in which options are limited and close monitoring can be provided. Other vasodilators such as prostacyclin analogs, endothelin receptor antagonists, and soluble guanylate cyclase modulators can also be considered[38,42]; however, there is very limited data for their use in the neonatal population. Currently, there is insufficient evidence on dosing, and when or how to stop these medications if they are initiated. Further collaborative studies and randomized trials are required to establish ideal disease treatment, including developing clear and practical diagnostic and classification criteria, the types of treatment, monitoring strategies, and duration of treatment. However, it is imperative to recognize that the vascular maldevelopment component of BPD, especially early in the NICU course, is crucial to understanding this "new" comorbidity effect of prematurity on lung development seen now in babies with and without BPD.[5] It is also becoming clear that while BPD is a significant risk factor, non-BPD premature infants also are at risk for late-onset PHTN.[43]

SUMMARY

BPD is a complex disease, with some of its manifestations driven strictly by the altered biology dictated by being born too soon, and others driven by our own necessary therapies. We have not discussed the dramatic changes, for example, in how aggressive or less aggressive we have been in mechanical ventilation versus noninvasive approaches, i.e., the changes which have occurred over the past 30 years. Our animal models are good for modeling alveolar simplification but rely primarily on hyperoxia effects. The lack of human neonatal lung tissue availability has been identified as an important research target,[14] and should continue to be pursued. When we do not have adequate evidence-based data to drive clinical practice, at least registry data should be collected which may be able to help in guiding future questions. One of the important lessons from the PROP cohort is the need for neonatologists and pulmonologists to work together across disciplines to improve our understanding, and management of babies with BPD. Studies of race and involvement of other genetic/"-omic" factors may be informative as to BPD pathophysiology in the future. Inflammation and immunology components also remain important areas of investigation. There is still much work to be done to truly protect the lung from the effects of prematurity and the NICU environment.

REFERENCES

1. MV F, S G. Lung development. In: CA G, SU D, eds. *Avery's Diseases of the Newborn*. 9th ed. Philadelphia PA: Elsevier; 2012.
2. CL D, JE B, RM R. *Fetal lung development. Encyclopedia of reproduction*. 2nd ed 2018.
3. Thébaud B, Abman SH. Bronchopulmonary dysplasia: where have all the vessels gone? Roles of angiogenic growth factors in chronic lung disease. *Am J Respir Crit Care Med*. 2007;175(10):978–985.
4. Stoll BJ, Hansen NI, Bell EF, et al. Trends in care practices, morbidity, and mortality of extremely preterm neonates, 1993–2012. *JAMA*. 2015;314(10):1039–1051.
5. Day CL, Ryan RM. Bronchopulmonary dysplasia: new becomes old again!. *Pediatr Res*. 2017;81(1–2):210–213.
6. Northway WH, Rosan RC, Porter DY. Pulmonary disease following respirator therapy of hyaline-membrane disease. Bronchopulmonary dysplasia. *N Engl J Med*. 1967;276(7): 357–368.
7. Shennan AT, Dunn MS, Ohlsson A, Lennox K, Hoskins EM. Abnormal pulmonary outcomes in premature infants: prediction from oxygen requirement in the neonatal period. *Pediatrics*. 1988;82(4):527–532.
8. Jobe AJ. The new BPD: an arrest of lung development. *Pediatr Res*. 1999;46(6):641–643.
9. Jobe AH, Bancalari E. Bronchopulmonary dysplasia. *Am J Respir Crit Care Med*. 2001;163(7):1723–1729.
10. Walsh MC, Wilson-Costello D, Zadell A, Newman N, Fanaroff A. Safety, reliability, and validity of a physiologic definition of bronchopulmonary dysplasia. *J Perinatol*. 2003;23(6):451–456.
11. Gomez Pomar E, Concina VA, Samide A, Westgate PM, Bada HS. Bronchopulmonary dysplasia: comparison between the two most used diagnostic criteria. *Front Pediatr*. 2018;6:397.
12. Ryan RM. A new look at bronchopulmonary dysplasia classification. *J Perinatol*. 2006;26(4):207–209.
13. Isayama T, Lee SK, Yang J, et al. Revisiting the definition of bronchopulmonary dysplasia: effect of changing panoply of respiratory support for preterm neonates. *JAMA Pediatr*. 2017;171(3):271–279.
14. Higgins RD, Jobe AH, Koso-Thomas M, et al. Bronchopulmonary dysplasia: executive summary of a workshop. *J Pediatr*. 2018;197:300–308.
15. Bhatt AJ, Pryhuber GS, Huyck H, Watkins RH, Metlay LA, Maniscalco WM. Disrupted pulmonary vasculature and decreased vascular endothelial growth factor, Flt-1, and TIE-2 in human infants dying with bronchopulmonary dysplasia. *Am J Respir Crit Care Med*. 2001;164(10 Pt 1): 1971–1980.
16. Abman SH. Bronchopulmonary dysplasia: "a vascular hypothesis. *Am J Respir Crit Care Med*. 2001;164(10 Pt 1): 1755–1756.
17. Maitre NL, Ballard RA, Ellenberg JH, et al. Respiratory consequences of prematurity: evolution of a diagnosis and development of a comprehensive approach. *J Perinatol*. 2015;35(5):313–321.
18. Pryhuber GS, Maitre NL, Ballard RA, et al. Prematurity and respiratory outcomes program (PROP): study protocol of a prospective multicenter study of respiratory outcomes of preterm infants in the United States. *BMC Pediatr*. 2015; 15:37.
19. Poindexter BB, Feng R, Schmidt B, et al. Comparisons and limitations of current definitions of bronchopulmonary dysplasia for the prematurity and respiratory outcomes program. *Ann Am Thorac Soc*. 2015;12(12):1822–1830.
20. Keller RL, Feng R, DeMauro SB, et al. Bronchopulmonary dysplasia and perinatal characteristics predict 1-year respiratory outcomes in newborns born at extremely low gestational age: a prospective cohort study. *J Pediatr*. 2017;187: 89–97. e83.
21. Ryan RM, Keller RL, Poindexter BB, et al. Respiratory medications in infants <29 Weeks during the first year postdischarge: the prematurity and respiratory outcomes program (PROP) consortium. *J Pediatr*. 2019;208: 148–155. e143.
22. Blaisdell CJ, Troendle J, Zajicek A, Prematurity and Respiratory Outcomes Program. Acute responses to diuretic therapy in extremely low gestational age newborns: results from the prematurity and respiratory outcomes program cohort study. *J Pediatr*. 2018;197:42–47. e41.
23. Ren CL, Feng R, Davis SD, et al. Tidal breathing measurements at discharge and clinical outcomes in extremely low gestational age neonates. *Ann Am Thorac Soc*. 2018;15(11): 1311–1319.
24. Morrow LA, Wagner BD, Ingram DA, et al. Antenatal determinants of bronchopulmonary dysplasia and late respiratory disease in preterm infants. *Am J Respir Crit Care Med*. 2017;196(3):364–374.
25. Jobe AH. Mechanisms of lung injury and bronchopulmonary dysplasia. *Am J Perinatol*. 2016;33(11):1076–1078.
26. Ryan RM, Feng R, Bazacliu C, et al. Black race is associated with a lower risk of bronchopulmonary dysplasia. *J Pediatr*. 2019.
27. McDowell KM, Jobe AH, Fenchel M, et al. Pulmonary morbidity in infancy after exposure to chorioamnionitis in late preterm infants. *Ann Am Thorac Soc*. 2016;13(6): 867–876.
28. Stocks J, Henschen M, Hoo AF, Costeloe K, Dezateux C. Influence of ethnicity and gender on airway function in preterm infants. *Am J Respir Crit Care Med*. 1997;156(6): 1855–1862.
29. Yüksel B, Greenough A. Ethnic origin and lung function of infants born prematurely. *Thorax*. 1995;50(7):773–776.
30. Hoo AF, Gupta A, Lum S, et al. Impact of ethnicity and extreme prematurity on infant pulmonary function. *Pediatr Pulmonol*. 2014;49(7):679–687.
31. Scheible KM, Emo J, Laniewski N, et al. T cell developmental arrest in former premature infants increases risk of respiratory morbidity later in infancy. *JCI Insight*. 2018;3(4).
32. Misra R, Shah S, Fowell D, et al. Preterm cord blood $CD4^+$ T cells exhibit increased IL-6 production in chorioamnionitis and decreased $CD4^+$ T cells in bronchopulmonary dysplasia. *Hum Immunol*. 2015;76(5):329–338.

33. Benjamin JT, van der Meer R, Slaughter JC, et al. Inverse relationship between soluble RAGE and risk for bronchopulmonary dysplasia. *Am J Respir Crit Care Med.* 2018;197(8):1083–1086.
34. Rivera L, Siddaiah R, Oji-Mmuo C, Silveyra GR, Silveyra P. Biomarkers for bronchopulmonary dysplasia in the preterm infant. *Front Pediatr.* 2016;4:33.
35. van Tuyl M, Liu J, Wang J, Kuliszewski M, Tibboel D, Post M. Role of oxygen and vascular development in epithelial branching morphogenesis of the developing mouse lung. *Am J Physiol Lung Cell Mol Physiol.* 2005;288(1):L167–L178.
36. Altit G, Dancea A, Renaud C, Perreault T, Lands LC, Sant'Anna G. Pathophysiology, screening and diagnosis of pulmonary hypertension in infants with bronchopulmonary dysplasia – a review of the literature. *Paediatr Respir Rev.* 2017;23:16–26.
37. Khemani E, McElhinney DB, Rhein L, et al. Pulmonary artery hypertension in formerly premature infants with bronchopulmonary dysplasia: clinical features and outcomes in the surfactant era. *Pediatrics.* 2007;120(6):1260–1269.
38. Hilgendorff A, Apitz C, Bonnet D, Hansmann G. Pulmonary hypertension associated with acute or chronic lung diseases in the preterm and term neonate and infant. The European Paediatric Pulmonary Vascular Disease Network, endorsed by ISHLT and DGPK. *Heart.* 2016;102(Suppl 2):ii49–56.
39. Abman SH, Hansmann G, Archer SL, et al. Pediatric pulmonary hypertension: guidelines from the American heart association and American thoracic society. *Circulation.* 2015;132(21):2037–2099.
40. Nyp M, Sandritter T, Poppinga N, Simon C, Truog WE. Sildenafil citrate, bronchopulmonary dysplasia and disordered pulmonary gas exchange: any benefits? *J Perinatol.* 2012;32(1):64–69.
41. Mourani PM, Sontag MK, Ivy DD, Abman SH. Effects of long-term sildenafil treatment for pulmonary hypertension in infants with chronic lung disease. *J Pediatr.* 2009;154(3), 379-384, 384.e371-372.
42. Lai MY, Chu SM, Lakshminrusimha S, Lin HC. Beyond the inhaled nitric oxide in persistent pulmonary hypertension of the newborn. *Pediatr Neonatol.* 2018;59(1):15–23.
43. Mehler K, Udink Ten Cate FE, Keller T, Bangen U, Kribs A, Oberthuer A. An echocardiographic screening program helps to identify pulmonary hypertension in extremely low birthweight infants with and without bronchopulmonary dysplasia: a single-center experience. *Neonatology.* 2018;113(1):81–88.

CHAPTER 2

Histologic Phenotypes of Bronchopulmonary Dysplasia and Childhood Interstitial and Diffuse Lung Disease

GAIL H. DEUTSCH, MD

INTRODUCTION

As manifested by the histology, the lung undergoes significant morphologic alterations during fetal development to provide adequate respiration and gas exchange required at birth (Fig. 2.1). While lung development is a continuous process, five developmental stages have been delineated based on anatomical and histologic characteristics.[4] The early embryonic and pseudoglandular stages elaborate the conducting airways down to the terminal bronchioles; the latter canalicular, saccular, and alveolar stages are characterized by formation and remodeling of the acinus, the future site of gas exchange, with progressive vascularization and reduction of mesenchyme to form a thin air/blood barrier.[5] Birth does not signal the end of lung development. There is a continuing complex process of lung growth after birth with alterations in airway size, alveolar size, surface area, and vascularization.[6–9] Although there is significant variation, the newborn infant has an average of 50 million alveoli at birth, with potential to add another 250–650 million alveoli by the end of somatic growth[10,11]; the most rapid growth occurs in the first 2 years of life concomitant with septal maturation.[7,12]

Given the complexity of these developmental processes it becomes evident how a variety of pre and postnatal insults can impact lung maturation and growth. Chronic neonatal lung disease (CNLD) exemplifies how susceptible the immature lung is to exogenous stimuli, resulting in interruption of development, inflammation, and structural abnormalities that vary depending on the underlying disease process, comorbidities, and treatment modalities.

HISTOLOGIC PHENOTYPES OF BRONCHOPULMONARY DYSPLASIA/ CHRONIC NEONATAL LUNG DISEASE

Since its original description by Northway et al.,[13] the histologic picture of lung disease related to prematurity and its therapy has been well-characterized over the last decades, reflecting the high morbidity and mortality in these patients. Late preterm and term infants are also at risk for similar complications in the setting of perinatal asphyxia, fetal growth restriction, infection, meconium aspiration, and other entities that result in injury to the developing lung.[14–19] As such the term "chronic neonatal lung disease" has been favored by many to reflect the common phenotype of lung disease in infants who require prolonged support for respiratory dysfunction, regardless of etiology.[2,20]

Chronic neonatal lung disease (CNLD) is a disorder of lung injury and repair, which follows some form of acute insult or disorder that requires treatment with high concentrations of oxygen and mechanical ventilation.[21] Bronchopulmonary dysplasia (BPD) in the presurfactant era occurred in stages, advancing from acute infantile respiratory distress syndrome (RDS) to fibrotic lung disease.[13] Acute lung injury in the neonate frequently manifests histologically as hyaline membrane disease (HMD), the pathologic correlate of infantile RDS.[22] The pathology of HMD, including the early exudative and following reparative process, is analogous to that of diffuse alveolar damage as occurs in acute respiratory distress syndrome (ARDS) in older patients. HMD results from surfactant deficiency or dysfunction in the context of lung immaturity or pulmonary epithelial injury.[13,16] As a consequence of

Updates on Neonatal Chronic Lung Disease. https://doi.org/10.1016/B978-0-323-68353-1.00002-6

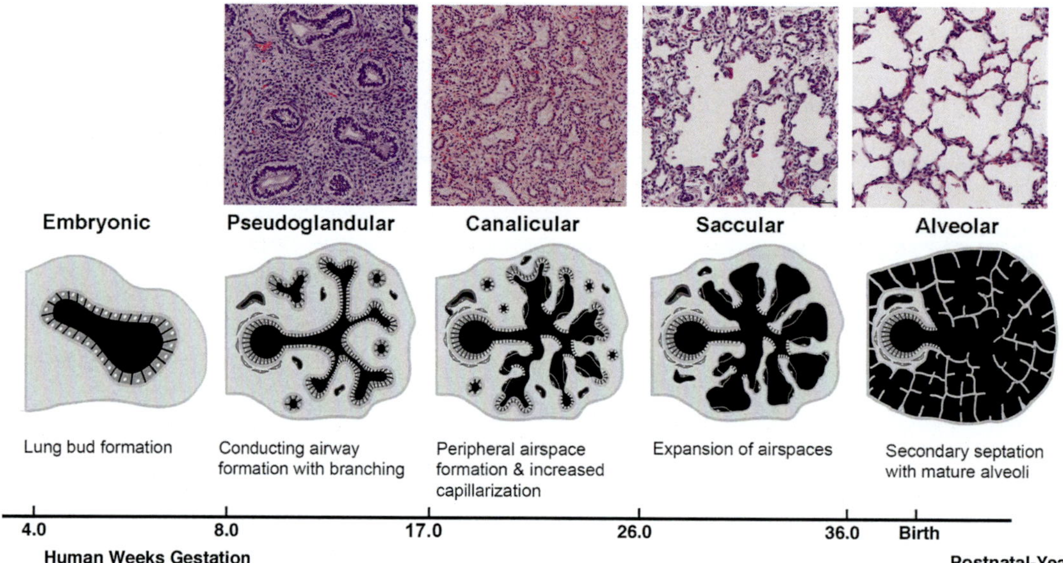

FIG. 2.1 **Morphologic stages during human lung development.** Images of normal fetal lung at different gestational ages demonstrate significant variation in appearance, corresponding to designated stages of lung development.[4] (All images original magnification ×100).

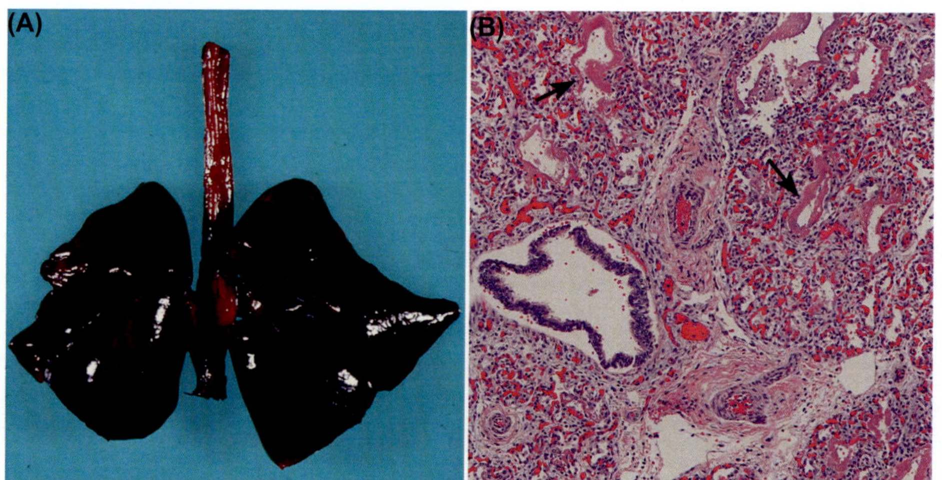

FIG. 2.2 **Hyaline membrane disease. (A)** In hyaline membrane disease marked congestion and atelectasis impart a "liver-like" appearance to the lungs. **(B)** Hyaline membranes are seen lining dilated alveolar ducts (*arrows*). There is congestion and collapse of the surrounding parenchyma. Lymphatics (*asterisks*) are dilated.

surfactant insufficiency there is increased surface tension at the air-liquid interface of the alveolus during expiration, leading to alveolar collapse, increased work of breathing, capillary leak, decreased gas exchange, and severe hypoxia. Grossly the poorly aerated lungs are firm, red, and consolidated (Fig. 2.2A). Microscopic examination demonstrates distal airspace collapse with more proximal airspaces lined by homogenous, dense, eosinophilic membranes from which the disorder was named (Fig. 2.2B).[23] These membranes may be bright yellow from bilirubin staining in infants with severe hyperbilirubinemia.[24] Hyaline membranes are composed of cellular debris, fibrin, plasma transudate, and residual amniotic fluid.[23] They form within 3–4 h after development of symptoms and are most prominent at approximately 12 h. As well as airspace collapse, the surrounding lung shows congestion, edema, focal hemorrhage, and lymphatic dilatation.[23] There may be epithelial necrosis in the airways with bronchiolar plugging. As most infants with RDS are premature, there is lung immaturity, which correlates with gestational age. If the process does not resolve, progression to more classic CNLD, with airway and interstitial fibrosis, may be seen as early as 36 h after birth. With current neonatal practices, including surfactant replacement, use of early continuous positive airway pressure (CPAP) and refined ventilatory strategies, HMD is less frequent but still seen in infants with severe prematurity, immaturity for age, pulmonary hypoplasia, superimposed infection, and other entities more refractory to therapeutic intervention.

CNLD of the presurfactant era is typified by variable inflation of the lung with a combination of airway injury, parenchymal fibrosis, and hypertensive vascular lesions.[13,25,26] Severity of pathologic injury frequently correlates with severity of clinical disease. As detailed with HMD, the acute phase of CNLD is characterized by extensive epithelial injury involving both the alveoli and airways. Reparative changes in the subsequent days to weeks may lead to lobular remodeling with fibrosis, evident at autopsy by the cobblestone appearance of the lung (Fig. 2.3A and B). Patchy airway obstruction from tracheobronchomalacia results in the alternating areas of atelectasis and hyperinflation seen on imaging and at gross exam (Figs. 2.3B and 2.4A).[26,27] Histologically, the early organizing phase of alveolar remodeling is characterized by hyperplasia of bronchiolar smooth muscle with extension into the lobule, hyperplasia of alveolar pneumocytes, and early fibrosis (2.4b). The trachea and more distal airways may show squamous metaplasia and scarring which could lead to stenosis (2.4c). Arterial wall thickening is common and may correlate with clinical pulmonary hypertension. By the chronic stage (>1 month), there is significant lung distortion with a combination of large simplified alveoli and dense interstitial fibrosis (Fig. 2.4D). Alveolar remodeling can be so severe as to mimic a primary disorder of lung development, such as congenital alveolar dysplasia (see below). Correlation of the pathology with prenatal and clinical course, including imaging and possibly molecular testing, may be needed to arrive at a specific diagnosis.

In contrast to the inflammation, fibrosis, and scarring that characterized "classic BPD", CNLD in the current/postsurfactant era is conceptualized as a consequence of disrupted and impaired lung alveolization, termed "new BPD".[28–30] Due to the use of antenatal steroids and surfactant replacement, infants who now develop prematurity-associated CNLD are much younger than those in prior years, born in the

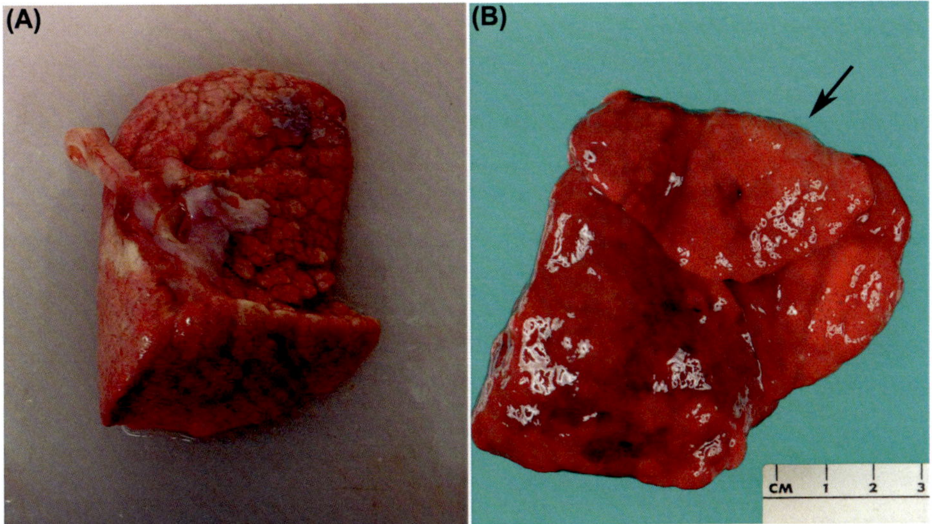

FIG. 2.3 Chronic neonatal lung disease/"Old" bronchopulmonary dysplasia: Gross appearance. (A) Pleural surface of left upper and lower lobes at 3.8 months of age following birth at 23 weeks gestation and chronic ventilation. The outer pleural surface has cobblestone appearance due to parenchymal collapse with fibrosis. (LungMAP BRINDL;D029) **(B)** Alternating areas of atelectasis and hyperinflation (*arrow*).

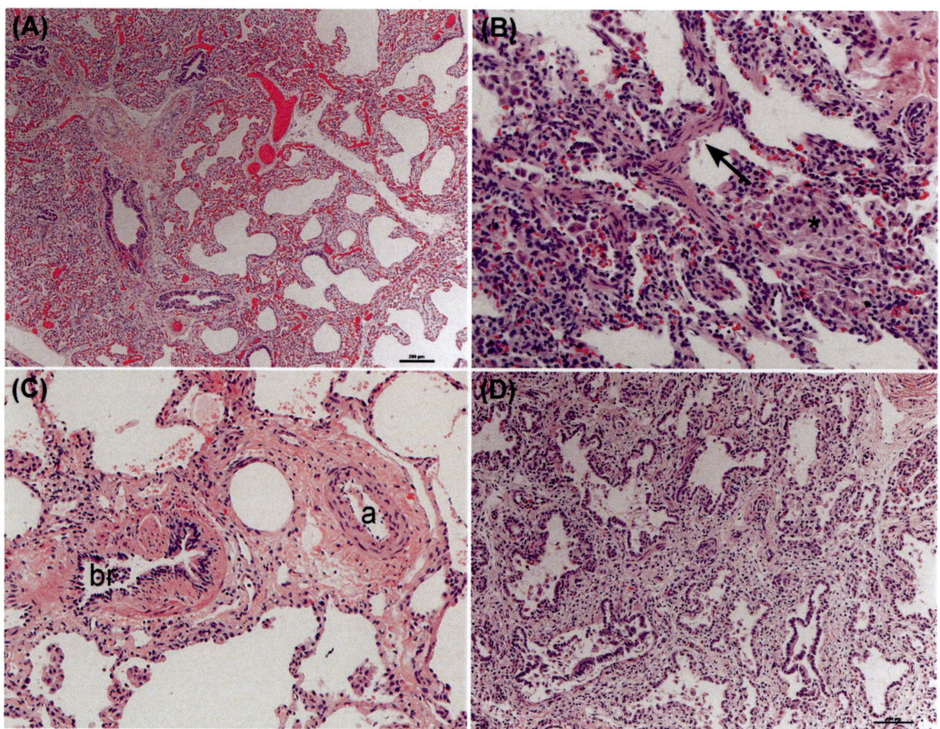

FIG. 2.4 **Chronic neonatal lung disease/"Old" bronchopulmonary dysplasia: Histologic appearance.** **(A)** Regions of atelectasis (left side) alternate with regions of alveolar duct expansion (right side) (X40). **(B)** The early reparative phase of alveolar injury in this infant (born at 28 weeks) who lived for 16 days shows accumulation of alveolar macrophages (*) due to poor airway clearance, and prominent hyperplasia of airway smooth muscle (*arrow*). **(C)** The bronchiole (br) has luminal narrowing from subepithelial fibrosis (a, pulmonary artery; original magnification ×100). **(D)** Severe interstitial fibrosis with abnormal remodeled distal airspaces from an infant born at 24 weeks who lived for 86 days.

canalicular versus saccular stage of human lung development. In conjunction with diminished oxygen exposure and less damaging ventilation, the pathology of "new BPD" is less reflective of injury than an interruption in normal alveolar development, with more uniform expansion of the lung and larger than normal air spaces which appear "emphysematous" (Fig. 2.5).[28,29] Morphometric assessment of the lung demonstrates fewer alveoli and decreased internal surface area compared to age-matched controls.[29,31–33] Acinar spaces are simplified with decreased secondary crests, irregularly distributed elastic fibers in the alveolar walls, and an abnormal capillary distribution (Fig. 2.6).[34–36] Airways show less injury than that seen in classic CNLD, but frequently have bronchiolar smooth muscle hypertrophy and a mild increase in seromucinous glands (Fig. 2.5B).[32,37] Hypertensive changes of the arteries are typically less severe than previously seen.[29] Simplified lung architecture with reduced alveolarization is also evident months to years later at autopsy or on lung biopsy, albeit often selected for patients with persistent/severe respiratory dysfunction.[1,32,38] In lung biopsy cases, clinical pulmonary hypertension or severity of lung growth abnormality, as judged by degree of alveolar enlargement and simplification, is associated with a high mortality.[1] Availability of a large number of neonatal and pediatric lungs through The LungMAP Consortium (U01HL122638; LungMAP.net) provides a unique opportunity to assess the natural history of lung growth in premature infants with a history of BPD, including those who died of nonrespiratory causes.[39,40] Assessment of lung in these former premature infants demonstrates that abnormalities in alveolarization and airways may persist, even if respiratory symptoms clinically resolve (Fig. 2.7, Fig. 2.9).[33]

As with HMD, the severe pathology of classic CNLD is less frequently seen with current neonatal practices, but still occurs to a variable degree, especially in cases where neonates need aggressive support or have superimposed processes.[43]

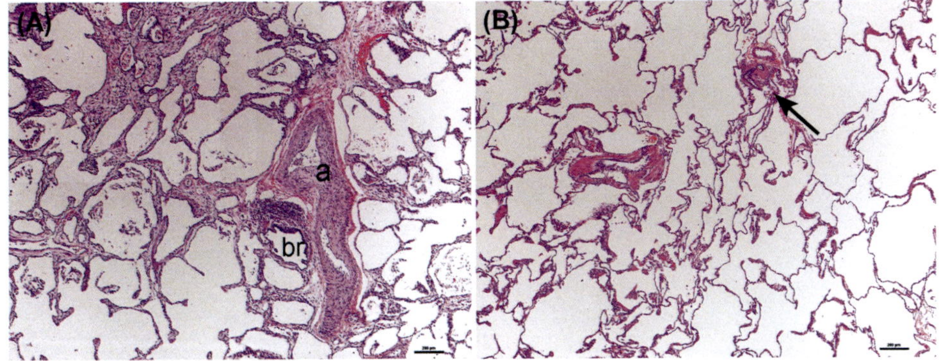

FIG. 2.5 **"Old" bronchopulmonary dysplasia (BPD) in comparison to "New" BPD. (A)** Characteristic findings of "Old" BPD with patchy interstitial fibrosis (upper left) and marked medial hypertrophy of pulmonary arteries (a) (LungMAP BRINDL; D115-RLL). **(B)** "New" BPD in comparison has similar large simplified alveolar spaces but no significant fibrosis or significant vascular alterations; there is bronchiolar wall smooth muscle hyperplasia (arrow) (LungMAP BRINDL; D141-RLL). Both children were born at 25–26 weeks gestational age and died from respiratory failure and pulmonary hypertension in the second year of life. *br*, bronchiole.

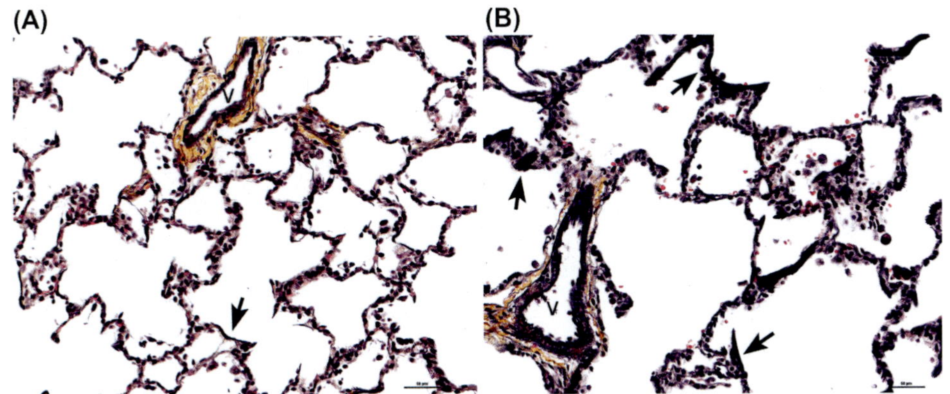

FIG. 2.6 **Elastic fiber deposition in chronic neonatal lung disease (CNLD).** Compared to an age-match control **(A)**, there is marked increase in black elastic fiber deposition (arrows) within the alveolar ducts and septa in a child with CNLD **(B)** (v, vein. Movat pentachrome stain).

OTHER ALVEOLAR GROWTH ABNORMALITIES

While abnormalities of lung growth are traditionally considered in the context of prematurity and prenatal onset pulmonary hypoplasia, they also occur in the setting of congenital heart disease, chromosomal abnormalities (particularly Trisomy 21), and other chronic conditions interfering with postnatal alveolarization (Table 2.1).[1,2,44] Monogenetic disorders presenting with deficient lung growth are being identified in neonates with idiopathic respiratory failure as genetic testing is more accessible. Such genetic disorders also frequently have other notable anomalies.[45,46] Regardless of the etiology, the pathology of alveolar growth abnormalities overlaps considerably; especially as neonatal lung disease often occurs in the context of several comorbid conditions which cannot be easily separated. Similar to the pathology of "new BPD", a final common appearance is lobular simplification with enlarged alveolar spaces which lack complexity (Fig. 2.8).

Prenatal onset pulmonary hypoplasia ranges from mild to severe, depending on the mechanism of hypoplasia and timing of the insult in relation to the stage of lung development.[47] As distension of the lung with liquid and fetal respiratory movements is required for prenatal lung growth, any mechanism that interferes with these processes can result in pulmonary

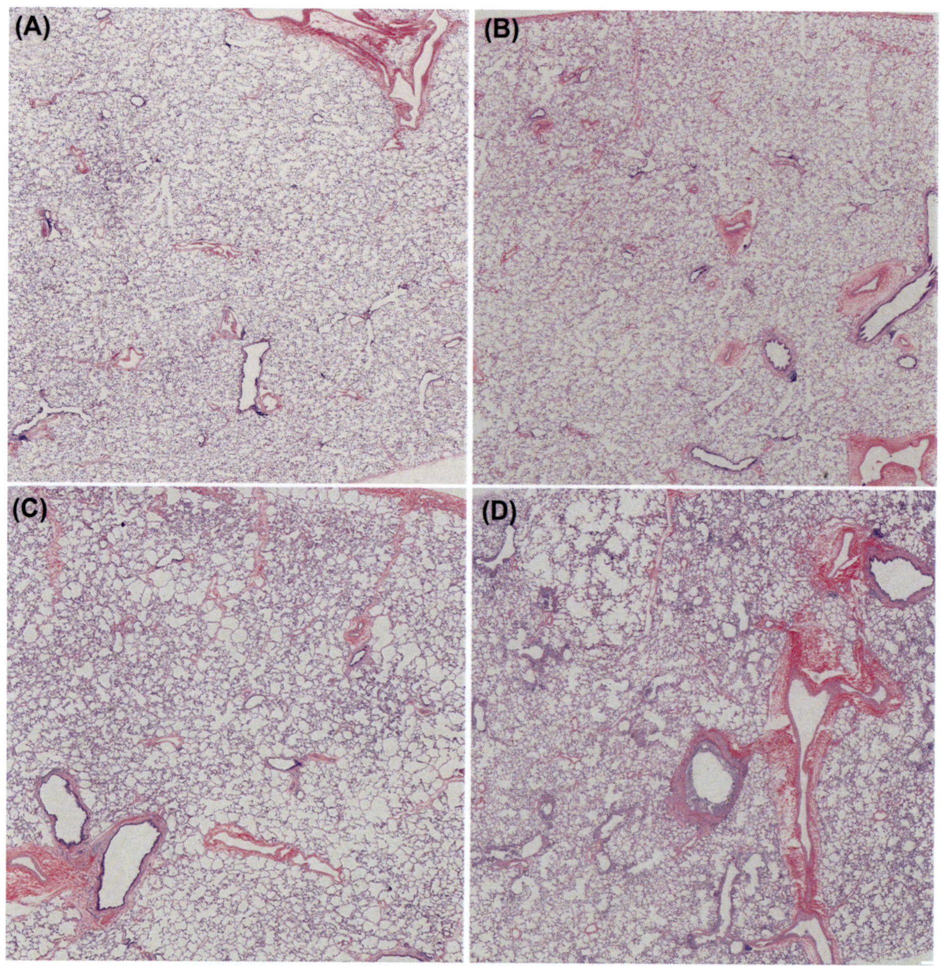

FIG. 2.7 **Persistence of chronic neonatal lung disease at 3 years of age.** Compared to age-match controls (**A, B**: LungMAP BRINDL; D32-RLL, D46-RLL), lung from 3-year-old infants born at 23 weeks gestational age and 25 weeks gestational age (**C, D**: LungMAP BRINDL; D39-RLL, D15-RLL) shows patchy alveolar enlargement with diminished spaces by radial alveolar count.

hypoplasia. Early insults that take place before 16 weeks gestation (renal anomalies, congenital diaphragmatic hernia) may interfere with airway branching as well as acinar development, while later events (premature rupture of membranes) will exclusively impact acinar development.[48–50] In prenatal onset pulmonary hypoplasia, there is diffuse reduction and simplification of alveolar spaces, which is often accompanied by prominence of the bronchovascular structures and a widened interstitium (Fig. 2.8A). Pulmonary vascular changes are common and especially prominent in infants with a severe lung growth abnormality or Down syndrome, the latter with or without associated cardiac abnormalities.[51] These vascular changes include a primary reduction in the cross-sectional area of the pulmonary vascular bed and an increase in pulmonary arterial medial smooth muscle.[52,53] Similar to the pathology of idiopathic persistent pulmonary hypertension of the newborn (PPHN), there may be abnormal extension of arterial smooth muscle into normally nonmuscularized intraacinar vessels (Fig. 2.8B).[53] This increase in smooth muscle may result in clinically significant reactive or relatively fixed pulmonary vasoconstriction.[52]

Postnatal onset growth abnormalities impact late alveolarization, most evident in the subpleural space, which is theorized to be the predominant site for late alveolar formation (Fig. 2.8D).[54,55] The imaging appearance of subpleural cysts along the lung periphery, pulmonary fissures, and bronchovascular bundles

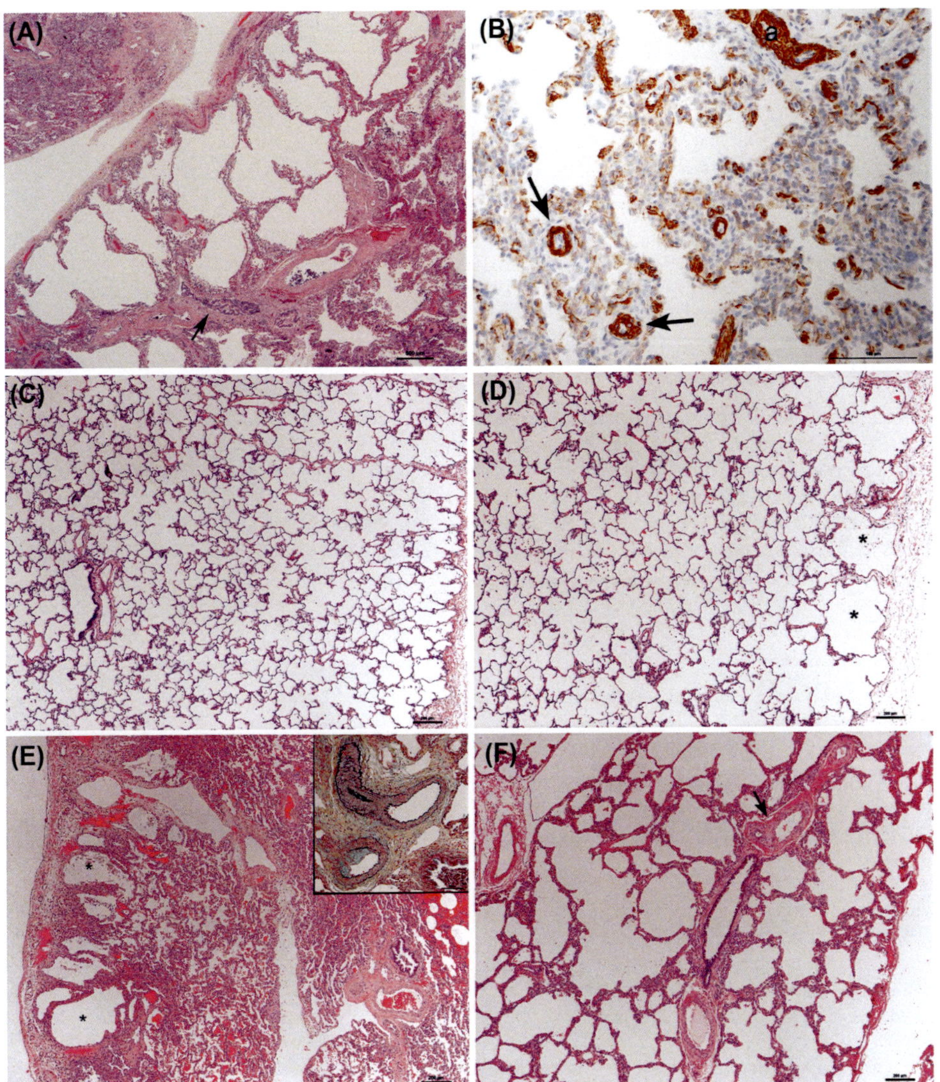

FIG. 2.8 **Deficient alveolar growth outside of prematurity.** **(A)** In this infant who died from severe pulmonary hypoplasia from bladder outlet obstruction, there is marked enlargement and simplification of alveoli which normally are smaller in size than bronchioles (*arrow*). **(B)** Muscularization of normally nonmuscularized small vessels (arrows) in the alveolar parenchyma is highlighted by smooth-muscle actin immunostaining; small arteries (a) also have increased smooth muscle. **(C)** Compared to a normal age-match control lung (LungMAP BRINDL; D072-RLL), **(D)**, the lung biopsy from an infant with Noonan syndrome and chronic pleural effusions has deficient alveolarization most visible in the subpleural space (*asterisks*). **(E)** Deficient alveolarization in Trisomy 21 is also most prominent in the subpleural space (*asterisks*), and may be accompanied by marked hypertensive changes of the pulmonary arteries characterized by medial hypertrophy and intimal hyperplasia (inset, Movat pentachrome stain). **(F)** A 36-week infant with a hypoplastic aortic arch and early-onset respiratory distress was found to have a mutation in Filamin-A (*FLNA*) after lung biopsy, which demonstrated diffuse airspace enlargement and medial hypertrophy of the pulmonary arteries (*arrow*).

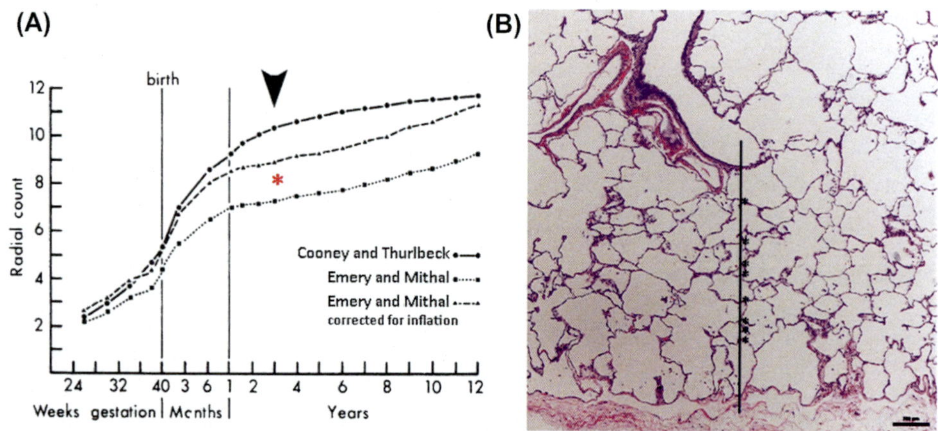

FIG. 2.9 Assessment of lung growth by radial alveolar count. (A) Normative radial alveolar counts for postnatal lung growth by Cooney and Thurbeck (top line)[41] in comparison with those of Emery and Mithal,[42] which were performed on limited areas in the lung and not inflated before fixation. **(B)** Radial alveolar count is estimated by drawing a perpendicular line from the geometric center of the bronchiole to the nearest connective tissue septum or pleura, and counting the points of intersection (*asterisks*); red asterisk in (A) reflects the radial alveolar count of a 3-year-old child with a history of BPD who died from nonpulmonary causes (LungMAP BRINDL; D053-RLL).

TABLE 2.1
Entities Presenting With Deficient Alveolar Growth on Pathology.

I. Chronic lung disease of prematurity (clinical-bronchopulmonary dysplasia)
II. Pulmonary hypoplasia (deficient prenatal lung growth)
   - Oligohydramnios (e.g., prolonged rupture of membranes, genitourinary anomalies)
   - Restriction of thoracic volume (e.g., pleural effusions, diaphragmatic hernia, thoracic deformity including skeletal malformations)
   - Central nervous system and neuromuscular disorders affecting fetal respiration
III. Congenital heart disease
   - Cardiac anomalies associated with reduced pulmonary blood flow (e.g., Tetralogy of Fallot, pulmonary artery stenosis/ atresia, tricuspid atresia)
   - Cyanotic heart disease impairing postnatal alveolar growth
IV. Chromosomal disorders
   - Trisomy 21 with deficient postnatal alveolar growth (may manifest with subpleural cysts on imaging)
   - Other chromosomal defects
V. Monogenetic disorders
   - *FLNA* (Filamin A; also associated with brain, cardiovascular, and gastrointestinal anomalies)
   - *NKX2.1* (NKX2.1; associated with brain-thyroid-lung syndrome)

can be the first indication of an alveolar growth abnormality, and is particularly characteristic of deficient alveolar growth associated with Trisomy 21 (Fig. 2.8E).[1,56] This finding correlates well with the subpleural accentuation of cystically dilated alveoli frequently seen on lung biopsy.[57] Multiple factors likely lead to deficient alveolarization in infants with congenital heart disease, including hypoxia and abnormal pulmonary blood flow.[47,57]

Diffuse alveolar simplification on lung biopsy can also be the first indication of a genetic disorder in infants with idiopathic respiratory dysfunction.[45,58,59] Haploinsufficiency of *NKX2.1* due to gene deletions or loss-of-function mutations results in "brain-thyroid-lung" syndrome, with affected individuals having a variable degree of pulmonary disease, thyroid dysfunction, and neurologic abnormalities.[45,60] *NKX2.1* encodes a homeobox protein (TTF-1) critical for development and function of the lung, brain, and thyroid.[61,62] Onset of pulmonary disease in these patients is often in the newborn period or early childhood with RDS progressing to interstitial lung disease, and frequent pulmonary infections.[45] Pathologic findings in symptomatic patients are extremely variable and include, as well as deficient alveolarization, alveolar proteinosis, nonspecific interstitial pneumonitis, and fibrous remodeling.[45,59,63]

Heterozygous loss-of-function mutations in *FLNA*, which encodes the actin cross-linking protein filamin A, cause an X-linked dominant disorder with often multiorgan involvement, including brain (periventricular nodular heterotopia), cardiovascular abnormalities, intestinal pseudo-obstruction, Ehlers-Danlos syndrome–like features, and pulmonary disease of varying severity.[46,64–66] Respiratory symptoms are usually progressive and accompanied by severe clinical pulmonary hypertension. The age of pulmonary disease onset occurs over a wide range but frequently presents in the first few months of life.[46,67] Characteristic chest CT imaging shows severe hyperinflation with hyperlucent cystic areas alternating with areas of atelectasis and thickening of the interlobular septa.[46,67] Histologic assessment of lung reveals marked alveolar enlargement and simplification reflective of a lung growth abnormality, as well as pulmonary arterial wall thickening: Abnormal muscularization of pulmonary veins and lymphatics is also common (Fig. 2.8F).[58,67]

PATHOLOGIC ASSESSMENT OF LUNG GROWTH

As evident, there is a need for accurate, objective, and practical techniques for pathologists to assess lung growth. The most widely used parameters are lung weight normalized to body weight and radial alveolar account (RAC). Lung volume, measured after inflation of the lungs at a transpulmonary pressure of 25 cm H2O, correlates well with imaging derived formulas for prediction of fetal lung volume age, but is also subject to variations in inflation, either technical or intrinsic to the lung such as atelectasis, alveolar filling processes, or airway obstruction.[68] The ratio of lung weight to body weight is the most reliable parameter of lung growth, especially in preterm infants.[49,69] Use of lung weight alone as a measure of growth is of limited value because of the wide distribution of normal weights and impact of fluid shifts. As these criterion are not useful for lung biopsies, and standardized charts are limited for patients beyond infancy, microscopic criteria to assess lung growth are employed. RAC was first described by Emery and Mithal as a measure of complexity of the acinus.[42] RAC is derived from the number of alveoli or alveolar septa transected by a perpendicular line drawn from the center of a respiratory bronchiole to the nearest septal division or pleural margin (Fig. 2.9). The radial alveolar count in a full-term infant should average 5 alveolar spaces and approximates 12 alveolar spaces by early adolescence. While a valuable tool to evaluate lung complexity and growth, this method requires standardized inflation of the lung, as the radial alveolar count is substantially reduced in uninflated lungs[41,70]; it also requires multiple measurements to be taken as there is variation throughout the lung. As detailed above, moderate to severe deficient lung growth can be recognized without formal assessment by the enlarged size of the alveoli (comparable to bronchioles) and lack of complexity (Figs. 2.5 and 2.7)

PATHOLOGIC ENTITIES FREQUENT IN BPD/CNLD

Pulmonary Interstitial Glycogenosis

Pulmonary interstitial glycogenosis (PIG), previously referred to as cellular interstitial pneumonitis,[71] is an idiopathic lung disorder that is characterized histologically by expansion of the interstitium by glycogen-laden mesenchymal cells (Fig. 2.10A).[72] PIG commonly occurs in the setting of deficient alveolar growth, including CNLD of prematurity, but is also observed in various conditions associated with neonatal hypoxemia and injury, including pulmonary hypertension, meconium aspiration, and even congenital lung malformations.[1,73–75] The clinical presentation can be variable, ranging from mild tachypnea and hypoxemia to refractory pulmonary hypertension and acute respiratory failure requiring nitric oxide and mechanical ventilation. There is clinical and pathologic evidence to support that PIG is often a self-limited disorder, which may be responsive to high-dose pulse corticosteroids, as well as spontaneously resolve over time.[72,76,77] Ultimately, however, the prognosis is related to the presence of comorbidities, particularly deficient lung growth or congenital heart disease.[1] Patients may remain symptomatic for months and require supplemental oxygen.

The impetus for mesenchymal cell proliferation, marked by mitotic activity and positive Ki67 immunostaining, in PIG is unknown, but identification of lipofibroblasts in a subset of these cells implies that this idiopathic disorder is related to lung development (Fig. 2.10B).[78] In the rodent lung, lipofibroblasts play a critical role in postnatal alveolarization by mediating

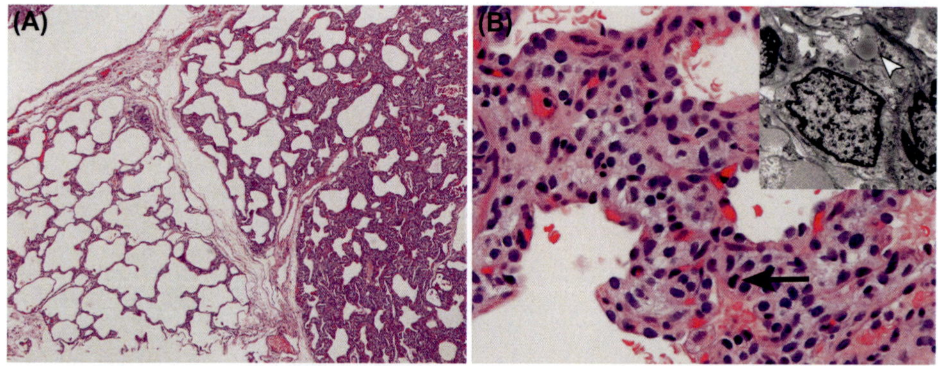

FIG. 2.10 Pulmonary interstitial glycogenosis. **(A)** This condition is typically patchy (right side of panel) and associated with a concurrent alveolar growth abnormality (original magnification x40). **(B)** The alveolar septa are expanded by mesenchymal cells which have vacuolated cytoplasm reflecting glycogen; mitotic activity is frequently seen (*arrow*; original magnification x200). Electron microscopy (inset) demonstrates immature mesenchymal cells containing monoparticulate glycogen and lipid (*arrowhead*).

lipid transfer to type 2 alveolar epithelial cells for surfactant phospholipid synthesis and protecting against oxidant injury.[79] Disruption of lipofibroblast differentiation via Thy-1 and peroxisome proliferator-activated receptor-γ (PPAR γ) results in a myofibroblast phenotype, as seen in models of neonatal hyperoxic lung injury.[79,80] Lipofibroblasts have been documented in normal developing human lung.[81,82]

Pulmonary Interstitial Emphysema

Pulmonary interstitial emphysema (PIE) is an acquired condition in which air gains access to the lung via rupture of small bronchioles or alveoli, dissecting along connective tissue sheaths of the bronchovascular bundles, interlobular septa, and pleura.[83,84] PIE most frequently occurs in the setting of respiratory distress of the newborn, in which there is reduced lung compliance and the patient is being mechanically ventilated.[83] PIE can further compromise an already critically ill neonate by compressing adjacent functional lung tissue and vascular structures, impeding oxygenation, ventilation, and blood flow. Subpleural blebs may rupture into the pleural space resulting in a pneumothorax. The extent of PIE can vary, with single or numerous cysts, diffusely involving the lungs or localized to one or multiple lobes (Fig. 2.11A). Radiographically it may be confused with a lung growth disorder or a congenital cystic lung malformation.[85] On histology there are round to elongated empty spaces of variable size present beneath the pleura and along bronchovascular bundles and interlobular septa (Fig. 2.11B). If prolonged, the presence of air elicits a foreign body reaction with multinucleated giant cells lining the cystic spaces.

Neuroendocrine Cell Hyperplasia

Pulmonary neuroendocrine cells (PNECs) are specialized epithelial cells scattered throughout the airways and as innervated clusters in the alveolar ducts, termed neuroepithelial bodies (NEBs). Neuroendocrine cells produce potent bioactive products, including serotonin, bombesin-like peptide in humans, and calcitonin gene–related peptide (CGRP) in rodents.[86] PNEC/NEBs are most numerous during fetal and neonatal life, and in experimental models have been shown to promote branching morphogenesis, epithelial and mesenchymal cell proliferation, and surfactant production.[87–89] During postnatal life they are thought to function as airway chemosensors, releasing proinflammatory, vasoactive, and bronchoconstrictive factors in response to hypoxia and other stimuli.[90] While PNEC/NEBs decline rapidly after the neonatal period, they have been shown to be abnormally increased in a number of pediatric lung disorders, including BPD, sudden infant death syndrome, cystic fibrosis, asthma, and most recently neuroendocrine cell hyperplasia of infancy (NEHI).[91] The role of PNEC/NEBs in BPD has been extensively studied using a baboon model of BPD and transgenic mice lacking bombesin/GRP receptors.[92–95] These studies demonstrated a positive relationship between bombesin/GRP and mast cell recruitment, suggesting PNEC/NEBs are proinflammatory. Urine bombesin-like peptide levels are elevated in premature newborns who later developed BPD and postnatal administration of anti-BLP antibody in the hyperoxic baboon model attenuated clinical and pathological evidence of chronic lung disease[92,96]; treatment with antioxidant compounds had a similar effect.[97]

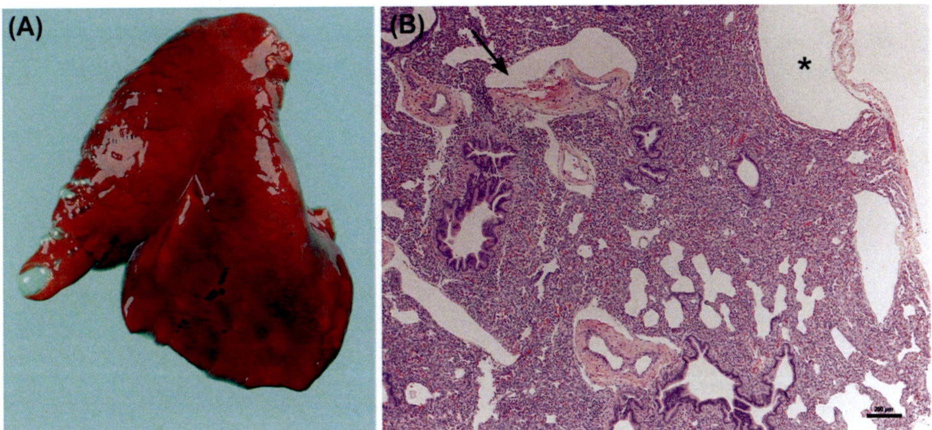

FIG. 2.11 **Pulmonary interstitial emphysema.** **(A)** Pulmonary interstitial emphysema superimposed on hyaline membrane disease in a premature infant with respiratory distress syndrome. **(B)** Histologically, there are empty cystic spaces in the subpleural space (*asterisk*) and around bronchovascular bundles (*arrow*).

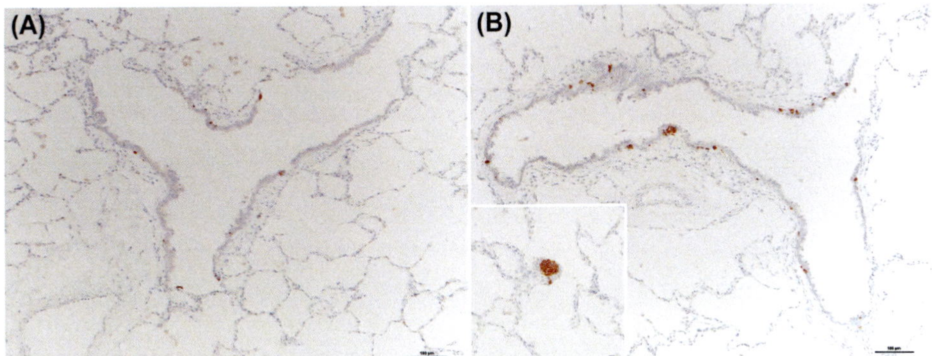

FIG. 2.12 **Increased neuroendocrine cells in chronic neonatal lung disease.** Compared to lung from an age-matched control **(A)** there are increased bombesin-immunopositive neuroendocrine cells in a 13-month-old with bronchopulmonary dysplasia **(B)**; insert demonstrates a prominent neuroepithelial body.

PNEC/NEB increase is also observed in postsurfactant BPD, compared to age-matched controls with upregulation of Mash 1, a transcription factor essential for PNEC/NEB development[91,98] (Fig. 2.12).

OTHER CHILD DISORDERS PRESENTING IN EARLY INFANCY

In the differential of diffuse lung disease presenting in infancy are a diverse group of rare disorders associated with significant morbidity and mortality.[1] Many of the disorders have a genetic basis, allowing noninvasive diagnosis when feasible and in the appropriate clinical context.[3,99] As well as deficient lung growth/CNLD, major categories of neonatal diffuse lung disease include diffuse developmental disorders, surfactant dysfunction disorders, PIG (see discussion above), and vascular disorders including persistent PPHN, pulmonary arterial, and venous hypertension and lymphangiectasia (Table 2.2). While the disorder NEHI is included in infant lung disease, it is unlikely to present in the setting in which CNLD is in the differential as these infants are born term or near-term, and are rarely symptomatic at birth.[100]

DIFFUSE DEVELOPMENTAL DISORDERS

Disorders that disrupt early lung development present in term infants with hypoxemic respiratory failure refractory to medical intervention. These disorders include acinar dysplasia, congenital alveolar dysplasia, and alveolar capillary dysplasia with misalignment of

TABLE 2.2
Other Forms of Childhood Interstitial and Diffuse Lung Disease Presenting in Early Infancy.

Category	Diffuse Developmental Disorders	Pulmonary Interstitial Glycogenosis	Genetic Disorders of Surfactant Metabolism	Pulmonary Vascular Disorders
Included entities; hereditary basis	• acinar dysplasia; *TBX4* • Congenital alveolar dysplasia; *FGF10* • Alveolar capillary dysplasia with misalignment of pulmonary veins; *FOXF1*	Frequent in entities with deficient alveolar growth	• *SFTPB*; autosomal recessive • *SFTPC*; autosomal dominant • *ABCA3*; autosomal recessive • *NKX2.1*; autosomal dominant	Persistent pulmonary hypertension of the newborn PHTN Venous hypertension Lymphangiectasia
Associated features	Other congenital anomalies PHTN	Prematurity Congenital heart disease Injury (e.g., meconium) PHTN	*NKX2.1*—Hypothyroidism, hypotonia, chorea	Congenital heart disease Genetic syndromes
Outcome	Usually fatal without lung transplant	Variable depending on comorbidities	Variable depending on mutation	Variable depending on underlying etiology

TBX4, gene encoding T-box transcription factor 4; *FGF10*, gene encoding fibroblast growth factor 10; *FOXF1*, gene encoding Forkhead Box F1; PHTN, pulmonary arterial hypertension; *SFTPB*, gene encoding surfactant protein B; *SFTPC*, gene encoding surfactant protein C; *ABCA3*, gene encoding adenosine 5'triphosphate-binding cassette family member A-3; *NKX2.1*, gene coding thyroid transcription factor 1 (TTF-1).

pulmonary veins (ACDMPV).[2] Characterization of these rare entities has been based on their histopathologic appearance on lung biopsy or at autopsy. Acinar dysplasia (inappropriately termed in the past Type 0 cystic pulmonary airway malformation) represents the most extreme form of lung developmental arrest, being comprised predominantly of bronchi and bronchioles, with only rare acinar structures present (Fig. 2.13A).[101–103] The histologic appearance is that of the late pseudoglandular stage of lung development. In contrast to acinar dysplasia, the disorder congenital alveolar dysplasia contains more easily identifiable distal acinar spaces, resembling maturational arrest in the canalicular to early saccular stage of development.[104–106] While not dissimilar in appearance to severe pulmonary hypoplasia, infants with congenital alveolar dysplasia are born at term and have normal to increased lung weight. Clinical history and the absence of other anomalies limiting lung growth should be used to distinguish between the entities. Due to similar lung immaturity, the diagnosis of congenital alveolar dysplasia cannot be made with certainty in premature infants. While multiple reports of familial cases of acinar dysplasia suggest an underlying genetic mechanism, until recently no single candidate gene has been isolated. A comprehensive genetic analysis of a large number of cases of acinar dysplasia, congenital alveolar dysplasia, and other idiopathic lethal lung hypoplasias by Karolak et al. demonstrated disruption in *TBX4* or *FGF10* in over 50%, with compound heterozygosity of both coding and noncoding variant alleles.[107] Disruption of the TBX-FGF pathway in acinar dysplasia has been substantiated in other case reports.[108–110]

ACDMPV presents similarly to infants with acinar dysplasia and congenital alveolar dysplasia, with respiratory distress and severe pulmonary hypertension within a few hours or days after birth. They demonstrate no sustained response to extensive therapeutic interventions, including inhaled nitric oxide and ECMO, and usually die within the first few weeks of life. A few cases of delayed presentation to weeks or months with longer survival have rarely been described.[111–114] Many infants with ACDMPV have additional congenital malformations with cardiac, gastrointestinal, and renal abnormalities the most frequent.[115–117] ACDMPV is

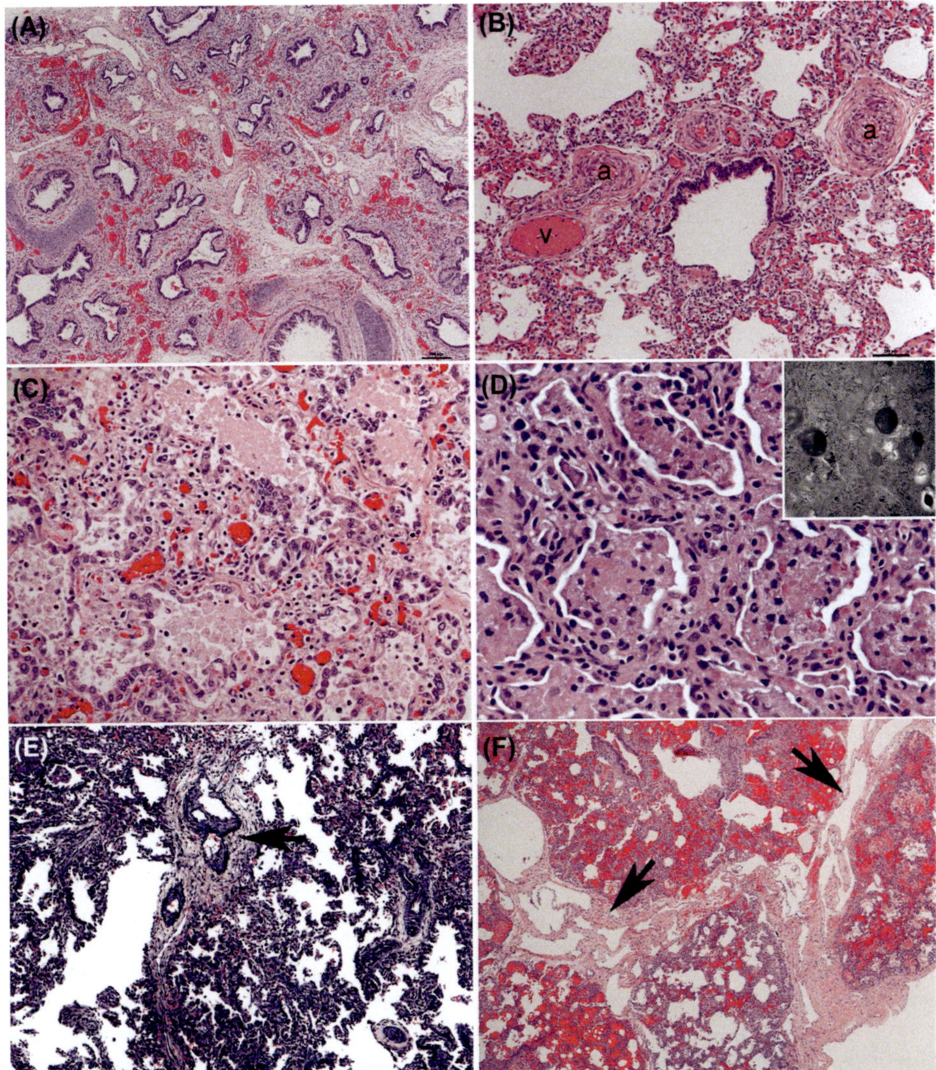

FIG. 2.13 **Other chronic neonatal lung disease disorders in the differential of chronic neonatal lung disease.** **(A)** Acinar dysplasia shows only proximal airway development composed of bronchial and bronchiolar structures; this infant was found to have a mutation in *TBX-4.* **(B)** Aberrant location of pulmonary veins adjacent to arteries is pathognomonic of the disorder alveolar capillary dysplasia with misalignment of pulmonary veins (v, vein; a, artery). **(C)** A term infant with idiopathic respiratory distress syndrome at birth was found to have an *NKX2.1* mutation at autopsy, suspected due to the presence of diffuse alveolar damage with proteinosis and absence of prosurfactant C staining in Type II alveolar cells. **(D)** Coarse pulmonary alveolar proteinosis in an infant with an *ABCA3* mutation; insert demonstrates the distinctive appearance of the lamellar bodies in this mutation, which are small and contain eccentric electron-dense inclusion bodies. **(E)** A rare case of idiopathic veno-occlusive disease in a former 32-week gestation infant who succumbed at 7 weeks to severe pulmonary hypertension (Movat pentachrome stain; *arrow* denotes vein with occlusive fibrosis). **(F)** Pulmonary lymphangiectasia (*arrows* point to dilated lymphatics in the interlobular septa) in an infant with total anomalous pulmonary venous return; congestion and hemorrhage is also present.

defined by its characteristic constellation of histologic features, of which anomalously situated pulmonary veins accompanying bronchioles and small pulmonary arteries in the same adventitial sheath is essential (Fig. 2.13B). Normally, pulmonary veins are positioned in the interlobular septa, arising from small veins which drain pulmonary lobules. In conjunction with the abnormally positioned veins, there is marked medial hypertrophy of pulmonary arteries and often abnormal lung growth. The origin of these misaligned vessels is not well understood, but three-dimensional reconstruction of the vasculature in cases of ACDMPV has demonstrated they are abnormal vascular shunts between the systemic and pulmonary circulations.[118] Mutations and deletions involving the *FOXF1* gene, which encodes a transcription factor important in vascular development, have been identified in the majority of infants with ACDMPV.[119–121] Approximately 10% of cases have a familial association, with the remaining being sporadic.

GENETIC DISORDERS OF SURFACTANT METABOLISM

Mutations in genes encoding proteins necessary for production, function, and metabolism of pulmonary surfactant are becoming a frequent cause of unexplained RDS in otherwise normal term infants.[1,45,122–124] These disorders include mutations in adenosine 5′triphosphate-binding cassette family member A-3 *(ABCA3)*, surfactant protein B (*SFTPB*), surfactant protein C (*SFTPC*), and mutations or deletions in *NKX2.1*. Inheritance patterns depend on the underlying genetic defect with variable age of presentation (Table 2.2). Infants with surfactant protein B deficiency and certain subtypes of ABCA3 deficiency (nonsense or frameshift mutations) develop respiratory distress shortly after birth that is rapidly fatal without transplant.[125] Partial SP-B deficiency and other forms of ABCA3 deficiency (missense mutations), however, can present latter in life and with variable degrees of clinical manifestation.[125–128] Cough, tachypnea, hypoxemia, and failure to thrive are frequently reported. *SFTPC* mutations have even more variable age of onset of symptoms with generally milder disease and prolonged survival.[129] *SFTPC* mutations are a recognized cause of idiopathic and familial pulmonary fibrosis in older children and adults. Mutations and deletions in *NKX2.1* result in "brain-thyroid-lung" syndrome, with a large spectrum of presentations from RDS in infancy, chronic lung disease, and recurrent infections (Fig. 2.13C).[45] The pathology of these disorders on lung biopsy can present with a variety of histologic patterns including pulmonary alveolar proteinosis (PAP), chronic pneumonitis of infancy, desquamative interstitial pneumonia, and nonspecific interstitial pneumonia (NSIP) (Fig. 2.13D).[1,128] Electron microscopy may be helpful as mutations in *SFTPB* and *ABCA3* that present in infancy have characteristic findings.[123,124,130] Lung from older children and adults with *ABCA3* and *SFTPC* mutations tend to show more fibrosis, with the pattern of NSIP or even UIP, although a degree of proteinosis is usually present.[128,131,132] The histology in individuals with NKX2.1 mutations is notably heterogeneous and includes HMD, PAP, deficient lung growth, NSIP, and even normal.[45]

PULMONARY VASCULAR DISORDERS

As well as pulmonary arterial hypertension being a component of many of the disorders described above, primary arterial, venous, and lymphatic disorders may masquerade as ILD by clinical and imaging criteria.[1,133] Distinguishing these conditions from those associated with ILD requires high-quality high-resolution CT images in conjunction with echocardiography to rule out structural cardiovascular disease.[3] Genetic testing for chromosomal disorders (Trisomy 21, Turner syndrome) or specific mutations (*FOXF1, PTPN11)* is often required to put the vascular disease in context.

Persistent PPHN is a clinical syndrome defined by severe hypoxemia and pulmonary hypertension from failure of the normal fetal to neonatal circulatory transition.[134] Affected infants are typically late-preterm or full-term and present with cyanosis and respiratory distress at or shortly after birth. By echocardiogram they have evidence of a right-to-left shunt with elevated pulmonary artery pressures. There are many known etiologies of PPHN, which may be classified as primary or secondary.[135] Primary PPHN is related to a decrease in the cross-sectional area of the pulmonary vasculature, as in the case of pulmonary hypoplasia or alveolar capillary dysplasia with misalignment of the pulmonary veins. Secondary PPHN commonly occurs in the context of congenital heart disease or severe acquired pulmonary disease (i.e., meconium aspiration, neonatal pneumonia) resulting in clinically significant pulmonary vasoconstriction. PPHN may also result from decreased in utero perfusion/oxygenation or intrapartum asphyxia. Histologically, it is characterized by increased muscularization of the small pulmonary arteries and abnormal extension of smooth muscle into normally nonmuscularized intraacinar vessels, which account for increased pulmonary vascular resistance and reduced compliance.[136] As PPHN is a component of many of the hypoxic neonatal lung disorders described above (diffuse developmental disorders, deficient lung alveolarization, PIG, congenital abnormalities of surfactant metabolism), it is critical to define pathologically as well as clinically the potential underlying etiology of vascular remodeling. In the past few years a number of genes associated with inheritable and sporadic pulmonary arterial hypertension have been discovered, but this remains a rare etiology of vascular disease presenting in the neonate.[137]

Congestive vasculopathy is a term applied to a variety of conditions related to pulmonary veins and pulmonary venous hypertension. These include left-sided cardiac disease, pulmonary vein stenosis or atresia, extrinsic pulmonary venous compression, and rarely in a neonate pulmonary veno-occlusive disease.[138] Congestive vasculopathy is characterized pathologically by pulmonary vein wall thickening and arterialization, lymphatic dilatation, congested capillaries, accumulation of hemosiderin-laden macrophages, and pulmonary arterial hypertension (Fig. 2.13E).

Lymphangiectasia, either isolated to the lung or associated with involvement of other organs, presents in the neonate with severe respiratory distress and chylous pleural effusions.[139] Lymphangiectasia may be primary/congenital or secondary to conditions that increase lymph production or impair lymph drainage. Primary lymphangiectasia may be sporadic or a component of a chromosomal (Down syndrome, Turner syndrome) or genetic disorder (Noonan syndrome, Ehlers-Danlos syndrome).[140,141] Secondary lymphangiectasia occurs if there is obstruction to lymphatic drainage (surgery, radiation, infection) or increased lymphatic circulation, the latter predominantly in children with congenital heart disease (e.g., total anomalous pulmonary venous return, hypoplastic left heart, congenital mitral stenosis). On histology there is diffuse dilatation of lymphatic channels adjacent to blood vessels in the bronchovascular space and the connective tissue of interlobular septa and the pleura, with no discernible difference between primary or secondary etiology (Fig. 2.13F). As pulmonary lymphangiectasia may be confused with PIE, a lymphatic immunostain may be required.

ACKNOWLEDGMENTS

Many of the lungs illustrated were obtained through the Biorepository for Investigation of Neonatal Diseases of the Lung (BRINDL) established through the LungMAP Consortium [U01HL122642; lungmap.net], funded by the National Heart, Lung, and Blood Institute (NHLBI).

REFERENCES

1. Deutsch GH, Young LR, Deterding RR, et al. Diffuse lung disease in young children: application of a novel classification scheme. *Am J Respir Crit Care Med*. 2007;176: 1120–1128.
2. Langston C, Dishop MK. Diffuse lung disease in infancy: a proposed classification applied to 259 diagnostic biopsies. *Pediatr Dev Pathol*. 2009;12:421–437.
3. Kurland G, Deterding RR, Hagood JS, et al. An official American Thoracic Society clinical practice guideline: classification, evaluation, and management of childhood interstitial lung disease in infancy. *Am J Respir Crit Care Med*. 2013;188:376–394.
4. Burri PH. Fetal and postnatal development of the lung. *Annu Rev Physiol*. 1984;46:617–628.
5. Langston C, Kida K, Reed M, et al. Human lung growth in late gestation and in the neonate. *Am Rev Respir Dis*. 1984; 129:607–613.
6. Burri PH. Structural aspects of postnatal lung development - alveolar formation and growth. *Biol Neonate*. 2006;89:313–322.
7. Zeltner TB, Burri PH. The postnatal development and growth of the human lung. II. Morphology. *Respir Physiol*. 1987;67:269–282.
8. Zeltner TB, Caduff JH, Gehr P, et al. The postnatal development and growth of the human lung. I. Morphometry. *Respir Physiol*. 1987;67:247–267.
9. Davies G, Reid L. Growth of the alveoli and pulmonary arteries in childhood. *Thorax*. 1970;25:669–681.
10. Ochs M, Nyengaard JR, Jung A, et al. The number of alveoli in the human lung. *Am J Respir Crit Care Med*. 2004;169:120–124.
11. Herring MJ, Putney LF, Wyatt G, et al. Growth of alveoli during postnatal development in humans based on stereological estimation. *Am J Physiol Lung Cell Mol Physiol*. 2014;307:L338–L344.
12. Thurlbeck WM. Postnatal human lung growth. *Thorax*. 1982;37:564–571.
13. Northway Jr WH, Rosan RC, Porter DY. Pulmonary disease following respirator therapy of hyaline-membrane disease. Bronchopulmonary dysplasia. *N Engl J Med*. 1967;276:357–368.
14. Northway Jr WH. Observations on bronchopulmonary dysplasia. *J Pediatr*. 1979;95:815–818.
15. O'Brodovich HM, Mellins RB. Bronchopulmonary dysplasia. Unresolved neonatal acute lung injury. *Am Rev Respir Dis*. 1985;132:694–709.
16. Pfenninger J, Tschaeppeler H, Wagner BP, et al. The paradox of adult respiratory distress syndrome in neonates. *Pediatr Pulmonol*. 1991;10:18–24.
17. Hung HY, Huang FY, Ho MY, et al. Adult respiratory distress syndrome in full term neonates. *Zhonghua Min Guo Xiao Er Ke Yi Xue Hui Za Zhi*. 1994;35:36–44.

18. Faix RG, Viscardi RM, DiPietro MA, et al. Adult respiratory distress syndrome in full-term newborns. *Pediatrics.* 1989;83:971–976.
19. Charafeddine L, D'Angio CT, Phelps DL. Atypical chronic lung disease patterns in neonates. *Pediatrics.* 1999;103: 759–765.
20. Allen J, Zwerdling R, Ehrenkranz R, et al. Statement on the care of the child with chronic lung disease of infancy and childhood. *Am J Respir Crit Care Med.* 2003;168:356–396.
21. Comroe Jr JH. Premature science and immature lungs. Part III. The attack on immature lungs. *Am Rev Respir Dis.* 1977;116:497–518.
22. Farrell PM, Avery ME. Hyaline membrane disease. *Am Rev Respir Dis.* 1975;111:657–688.
23. Lauweryns JM. Hyaline membrane disease" in newborn infants. Macroscopic, radiographic, and light and electron microscopic studies. *Hum Pathol.* 1970;1:175–204.
24. Morgenstern B, Klionsky B, Doshi N. Yellow hyaline membrane disease. Identification of the pigment and bilirubin binding. *Lab Investig.* 1981;44:514–518.
25. Stocker JT. Pathologic features of long-standing "healed" bronchopulmonary dysplasia: a study of 28 3- to 40-month-old infants. *Hum Pathol.* 1986;17:943–961.
26. Bonikos DS, Bensch KG, Northway Jr WH, et al. Bronchopulmonary dysplasia: the pulmonary pathologic sequel of necrotizing bronchiolitis and pulmonary fibrosis. *Hum Pathol.* 1976;7:643–666.
27. Miller RW, Woo P, Kellman RK, et al. Tracheobronchial abnormalities in infants with bronchopulmonary dysplasia. *J Pediatr.* 1987;111:779–782.
28. Husain AN, Siddiqui NH, Stocker JT. Pathology of arrested acinar development in postsurfactant bronchopulmonary dysplasia. *Hum Pathol.* 1998;29:710–717.
29. Coalson JJ. Pathology of new bronchopulmonary dysplasia. *Semin Neonatol.* 2003;8:73–81.
30. Jobe AJ. The new BPD: an arrest of lung development. *Pediatr Res.* 1999;46:641–643.
31. De Paepe ME, Mao Q, Powell J, et al. Growth of pulmonary microvasculature in ventilated preterm infants. *Am J Respir Crit Care Med.* 2006;173:204–211.
32. Margraf LR, Tomashefski Jr JF, Bruce MC, et al. Morphometric analysis of the lung in bronchopulmonary dysplasia. *Am Rev Respir Dis.* 1991;143:391–400.
33. Aguayo SM, Schuyler WE, Murtagh Jr JJ, et al. Regulation of lung branching morphogenesis by bombesin-like peptides and neutral endopeptidase. *Am J Respir Cell Mol Biol.* 1994;10:635–642.
34. Thibeault DW, Mabry SM, Norberg M, et al. Lung microvascular adaptation in infants with chronic lung disease. *Biol Neonate.* 2004;85:273–282.
35. Thibeault DW, Mabry SM, Ekekezie II , et al. Lung elastic tissue maturation and perturbations during the evolution of chronic lung disease. *Pediatrics.* 2000;106:1452–1459.
36. Bhatt AJ, Pryhuber GS, Huyck H, et al. Disrupted pulmonary vasculature and decreased vascular endothelial growth factor, Flt-1, and TIE-2 in human infants dying with bronchopulmonary dysplasia. *Am J Respir Crit Care Med.* 2001;164:1971–1980.
37. Chambers HM, van Velzen D. Ventilator-related pathology in the extremely immature lung. *Pathology.* 1989;21:79–83.
38. Fan LL, Dishop MK, Galambos C, et al. Diffuse lung disease in biopsied children 2 to 18 Years of age. Application of the chILD classification scheme. *Ann Am Thorac Soc.* 2015;12:1498–1505.
39. Ardini-Poleske ME, Clark RF, Ansong C, et al. LungMAP: the molecular atlas of lung development program. *Am J Physiol Lung Cell Mol Physiol.* 2017;313:L733–L740.
40. Bandyopadhyay G, Huyck HL, Misra RS, et al. Dissociation, cellular isolation, and initial molecular characterization of neonatal and pediatric human lung tissues. *Am J Physiol Lung Cell Mol Physiol.* 2018;315:L576–L583.
41. Cooney TP, Thurlbeck WM. The radial alveolar count method of Emery and Mithal: a reappraisal 1–postnatal lung growth. *Thorax.* 1982;37:572–579.
42. Emery JL, Mithal A. The number of alveoli in the terminal respiratory unit of man during late intrauterine life and childhood. *Arch Dis Child.* 1960;35:544–547.
43. Coalson JJ. Pathology of bronchopulmonary dysplasia. *Semin Perinatol.* 2006;30:179–184.
44. Page DV, Stocker JT. Anomalies associated with pulmonary hypoplasia. *Am Rev Respir Dis.* 1982;125:216–221.
45. Hamvas A, Deterding RR, Wert SE, et al. Heterogeneous pulmonary phenotypes associated with mutations in the thyroid transcription factor gene NKX2-1. *Chest.* 2013;144:794–804.
46. Shelmerdine SC, Semple T, Wallis C, et al. Filamin A (FLNA) mutation-A newcomer to the childhood interstitial lung disease (Child) classification. *Pediatr Pulmonol.* 2017;52:1306–1315.
47. Sherer DM, Davis JM, Woods Jr JR. Pulmonary hypoplasia: a review. *Obstet Gynecol Surv.* 1990;45:792–803.
48. Nakamura Y, Harada K, Yamamoto I, et al. Human pulmonary hypoplasia. Statistical, morphological, morphometric, and biochemical study. *Arch Pathol Lab Med.* 1992;116:635–642.
49. Wigglesworth JS, Desai R, Guerrini P. Fetal lung hypoplasia: biochemical and structural variations and their possible significance. *Arch Dis Child.* 1981;56:606–615.
50. Reale FR, Esterly JR. Pulmonary hypoplasia: a morphometric study of the lungs of infants with diaphragmatic hernia, anencephaly, and renal malformations. *Pediatrics.* 1973;51:91–96.
51. Chi TPLKJ. The pulmonary vascular bed in children with Down syndrome. *J Pediatr.* 1975;86:533–538.
52. Rudolph AM. High pulmonary vascular resistance after birth: I. Pathophysiologic considerations and etiologic classification. *Clin Pediatr.* 1980;19:585–590.
53. Geggel RL, Reid LM. The structural basis of PPHN. *Clin Perinatol.* 1984;11:525–549.
54. Massaro GD, Massaro D. Postnatal lung growth: evidence that the gas-exchange region grows fastest at the periphery. *Am J Physiol.* 1993;265:L319–L322.
55. Narayanan M, Owers-Bradley J, Beardsmore CS, et al. Alveolarization continues during childhood and adolescence: new evidence from helium-3 magnetic resonance. *Am J Respir Crit Care Med.* 2012;185:186–191.

56. Biko DM, Schwartz M, Anupindi SA, et al. Subpleural lung cysts in Down syndrome: prevalence and association with coexisting diagnoses. *Pediatr Radiol.* 2008;38: 280–284.
57. Cooney TP, Thurlbeck WM. Pulmonary hypoplasia in Down's syndrome. *N Engl J Med.* 1982;307: 1170–1173.
58. Lord A, Shapiro AJ, Saint-Martin C, et al. Filamin A mutation may be associated with diffuse lung disease mimicking bronchopulmonary dysplasia in premature newborns. *Respir Care.* 2014;59:e171–177.
59. Galambos C, Levy H, Cannon CL, et al. Pulmonary pathology in thyroid transcription factor-1 deficiency syndrome. *Am J Respir Crit Care Med.* 2010;182: 549–554.
60. Krude H, Schutz B, Biebermann H, et al. Choreoathetosis, hypothyroidism, and pulmonary alterations due to human NKX2-1 haploinsufficiency. *J Clin Investig.* 2002; 109:475–480.
61. Kimura S, Hara Y, Pineau T, et al. The T/ebp null mouse: thyroid-specific enhancer-binding protein is essential for the organogenesis of the thyroid, lung, ventral forebrain, and pituitary. *Genes Dev.* 1996;10:60–69.
62. Guillot L, Carre A, Szinnai G, et al. NKX2-1 mutations leading to surfactant protein promoter dysregulation cause interstitial lung disease in "Brain-Lung-Thyroid Syndrome". *Hum Mutat.* 2010;31:E1146–E1162.
63. Thorwarth A, Schnittert-Hubener S, Schrumpf P, et al. Comprehensive genotyping and clinical characterisation reveal 27 novel NKX2-1 mutations and expand the phenotypic spectrum. *J Med Genet.* 2014;51: 375–387.
64. Robertson SP, Twigg SR, Sutherland-Smith AJ, et al. Localized mutations in the gene encoding the cytoskeletal protein filamin A cause diverse malformations in humans. *Nat Genet.* 2003;33:487–491.
65. Sole G, Coupry I, Rooryck C, et al. Bilateral periventricular nodular heterotopia in France: frequency of mutations in FLNA, phenotypic heterogeneity and spectrum of mutations. *J Neurol Neurosurg Psychiatry.* 2009;80: 1394–1398.
66. Masurel-Paulet A, Haan E, Thompson EM, et al. Lung disease associated with periventricular nodular heterotopia and an FLNA mutation. *Eur J Med Genet.* 2011; 54:25–28.
67. Burrage LC, Guillerman RP, Das S, et al. Lung transplantation for FLNA-associated progressive lung disease. *J Pediatr.* 2017;186, 118–123 e116.
68. De Paepe ME, Carr SR, Cassese JA. Postmortem validation of imaging-derived formulas for prediction of fetal lung volume. *Fetal Diagn Ther.* 2003;18:353–359.
69. De Paepe ME, Friedman RM, Gundogan F, et al. Postmortem lung weight/body weight standards for term and preterm infants. *Pediatr Pulmonol.* 2005;40:445–448.
70. Cooney TP, Thurlbeck WM. The radial alveolar count method of Emery and Mithal: a reappraisal 2–intrauterine and early postnatal lung growth. *Thorax.* 1982;37:580–583.
71. Schroeder SA, Shannon DC, Mark EJ. Cellular interstitial pneumonitis in infants. A clinicopathologic study. *Chest.* 1992;101:1065–1069.
72. Canakis AM, Cutz E, Manson D, et al. Pulmonary interstitial glycogenosis: a new variant of neonatal interstitial lung disease. *Am J Respir Crit Care Med.* 2002;165: 1557–1565.
73. Castillo, M., A. Vade, J.E. Lim-Dunham, et al., Pulmonary interstitial glycogenosis in the setting of lung growth abnormality: radiographic and pathologic correlation. Pediatr Radiol 40:1562-1565.
74. Deutsch, G.H. and L.R. Young, Pulmonary interstitial glycogenosis: words of caution. Pediatr Radiol 40:1471-1475.
75. Cutz E, Chami R, Dell S, et al. Pulmonary interstitial glycogenosis associated with a spectrum of neonatal pulmonary disorders. *Hum Pathol.* 2017;68:154–165.
76. Deutsch GH, Young LR. Histologic resolution of pulmonary interstitial glycogenosis. *Pediatr Dev Pathol.* 2009;12: 475–480.
77. Lanfranchi, M., S.M. Allbery, L. Wheelock, et al., Pulmonary interstitial glycogenosis. Pediatr Radiol 40:361-365.
78. Deutsch GH, Young LR. Lipofibroblast phenotype in pulmonary interstitial glycogenosis. *Am J Respir Crit Care Med.* 2016;193:694–696.
79. Rehan VK, Torday JS. PPARgamma signaling mediates the evolution, development, homeostasis, and repair of the lung. *PPAR Res.* 2012;2012:289867.
80. Varisco BM, Ambalavanan N, Whitsett JA, et al. Thy-1 signals through PPARgamma to promote lipofibroblast differentiation in the developing lung. *Am J Respir Cell Mol Biol.* 2012;46:765–772.
81. Rehan VK, Sugano S, Wang Y, et al. Evidence for the presence of lipofibroblasts in human lung. *Exp Lung Res.* 2006;32:379–393.
82. Kyle JE, Clair G, Bandyopadhyay G, et al. Cell type-resolved human lung lipidome reveals cellular cooperation in lung function. *Sci Rep.* 2018;8:13455.
83. Stocker JT, Madewell JE. Persistent interstitial pulmonary emphysema: another complication of the respiratory distress syndrome. *Pediatrics.* 1977;59:847–857.
84. Brewer LL, Moskowitz PS, Carrington CB, et al. Pneumatosis pulmonalis: a complication of the idiopathic respiratory distress syndrome. *Am J Pathol.* 1979;95:171–190.
85. Shieh SY, Ikeda M, Taya Y, et al. DNA damage-induced phosphorylation of p53 alleviates inhibition of MDM2. *Cell.* 1997;91:325–334.
86. Linnoila RI. Functional facets of the pulmonary neuroendocrine system. *Lab Investig.* 2006;86:425–444.
87. Willey JC, Lechner JF, Harris CC. Bombesin and the C-terminal tetradecapeptide of gastrin-releasing peptide are growth factors for normal human bronchial epithelial cells. *Exp Cell Res.* 1984;153:245–248.
88. Sunday ME, Hua J, Dai HB, et al. Bombesin increases fetal lung growth and maturation in utero and in organ culture. *Am J Respir Cell Mol Biol.* 1990;3:199–205.
89. King KA, Torday JS, Sunday ME. Bombesin and [Leu8] phyllolitorin promote fetal mouse lung branching

morphogenesis via a receptor-mediated mechanism. *Proc Natl Acad Sci USA*. 1995;92:4357–4361.

90. Cutz E, Yeger H, Pan J. Pulmonary neuroendocrine cell system in pediatric lung disease-recent advances. *Pediatr Dev Pathol*. 2007;10:419–435.
91. Cutz E. Hyperplasia of pulmonary neuroendocrine cells in infancy and childhood. *Semin Diagn Pathol*. 2015;32: 420–437.
92. Sunday ME, Yoder BA, Cuttitta F, et al. Bombesin-like peptide mediates lung injury in a baboon model of bronchopulmonary dysplasia. *J Clin Investig*. 1998;102: 584–594.
93. Subramaniam M, Sugiyama K, Coy DH, et al. Bombesin-like peptides and mast cell responses: relevance to bronchopulmonary dysplasia? *Am J Respir Crit Care Med*. 2003;168:601–611.
94. Ashour K, Shan L, Lee JH, et al. Bombesin inhibits alveolarization and promotes pulmonary fibrosis in newborn mice. *Am J Respir Crit Care Med*. 2006;173: 1377–1385.
95. Subramaniam M, Bausch C, Twomey A, et al. Bombesin-like peptides modulate alveolarization and angiogenesis in bronchopulmonary dysplasia. *Am J Respir Crit Care Med*. 2007;176:902–912.
96. Cullen A, Van Marter LJ, Allred EN, et al. Urine bombesin-like peptide elevation precedes clinical evidence of bronchopulmonary dysplasia. *Am J Respir Crit Care Med*. 2002;165:1093–1097.
97. Chang LY, Subramaniam M, Yoder BA, et al. A catalytic antioxidant attenuates alveolar structural remodeling in bronchopulmonary dysplasia. *Am J Respir Crit Care Med*. 2003;167:57–64.
98. Borges M, Linnoila RI, van de Velde HJ, et al. An achaete-scute homologue essential for neuroendocrine differentiation in the lung. *Nature*. 1997;386:852–855.
99. Nogee LM. Interstitial lung disease in newborns. *Semin Fetal Neonatal Med*. 2017;22:227–233.
100. Deterding RR, Pye C, Fan LL, et al. Persistent tachypnea of infancy is associated with neuroendocrine cell hyperplasia. *Pediatr Pulmonol*. 2005;40:157–165.
101. Stocker JT, Drake RM, Madewell JE. Cystic and congenital lung disease in the newborn. *Perspect Pediatr Pathol*. 1978; 4:93–154.
102. Rutledge JC, Jensen P. Acinar dysplasia: a new form of pulmonary maldevelopment. *Hum Pathol*. 1986;17: 1290–1293.
103. Chambers HM. Congenital acinar aplasia: an extreme form of pulmonary maldevelopment. *Pathology*. 1991; 23:69–71.
104. Davidson LA, Batman P, Fagan DG. Congenital acinar dysplasia: a rare cause of pulmonary hypoplasia. *Histopathology*. 1998;32:57–59.
105. Langenstroer M, Carlan SJ, Fanaian N, et al. Congenital acinar dysplasia: report of a case and review of literature. *AJP Rep*. 2013;3:9–12.
106. Mac MH. Congenital alveolar dysplasia; a developmental anomaly involving pulmonary alveoli. *Pediatrics*. 1948;2: 43–57.
107. Karolak JA, Vincent M, Deutsch G, et al. Complex compound inheritance of lethal lung developmental disorders due to disruption of the TBX-FGF pathway. *Am J Hum Genet*. 2019;104:213–228.
108. Barnett CP, Nataren NJ, Klingler-Hoffmann M, et al. Ectrodactyly and lethal pulmonary acinar dysplasia associated with homozygous FGFR2 mutations identified by exome sequencing. *Hum Mutat*. 2016;37:955–963.
109. Szafranski P, Coban-Akdemir ZH, Rupps R, et al. Phenotypic expansion of TBX4 mutations to include acinar dysplasia of the lungs. *Am J Med Genet A*. 2016;170: 2440–2444.
110. Suhrie K, Pajor NM, Ahlfeld SK, et al. Neonatal lung disease associated with TBX4 mutations. *J Pediatr*. 2018.
111. Licht C, Schickendantz S, Sreeram N, et al. Prolonged survival in alveolar capillary dysplasia syndrome. *Eur J Pediatr*. 2004;163:181–182.
112. Shankar V, Haque A, Johnson J, et al. Late presentation of alveolar capillary dysplasia in an infant. *Pediatr Crit Care Med*. 2006;7:177–179.
113. Ahmed S, Ackerman V, Faught P, et al. Profound hypoxemia and pulmonary hypertension in a 7-month-old infant: late presentation of alveolar capillary dysplasia. *Pediatr Crit Care Med*. 2008;9:e43–46.
114. Al-Hathlol K, Phillips S, Seshia MK, et al. Alveolar capillary dysplasia. Report of a case of prolonged life without extracorporeal membrane oxygenation (ECMO) and review of the literature. *Early Hum Dev*. 2000;57:85–94.
115. Rabah R, Poulik JM. Congenital alveolar capillary dysplasia with misalignment of pulmonary veins associated with hypoplastic left heart syndrome. *Pediatr Dev Pathol*. 2001;4:167–174.
116. Sen P, Thakur N, Stockton DW, et al. Expanding the phenotype of alveolar capillary dysplasia (ACD). *J Pediatr*. 2004;145:646–651.
117. Antao B, Samuel M, Kiely E, et al. Congenital alveolar capillary dysplasia and associated gastrointestinal anomalies. *Fetal Pediatr Pathol*. 2006;25:137–145.
118. Galambos C, Sims-Lucas S, Abman SH. Three-dimensional reconstruction identifies misaligned pulmonary veins as intrapulmonary shunt vessels in alveolar capillary dysplasia. *J Pediatr*. 2014;164:192–195.
119. Stankiewicz P, Sen P, Bhatt SS, et al. Genomic and genic deletions of the FOX gene cluster on 16q24.1 and inactivating mutations of FOXF1 cause alveolar capillary dysplasia and other malformations. *Am J Hum Genet*. 2009;84:780–791.
120. Yu, S., L. Shao, H. Kilbride, et al., Haploinsufficiencies of FOXF1 and FOXC2 genes associated with lethal alveolar capillary dysplasia and congenital heart disease. Am J Med Genet A 152A:1257-1262.
121. Szafranski P, Dharmadhikari AV, Wambach JA, et al. Two deletions overlapping a distant FOXF1 enhancer unravel the role of lncRNA LINC01081 in etiology of alveolar capillary dysplasia with misalignment of pulmonary veins. *Am J Med Genet A*. 2014;164A:2013–2019.
122. Nogee LM, Garnier G, Dietz HC, et al. A mutation in the surfactant protein B gene responsible for fatal neonatal

respiratory disease in multiple kindreds. *J Clin Investig.* 1994;93:1860–1863.
123. Shulenin S, Nogee LM, Annilo T, et al. ABCA3 gene mutations in newborns with fatal surfactant deficiency. *N Engl J Med.* 2004;350:1296–1303.
124. Wert SE, Whitsett JA, Nogee LM. Genetic disorders of surfactant dysfunction. *Pediatr Dev Pathol.* 2009;12: 253–274.
125. Wambach JA, Casey AM, Fishman MP, et al. Genotype-phenotype correlations for infants and children with ABCA3 deficiency. *Am J Respir Crit Care Med.* 2014;189: 1538–1543.
126. Ballard PL, Nogee LM, Beers MF, et al. Partial deficiency of surfactant protein B in an infant with chronic lung disease. *Pediatrics.* 1995;96:1046–1052.
127. Dunbar 3rd AE, Wert SE, Ikegami M, et al. Prolonged survival in hereditary surfactant protein B (SP-B) deficiency associated with a novel splicing mutation. *Pediatr Res.* 2000;48:275–282.
128. Doan ML, Guillerman RP, Dishop MK, et al. Clinical, radiological and pathological features of ABCA3 mutations in children. *Thorax.* 2008;63:366–373.
129. Hamvas A, Cole FS, Nogee LM. Genetic disorders of surfactant proteins. *Neonatology.* 2007;91:311–317.
130. Tryka AF, Wert SE, Mazursky JE, et al. Absence of lamellar bodies with accumulation of dense bodies characterizes a novel form of congenital surfactant defect. *Pediatr Dev Pathol.* 2000;3:335–345.
131. Chibbar R, Shih F, Baga M, et al. Nonspecific interstitial pneumonia and usual interstitial pneumonia with mutation in surfactant protein C in familial pulmonary fibrosis. *Mod Pathol.* 2004;17:973–980.
132. Young LR, Nogee LM, Barnett B, et al. Usual interstitial pneumonia in an adolescent with ABCA3 mutations. *Chest.* 2008;134:192–195.
133. Sondheimer HM, Lung MC, Brugman SM, et al. Pulmonary vascular disorders masquerading as interstitial lung disease. *Pediatr Pulmonol.* 1995;20:284–288.
134. Morin 3rd FC, Stenmark KR. Persistent pulmonary hypertension of the newborn. *Am J Respir Crit Care Med.* 1995; 151:2010–2032.
135. Haworth SG. Primary and secondary pulmonary hypertension in childhood: a clinicopathological reappraisal. *Curr Top Pathol.* 1983;73:91–152.
136. Murphy JD, Rabinovitch M, Goldstein JD, et al. The structural basis of persistent pulmonary hypertension of the newborn infant. *J Pediatr.* 1981;98:962–967.
137. Chew JD, Loyd JE, Austin ED. Genetics of pulmonary arterial hypertension. *Semin Respir Crit Care Med.* 2017; 38:585–595.
138. Abman SH, Hansmann G, Archer SL, et al. Pediatric pulmonary hypertension: guidelines from the American heart association and American thoracic society. *Circulation.* 2015;132:2037–2099.
139. Faul JL, Berry GJ, Colby TV, et al. Thoracic lymphangiomas, lymphangiectasis, lymphangiomatosis, and lymphatic dysplasia syndrome. *Am J Respir Crit Care Med.* 2000;161:1037–1046.
140. Bellini C, Boccardo F, Campisi C, et al. Congenital pulmonary lymphangiectasia. *Orphanet J Rare Dis.* 2006;1: 43.
141. Barker PM, Esther Jr CR, Fordham LA, et al. Primary pulmonary lymphangiectasia in infancy and childhood. *Eur Respir J.* 2004;24:413–419.

CHAPTER 3

Animal Models of Bronchopulmonary Dysplasia

SEAN LEARY, BS • VINEET BHANDARI, MBBS, MD, DM

INTRODUCTION

The clinical definition and pathological characteristics of bronchopulmonary dysplasia (BPD) have evolved over time, and because of this, through the years, there has been a need for a developmentally appropriate animal model that can recapitulate the changing pathogenesis. The first animal model that could be considered a model for BPD was rats that were exposed to elevated oxygen levels in the 1930s.[1] Since then, models have become more specific in their targeting of the critical saccular stage of lung development and the experimental conditions exposed to the animals designed to recreate the factors contributing to the progression of BPD.

Throughout this chapter, the body of literature surrounding the various animal models of BPD will be explored, detailing parameters, benefits, and drawbacks of the rodent, large mammal, and primate models of BPD and their contributions to our understanding of the pathogenesis of BPD.

RODENT MODELS

Mouse

The mouse model is the most extensively researched animal model of BPD and the availability of literature is very broad. Because of the wide-ranging use of mice in BPD research, there are many significant and subtle differences in the models. Some of the models used include hyperoxia-induced lung injury, hypoxia, combined hypoxia/hyperoxia, inflammation-induced, and transgenic models.[2]

The small size, short life cycle, ease of breeding, low cost of purchase, and broad commercial availability of research products such as antibodies contribute to the widespread use of mice in BPD research.[2] These characteristics of mice allow for larger sample sizes to be utilized and make mice one of the easiest animal models to work with for BPD modeling. Mice born at term, like human infants born preterm, are in the saccular stage of pulmonary development. This stage begins at ~ embryonic (E) day 18 (~E18) and continues through postnatal (PN) day 5 (PN5).[3] Despite being born at the more immature stage where preterm humans regularly require invasive and intensive neonatal care for survival, mouse pups born in the saccular stage are perfectly viable without any care due to functionally mature pulmonary surfactant systems.[4] These functional qualities of mouse pup lungs show strong comparability to a preterm human after receiving a complete course of antenatal steroid treatment.[2]

Hyperoxia is used in a majority of studies modeling BPD because of the injurious effects of oxygen via direct injury to cells through reactive oxygen species and propagation of the inflammatory cascade.[5] Earlier studies used continuous oxygen exposure, sometimes up to 14, 21, or 28 days, with high fractions of inspired oxygen (FiO_2) to induce significant hyperoxic damage.[6–8] Pulmonary damage worsened over time and resulted in decreased septation, enlarged terminal air sacs, and prominent pulmonary fibrosis, and these morphologic damages were seen as early as 7 days after exposure to high concentrations of O_2. Because of the significant pulmonary fibrosis, the extended hyperoxia model is probably better at recapitulating "old BPD", rather than "new" BPD.[9] The most successful models that most accurately represent "new BPD" involve those that limit the hyperoxia exposure to the saccular stage of lung development.[2] Exposure to hyperoxia for PN1-4 followed by recovery in room air until week 8 shows a dose-dependent response to degrees of hyperoxia.[10] This model accurately simulates a clinical scenario of premature humans exposed to supplemental oxygen therapy immediately after birth but then weaned off through their recovery and further development.[2] More recently, researchers have fairly accurately recreated the morphologic pathology of BPD by

Updates on Neonatal Chronic Lung Disease. https://doi.org/10.1016/B978-0-323-68353-1.00003-8

exposing the newborn pups to hyperoxia from PN1-4 followed by the next 10 days of recovery in room air.[10–12]

Hypoxia used in BPD research has involved exposing the pups to hypoxia in either the prenatal or postnatal period.[2] Postnatal hypoxia models have been successful in disrupting alveolar architecture in a similar manner as BPD. Investigators have exposed newborn pups to FiO_2 of 0.12 for 14 days and the animals showed evidence of impaired alveolarization, increased pulmonary artery thickness, and right ventricular hypertrophy—all pathological signs of BPD.[13] Despite this model accurately recreating the morphological pathology of BPD, this model fails to recreate the clinical setting of hyperoxia.[2]

The hyperoxia with intermittent hypoxia model was created to recapitulate the clinical setting of preterm infants in a hyperoxic environment that are exposed to periodic episodes of apnea and hypoxemia.[2] One such study exposed mouse pups to FiO_2 0.8 for 4 weeks with intermittent hypoxemic episodes of 10 minutes at FiO_2 0.08 and found that the mice that experienced the intermittent hypoxia had fewer alveoli, increased granulocytes, and greater oxidative damage than the purely hyperoxia-exposed mice.[14] These data suggest that the bouts of hypoxemia clinically worsen the already deleterious effects of hyperoxia.[2] Other researchers have developed models of prenatal hypoxia and postnatal hyperoxia and revealed the occurrence of significant growth restriction, in addition to the typical morphologic manifestations of BPD.[15]

Another contributing cause in the multifactorial development of BPD is volutrauma and barotrauma due to invasive mechanical ventilation. Because of the small size of mouse pups, long-term invasive ventilation is extremely difficult.[2] Beginning ventilation before PN5 is extremely challenging, limiting the exposure window to the alveolar stage of lung development and thus, limiting the applicability of the invasive mechanical ventilation model.[2,16]

Investigators have successfully created models of BPD by creating prenatal inflammation with bacterial lipopolysaccharide (LPS).[17] Studies have shown decreased levels of the bronchial development protein fibroblast growth factor-10 (FGF-10), altered location of myofibroblasts, and increased levels of proangiogenic chemokines after treatment with prenatal LPS.[17,18] Combining prenatal inflammation with postnatal hyperoxia attempts to better recapitulate the multifactorial nature of BPD and results in impaired alveolarization and widespread fibrosis.[19]

The transgenic model of BPD allows single-gene overexpression or knockout to elucidate a more precise role of various genes in the pathogenesis of BPD. While the development and progression of BPD is multifactorial, the applicability of transgenic models to the BPD phenotype may allow greater understanding of specific molecular signaling pathways. Transgenic models can provide deep insight into the unique roles various genes, cytokines, and inflammatory markers play in the development of BPD, especially when combined with additional factors such as hyperoxia, hypoxia, or prenatal inflammation.[2] Transgenic mouse models have elucidated the roles of various markers and cytokines in the pathogenesis of BPD such as interleukin (IL)-1, cellular retinoic acid binding proteins, nuclear retinoic acid binding proteins, interferon gamma, angiopoietin 2, matrix metalloproteinases, cyclooxygenase-2, transforming growth factor (TGF)-β, c-Jun N-terminal kinase (JNK) pathways, macrophage migration inhibitory factor, and many others.[2,20–30]

Besides molecular signaling pathways, hyperoxia-exposed mouse models of BPD can also provide information of pulmonary function[31,32] as well as neurodevelopment[33,34]—which would bring it closer for clinical correlation with human infants with BPD.

Overall, the mouse model provides great utility in BPD research because of the accuracy of pathology recreated, the ease of working with mice, the low cost of colony maintenance, and the wide-ranging options for specific models utilizing hyperoxia, hypoxia, inflammatory insults, and transgenic animals.

Rat

The rat model of BPD has been used extensively to study the pathophysiology of BPD, in addition to various therapeutic strategies. Various different hyperoxia exposure protocols have been used ranging typically up to 14 days using oxygen concentrations above 90%, resulting in a severe oxygen-induced injury phenotype.[35] Because of a closer relation to the treatment of premature infants in the NICU, some studies have used 0.6 FiO_2 models that produce variable changes in BPD phenotype.[35–38] The pathology of BPD observed in human infants, such as impaired alveolarization, pulmonary hypertension, disrupted vascular growth, vascular leak, accumulation of plasma proteins and inflammatory cells, extravascular fibrin deposition, and disorganized elastin deposition can be recapitulated using the rat model of BPD.[35,38–41]

At term gestation, like mice, rats are still in the saccular stage of lung development at birth and complete alveolarization *ex utero*, similar to preterm infants.[35] Despite structural immaturity, the lungs are functionally mature due to adequate surfactant production, thus eliminating the need for intensive intervention to ensure survival.[35,42] Other advantages include short estrous cycles and gestation, large litter sizes, short life span, and commercial availability of analysis products. An additional benefit of the rat model over the mouse model is the possibility to deliver the pups 0.5–1 day prematurely.[35]

Despite many benefits, there are various disadvantages of the rat model of BPD. It has been documented that the occurrence of postnatal growth restriction can negatively influence the development of the lung resulting in enlarged alveoli, thicker septa, and reduced elastin deposition in the lung parenchyma, although this can be partially mitigated through dam rotation.[43] Another disadvantage that limits the relevance of the rat model are the oxygen concentrations used, which are almost always are over 0.6 FiO_2, which are much higher than those often used in clinical practice.[35] In addition, unlike preterm infants, rats have mature antioxidant enzyme activity that can increase the tolerance to hyperoxia.[44,45]

The rat model of BPD has contributed to our understanding of the BPD phenotype. The role of vascular endothelial growth factor (VEGF) in normal lung development, its impairment in BPD, and the beneficial effect of supplementation have been studied in the rat model.[46,47] In addition, the benefits of inhaled nitric oxide (iNO), phosphodiesterase (PDE) type 5 (PDE5) and PDE4 inhibition, L-citrulline, endothelin receptor type A inhibition, and apelin, adrenomedullin, and recombinant human erythropoietin administration have been studied.[48–56] Growth factors such as keratinocyte growth factor (KGF), platelet-derived GF (PDGF), insulin-like GF (IGF), and connective tissue GF (CTGF) have also been studied in the rat models.[57–60] The rat model of BPD has also contributed to our understanding of inflammatory pathways in BPD such as glycogen synthase kinase regulation of nuclear factor (NF)-κB, treatment with pentoxifylline, administration of curcumin, the effects of resveratrol, the role of chemokine receptor 2 antagonist, and various cell line studies.[35,36,38,61–63]

Overall, the rat model has greatly contributed to our understanding of BPD. The low cost of study, ease of use, and biological applicability highlight this model's usefulness in future studies.

Guinea Pig

The guinea pig is a small animal model, like the mouse and rat, but provides a unique advantage in that the pups can be studied after preterm delivery with significant viability. Term gestation typically lasts 68 days, but the pups can be delivered prematurely via Cesarean section at gestational day (GD) 65. Preterm pups experience transient respiratory distress and significantly higher mortality than term pups (42% vs. 79% respectively) when exposed to hyperoxia postdelivery.[64] Histologically, preterm pups exposed to hyperoxia show phenotypically similar, but more severe, acute pulmonary lung damage than term pups including areas of atelectasis, pulmonary edema, fibrin deposition, and inflammatory cell infiltration.[65] Additional studies with preterm guinea pigs have shown the role leukotriene B4 plays in pulmonary neutrophil recruitment and the role of hydroxyl radicals in oxidative lung injury.[65,66]

Term guinea pig models allow spontaneous delivery around GD 68. Investigators have used an FiO_2 ranging from 0.7 to 0.95 for between 3.5 and 5 days.[67–69] Compared to the preterm model, allowing the pups to mature to term provides an added mortality benefit, and studies have been done investigating airway hyperreactivity and the role of iNO in the pathogenesis of BPD. Other more recent studies have investigated the role of glutathione in the prevention of alveolar loss.[70,71]

Overall, the guinea pig model of BPD provides many of the benefits of mouse and rat models with the added benefit of the possibility of preterm delivery. Preterm delivery of guinea pigs exacerbates the hyperoxia-associated pulmonary damage compared to term delivery, so this model provides an economical method of more accurately representing the clinical scenario of preterm birth and BPD.

Rabbit

Rabbits, in their use for BPD research, have many inherent advantages, including viability of preterm animals, the size being large enough to permit invasive procedures, and the relatively low cost.[72] Studies have shown relevant physiological and biochemical similarities to human newborns including pulmonary function, lung architecture, the development of fibrosis, the acute inflammatory response, and cytokine and growth factor production.[73–76] Term rabbits are delivered at 31 days gestation. Kittens born at this stage are in the alveolar stage of lung development and have mature surfactant and antioxidant systems.[77,78]

Short-term hyperoxia exposure in the term rabbit model involves exposing the kittens to $FiO_2 > 0.95$ for 48–96 hours. The data from these experiments suggest that newborn kittens are more resistant to hyperoxia than adults and the physiological response to the hyperoxia exposure mimics that of preterm human infants. This model highlights the feasibility of performing morphometric analysis, collecting bronchoalveolar lavage fluid (BALF) and pulmonary function data, and testing interventions in newborn rabbits.[72]

The term rabbit model involving long-term hyperoxia exposure involves the newborn kittens being exposed to an FiO_2 ranging from 0.55 to >0.95 for up to 11 days.[72] This exposure has been shown to restrict growth and development, impair immune-mediated killing of inhaled *Staphylococci*, and elicit various inflammatory responses such as increased immunostaining for NFκ-B, higher peak levels of TGF-β, and increased alveolar macrophages.[79,80] Overall, the extended hyperoxia exposure model allows the study of the inflammatory response and the effect of weight gain and development.

These models provide quality insight into the pathology of hyperoxia-mediated damage but fail to accurately represent the setting of human infants exposed to acute injury followed by a period of recovery. For this, another model is needed. Newborn kittens are exposed to FiO_2>0.95 for 8–9 days followed by exposure to FiO_2 0.6 for up to 36 subsequent days. Studies found that overall these rabbits gained weight poorly. By day 10, the kittens show moderate alveolar edema, significant alveolitis, increased cellular infiltrates and septal edema, Type II alveolar epithelial hyperplasia, and simplified alveolar structure. By day 14, the septal edema begins to resolve while the alveolitis persists. In addition, alveolar septal thickness and septal collagen content remained elevated at 22 days. By day 36, cellular infiltrates are largely resolved, and the average septal thickness is no longer significantly different than control animals, although patchy septal thickness changes still may remain.[81,82] In terms of the biochemical and immunological response, proinflammatory cytokines, interleukins, growth-regulated proteins, and growth factors all peak between 6 and 10 days of hyperoxia exposure but then decrease rapidly once the degree of hyperoxia is reduced.[83] Overall, this model reveals connections between histological and physiological changes and changes in proinflammatory cytokines and growth factors but fails to recreate the apparent long-term changes in alveolar size and structure seen in BPD.

In an attempt to more accurately represent the clinical scenario of preterm neonates, the preterm rabbit model of BPD was created. Rabbits are delivered via Cesarean section at 28–29 days gestation. These animals are in the saccular stage of lung development, have immature surfactant and antioxidant systems, and present with an increased sensitivity to hyperoxia when compared to term rabbits.[77,78,84] Short-term hyperoxia experiments involve exposing the preterm rabbits to FiO_2>0.95 for 48–96 hours. These kittens show increased BALF protein content, more severe lung pathology, and increased areas of atelectasis and hyperexpansion.[85,86] Long-term hyperoxia experiments expose the preterm kittens to hyperoxia for 7–11 days. Because of the high mortality, around 90%, experiments are difficult to execute using this model.[87–89] Despite this burden, studies have shown multiple lung function abnormalities including decreased minute volume, total lung capacity, and static compliance in addition to increased tissue elasticity and pH.[89,90]

Overall, the neonatal rabbit model of hyperoxia exposure recreates many of the patterns seen in human BPD including acute inflammatory response, abnormal pulmonary function, disordered lung architecture, alveolar simplification, development of fibrosis, and abnormal vascular growth factor expression, although many of these findings resolve when exposed to a period of recovery.[73–76] These findings become more important when considering the fact that rabbits are more similar to humans at term compared to both mice and rats, but the term model has been called into question due to the majority of BPD cases occurring in preterm infants in the saccular stage of lung development.

LARGE MAMMAL MODELS

Lamb

Lambs, like humans, born at term are in the beginning of the alveolar stage of lung development. The lamb model of BPD allows a unique insight into the complex pathogenesis of preterm neonates under intensive care.[91] Delivering the lambs preterm via Cesarean section at 125–131 days out of a typical 147-day term gestation puts the lambs in the saccular stage of lung development, similar to humans born preterm.[92] Because of the combination of physical size developmental stage of neonatal lambs, it is possible to reproduce a clinical setting of preterm birth and respiratory failure associated with mechanical ventilation. Compared to rodents and their small size, investigators are able to conduct frequent blood sampling and subject the animals to invasive mechanical ventilation.[92]

There has been evidence of an association between less invasive methods of mechanical ventilation and lower incidence and severity of BPD in human preterm infants.[93] Similarly, studies on preterm lambs have shown that less invasive mechanical ventilation, such as high-frequency nasal ventilation (HFNV) leads to decreased biochemical and morphological evidence of pulmonary damage[94–97] and allows for significantly lower applied O_2 levels and respiratory pressures.[98] Recent studies have explored the role of vitamin A and its protective role in the pathogenesis of BPD[99] and epithelial repair mechanisms after brief mechanical ventilation.[100] Within the lamb model, the effect of chronic ventilation has also been explored for cardiac complications. Pulmonary hypertension is a frequent complication of BPD in human infants despite the molecular basis being poorly understood.[101–103] When ventilated with chronic invasive methods, pulmonary vascular resistance does not decrease after birth as it does in reference lambs, and significant muscularization of the pulmonary arterioles adjacent to the terminal bronchioles is seen.[104]

Overall, the preterm lamb model provides mechanistic insights into the biochemical and molecular factors leading to BPD. The pulmonary injury associated with invasive mechanical ventilation in the clinical setting can be recreated in the preterm lamb model, and the similarities in developmental stage between preterm humans and preterm lambs highlight the relevance of this model to BPD.

Pig

The preterm pig model of BPD, like the lamb model, is a large animal model that is clinically relevant due to the ability to subject the piglets to premature birth and invasive mechanical ventilation. This compatibility with intensive care equipment combined with the wide availability of pregnant sows increases that relevance and availability of the pig model of BPD. Various gestational ages of piglets have been used in the literature. Term gestation typically lasts 114 days, but preterm delivery at gestational ages of 98, 100, 102, and 104 days have been explored. Piglets born before 97 days gestation typically experience 100% mortality, thus setting the lower limit of gestational age used for this model of BPD. Piglets born in this 98–104 GD window are in the saccular stage of lung development, similar to humans born preterm, highlighting the relevance.[105]

Piglets delivered at GD 104 are at the border of the saccular and alveolar phases of lung development and reflect the development of a 32-week infant. At this age, survival is over 80% and distinct thin-walled alveoli become abundant, while minimal areas of atelectasis are observed. The risk for respiratory distress syndrome (RDS) and BPD also is significantly decreased compared to delivery at more immature gestational ages, which is also reflected in human infants born between 32 and 34 weeks. At this stage, invasive mechanical ventilation is not needed, and the piglets thrived after receiving supplemental oxygen through an open mask for a short period.[105] This stage of development reflects a near-term human who still might require minimal, noninvasive mechanical ventilation.

Piglets born on GD 102 are in the saccular stage of lung development and reflect the development of a 28–30 week human. At this stage, alveoli are beginning to develop, the capacity for gas exchange starting to function, and the risk of RDS and need for mechanical ventilation is higher than piglets born later. Survival of piglets born at this age is 100% if mechanical ventilation is provided within 2 hours after birth. Thin-walled alveoli are noted, but areas of consolidation also start to be found.[105]

Delivering the piglets at GD 100 coincides with a preterm human delivered at 26 weeks, the age considered appropriate for pulmonary viability.[105] This age range represents the span when human infants spontaneously breathe and blood gasses remain within acceptable ranges with noninvasive ventilation, although ultimately, many of these infants will require invasive mechanical ventilation for survival.[106] In terms of the piglets, many were able to survive 8–24 hours without any mechanical ventilation, and initiation of mechanical ventilation within 2 hours of birth resulted in 100% survival. Piglets provided with ventilation show some histological changes concordant with typical findings of premature lungs. These lungs appear extensively consolidated with an absence of developed alveoli, and general lung immaturity, although they do not show any signs of inflammatory infiltrates.[105]

Piglets delivered at 98 days gestation are at the border of viability, in the early saccular stage of lung development, and represent a human born at 24 weeks.[105] Significant mortality of the piglets is seen at this gestational age as they require immediate intensive care at birth, including invasive mechanical ventilation and surfactant administration. Even despite these aggressive measures, survival is limited to around 3 hours. Morphologically, these lungs show obvious signs of atelectasis and trauma, and the alveoli that were present were not uniformly open. This gestational age mimics the age of humans born in the saccular stage of lung development, but the significant respiratory distress and short-term mortality limit the model's usefulness.[105]

PRIMATE MODELS

Baboon

Despite various drawbacks, the baboon model of BPD is of increased relevance due to the close phylogenic relation to humans. In order to understand the uses of the two distinct baboon models for BPD, one must look to history to gather information about the historical differences in the definition of BPD. The concept of "old BPD" emerged at a time when surfactant replacement therapy had not been approved for human use and antenatal steroids were provided to a minority of women with an elevated chance for preterm birth. BPD was largely confined to large premature infants with moderate to severe RDS managed with high pressure and high tidal volume mechanical ventilation.[107]

During the 1980s, the first baboon model was designed to represent this example of "old BPD".[108,109] Term gestation for baboons typically lasts 183 days, but the animals were prematurely delivered at 140 days and provided invasive mechanical ventilation with FiO_2>0.95. At this point in gestation, the animals were at the transition between saccular and alveolar phases, and those exposed to this model began to develop the clinical feature of BPD after 8–9 days. If the animals survived, they showed the classic signs of clinical "old BPD" including increased areas of atelectasis, emphysema, bronchiolar necrosis, early alveolar wall and peribronchial fibrosis, and squamous metaplasia of the airways.[107] In later studies and upon further revision of the model, pro re nata (PRN) O_2 therapy given to these preterm baboons allowed for complete recovery from RDS without the developing signs of BPD.[110–112] Additional studies showed that abnormal surfactant protein A metabolism and postnatal infection were important cofactors in the manifestation of the BPD phenotype in this model.[113]

Clinically, improvements in pre- and postnatal care, such as early surfactant replacement, low tidal volume ventilation, tolerance to moderate elevation in PCO_2, and limiting exposure to high FiO_2 levels, allowed for increased survival for extremely preterm infants. Because of these advancements, there became a need for a new model of BPD that more accurately reflected the current clinical manifestations. Early and sustained invasive mechanical ventilation appears to be a key risk factor, and severe RDS is no longer a prerequisite for the disease.[107] Pathologically, the findings emphasized an interruption in alveolarization including decreased secondary crest formation, disrupted elastin-collagen deposition, and altered microvascular development, and shifted away from severe airway lesions and atelectasis/emphysema.[114–116] These new pathological findings are known as "new BPD" and are prominently found in a 125-day gestation baboon managed with antenatal steroids, surfactant replacement, low tidal volume ventilation, and PRN O_2.[117,118]

This newer and modified model of BPD allowed for administration of various interventions with pathological and developmental features similar to what is done in the neonatal intensive care unit (NICU) setting, such as provision of antenatal steroids and the ability to induce intrauterine infection.[107] Many approaches to prevent BPD have been investigated such as upregulation of hypoxia-inducible factor 1, superoxide dismutase mimetics, antibombesin antibodies, iNO, retinoic acid, patent ductus arteriosus closure, HFV, and the early transition to nasal continuous positive airway pressure (NCPAP) support.[107,119,120] Recent studies have identified the role of nucleotide-binding domain, leucine-rich repeat protein 3 (NLRP3) inflammasome, impairment of L-type amino acid transporter-1 expression, and the oxidative inactivation of alpha 1-antitrypsin as key components to the mechanism of BPD.[121–123]

Of all the models of BPD, the baboon shares the closest phylogeny to humans and therefore holds a high clinical relevance. Preterm baboons accurately represent human preterm infants in terms of viability and health-related consequences of being born preterm and are compatible with most intensive care equipment. Disadvantages of the preterm baboon model include limited access to baboon colonies and a very high cost per animal. Expenses also begin to accumulate when the costs to provide intensive care in an NICU setting are factored into the equation. Because of these reasons, very few recent studies have been completed and the baboon research program has mainly been discontinued or functioning intermittently, but future studies (if done) do have the potential to provide insight into many pathological and histological processes attributed to BPD.

Rhesus Monkey

The rhesus monkey has been briefly studied in relation to BPD, pulmonary fibrosis, and choriodecidual infection. Historically, some early research into aggressive ventilation in full-term monkeys was produced throughout the 1980s. In one study, 6-month old rhesus monkeys born at term were positive pressure ventilated with FiO_2>0.95 or room air, designed to closely mimic pediatric intensive care.[124] Lung tissue gastrin releasing peptide, peptide YY, calcitonin, and vasoactive intestinal peptide were all studied using this O_2

exposure model. Another study used positive pressure ventilated term rhesus monkeys exposed to either FiO_2>0.95 or room air for 24 hours.[125] After 24 hours of ventilation, interstitial edema accompanied by morphologic signs of O_2 toxicity such as swelling and disruption of the vascular endothelium and swelling of alveolar Type II pneumocytes were observed. In addition, certain monkeys were also treated with *E. coli* endotoxin which was associated with exacerbation of the morphological damages seen in hyperoxia-treated animals.

More recently, the effects of variable expression of TGF-β have been explored in the rhesus monkey model.[126] Developing monkeys were injected with biologically active human TGF-β into one lung. Injections were done either in the canalicular stage at GD 100 or the saccular stage at GD 140, as term gestation in rhesus monkeys typically lasts 165 days. The overexpression of

TABLE 3.1
Summary Information of Animal Models of BPD.

Model	Invasive Ventilation	Preterm Model	Advantages	Disadvantages
Mouse	No	No	Low cost and rapid life cycle/development allow for larger sample sizes Delivered at term in the saccular stage of lung development	Incompatible with long-term invasive ventilation Surfactant sufficient at term, despite an immature stage of lung development
Rat	No	Yes	Low cost and rapid life cycle/development allow for larger sample sizes Delivered at term in the saccular stage of lung development	Fewer transgenic models Research technologies, reagents etc. less available than mouse
Guinea pig	No	Yes	Same small animal model advantages as mice/rat Ability to deliver animals preterm	Longer gestation than mouse/rat Fewer established models available in the literature
Rabbit	Yes	Yes	Preterm models mimic preterm human development Larger size than small rodent models	High preterm mortality Lack of a standardized model
Lamb	Yes	Yes	Larger size allows invasive ventilation and blood sampling Preterm models mimic preterm human development	Require intensive life support care Smaller sample sizes
Piglet	Yes	Yes	Compatible with intensive care equipment Various age models can focus studies on certain developmental stages	Require intensive life support care Increased cost
Baboon	Yes	Yes	Close phylogeny to humans and developmentally similar Ability to provide antenatal steroids and mechanical ventilation	Cost prohibitive Limited recent studies available in the literature
Rhesus Monkey	Yes	Yes	Close phylogeny to humans and developmentally similar Ability to provide antenatal steroids and mechanical ventilation	Models represent "old BPD" Sparse studies available in the literature

TGF-β within the developing fetal monkey resulted in severe pulmonary fibrosis and hypoplasia which appeared at both injection ages. Choriodecidual infection has also been studied in the context of the rhesus monkey model. In one study, pregnant monkeys were injected with group B streptococcus and microRNA (miR)-155-5p was shown to be upregulated, which may be acting as a compensatory mechanism to provide a protective benefit.[127] Another study from the same group showed that choriodecidual infection downregulated angiogenesis and morphogenesis pathways while increasing many proinflammatory cytokines.[128]

Overall, studies on rhesus monkeys surrounding BPD have been sparse. Because of the developmental similarities, such as branching morphogenesis and alveolarization, among humans and nonhuman primates, the nonhuman primate model of BPD provides beneficial insight, but the combination of prohibitory cost and the results having a closer relation to "old BPD" proposes limits to the use of rhesus monkeys in BPD research that must be overcome.

SUMMARY

Knowledge of the specific applications, advantages, and limitations of each animal model of BPD (Table 3.1) aids investigators in tailoring their approaches to evaluate specific aspects of the pathogenesis of BPD and the efficacy of various therapeutic modalities. Rodent models, including the mouse, rat, and guinea pig models, have played a tremendous role in BPD research throughout history. This model is most successful when the animals are subjected to the triggering stimuli in the saccular stage of lung development. Mouse models have the broadest diversity of models including hyperoxia, hypoxia, combined hyperoxia/hyperoxia, inflammation, and many transgenic models, while rats and guinea pigs are typically only subjected to hyperoxia, although transgenic rat models are coming into consideration. Rabbit models of BPD have used varying durations of hyperoxia and recovery in room air in addition to experimenting with preterm delivery. The preterm lamb model is a large animal model that allows for the exploration of mechanistic insights into various morphological, biochemical, and immunological factors leading to BPD due to mechanical ventilation. Despite these benefits, being a large animal model, the lamb model suffers from similar drawbacks as the other large animal models such a higher cost of maintaining animals and intensive life support required. The preterm piglet model of BPD allows researchers to study various time points in development through the early saccular to late alveolar stage of pulmonary development while the primate models take advantage of the close phylogeny to humans.

Overall, the tremendous diversity in the animal models used to recreate the pathogenesis of BPD contributes to our current knowledge of the disease and will continue to direct our clinical research into therapeutics designed to mitigate its deleterious and permanent sequelae.

REFERENCES

1. Smith FJ, Bennett GA, Heim JW, Thomson RM, Drinker CK. Morphological changes in the lungs of rats living under compressed air conditions. *J Exp Med.* 1932;56:79–89.
2. Berger J, Bhandari V. Animal models of bronchopulmonary dysplasia. The term mouse models. *Am J Physiol Lung Cell Mol Physiol.* 2014;307:L936–L947.
3. Maeda Y, Dave V, Whitsett JA. Transcriptional control of lung morphogenesis. *Physiol Rev.* 2007;87:219–244.
4. Kramer EL, Deutsch GH, Sartor MA, et al. Perinatal increases in TGF-{alpha} disrupt the saccular phase of lung morphogenesis and cause remodeling: microarray analysis. *Am J Physiol Lung Cell Mol Physiol.* 2007;293: L314–L327.
5. Bhandari V. Hyperoxia-derived lung damage in preterm infants. *Semin Fetal Neonatal Med.* 2010;15:223–229.
6. Warner BB, Stuart LA, Papes RA, Wispe JR. Functional and pathological effects of prolonged hyperoxia in neonatal mice. *Am J Physiol.* 1998;275:L110–L117.
7. Zhang X, Peng W, Zhang S, et al. MicroRNA expression profile in hyperoxia-exposed newborn mice during the development of bronchopulmonary dysplasia. *Respir Care.* 2011;56:1009–1015.
8. Zhang X, Wang H, Shi Y, et al. Role of bone marrow-derived mesenchymal stem cells in the prevention of hyperoxia-induced lung injury in newborn mice. *Cell Biol Int.* 2012;36:589–594.
9. Bhandari A, Bhandari V. "New" bronchopulmonary dysplasia. *Clin Pulm Med.* 2011;18:137–143.
10. Yee M, Chess PR, McGrath-Morrow SA, et al. Neonatal oxygen adversely affects lung function in adult mice without altering surfactant composition or activity. *Am J Physiol Lung Cell Mol Physiol.* 2009;297:L641–L649.
11. Sun H, Choo-Wing R, Fan J, et al. Small molecular modulation of macrophage migration inhibitory factor in the hyperoxia-induced mouse model of bronchopulmonary dysplasia. *Respir Res.* 2013;14:27.
12. Syed MA, Shah D, Das P, Andersson S, Pryhuber G, Bhandari V. TREM-1 attenuates RIPK3 mediated necroptosis in hyperoxia induced lung injury in neonatal mice. *Am J Respir Cell Mol Biol.* 2019;60:308–322.
13. Ambalavanan N, Nicola T, Hagood J, et al. Transforming growth factor-beta signaling mediates hypoxia-induced pulmonary arterial remodeling and inhibition of alveolar

development in newborn mouse lung. *Am J Physiol Lung Cell Mol Physiol*. 2008;295:L86–L95.

14. Ratner V, Slinko S, Utkina-Sosunova I, Starkov A, Polin RA, Ten VS. Hypoxic stress exacerbates hyperoxia-induced lung injury in a neonatal mouse model of bronchopulmonary dysplasia. *Neonatology*. 2009;95: 299–305.
15. Gortner L, Monz D, Mildau C, et al. Bronchopulmonary dysplasia in a double-hit mouse model induced by intrauterine hypoxia and postnatal hyperoxia: closer to clinical features? *Ann Anat*. 2013;195:351–358.
16. Mokres LM, Parai K, Hilgendorff A, et al. Prolonged mechanical ventilation with air induces apoptosis and causes failure of alveolar septation and angiogenesis in lungs of newborn mice. *Am J Physiol Lung Cell Mol Physiol*. 2010;298:L23–L35.
17. Benjamin JT, Smith RJ, Halloran BA, Day TJ, Kelly DR, Prince LS. FGF-10 is decreased in bronchopulmonary dysplasia and suppressed by toll-like receptor activation. *Am J Physiol Lung Cell Mol Physiol*. 2007;292: L550–L558.
18. Miller JD, Benjamin JT, Kelly DR, Frank DB, Prince LS. Chorioamnionitis stimulates angiogenesis in saccular stage fetal lungs via CC chemokines. *Am J Physiol Lung Cell Mol Physiol*. 2010;298:L637–L645.
19. Velten M, Heyob KM, Rogers LK, Welty SE. Deficits in lung alveolarization and function after systemic maternal inflammation and neonatal hyperoxia exposure. *J Appl Physiol*. 2010;108:1347–1356.
20. Bry K, Whitsett JA, Lappalainen U. IL-1beta disrupts postnatal lung morphogenesis in the mouse. *Am J Respir Cell Mol Biol*. 2007;36:32–42.
21. Hogmalm A, Backstrom E, Bry M, Lappalainen U, Lukkarinen HP, Bry K. Role of CXC chemokine receptor-2 in a murine model of bronchopulmonary dysplasia. *Am J Respir Cell Mol Biol*. 2012;47:746–758.
22. Bry K, Lappalainen U. Pathogenesis of bronchopulmonary dysplasia: the role of interleukin 1beta in the regulation of inflammation-mediated pulmonary retinoic acid pathways in transgenic mice. *Semin Perinatol*. 2006;30: 121–128.
23. Aghai ZH, Saslow JG, Mody K, et al. IFN-gamma and IP-10 in tracheal aspirates from premature infants: relationship with bronchopulmonary dysplasia. *Pediatr Pulmonol*. 2013;48:8–13.
24. Aghai ZH, Faqiri S, Saslow JG, et al. Angiopoietin 2 concentrations in infants developing bronchopulmonary dysplasia: attenuation by dexamethasone. *J Perinatol*. 2008;28:149–155.
25. Harijith A, Choo-Wing R, Cataltepe S, et al. A role for matrix metalloproteinase 9 in IFNgamma-mediated injury in developing lungs: relevance to bronchopulmonary dysplasia. *Am J Respir Cell Mol Biol*. 2011;44:621–630.
26. Bhandari V, Choo-Wing R, Lee CG, et al. Hyperoxia causes angiopoietin 2-mediated acute lung injury and necrotic cell death. *Nat Med*. 2006;12:1286–1293.
27. Choo-Wing R, Syed MA, Harijith A, et al. Hyperoxia and interferon-gamma-induced injury in developing lungs occur via cyclooxygenase-2 and the endoplasmic reticulum stress-dependent pathway. *Am J Respir Cell Mol Biol*. 2013;48:749–757.
28. Vicencio AG, Lee CG, Cho SJ, et al. Conditional overexpression of bioactive transforming growth factor-beta1 in neonatal mouse lung: a new model for bronchopulmonary dysplasia? *Am J Respir Cell Mol Biol*. 2004;31: 650–656.
29. Li Z, Choo-Wing R, Sun H, et al. A potential role of the JNK pathway in hyperoxia-induced cell death, myofibroblast transdifferentiation and TGF-beta1-mediated injury in the developing murine lung. *BMC Cell Biol*. 2011;12: 54.
30. Kevill KA, Bhandari V, Kettunen M, et al. A role for macrophage migration inhibitory factor in the neonatal respiratory distress syndrome. *J Immunol*. 2008;180:601–608.
31. James ML, Ross AC, Nicola T, Steele C, Ambalavanan N. VARA attenuates hyperoxia-induced impaired alveolar development and lung function in newborn mice. *Am J Physiol Lung Cell Mol Physiol*. 2013;304:L803–L812.
32. Olave N, Lal CV, Halloran B, Bhandari V, Ambalavanan N. Iloprost attenuates hyperoxia-mediated impairment of lung development in newborn mice. *Am J Physiol Lung Cell Mol Physiol*. 2018;315: L535–L544.
33. Ratner V, Kishkurno SV, Slinko SK, et al. The contribution of intermittent hypoxemia to late neurological handicap in mice with hyperoxia-induced lung injury. *Neonatology*. 2007;92:50–58.
34. Ramani M, van Groen T, Kadish I, Bulger A, Ambalavanan N. Neurodevelopmental impairment following neonatal hyperoxia in the mouse. *Neurobiol Dis*. 2013;50:69–75.
35. O'Reilly M, Thebaud B. Animal models of bronchopulmonary dysplasia. The term rat models. *Am J Physiol Lung Cell Mol Physiol*. 2014;307:L948–L958.
36. Almario B, Wu S, Peng J, Alapati D, Chen S, Sosenko IR. Pentoxifylline and prevention of hyperoxia-induced lung -injury in neonatal rats. *Pediatr Res*. 2012;71:583–589.
37. Jankov RP, Luo X, Belcastro R, et al. Gadolinium chloride inhibits pulmonary macrophage influx and prevents O(2)-induced pulmonary hypertension in the neonatal rat. *Pediatr Res*. 2001;50:172–183.
38. Yi M, Jankov RP, Belcastro R, et al. Opposing effects of 60% oxygen and neutrophil influx on alveologenesis in the neonatal rat. *Am J Respir Crit Care Med*. 2004;170: 1188–1196.
39. Chen CM, Wang LF, Chou HC, Lang YD, Lai YP. Up-regulation of connective tissue growth factor in hyperoxia-induced lung fibrosis. *Pediatr Res*. 2007;62: 128–133.
40. Wagenaar GT, ter Horst SA, van Gastelen MA, et al. Gene expression profile and histopathology of experimental bronchopulmonary dysplasia induced by prolonged oxidative stress. *Free Radic Biol Med*. 2004;36: 782–801.
41. Waszak P, Alphonse R, Vadivel A, Ionescu L, Eaton F, Thebaud B. Preconditioning enhances the paracrine effect

of mesenchymal stem cells in preventing oxygen-induced neonatal lung injury in rats. *Stem Cells Dev.* 2012;21: 2789–2797.
42. Schmiedl A, Ochs M, Muhlfeld C, Johnen G, Brasch F. Distribution of surfactant proteins in type II pneumocytes of newborn, 14-day old, and adult rats: an immunoelectron microscopic and stereological study. *Histochem Cell Biol.* 2005;124:465–476.
43. Das RM. The effects of intermittent starvation on lung development in suckling rats. *Am J Pathol.* 1984;117: 326–332.
44. Tanswell AK, Freeman BA. Pulmonary antioxidant enzyme maturation in the fetal and neonatal rat. I. Developmental profiles. *Pediatr Res.* 1984;18:584–587.
45. Yam J, Frank L, Roberts RJ. Oxygen toxicity: comparison of lung biochemical responses in neonatal and adult rats. *Pediatr Res.* 1978;12:115–119.
46. Kunig AM, Balasubramaniam V, Markham NE, et al. Recombinant human VEGF treatment enhances alveolarization after hyperoxic lung injury in neonatal rats. *Am J Physiol Lung Cell Mol Physiol.* 2005;289:L529–L535.
47. Thebaud B, Ladha F, Michelakis ED, et al. Vascular endothelial growth factor gene therapy increases survival, promotes lung angiogenesis, and prevents alveolar damage in hyperoxia-induced lung injury: evidence that angiogenesis participates in alveolarization. *Circulation.* 2005; 112:2477–2486.
48. ter Horst SA, Walther FJ, Poorthuis BJ, Hiemstra PS, Wagenaar GT. Inhaled nitric oxide attenuates pulmonary inflammation and fibrin deposition and prolongs survival in neonatal hyperoxic lung injury. *Am J Physiol Lung Cell Mol Physiol.* 2007;293:L35–L44.
49. de Visser YP, Walther FJ, Laghmani el H, Boersma H, van der Laarse A, Wagenaar GT. Sildenafil attenuates pulmonary inflammation and fibrin deposition, mortality and right ventricular hypertrophy in neonatal hyperoxic lung injury. *Respir Res.* 2009;10:30.
50. Ladha F, Bonnet S, Eaton F, Hashimoto K, Korbutt G, Thebaud B. Sildenafil improves alveolar growth and pulmonary hypertension in hyperoxia-induced lung injury. *Am J Respir Crit Care Med.* 2005;172:750–756.
51. de Visser YP, Walther FJ, Laghmani el H, et al. Phosphodiesterase 4 inhibition attenuates persistent heart and lung injury by neonatal hyperoxia in rats. *Am J Physiol Lung Cell Mol Physiol.* 2012;302:L56–L67.
52. Vadivel A, Aschner JL, Rey-Parra GJ, et al. L-citrulline attenuates arrested alveolar growth and pulmonary hypertension in oxygen-induced lung injury in newborn rats. *Pediatr Res.* 2010;68:519–525.
53. Wagenaar GT, Laghmani el H, de Visser YP, et al. Ambrisentan reduces pulmonary arterial hypertension but does not stimulate alveolar and vascular development in neonatal rats with hyperoxic lung injury. *Am J Physiol Lung Cell Mol Physiol.* 2013;304:L264–L275.
54. Visser YP, Walther FJ, Laghmani el H, Laarse A, Wagenaar GT. Apelin attenuates hyperoxic lung and heart injury in neonatal rats. *Am J Respir Crit Care Med.* 2010; 182:1239–1250.
55. Vadivel A, Abozaid S, van Haaften T, et al. Adrenomedullin promotes lung angiogenesis, alveolar development, and repair. *Am J Respir Cell Mol Biol.* 2010;43:152–160.
56. Ozer EA, Kumral A, Ozer E, et al. Effects of erythropoietin on hyperoxic lung injury in neonatal rats. *Pediatr Res.* 2005;58:38–41.
57. Franco-Montoya ML, Bourbon JR, Durrmeyer X, Lorotte S, Jarreau PH, Delacourt C. Pulmonary effects of keratinocyte growth factor in newborn rats exposed to hyperoxia. *Am J Physiol Lung Cell Mol Physiol.* 2009; 297:L965–L976.
58. Buch S, Han RN, Cabacungan J, et al. Changes in expression of platelet-derived growth factor and its receptors in the lungs of newborn rats exposed to air or 60% O(2). *Pediatr Res.* 2000;48:423–433.
59. Han RN, Buch S, Tseu I, et al. Changes in structure, mechanics, and insulin-like growth factor-related gene expression in the lungs of newborn rats exposed to air or 60% oxygen. *Pediatr Res.* 1996;39:921–929.
60. Alapati D, Rong M, Chen S, et al. Connective tissue growth factor antibody therapy attenuates hyperoxia-induced lung injury in neonatal rats. *Am J Respir Cell Mol Biol.* 2011;45:1169–1177.
61. Hummler SC, Rong M, Chen S, Hehre D, Alapati D, Wu S. Targeting glycogen synthase kinase-3beta to prevent hyperoxia-induced lung injury in neonatal rats. *Am J Respir Cell Mol Biol.* 2013;48:578–588.
62. Sakurai R, Li Y, Torday JS, Rehan VK. Curcumin augments lung maturation, preventing neonatal lung injury by inhibiting TGF-beta signaling. *Am J Physiol Lung Cell Mol Physiol.* 2011;301:L721–L730.
63. Ozdemir OM, Gozkeser E, Bir F, Yenisey C. The effects of resveratrol on hyperoxia-induced lung injury in neonatal rats. *Pediatr Neonatol.* 2014;55:352–357.
64. Kelly FJ, Town GI, Phillips GJ, Holgate ST, Roche WR, Postle AD. The pre-term Guinea-pig: a model for the study of neonatal lung disease. *Clin Sci.* 1991;81: 439–446.
65. Kelly FJ, Lubec G. Hyperoxic injury of immature Guinea pig lung is mediated via hydroxyl radicals. *Pediatr Res.* 1995;38:286–291.
66. Phillips GJ, Mohammed W, Kelly FJ. Oxygen-induced lung injury in the pre-term Guinea pig: the role of leukotriene B4. *Respir Med.* 1995;89:607–613.
67. Gries DM, Tam EK, Blaisdell JM, et al. Differential effects of inhaled nitric oxide and hyperoxia on pulmonary dysfunction in newborn Guinea pigs. *Am J Physiol Regul Integr Comp Physiol.* 2000;279:R1525–R1530.
68. Schulman SR, Canada AT, Fryer AD, Winsett DW, Costa DL. Airway hyperreactivity produced by short-term exposure to hyperoxia in neonatal Guinea pigs. *Am J Physiol.* 1997;272:L1211–L1216.
69. Uyehara CF, Pichoff BE, Sim HH, Uemura HS, Nakamura KT. Hyperoxic exposure enhances airway reactivity of newborn Guinea pigs. *J Appl Physiol.* 1993;74: 2649–2654.
70. Elremaly W, Mohamed I, Mialet-Marty T, Rouleau T, Lavoie JC. Ascorbylperoxide from parenteral nutrition

induces an increase of redox potential of glutathione and loss of alveoli in newborn Guinea pig lungs. *Redox Biol.* 2014;2:725–731.
71. Elremaly W, Mohamed I, Rouleau T, Lavoie JC. Adding glutathione to parenteral nutrition prevents alveolar loss in newborn Guinea pig. *Free Radic Biol Med.* 2015; 87:274–281.
72. D'Angio CT, Ryan RM. Animal models of bronchopulmonary dysplasia. The preterm and term rabbit models. *Am J Physiol Lung Cell Mol Physiol.* 2014;307: L959–L969.
73. Ambalavanan N, Carlo WA, D'Angio CT, et al. Human Development Neonatal Research N: cytokines associated with bronchopulmonary dysplasia or death in extremely low birth weight infants. *Pediatrics.* 2009;123: 1132–1141.
74. Chess PR, D'Angio CT, Pryhuber GS, Maniscalco WM. Pathogenesis of bronchopulmonary dysplasia. *Semin Perinatol.* 2006;30:171–178.
75. D'Angio CT, Basavegowda K, Avissar NE, Finkelstein JN, Sinkin RA. Comparison of tracheal aspirate and bronchoalveolar lavage specimens from premature infants. *Biol Neonate.* 2002;82:145–149.
76. D'Angio CT, Maniscalco WM, Ryan RM, Avissar NE, Basavegowda K, Sinkin RA. Vascular endothelial growth factor in pulmonary lavage fluid from premature infants: effects of age and postnatal dexamethasone. *Biol Neonate.* 1999;76:266–273.
77. Frank L. Developmental aspects of experimental pulmonary oxygen toxicity. *Free Radic Biol Med.* 1991;11: 463–494.
78. Kovar J, Sly PD, Willet KE. Postnatal alveolar development of the rabbit. *J Appl Physiol.* 2002;93:629–635.
79. Sherman MP, Condiotti R. Hyperoxia damages phagocytic defenses of neonatal rabbit lung. *J Appl Physiol.* 1987;62:684–690.
80. Ahmed MN, Codipilly C, Hogg N, Auten RL. The protective effect of overexpression of extracellular superoxide dismutase on nitric oxide bioavailability in the lung after exposure to hyperoxia stress. *Exp Lung Res.* 2011;37: 10–17.
81. D'Angio CT, Finkelstein JN, Lomonaco MB, et al. Changes in surfactant protein gene expression in a neonatal rabbit model of hyperoxia-induced fibrosis. *Am J Physiol.* 1997;272:L720–L730.
82. D'Angio CT, LoMonaco MB, Chaudhry SA, Paxhia A, Ryan RM. Discordant pulmonary proinflammatory cytokine expression during acute hyperoxia in the newborn rabbit. *Exp Lung Res.* 1999;25:443–465.
83. Varughese R, Nayak JL, LoMonaco M, O'Reilly MA, Ryan RM, D'Angio CT. Effects of hyperoxia on tumor necrosis factor alpha and Grobeta expression in newborn rabbit lungs. *Lung.* 2003;181:335–346.
84. Ogawa J, Saito H. Hyaline membrane in the lung of premature newborn mammals. Study on the etiological factors. *Nagoya Med J.* 1961;7:44–49.
85. Frank L, Sosenko IR. Failure of premature rabbits to increase antioxidant enzymes during hyperoxic exposure: increased susceptibility to pulmonary oxygen toxicity compared with term rabbits. *Pediatr Res.* 1991;29: 292–296.
86. Wender DF, Thulin GE, Smith GJ, Warshaw JB. Vitamin E affects lung biochemical and morphologic response to hyperoxia in the newborn rabbit. *Pediatr Res.* 1981;15: 262–268.
87. Manzano RM, Mascaretti RS, Carrer V, et al. A hyperoxic lung injury model in premature rabbits: the influence of different gestational ages and oxygen concentrations. *PLoS One.* 2014;9:e95844.
88. Mascaretti RS, Mataloun MM, Dolhnikoff M, Rebello CM. Lung morphometry, collagen and elastin content: changes after hyperoxic exposure in preterm rabbits. *Clinics.* 2009;64:1099–1104.
89. Richter J, Toelen J, Vanoirbeek J, et al. Functional assessment of hyperoxia-induced lung injury after preterm birth in the rabbit. *Am J Physiol Lung Cell Mol Physiol.* 2014;306:L277–L283.
90. Jimenez J, Richter J, Nagatomo T, et al. Progressive vascular functional and structural damage in a bronchopulmonary dysplasia model in preterm rabbits exposed to hyperoxia. *Int J Mol Sci.* 2016;17.
91. Madurga A, Mizikova I, Ruiz-Camp J, Morty RE. Recent advances in late lung development and the pathogenesis of bronchopulmonary dysplasia. *Am J Physiol Lung Cell Mol Physiol.* 2013;305:L893–L905.
92. Albertine KH. Utility of large-animal models of BPD: chronically ventilated preterm lambs. *Am J Physiol Lung Cell Mol Physiol.* 2015;308:L983–L1001.
93. Van Marter LJ, Allred EN, Pagano M, et al. Do clinical markers of barotrauma and oxygen toxicity explain interhospital variation in rates of chronic lung disease? The Neonatology Committee for the Developmental Network. *Pediatrics.* 2000;105:1194–1201.
94. Jobe AH, Kramer BW, Moss TJ, Newnham JP, Ikegami M. Decreased indicators of lung injury with continuous positive expiratory pressure in preterm lambs. *Pediatr Res.* 2002;52:387–392.
95. Mulrooney N, Champion Z, Moss TJ, Nitsos I, Ikegami M, Jobe AH. Surfactant and physiologic responses of preterm lambs to continuous positive airway pressure. *Am J Respir Crit Care Med.* 2005;171: 488–493.
96. Null DM, Alvord J, Leavitt W, et al. High-frequency nasal ventilation for 21 d maintains gas exchange with lower respiratory pressures and promotes alveolarization in preterm lambs. *Pediatr Res.* 2014;75:507–516.
97. Reyburn B, Li M, Metcalfe DB, et al. Nasal ventilation alters mesenchymal cell turnover and improves alveolarization in preterm lambs. *Am J Respir Crit Care Med.* 2008;178:407–418.
98. Lucangelo U, Fontanesi L, Antonaglia V, et al. High frequency percussive ventilation (HFPV). Principles and technique. *Minerva Anestesiol.* 2003;69, 841–8, 8-51.
99. Song Y, Dahl M, Leavitt W, et al. Vitamin A protects the preterm lamb diaphragm against adverse effects of mechanical ventilation. *Front Physiol.* 2018;9:1119.

100. Deptula N, Royse E, Kemp MW, et al. Brief mechanical ventilation causes differential epithelial repair along the airways of fetal, preterm lambs. *Am J Physiol Lung Cell Mol Physiol*. 2016;311:L412–L420.
101. Abman SH, Wolfe RR, Accurso FJ, Koops BL, Bowman CM, Wiggins Jr JW. Pulmonary vascular response to oxygen in infants with severe bronchopulmonary dysplasia. *Pediatrics*. 1985;75:80–84.
102. Berman Jr W, Yabek SM, Dillon T, Burstein R, Corlew S. Evaluation of infants with bronchopulmonary dysplasia using cardiac catheterization. *Pediatrics*. 1982;70:708–712.
103. Bush A, Busst CM, Knight WB, Hislop AA, Haworth SG, Shinebourne EA. Changes in pulmonary circulation in severe bronchopulmonary dysplasia. *Arch Dis Child*. 1990; 65:739–745.
104. Bland RD, Albertine KH, Carlton DP, et al. Chronic lung injury in preterm lambs: abnormalities of the pulmonary circulation and lung fluid balance. *Pediatr Res*. 2000;48: 64–74.
105. Caminita F, van der Merwe M, Hance B, et al. A preterm pig model of lung immaturity and spontaneous infant respiratory distress syndrome. *Am J Physiol Lung Cell Mol Physiol*. 2015;308:L118–L129.
106. Sun H, Xu F, Xiong H, et al. Characteristics of respiratory distress syndrome in infants of different gestational ages. *Lung*. 2013;191:425–433.
107. Yoder BA, Coalson JJ. Animal models of bronchopulmonary dysplasia. The preterm baboon models. *Am J Physiol Lung Cell Mol Physiol*. 2014;307:L970–L977.
108. Coalson JJ, Kuehl TJ, Escobedo MB, et al. A baboon model of bronchopulmonary dysplasia. II. Pathologic features. *Exp Mol Pathol*. 1982;37:335–350.
109. Escobedo MB, Hilliard JL, Smith F, et al. A baboon model of bronchopulmonary dysplasia. I. Clinical features. *Exp Mol Pathol*. 1982;37:323–334.
110. Coalson JJ, Winter VT, Gerstmann DR, Idell S, King RJ, Delemos RA. Pathophysiologic, morphometric, and biochemical studies of the premature baboon with bronchopulmonary dysplasia. *Am Rev Respir Dis*. 1992;145: 872–881.
111. Delemos RA, Coalson JJ, Gerstmann DR, Kuehl TJ, Null Jr DM. Oxygen toxicity in the premature baboon with hyaline membrane disease. *Am Rev Respir Dis*. 1987;136:677–682.
112. Gerstmann DR, deLemos RA, Coalson JJ, et al. Influence of ventilatory technique on pulmonary baroinjury in baboons with hyaline membrane disease. *Pediatr Pulmonol*. 1988;5:82–91.
113. Awasthi S, Coalson JJ, Crouch E, Yang F, King RJ. Surfactant proteins A and D in premature baboons with chronic lung injury (Bronchopulmonary dysplasia). Evidence for an inhibition of secretion. *Am J Respir Crit Care Med*. 1999;160:942–949.
114. Chambers HM, van Velzen D. Ventilator-related pathology in the extremely immature lung. *Pathology*. 1989;21: 79–83.
115. Husain AN, Siddiqui NH, Stocker JT. Pathology of arrested acinar development in postsurfactant bronchopulmonary dysplasia. *Hum Pathol*. 1998;29:710–717.
116. Herring MJ, Putney LF, Wyatt G, Finkbeiner WE, Hyde DM. Growth of alveoli during postnatal development in humans based on stereological estimation. *Am J Physiol Lung Cell Mol Physiol*. 2014;307:L338–L344.
117. Coalson JJ, Winter VT, Siler-Khodr T, Yoder BA. Neonatal chronic lung disease in extremely immature baboons. *Am J Respir Crit Care Med*. 1999;160:1333–1346.
118. Maniscalco WM, Watkins RH, Pryhuber GS, Bhatt A, Shea C, Huyck H. Angiogenic factors and alveolar vasculature: development and alterations by injury in very premature baboons. *Am J Physiol Lung Cell Mol Physiol*. 2002; 282:L811–L823.
119. Thomson MA, Yoder BA, Winter VT, et al. Treatment of immature baboons for 28 days with early nasal continuous positive airway pressure. *Am J Respir Crit Care Med*. 2004;169:1054–1062.
120. Thomson MA, Yoder BA, Winter VT, Giavedoni L, Chang LY, Coalson JJ. Delayed extubation to nasal continuous positive airway pressure in the immature baboon model of bronchopulmonary dysplasia: lung clinical and pathological findings. *Pediatrics*. 2006;118: 2038–2050.
121. Liao J, Kapadia VS, Brown LS, et al. The NLRP3 inflammasome is critically involved in the development of bronchopulmonary dysplasia. *Nat Commun*. 2015;6:8977.
122. Bao EL, Chystsiakova A, Brahmajothi MV, et al. Bronchopulmonary dysplasia impairs L-type amino acid transporter-1 expression in human and baboon lung. *Pediatr Pulmonol*. 2016;51:1048–1056.
123. Karaaslan C, Hirakawa H, Yasumatsu R, et al. Elastase inhibitory activity of airway alpha1-antitrypsin is protected by treatment with a catalytic antioxidant in a baboon model of severe bronchopulmonary dysplasia. *Pediatr Res*. 2011;70:363–367.
124. Keith IM, Ekman R, Farrell PM. Oxygen toxicity in the infant rhesus monkey: effects on regulatory peptides in lung and blood. *Pediatr Pulmonol*. 1988;5:31–35.
125. Ainsworth DM, Keith IM, Lobas JG, Farrell PM, Eicker SW. Oxygen toxicity in the infant rhesus monkey lung. Light microscopic and ultrastructural studies. *Histol Histopathol*. 1986;1:75–87.
126. Tarantal AF, Chen H, Shi TT, et al. Overexpression of transforming growth factor-beta1 in fetal monkey lung results in prenatal pulmonary fibrosis. *Eur Respir J*. 2010;36:907–914.
127. McAdams RM, Bierle CJ, Boldenow E, et al. Choriodecidual group B streptococcal infection induces miR-155-5p in the fetal lung in *Macaca nemestrina*. *Infect Immun*. 2015;83:3909–3917.
128. McAdams RM, Vanderhoeven J, Beyer RP, et al. Choriodecidual infection downregulates angiogenesis and morphogenesis pathways in fetal lungs from *Macaca nemestrina*. *PLoS One*. 2012;7:e46863.

CHAPTER 4

Initiating Multiomics Approach to Understand Neonatal Chronic Lung Disease: the LungMAP Experience

MARYANNE E. ARDINI-POLESKE • THOMAS J. MARIANI, PHD • GLORIA S. PRYHUBER, MD • RAVI S. MISRA, PHD • THE LUNGMAP CONSORTIUM[a]

INTRODUCTION

Alveolar development (alveologenesis) is a critical stage of lung development when the lung begins to increase surface area to support gas exchange for air breathing. This stage involves complex cellular interactions and processes, some of which are recapitulated in response to lung injury or disease. Viable prematurely born infants, especially those at greatest risk for bronchopulmonary dysplasia (BPD), are born at the early alveolar and the preceding saccular stage of lung development. Lung structural and functional immaturity at birth is an inescapable element of lung diseases in infants and children that predisposes to early adult respiratory failure. Yet, knowledge of the molecular and cellular biology responsible for lung development and repair of injury from the third human trimester of gestation through the peak of lung function, occurring in early adulthood, is severely lacking. This pivotal phase of development requires multiple types of cellular differentiation driven by molecular processes linked to spatial context.

In 2014, an effort to develop a three-dimensional (3D) molecular, cellular, and structural atlas of normal human lung development from late gestation into late childhood, the Molecular Atlas of Lung Development Program (LungMAP), was initiated by the National Institutes of Health (NIH) in order to advance molecular, physiologic, and imaging research on the alveolar lung stage using normal, nondiseased human and mouse lung samples.[1] LungMAP in phase 1 had the important goal of looking across a diversity of data types to investigate the molecular and cellular interactions that result in alveologenesis. This nexus of molecules, cells, time, and place was explored by a set of research centers, using innovative methods that generate large-scale datasets. Studies initially focused upon normal fetal and postnatal development in the mouse, using defined time points to capture broad molecular information about lung developmental processes. The consortium also, uniquely, succeeded in collecting through the national organ transplant network a large quantity of pediatric human lungs free of overt respiratory diseases, ranging from late gestation through newborn, infant, and midchildhood ages. Data resulting from studies of these mouse and human samples are shared through an electronic atlas-based resource, namely, the Bioinformatics REsource ATlas for the Healthy lung (BREATH) database/repository. The data repository is available at www.LungMAP.net as a rich source of model and human experimental data and as a hub for exploration and interaction and is free to the research community as well as to consortium members. Data is presented for online browsing and can also be downloaded for local analysis. BREATH was developed by the Data

[a]Namasivayam Ambalavanan,[1] Charles Ansong,[2] Ziv Bar-Josph,[3] James P. Carson,[4] Robert F. Clark,[5] Richard A. Corley,[2] James S. Hagood,[6] Naftali Kaminski,[7] Scott M. Palmer,[8] Steven S. Potter,[9] Gloria S. Pryhuber,[10] David Warburton,[11] Jeffrey A. Whitsett,[9] and The LungMAP Consortium. [1]University of Alabama, Birmingham, Alabama; [2]Pacific Northwest National Laboratory, Richland, Washington; [3]Carnegie Mellon University; [4]Texas Advanced Computing Center, Austin, Texas; [5]RTI International, Research Triangle Park, North Carolina; [6]University of California, San Diego, California/University of North Carolina Chapel Hill; [7]Yale School of Medicine, New Haven, Connecticut; [8]Duke University School of Medicine, Durham, North Carolina; [9]Cincinnati Children's Hospital Medical Center, Cincinnati, Ohio; [10]University of Rochester Medical Center, Rochester, New York; [11]Children's Hospital of Los Angeles, Los Angeles, California.

Updates on Neonatal Chronic Lung Disease. https://doi.org/10.1016/B978-0-323-68353-1.00004-X

Coordinating Center at Duke University and RTI International, with data contributed by researchers across the LungMAP consortium. Together, the team has applied bioinformatics, statistical, and subject-matter expertise to develop tools, models, and a resource for the research community to support current work as well as to evolve over time as molecular biology techniques continue to rapidly develop. BREATH offers resources to the research user community, including tools for visualization and analysis of image and molecular data, thematic snapshot presentations, video tutorials, experimental protocols, and publications.

The National Heart, Lung, and Blood Institute (NHLBI) LungMAP program was the first effort to apply exploratory next-generation RNA sequencing, proteomic, and lipidomic ("omics") techniques to dissociated, flow cytometry "bulk" sorted, and single-cell captures of human pediatric lung cells, followed shortly thereafter by the privately funded international Human Cell Atlas (HCA),[2–5] the NIH Human BioMolecular Atlas Program (HuBMAP (https://commonfund.nih.gov/hubmap),[6] and the Brain Research through Advancing Innovative Neurotechnologies.[7] These programs, funded to move beyond animal models to normal human tissues and then to diseased human tissues, in combination with the rapid development of single-cell and single-nuclei gene expression, DNA chromatin conformation, and near single-cell proteomic analyses are uncovering new pulmonary cells,[8] subsets of cells, and inter- and intracellular communication pathways.[9] Studying these complex human organs requires unprecedented coordination and collaboration among researchers from a variety of fields, including cellular biology, molecular biology, bioinformatics, biostatistics, and data science. The datasets created and shared openly will revolutionize mechanistic knowledge and therapeutic, diagnostic, and personalized approaches to human health and disease. As many adult diseases can be traced back to pediatric and fetal origins, the emphasis on building molecular maps of normal human organ development has broad implications not only for understanding diseases of prematurity and neonatal onset, such as BPD, but also for predicting and preventing sequelae in adulthood.

CHALLENGE AND PROMISE OF BUILDING A MOLECULAR ATLAS OF LUNG DEVELOPMENT

In simplest terms, an atlas is a collection of maps, traditionally bound as a book yet now more frequently in digital multimedia formats and providing facts about population boundaries and statistics, details of natural resources, political and cultural data on the interactions, and life and work of area inhabitants. An effective atlas works in at least 3D, additionally with time or age often acting as the fourth dimension. Likewise, the LungMAP atlas was designed to be more than a collection of territorial maps or visual representations of cells in two dimensions (2D); the LungMAP strives to transcend and integrate dimensions and modalities. The atlas begins to bridge pulmonary geographic space as it transitions from anatomic features to cells differentiated through molecular processes of development, further into protein and lipid identification and localization, and ultimately to integrate ages, races, sex, and disease. Presentation of data that facilitates relating anatomic structure to molecules, without solely relying on *representation* of biological processes, offers a novel way to experience biology.

Image data are fundamental to any atlas. For LungMAP, the underlying "omics" data capturing molecular expression are equally critical. LungMAP has produced quantitative, graphic data demonstrating relative gene expression across cell types and developmental age as well as images that capture cellular activity in the form of RNA and protein expression. Integration of large complex datasets of expression and structure is a work in progress. LungMAP and similar programs including the Allen Brain Atlas[10] (www.brain-map.org), the HCA[2–4] (https://www.humancellatlas.org), and the HuBMAP[6] (https://hubmapconsortium.org), by necessity, continue to push boundaries to arrive at new methods of data visualization, analysis, and integration. Novel perspectives, tested on murine data, fueled the LungMAP vision, challenged by questions of how to present highly complex molecular data to reveal its previously underappreciated four-dimensional structure.[11] How can the combined presentation of expression levels and spatial information be encouraged to 'grow' in the minds of scientists, interested students, and the public into the shape of the unique lung tissue and the developmental timeline from which the tissue arose? Can an integrated model foster the identification of the mechanisms and regulation of development over time? Integration of RNA, proteins, lipids, their structures, locations, and regulatory elements, not grossly in homogenized whole tissue but in individual cells, was just recently highly speculative. But with advances in computational biology and multimodal methods of annotating distinct cell subsets, harmonizing such complex and diverse datasets is the current frontier of modern medicine.[12,13] Such exploration holds promise, for example, to identify methods to restart alveolarization arrested upon premature birth and to modulate the immune system to promote protection from viral infection while limiting bystander injury that contributes to BPD, asthma, and persistent symptomatic respiratory disease in children and adults.

LUNGMAP STANDARDS: TISSUE PROVISION FOR CONSORTIUM EXPERIMENTS

The mission of LungMAP was to provide data on both human and mouse tissues. High-quality, reliable experimental results begin with high-quality samples collected using standardized processes (see LungMAP.-net Resources and Standard Operating Procedures). For LungMAP mouse studies, a "Mouse Hub" was created at Cincinnati Children's Hospital Medical Center (CCHMC) to generate and provide tissue samples to be used by all LungMAP centers. The Mouse Hub at CCHMC generated 145 litters for postnatal tissue analysis as well as 143 litters of embryonic tissue (Table 4.1). Wherever possible, matched samples from a set of individual animals were distributed and studied, using multiple data collection modalities (e.g., proteomics, transcriptomics). However, sometimes this was not feasible due to the large amount of tissue, cells, or sections required, and new samples had to be dedicated to specific experiments. Examples are tissues used for RNA in situ hybridization and for laser capture microdissection.

TABLE 4.1
LungMAP I Mouse Tissue Samples and Assays Performed.

Material Produced	Assays	Ages
Whole lungs	Nano-DESI, proteomics, lipidomics metabolomics, single cell C1 Fluidigm RNA, DropSeq RNA	E16.5, E18.5, P01, P07, P10, P28
Sorted cells CD45 (immune), CD326 (epithelial), and CD31 (endothelial)	RNA seq	E16.5, E18.5, P01, P03, P07, P14, P28
CD140a (fibroblasts)	methylation, proteomics	E18.5, P01, P07, P28

While fulfilling requests for sort-purified cells, the Mouse Hub faced the challenges of obtaining sufficient numbers of specific cell types during the perinatal stages of development, specifically the stages of critical importance to alveolarization. To control for the pooling of multiple litters to obtain adequate numbers of rare cells, analyses and data were generally reported on at least two different pools of mouse lungs from different litters. Sample quality of sorted cells was assessed before distribution for analysis, with typical purities exceeding 95% for $CD45^+$ immune and $CD326^+$ epithelial cells and exceeding 80% for $CD31^+$ and $CD140^+$ endothelial cells. Ultimately, the important contributions of the Mouse Hub ensured that the generated experimental data were comparable across research centers and that differences in mouse breeding, handling, and processing that occur between research centers did not substantially confound the data or their interpretation. Future work will expand the analyses to identify differences based on sex and strain.

In addition, a major accomplishment of LungMAP was to establish a biorepository of human lung tissue samples obtained from pediatric lungs donated for research. Access to human, healthy, developing pediatric lungs is an extremely precious and a very limited resource. Development of the Biorepository for Investigation of Neonatal Diseases of the Lung (BRINDL) was the responsibility of the LungMAP Human Tissue Core (HTC) at the University of Rochester Medical Center (URMC). The HTC collected, preserved, and distributed embedded and nonembedded tissues, dissociated cells, and in rare circumstances, whole lung lobes to consortium investigators. The workflow for processing human lung samples is described in Fig. 4.1. As of this writing, at the completion of phase 1, the BRINDL inventory includes samples from over 230 cases. More than 80 of the cases are histopathologically normal in growth, structure, and health, whereas the others range from healthy with minor histopathologic abnormalities to overt known diseases.

Donor lungs were obtained with assistance from the US national Organ Procurement and Transplantation Network and the Research Recovery Organizations, namely, the International Institute for the Advancement of Medicine (IIAM) and the National Disease Research Interchange (NDRI). Organs were assessed by the HTC lead investigator and acceptance was based upon donor diagnoses, acute and past health history, and indicators of lung health including blood gases and chest radiography results. Cause of death and other medical

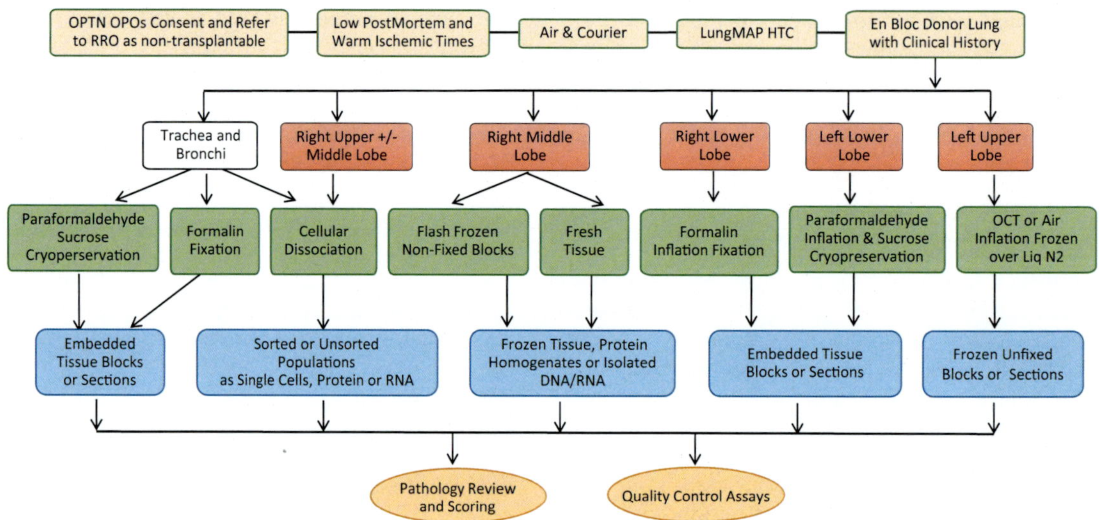

FIG. 4.1 The Biorepository for Investigation of Neonatal Diseases of the Lung LungMAP phase 1 identification, collection, and sample processing diagram of whole lungs to cells and tissues. HTC, Human Tissue Core; OPO, organ procurement organization; OPTN, Organ procurement and transplantation Network; pRRO, research recovery organization.

information were requested and added to the BRINDL database when available. Several criteria excluded donors: high-level infection in mother or infant; primary acute lung disease such as smoke inhalation, drowning with evidence of aspiration, or primary pneumonia and sepsis; more than 5 days on mechanical ventilation unless related to premature birth; more than 60 minutes of CPR; abnormal bronchoscopic results suggesting significant infection or hemorrhage; and evidence of significant lung trauma by radiographic imaging and/or placement of chest tubes. Some non-normal lungs were purposefully accepted when offered, including cases of premature births, asthma, interstitial lung disease, pulmonary hypoplasia, and pulmonary hypertension. Several cases with known chromosomal anomalies, for example, trisomy 21, have been accepted. LungMAP human lung tissue and related samples are available to the research community through an application process (https://www.youtube.com/watch?v=VBlUD9Qv1Ik). Consent was obtained from donor families to contribute to scientific investigation for the advancement of understanding the lung development and leading to cures for lung disease. In order to protect privacy and confidentiality, care was taken to provide only deidentified samples and metadata to investigators and to the BREATH database. All nonidentifiable human data is available for public access; only nucleic acid sequence data with the potential for reidentification is placed in the restricted database of Genotypes and Phenotypes (dbGaP) available to qualified investigators.

The HTC was asked to process samples in ways that were responsive to current research needs and to anticipate the evolving needs. Upon arrival at the HTC, ultrahigh-resolution computed tomography (CT) (Fig. 4.2) was performed on each air-inflated donor lung, providing an assessment of the parenchyma and airway structure, up to 15 generations. The HTC then processed each lung lobe to provide a variety of conditions for histologic analysis and created cellular suspensions by enzyme-mediated digestion of tissues.[14] All levels of airway structure with intact epithelium and submucosal glandular structures are present in the BRINDL repository (Fig. 4.3). The HTC demonstrated intact tissues suitable for multiphoton, multichannel imaging (Fig. 4.4). The cells were used in downstream protocols for generating RNA sequencing, proteomic, and lipidomic data from four sorted cell populations.[14] Utilizing these and other new technologies, the pace of discovery is steadily increasing and additional insights will capture the heterogeneity of the populations analyzed.[15,16]

From its inception, LungMAP has aspired to benefit the broader research community and to be a resource for feasibility information. A highly coordinated approach for studying both mouse and human tissues was critical for LungMAP to generate readily usable data. The Mouse Hub and HTC have ensured that

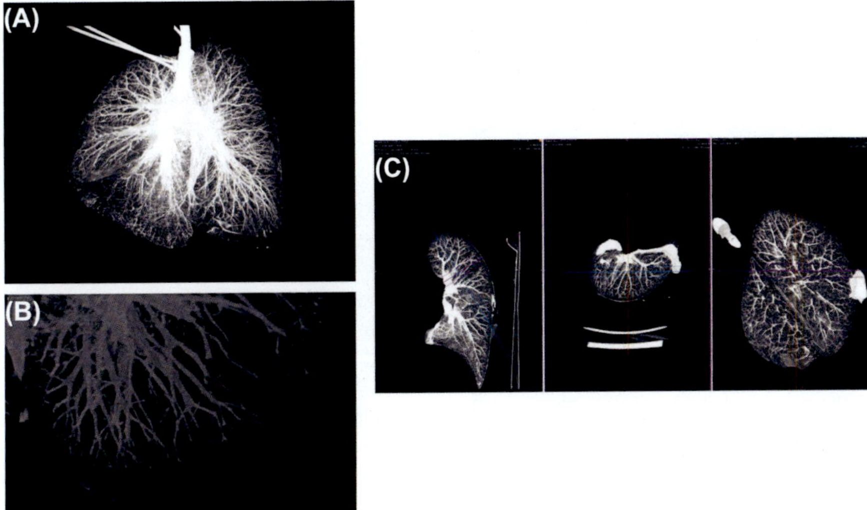

FIG. 4.2 Ultrahigh-resolution computed tomographic (CT) scans of air-inflated, whole, donor lungs. **(A)** Intact, intubated, air-inflated, no-contrast image of whole lungs; predominant structures are airways. **(B)** Projection of reconstructed CT scan focusing on airways just under the pleural surface. **(C)** CT scan of the left adult lung three-dimensional reconstruction in lateral, frontal, and transverse projections. (Courtesy of UR Medicine Department of Imaging Sciences, Dr. Tom Foster and Timothy Baran.)

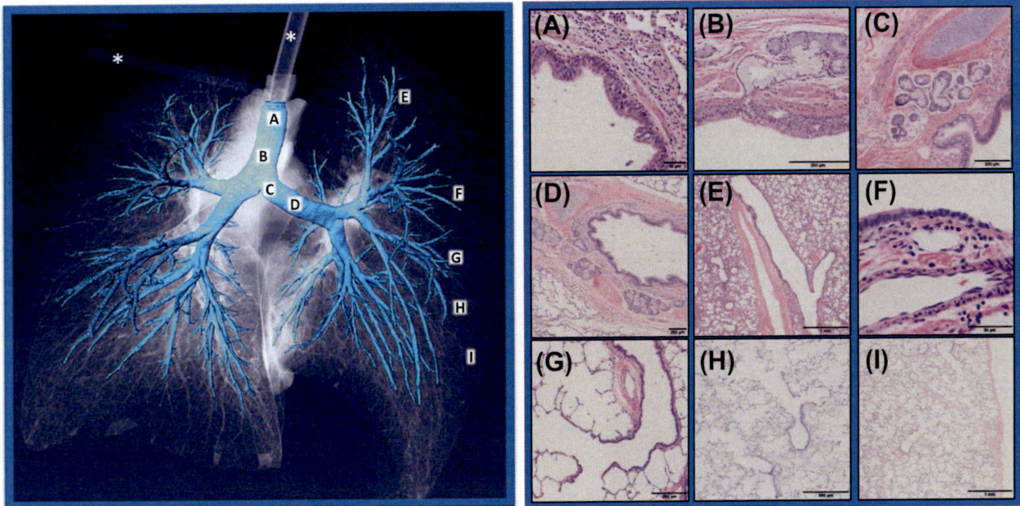

FIG. 4.3 Pediatric airways of a normal, 42-kg, 7-year-old boy demonstrated by three-dimensional volume rendering of **(A)** ex vivo computed tomographic scan and **(B)** representative histology from multiple, proximal to distal, levels **(A–I)**. **(A)** Trachea, **(B)** large submucosal gland, **(C,D)** submucosal glands with bronchial cartilage, **(E)** bronchiolar branch point (right) with pulmonary artery (left), **(F)** bronchiolar epithelium transition, **(G)** terminal to respiratory bronchiole, **(H)** respiratory bronchioles and alveoli, and **(I)** distal alveoli and pleura (hematoxylin-eosin staining). (Courtesy of UR Medicine Department of Imaging Sciences, Histology Courtesy of LungMAP HTC staff and Cory Poole.)

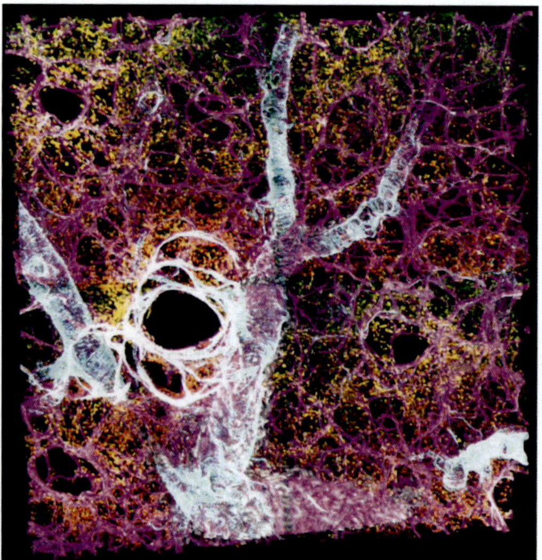

FIG. 4.4 Multiphoton microscopy of a normal 3-year-old lung, 200-μm-thick frozen section, cleared with a modified CUBIC (clear, unobstructed brain imaging cocktails and computational analysis) protocol. The central bronchiolar airway is defined by bands of collagen (second harmonic generation, *white*), elastin (Alexa Fluor 633 hydrazide, *magenta*), and thin smooth muscle actin (anti-ACTA2, *blue*) and it divides into respiratory bronchiole and alveolar structures as we go deeper into the section; angled above that airway and running to the right is a pulmonary artery with, at its largest diameters, collagen (*white*), elastin (*magenta*), and smooth muscle actin (*blue*) and then branching to "blue" thinner arteries with walls defined only by smooth muscle actin. Imaged tissue dimensions, 980 × 980 × 156 μm thick; two-dimensional image of a three-dimensional reconstruction. Nuclear DNA (Sytox green, *green*) and NKX2.1 (alveolar type II cell nuclear transcription factor, *yellow*). (Image acquired at the University of Rochester Medical Center multiphoton microscopy core, courtesy of LungMAP HTC staff and Cory Poole.)

standard methodologies used in obtaining, processing, and distributing tissues and cells yielded results that can be used to formulate hypotheses. Many of these protocols are available at LungMAP.net.

NOVEL CELLULAR AND MOLECULAR INSIGHTS INTO LUNG DEVELOPMENT

LungMAP has substantially increased data describing alveolar development, including both the spatial organization of alveoli and the critical molecular pathways and cell-cell interactions that mediate lung formation (Fig. 4.5). One critical achievement of LungMAP thus far is that it provides opportunities to develop and/or apply new methods of interrogating tissues and cells. Whole lung tissue and sorted cell proteomics, lipidomics, and metabolomics already in the LungMAP atlas characterize the activity of thousands of molecules throughout the developing lung and within key cell types.[9,17–19] The expression of hundreds of lipids, metabolites, and messenger RNA (mRNA) transcripts has been localized at high spatial resolution.[20–22] Additionally, new technologies have been developed that enable ultrasensitive mass-spectrometry-based proteomic analysis at the single-cell level.[23,24] These efforts resulted in LungMAP containing the most significant breadth of data available for the developing lung, both mouse and human, already in use to identify age-dependent cell subtypes and cell differentiation pathways.

It is worth noting that this progress was greatly facilitated by exceptional collaboration among the groups of investigators who comprise the LungMAP. This level of collaboration is evident in coauthorship of publications and in scientific presentations at national and international conferences. A successful approach was to identify 12–26 HTC cases that represented normal lung growth and development representing a range of ages from newborn to 10 years and to adulthood. These selected cases were distributed to each LungMAP Research Center to apply its method of analysis, including cellular transcriptomics, proteomics, high-throughput RNA in situ hybridization, and immunofluorescent imaging, to provide a package of data on each case that can be compared and combined. As an example of additional multicenter work, age-related gene expression was studied in four major lung cell types (epithelial, endothelial, immune, and mesenchymal) using high-throughput RNA sequencing,[25] and bioinformatics defined the unique and common patterns and pathways.[14] These data facilitated the identification and study of the spatial location of expression for over 500 genes using high-throughput in situ hybridization, with data available in over 10,000 images at BREATH.[21] In another example, time-dependent, cell-type-specific gene expression activity was resolved, integrated, and compared at the protein and transcript levels.[26]

Lipidomic, proteomic, and metabolomic analyses have been completed on the developing mouse lung from PN7, PN14, and adult mice, which identified over 900 different lipids, 8000 proteins, and over 175 metabolites, respectively.[17] This study is one of the deepest analyses of lipidomics in the field. Over 100 lipids appeared differentially expressed between each age epoch. An increase in the concentration of medium-chain saturated fatty acids that serve as rapid energy sources is higher in the lungs of pups than in those of adults. Conversely, adult lungs exhibit an

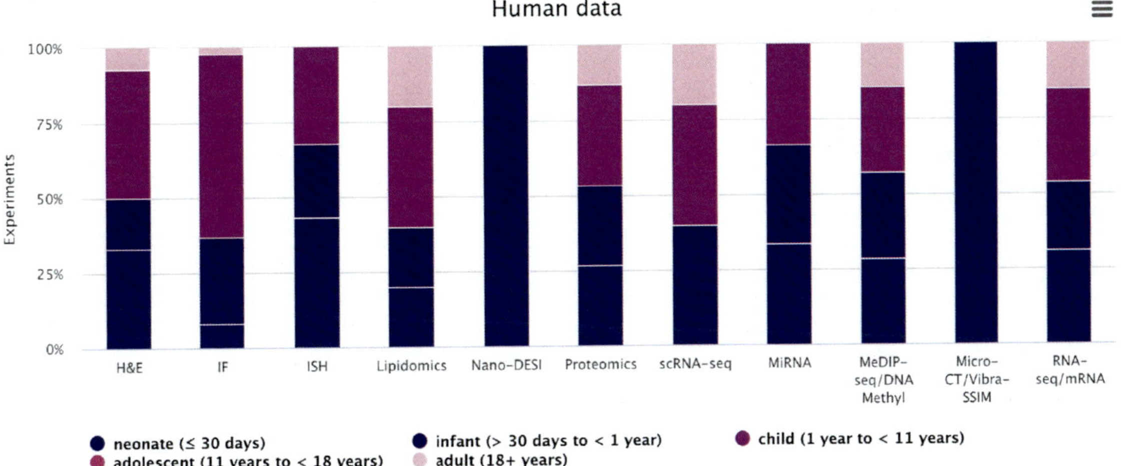

FIG. 4.5 Data from human lungs provided in LungMAP.net database in phase 1. *CT*, computed tomography; *H&E*, hematoxylin-eosin; *IF*, immunofluorescence; *ISH*, in situ hybridization; *MeDIP*, methylated DNA immunoprecipitation; *miRNA*, micro RNA; *mRNA*, messenger RNA; *Nano-DESI*, nanospray desorption electrospray ionization; *scRNA*, small conditional RNA; *Vibra-SSIM*, vibratome-assisted subsurface imaging microscopy.

increase in the level of enzymes that generate lipid mediators (e.g., lysophosphatidylcholine) that recruit T cells and inhibit surfactant production by epithelial cells. Thus this work further defines the tissue environment at different stages of lung development in the mouse that can then be applied to human samples.

Interestingly, recent integrated analyses of transcriptomic and proteomic data support the concept of post-transcriptional regulation playing a significant role in several aspects of lung formation and function.[26] In fact, the abundance of many proteins is anticorrelated with the abundance of their corresponding transcripts over the course of development, with concordance in only a minority of proteins. This is most apparent in relation to extracellular matrix proteins, immune processes, lipid metabolites, and transcription factors. The specific underlying mechanisms of these observed protein/transcript discrepancies remain to be elucidated. The value of integrating datasets is illustrated in a study that used proteomic and transcriptomic datasets in a mouse model of BPD to identify gene expression patterns that are disrupted in response to hyperoxia exposure.[27] The LungMAP group has demonstrated that human tissues, recovered by protocols used in organ transplant, transported, and stored in a repository, can be used to generate and integrate multianalyte datasets, whose analysis will advance the understanding of many developmental and other secondary diseases.

NOVEL INSIGHTS INTO TRANSCRIPTIONAL INFLUENCES ON LUNG DEVELOPMENT

Undoubtedly, the generation of comprehensive transcriptomic data from various biological paradigms has been accomplished, as the approaches are well developed and widely available. LungMAP has taken advantage of this opportunity to apply state-of-the-art methods to increase the understanding of transcriptional regulation orchestrated during mouse and human lung development. Investigators at CCHMC prioritized single-cell transcriptomic analyses, initially using the Fluidigm C1 platform[28,29] and later the Drop-seq-based system.[30] Initial efforts focused on in-depth characterization of the sorted epithelial, immune, mesenchymal, and endothelial cells obtained from mouse lung tissue into cell subtypes and gene expression networks. Using integrative analytic strategies, the cellular heterogeneity and adaptive responses were examined, focusing on the "first day of breathing" in the mouse.[15] Among the novel observations was the identification of unfolded protein response activation as an important cellular adaptation at birth. As temporal changes in lung cell proliferation and differentiation are highly dynamic during sacculation and alveolarization, cell transitional states and the transcriptional programs dynamically regulated at each stage of development were sought. SINCERA, a single-cell analysis tool developed at CCHMC,[31] was used to identify progenitor cells in alveoli and conducting airways, predicting mesenchymal cell lineage relationships that currently remain poorly defined. Complete datasets and descriptions of computational methods are available (https://research.cchmc.org/pbge/lunggens/SCLAB.html).

While many laboratories are applying single-cell transcriptomic analysis to the mouse lung, data from the perinatal and pediatric human lung is nearly absent. Using the tissues and cells in the LungMAP repository, a collaborative team of investigators has begun these explorations. Fig. 4.6 shows an example of Drop-seq analysis of cells dissociated from human lung tissue of two postnatal day 1 (P1) infants, one born at term and the other at 31 weeks of gestational age. Expression patterns of distal epithelial, endothelial, and myeloid cells are significantly shifted in preterm versus term cells (Fig. 4.6A and B). Differentially expressed genes in alveolar type 2 cells were identified and the predicted regulators were distinct in term versus preterm lungs (Fig. 4.6C and D).

Research led by a team composed of investigators from the University of Alabama at Birmingham, the University of California San Diego, the Yale University, and the Carnegie Mellon University generated a compendium of dynamic changes in epigenetic marks, microRNA (miRNA) and mRNA levels, DNA methylation, and protein levels that occur during alveolar septation. Initial efforts used data-intensive and computational methods to identify optimally informative time points to study during mouse lung development. Using the NanoString analysis of microdissected alveolar tissues, essentially from the time of lung formation to maturation (sampling every 12 hours), they developed the time point selection method to select a subset of the

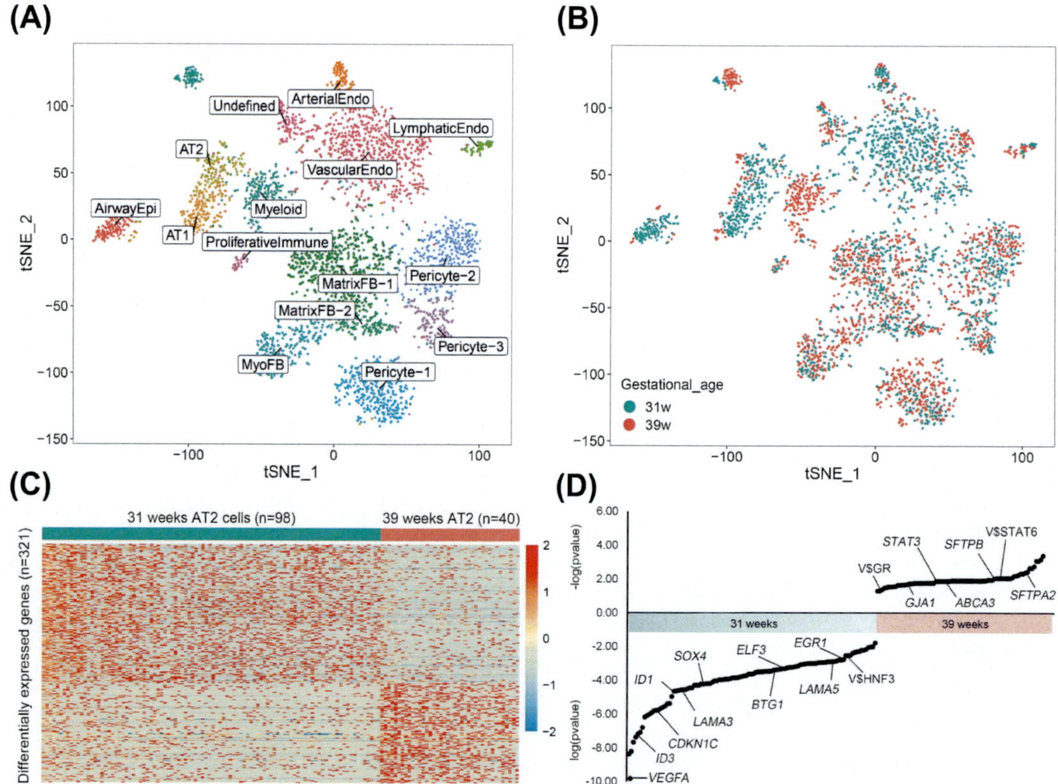

FIG. 4.6 scRNA-seq analyses of preterm versus term human lung 1 day after birth. **(A)** Fifteen distinct cell types were identified from Drop-seq analysis of full-term (39-week gestational age) and preterm (31-week gestational age) human donor lungs. A total of 3379 cells were used for this analysis. **(B)** Single cells were colored by the gestational ages of the donors. **(C)** Heat map of genes (n = 321) differentially expressed in alveolar type 2 (AT2) cells between the two donors. **(D)** Genes and transcription factor binding sites differentially enriched in AT2 cells of 31- and 39-week gestational age lungs. (Data available at LEGA (https://research.cchmc.org/pbge/lunggens/mainportal.html).)

points that provide maximal information for gene expression across mouse lung development.[32]

Following the identification of "critical" time points, complete mRNA, miRNA, proteomic, and DNA methylation profiles were generated from microdissected alveolar tissues. The resulting data are quite extensive: RNA sequencing data includes >24,000 expression profiles from mouse and the human lung AmpliSeq RNA profiling includes >25,000 expression profiles. NanoString profiles include >600 miRNA for mouse and >800 miRNA for human lung samples. DNA methylation was analyzed by MeDIP-seq for mouse and the Illumina Human Methylation EPIC chip for human samples, identifying approximately 60,000 differentially methylated regions in human lung development. Proteomic analysis (one-dimensional nLC-ESI-MS2 [nano-HPLC electrospray ionization multistage tandem mass spectrometry]) identified >1000 proteins differentially expressed in mouse and ~850 proteins differentially expressed in human lung development. This extensive dataset is available in BREATH at www.lungmap.net.

Finally, a computational analytic framework was developed for interactive visualization of dynamic regulatory networks, namely, the interactive Dynamic Regulatory Events Miner (iDREM). iDREM integrates mRNA, miRNA, DNA methylation, and proteomic data from multiple time points.[33] iDREM was used to model and visualize mouse and human lung development (tool ad model available at http://www.cs.cmu.edu/~jund/idrem_lung/ or http://www.cs.cmu.edu/~jund/idrem/).[34] Interestingly, iDREM facilitated "alignment" of data between mouse and human lung mRNA expression data, indicating human lung at birth corresponds to approximately P5 in mouse; 2 months in human lung, P15 in mouse; 3 years in human lung, P23 in mouse; and 9 years in human lung, P28 in mouse.

IMAGE-BASED ANALYSIS OF THE DEVELOPING LUNG

Any atlas is dependent on structural information to provide a geographic context to fine-resolution data. In the case of LungMAP, high-resolution data was needed at cellular and molecular levels, making imaging experiments a critical component to successfully complete the desired structural, cellular, and molecular atlas of lung development. Thus LungMAP has made multiple innovative advances for characterizing the structural development of the lung, including, but not limited to, (1) creating comprehensive structural and cellular ontologies,[35,36] (2) locating cell-type-specific heterogeneity within regions of the developing lung, (3) generating 3D "tours" of the developing respiratory system, and (4) providing insight into the dynamics of alveolar formation. The CCHMC research center prioritized generation and presentation of data from mouse lung from E16.5 to maturity (at approximately 4 weeks of age) and in human lung tissue from birth to adolescence. CCHMC and URMC produced high-resolution tile scans at various magnifications of tissue prepared for histology and stained with hematoxylin-eosin and alcian blue. High-resolution immunofluorescence confocal microscopy was used to identify known cell types in thin and thick sections. Methods of tissue preparation, including clearing of thick tissue sections, were applied. Second-harmonic laser confocal imaging was used to visualize the collagen matrices supporting the lung. Fig. 4.7 provides an example of the extensive data available.

On the macro scale, investigators at the Children's Hospital of Los Angeles (CHLA) worked to create digital 3D maps of lung and alveolar anatomy at key stages of

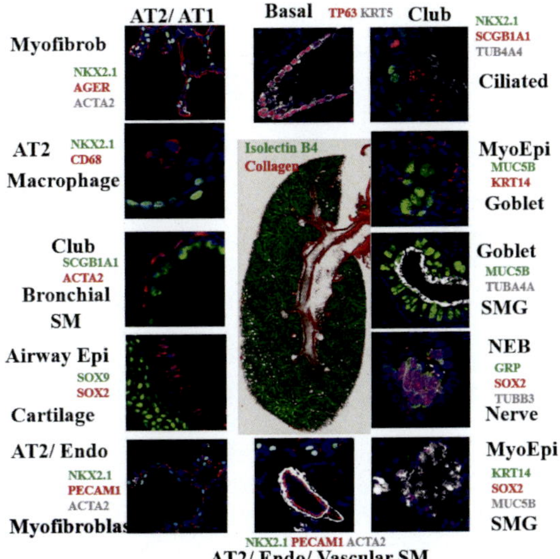

FIG. 4.7 Immunofluorescence confocal microscopy was used to image regions of the developing human lung. Cell-selective antibodies were used to identify distinct cell types in each region. Staining correlates to the color of the markers used to identify distinct cell types. Center image is the right lobe of a mouse lung indicating collagen (*red*), and the pulmonary microvasculature (*green*) is labeled after isolectin B injection. *SM*, smooth muscle; *SMG*, submandibular gland. (Adapted from Whitsett JA, Kalin TV, Xu Y, et al. Building and regenerating the lung cell by cell. *Physiol Rev*. 2019;99:513–554.)

development in vivo and in whole tissue pieces using micro-CT imaging and innovative postimage processing technology creating the 3D MicroCT/Microscopy Volume Renderer (MMVR) (see https://www.youtube.com/watch?v=5WOast-fuXU and https://www.youtube.com/watch?time_continue=456&v=2dvRXfdTb1o"https://www.youtube.com/watch?time_continue=456&v=2dvRXfdTb1o). This technique involved the development of automated measurement methods to define alveolar dimensions and volume and automated approaches for deconvoluting the lung structure, yielding 2D and 3D renderings of alveolar size, volume, and configuration. 3D MMVR brings image data into a 3D space allowing the user to navigate in real time through resolution levels from lower (i.e., large structure) to higher (i.e., cell level) and travel around the structures and "down" the airways. MMVR was used to create a video called "Fantastic Journey" that was featured on Francis Collins' NIH Director's Blog and has been viewed several million times (https://directorsblog.nih.gov/2015/02/05/cool-videos-a-look-inside-the-lung-of-a-mouse/). Fantastic Voyage was created with LightWave 3D animation software, which was a precursor to develop the MMVR tool. More recently, we produced a video of a journey into the lung of a newborn infant, a novel first-ever opportunity. In summary, this method resulted in some of the most striking videos produced during LungMAP phase 1, all of which are available to view and share (Lungmap.net).

The same group applied 3D "all-aqueous" extended volume imaging techniques to image postnatal mouse lung using vibratome-assisted subsurface imaging microscopy and serial two-photon tomography. This technique is a combination of a vibratome cutting device with a laser scanning microscope, in which a sample is imaged in depth, then a portion of the image depth is removed with the vibratome, and the next underlying volume is imaged. Importantly, the all-aqueous nature of this imaging technique preserves the tissue morphology, maintains native tissue geometries, and preserves the fluorescence of the expressed fluorescent proteins. A digitized volume rendering of the mouse lung reveals the entire airway and alveolar surface, as well as the arterial, venous, and capillary circulation (Fig. 4.8). This technique revealed previously unrecognized features of lung development, such as the separation between families of alveoli, with veins running between families of alveoli, whereas arteries follow the airways all the way to the final branch of prealveolar ducts. The generation of cast 3D-printed models of these images reveals novel features of the alveolar surface, showing that it is rugose and indented by the capillary plexus and that

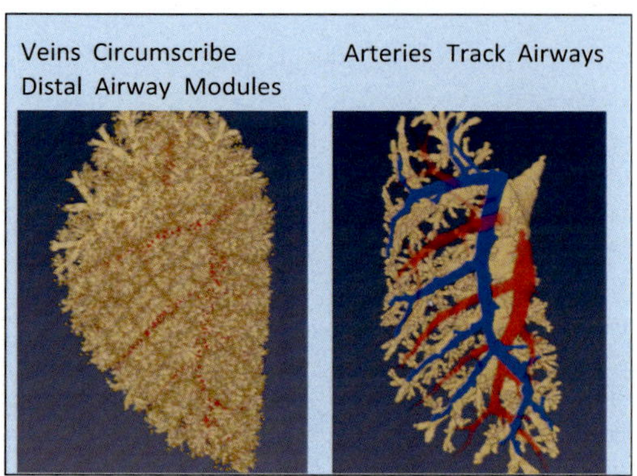

FIG. 4.8 A digitized volume rendering of the mouse lung using vibratome-assisted subsurface imaging microscopy (Vibra-SSIM) and serial two-photon tomography reveals the entire airway and alveolar surface, as well as the arterial, venous, and capillary circulation. (Courtesy of Dr. David Warburton and Children's Hospital of LA LungMAP team.)

the alveoli are arranged in clusters of five to seven at the terminal end of individual alveolar ducts adjacent to the pleura.

Investigators at CHLA also studied dynamic changes in extracellular matrix structures using whole mount protein immunofluorescence staining to visualize protein expression and distribution in 3D.[37] In the mouse, visualization of elastin fibers, the major protein structure underlying the recoiling mechanical property of lung, shows a network involving the alveolar wall connected to other structures, such as airways and vasculature. Elastin staining of human lungs also shows dynamic change of elastin fiber formation during alveolar growth with thinner and fewer fibers in the newborn and thicker and more numerous fibers at 3 years and after. In the mouse, visualization of laminin, a major component of the lung basement membrane, informed alveolar capillary development along the course of alveolar growth. Laminin staining was also consistent with a double capillary structure existing in the alveolar septa before P10 but a single capillary structure in the alveolar septa at maturity, P28. Interestingly, in the human lung, laminin staining appears as a continuous line in 2D imaging and an enlarged loop is always observed on the tip of alveolar septa during alveolarization, but not in adults. Moreover, dense and braided laminin structure was seen in the ages from 7 months to 8 years.[37] Together, knowledge of changes in noncellular components of the lung structure is critical to further understand the processes of alveolar growth and maturation.

ORGANIZATION AND INTEGRATION: THE LUNGMAP DIFFERENCE

The multiplicity of data generated by the LungMAP consortium includes RNA, proteins, metabolites, lipids, and epigenomics; high-resolution 2D and 3D imaging data of labeled and unlabeled tissues; experimental and sample metadata; protocols; and other supporting information. This diversity requires a flexible scalable system easily adapted to new data types with a built-in framework for linking datasets. Relational databases perform best when the data structure is known ahead of time, but graph databases are specifically designed as a structure that can change over time, as new types of data can be readily accommodated without the need to change the underlying object model. BREATH is a resource description framework triplestore graph database (OpenLink Virtuoso, OpenLink Software, Burlington, MA) that acts as the backbone of the LungMAP system.

Because of the flexible nature of the system, a robust ontology was needed to make the data findable and accessible. However, at the time of program initiation, no complete ontologies of the lung existed. Where existing ontologies were adequate to describe the data, these were used. But a group of investigators formed an Ontology Working Group and set out to fill the existing knowledge gaps by developing separate reference ontologies for both mouse and human lung development, highlighting similarities and differences. Separate ontology documents are currently available for human structure at the alveolar stage, mouse structure dynamically across all stages of development, and cellularity of the mature human and mature mouse lung (https://bioportal.bioontology.org/ontologies/LUNGMAP-HUMAN/).[35] Each of these separate ontologies contains over 300 terms, approximately 50% of which are novel, with 75%–80% overlap across species (S. Wert, H. Pan, personal communication). As new data types were added, the ontology was extended as needed. Additionally, standard ontologies used by BREATH are GO and LIPID MAPS, and interoperability is enhanced with identifiers from frequently used databases such as Entrez Gene. A related effort underway is the development of an *integrated application ontology* that combines these, along with modules for sample preparation, experimental platforms and analysis frameworks to support enhanced integration of diverse data types.

LUNGMAP.NET

The LungMAP website provides many ways for researchers to explore rich omics and imaging data. The tools range from basic charting and visualization to those that enable real-time upload and analyses of external data. Some tools were custom designed, whereas others effectively apply and adapt open source software. Powered by Highcharts (Vik i Sogn, Norway), users are enabled to dynamically generate charts of omics expression data with custom control of chart type (bar or line), choice of variable on each axis, groupings of variables (e.g., age groups), and transformations of the expression values (Fig. 4.9). The powerful, feature-rich Morpheus heat map visualization tool was chosen for its ability to group and sort variables, zoom, combine different datasets, run clustering analyses, and export heat map images and underlying datasets (see https://www.youtube.com/watch?time_continue=1&v=V0IaZ58FOxY) (Fig. 4.9).

A custom 2D image tool was developed using OpenLayers, an open-source JavaScript library that supports dynamic mapping of geographic locations, to enhance the viewing experience of 2D images. Users can zoom, pan, and rotate the images as well as view them in full-screen mode. LungMAP has also used this technology to map anatomic features on immunofluorescence confocal and histologic images of lung tissue. This visual histologic map is interactive; the assigned annotators identified and defined the locations within images using terms from the LungMAP ontologies. The markers linked to each term were stored in the BREATH database and rendered on the image upon loading. Machine annotation was also explored in a limited effort by the LungMAP Data Coordinating Center using a process of automated segmentation based on machine learning that uses an algorithm to outline structures. Machine learning requires a large set of manually annotated images to train and test the algorithm, thus automated annotation in phase 1 focused exclusively on immunofluorescent images of mouse lungs at embryonic age E16.5, which were abundant and had undergone manual annotation by lung development experts across the consortium.

LUNGMAP DATA: INSIGHTS INTO HUMAN LUNG DISEASE

One of the major long-term health concerns of premature birth is the development of lung disease, including but not limited to BPD. In order to understand and intervene in the lung disease that occurs in the immature lung, it is necessary to have comparative cellular and molecular data representing normal lung development. Lungs from infants with BPD exhibit an arrest in alveolar development, fibrosis, disrupted vasculature, and immune cell infiltration.[38–42]

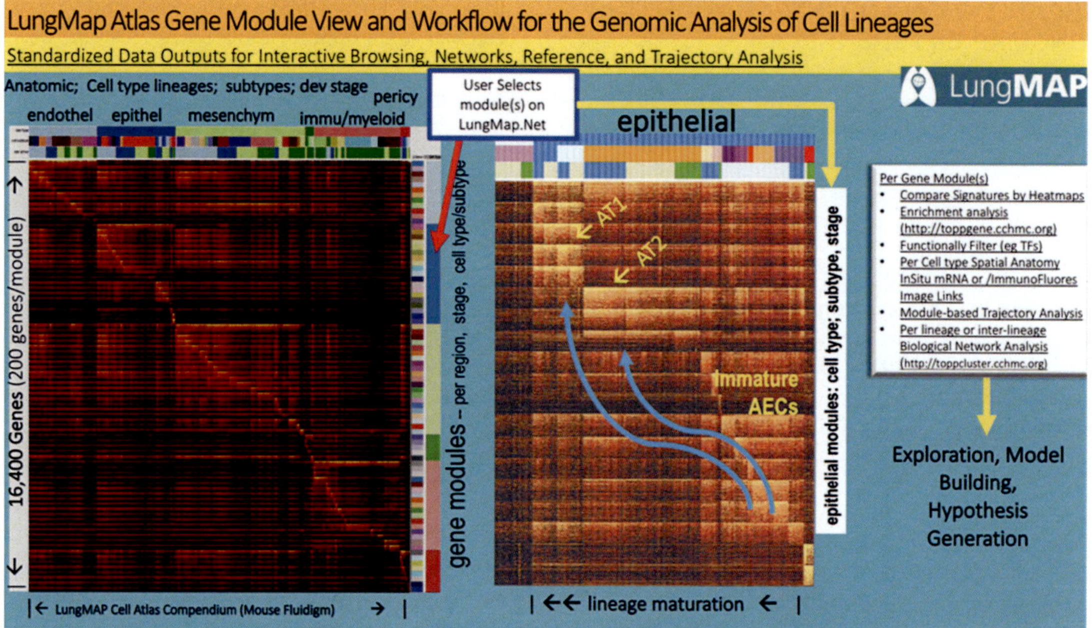

FIG. 4.9 An example of the use of LungMAP tools and workflow for genomic analysis of cell lineages using single-cell RNA sequencing data and refinement into gene expression modules defining cell types and subtypes correlating with age. *AECs*, alveolar epithelial cells. (Courtesy of Dr. Bruce Aronow, Cincinnati Children's Hospital Medical Center.)

Additional evidence suggests that less invasive respiratory support allows for alveolarization to continue, implying that either mechanical or oxidative stress contributes to impairment of alveolarization.[43] By applying advanced cellular and molecular techniques to study normal and diseased pediatric lungs, researchers will determine mechanisms for how hyperoxia and mechanically induced damage of the lung disrupts normal lung development.[44] Such information will be helpful for understanding and preventing progression of BPD.

It is known that multiple cell types and signaling pathways are affected in BPD. For instance, the WNT pathway, important for normal human lung development, is disrupted in mesenchymal cells isolated from lungs of patients with BPD.[45] Disruption of WNT pathways is also proposed to play a pathogenic role in adult lung diseases such as interstitial pulmonary fibrosis (IPF).[46,47] Molecular atlases such as LungMAP will provide a basis for determining (dis)similarities of WNT activity and regulation in IPF and BPD as compared to normal developmental programs.[48,49]

Abnormalities in the vasculature and endothelial cells are also observed in lungs of individuals with BPD.[39,50] A reduction in the concentration of proteins associated with the vascular endothelial growth factor signal transduction has been reported[41] and, like type I alveolar epithelial cells, endothelial cells are exquisitely sensitive to hyperoxia-induced damage in a sex-dependent manner.[51–53] Analysis of LungMAP data can reveal sexual dimorphisms in gene expression to inform studies of sex-dependent disease risk such as the increased incidence of BPD in premature male infants.[54] In order to promote lung healing, cell-based therapies have been proposed for treating BPD, but such treatments must be approached with caution.[40,55–58] LungMAP will assist in identifying molecular characteristics, gene and protein expression, and subsets of cells that either promote or protect from injury, expediting the development of optimized cell-based therapies.

CURRENT IMPACT AND FUTURE OPPORTUNITIES FOR LUNGMAP

LungMAP has had a substantial impact on the knowledge of lung development. As of May 2019, LungMAP has had at least 88 publications with over 1200 citations (https://lungmap.net/resources/publications/). LungMAP nucleic acid sequencing data is freely available through dbGaP and Gene Expression Omnibus and will integrate with newer initiatives such as NHLBI DataStage (https://www.nhlbi.nih.gov/science/

data-storage-toolspace-access-and-analytics-big-data-empowerment-datastage) and NIH Data Commons (https://commonfund.nih.gov/commons), both of which aim to increase the usability of complex biological data and tools across platforms with appropriate security and data provenance. Literally, tens of thousands of samples (tissue blocks, cells, etc.) are also available from the more than 230 lungs obtained and processed by the HTC. In July 2019, funding for the second phase of LungMAP was announced. Ongoing research will continue to address persistent knowledge gaps in our understanding of human lung development. A concerted effort will be made to expand sample collection, datasets, and data analyses to address newborn and pediatric lung disease. By tackling complex questions specific to the lung, LungMAP will continue to provide a one-of-a-kind resource to lung researchers, educators, and clinicians.

ACKNOWLEDGMENT

We thank all the members of the LungMAP consortium for assistance with this work: Sara Lin (National Heart Lung and Blood Institute Project Officer); Cecilia Ljungberg (Baylor College of Medicine); Denise Al Alam, Raul Figueroa, Scott Fraser, David Koos, Rusty Lansford, Rex Moats, Harvey Pollack, Wei Shi, Amelia Shirtz, and Clarence Wigfall (Children's Hospital of Los Angeles); Mike Adam, Bruce Aronow, Yina Du, Minzhe Guo, Joe Kitzmiller, Anne Perl, Andrew Potter, John Snowball, Susan Wert, Kathryn Wikenheiser-Brokamp, Jason Woods, and Yan Xu (Cincinnati Children's Hospital Medical Center); Cliburn Chan, Carol Hill, and Jerry Kirchner (Duke University); Geremy C. Clair, Julia Laskin, and Jason E. McDermott (Pacific Northwest National Laboratory); Christopher Ball, Martin Duparc, Nathan Gaddis, Michelle Krzyzanowski, Josh Levy, Grier Page, and Helen Pan (RTI International); Teodora Nicola (University of Alabama at Birmingham); Marilynn Chan, Divya Chhabra, and Celia Espinoza (University of California San Diego); Heidie Huyck, Cory Poole, Daria Krenitsky, Gautam Bandyopadhyay, Lisa Rogers, Amanda Howell, Mimi Moreland, Stephen Romas Timothy Bushnell, Jeanne Holden-Wiltse, Philip Katzman, Soumyaroop Bhattacharya, Tom Mariani, and Ravi Misra (University of Rochester Medical Center); Gail Deutsch, Charles Frevert, and Sina Gharib (University of Washington); and Farida Ahangari (Yale University School of Medicine). Special acknowledgment goes to the families of donors for their generous and irreplaceable contributions to this research coordinated by the efforts of the International Institute for the Advancement of Medicine (IIAM) and the National Disease Research Interchange (NDRI).

REFERENCES

1. Ardini-Poleske ME, Clark RF, Ansong C, et al. LungMAP: the molecular atlas of lung development program. *Am J Physiol Lung Cell Mol Physiol*. 2017;313:L733–L740.
2. Cool J, Conroy RS, Hanlon SE, et al. Spatial and temporal tools for building a human cell atlas. *Mol Biol Cell*. 2019; 30:2435–2438.
3. Ponting CP. The Human Cell Atlas: making 'cell space' for disease. *Dis Model Mech*. 2019;12.
4. Schiller HB, Montoro DT, Simon LM, et al. The human lung cell atlas: a high-resolution reference map of the human lung in health and disease. *Am J Respir Cell Mol Biol*. 2019;61:31–41.
5. Regev A, Teichmann SA, Lander ES, et al. The human cell atlas. *eLIFE*. 2017;6:e27041.
6. Snyder MP, Lin S, Posgai A, et al. *Mapping the Human Body at Cellular Resolution – the NIH Common Fund Human BioMolecular Atlas Program*. 2019. arXiv:190307231 [q-bioOT].
7. Koroshetz W, Gordon J, Adams A, et al. The state of the NIH BRAIN initiative. *J Neurosci*. 2018;38:6427–6438.
8. Plasschaert LW, Zilionis R, Choo-Wing R, et al. A single-cell atlas of the airway epithelium reveals the CFTR-rich pulmonary ionocyte. *Nature*. 2018;560:377–381.
9. Kyle JE, Clair G, Bandyopadhyay G, et al. Cell type-resolved human lung lipidome reveals cellular cooperation in lung function. *Sci Rep*. 2018;8:13455.
10. Sunkin SM, Ng L, Lau C, et al. Allen Brain Atlas: an integrated spatio-temporal portal for exploring the central nervous system. *Nucleic Acids Res*. 2013;41:D996–D1008.
11. Weinstein JA, Regev A, Zhang F. DNA microscopy: optics-free spatio-genetic imaging by a stand-alone chemical reaction. *Cell*. 2019;178:229–241 e216.
12. Stoeckius M, Zheng S, Houck-Loomis B, et al. Cell Hashing with barcoded antibodies enables multiplexing and doublet detection for single cell genomics. *Genome Biol*. 2018;19:224.
13. Stuart T, Butler A, Hoffman P, et al. Comprehensive integration of single-cell data. *Cell*. 2019;177:1888–1902 e1821.
14. Bandyopadhyay G, Huyck HL, Misra RS, et al. Dissociation, cellular isolation, and initial molecular characterization of neonatal and pediatric human lung tissues. *Am J Physiol Lung Cell Mol Physiol*. 2018;315:L576–L583.
15. Guo M, Du Y, Gokey JJ, et al. Single cell RNA analysis identifies cellular heterogeneity and adaptive responses of the lung at birth. *Nat Commun*. 2019;10:37.
16. Taylor DM, Aronow BJ, Tan K, et al. The pediatric cell atlas: defining the growth phase of human development at single-cell resolution. *Dev Cell*. 2019;49:10–29.
17. Dautel SE, Kyle JE, Clair G, et al. Lipidomics reveals dramatic lipid compositional changes in the maturing postnatal lung. *Sci Rep*. 2017;7:40555.
18. Moghieb A, Clair G, Mitchell HD, et al. Time-resolved proteome profiling of normal lung development. *Am J Physiol Lung Cell Mol Physiol*. 2018;315:L11–L24.
19. Stoddard EG, Volk RF, Carson JP, et al. Multifunctional activity-based protein profiling of the developing lung. *J Proteome Res*. 2018;17:2623–2634.

20. Nguyen SN, Sontag RL, Carson JP, et al. Towards high-resolution tissue imaging using nanospray desorption electrospray ionization mass spectrometry coupled to shear force microscopy. *J Am Soc Mass Spectrom*. 2018;29: 316–322.
21. Ljungberg MC, Sadi M, Wang Y, et al. Spatial distribution of marker gene activity in the mouse lung during alveolarization. *Data Brief*. 2019;22:365–372.
22. Nguyen SN, Kyle JE, Dautel SE, et al. Lipid coverage in nanospray desorption electrospray ionization mass spectrometry imaging of mouse lung tissues. *Anal Chem*. 2019;91(18):11629–11635. https://doi.org/10.1021/acs.analchem.9b02045. Epub 2019 Aug 27.
23. Clair G, Piehowski PD, Nicola T, et al. Spatially-resolved proteomics: rapid quantitative analysis of laser capture microdissected alveolar tissue samples. *Sci Rep*. 2016;6: 39223.
24. Zhu Y, Clair G, Chrisler WB, et al. Proteomic analysis of single mammalian cells enabled by microfluidic nanodroplet sample preparation and ultrasensitive nanolc-MS. *Angew Chem Int Ed Engl*. 2018;57:12370–12374.
25. Du Y, Kitzmiller JA, Sridharan A, et al. Lung gene expression analysis (LGEA): an integrative web portal for comprehensive gene expression data analysis in lung development. *Thorax*. 2017;72:481–484.
26. Du Y, Clair GC, Al Alam D, et al. Integration of transcriptomic and proteomic data identifies biological functions in cell populations from human infant lung. *Am J Physiol Lung Cell Mol Physiol*. 2019;317:L347–L360.
27. Shrestha AK, Gopal VYN, Menon RT, et al. Lung omics signatures in a bronchopulmonary dysplasia and pulmonary hypertension-like murine model. *Am J Physiol Lung Cell Mol Physiol*. 2018;315:L734–l741.
28. Durruthy-Durruthy R, Ray M. Using Fluidigm C1 to generate single-cell full-length cDNA libraries for mRNA sequencing. *Methods Mol Biol*. 2018;1706:199–221.
29. Gong H, Do D, Ramakrishnan R. Single-cell mRNA-seq using the Fluidigm C1 system and integrated fluidics circuits. *Methods Mol Biol*. 2018;1783:193–207.
30. Macosko EZ, Basu A, Satija R, et al. Highly parallel genome-wide expression profiling of individual cells using nanoliter droplets. *Cell*. 2015;161:1202–1214.
31. Guo M, Wang H, Potter SS, et al. Sincera: a pipeline for single-cell RNA-seq profiling analysis. *PLoS Comput Biol*. 2015;11:e1004575.
32. Kleyman M, Sefer E, Nicola T, et al. Selecting the most appropriate time points to profile in high-throughput studies. *eLIFE*. 2017;6:e18541.
33. Ding J, Hagood JS, Ambalavanan N, et al. iDREM: interactive visualization of dynamic regulatory networks. *PLoS Comput Biol*. 2018;14:e1006019.
34. Ding J, Ahangari F, Espinoza CR, et al. Integrating multiomics longitudinal data to reconstruct networks underlying lung development. *Am J Physiol Lung Cell Mol Physiol*. 2019. Published online 21 August.
35. Wert, S.E., G.H. Deutsch, H. Pan, et al. LungMAP Anatomic Ontologies. 2019; High-Resolution Ontologies Describe the Anatomical Structures, Tissues and Cells of the Developing Human and Mouse Lower Respiratory Tracts, Including the Trachea, Bronchi, Bronchioles, and Alveolar Parenchyma of the Lung, as Well as the Pulmonary and Bronchial Blood Vessels and the Autonomic Nervous and Immune Systems of the Lung. Available from: https://lungmap.net/resources/ontologies/.
36. Wert SE, Deutsch GH, Pan H, et al. Anatomic ontology for human lung maturation. In: *BioPortal*. 2019.
37. Luo Y, Li N, Chen H, et al. Spatial and temporal changes in extracellular elastin and laminin distribution during lung alveolar development. *Sci Rep*. 2018;8:8334.
38. Papagianis PC, Pillow JJ, Moss TJ. Bronchopulmonary dysplasia: pathophysiology and potential anti-inflammatory therapies. *Paediatr Respir Rev*. 2019;30:34–41.
39. Coalson JJ. Pathology of new bronchopulmonary dysplasia. *Semin Neonatol*. 2003;8:73–81.
40. Zhang X, Lu A, Li Z, et al. Exosomes secreted by endothelial progenitor cells improve the bioactivity of pulmonary microvascular endothelial cells exposed to hyperoxia in vitro. *Ann Transl Med*. 2019;7:254.
41. Bhatt AJ, Pryhuber GS, Huyck H, et al. Disrupted pulmonary vasculature and decreased vascular endothelial growth factor, Flt-1, and TIE-2 in human infants dying with bronchopulmonary dysplasia. *Am J Respir Crit Care Med*. 2001;164:1971–1980.
42. Taglauer E, Abman SH, Keller RL. Recent advances in antenatal factors predisposing to bronchopulmonary dysplasia. *Semin Perinatol*. 2018;42:413–424.
43. Coalson JJ. Pathology of bronchopulmonary dysplasia. *Semin Perinatol*. 2006;30:179–184.
44. Wang C, Zhu B, Chen M, et al. Revealing hub pathway cross-talk for premature newborns with bronchopulmonary dysplasia by the integration of pathway analysis and Monte Carlo cross-validation. *Exp Ther Med*. 2019; 17:2715–2719.
45. Popova AP. Mechanisms of bronchopulmonary dysplasia. *J Cell Commun Signal*. 2013;7:119–127.
46. Sucre JMS, Deutsch GH, Jetter CS, et al. A shared pattern of beta-catenin activation in bronchopulmonary dysplasia and idiopathic pulmonary fibrosis. *Am J Pathol*. 2018; 188:853–862.
47. Ota C, Baarsma HA, Wagner DE, et al. Linking bronchopulmonary dysplasia to adult chronic lung diseases: role of WNT signaling. *Mol Cell Pediatr*. 2016;3:34.
48. Xu Y, Mizuno T, Sridharan A, et al. Single-cell RNA sequencing identifies diverse roles of epithelial cells in idiopathic pulmonary fibrosis. *JCI Insight*. 2016;1:e90558.
49. Gokey JJ, Sridharan A, Xu Y, et al. Active epithelial Hippo signaling in idiopathic pulmonary fibrosis. *JCI Insight*. 2018;3.
50. Kalikkot Thekkeveedu R, Guaman MC, Shivanna B. Bronchopulmonary dysplasia: a review of pathogenesis and pathophysiology. *Respir Med*. 2017;132:170–177.
51. O'Reilly MA. DNA damage and cell cycle checkpoints in hyperoxic lung injury: braking to facilitate repair. *Am J Physiol Lung Cell Mol Physiol*. 2001;281:L291–L305.
52. Zhang Y, Dong X, Shirazi J, et al. Pulmonary endothelial cells exhibit sexual dimorphism in their response to

hyperoxia. *Am J Physiol Heart Circ Physiol*. 2018;315: H1287–H1292.
53. Kandasamy J, Olave N, Ballinger SW, et al. Vascular endothelial mitochondrial function predicts death or pulmonary outcomes in preterm infants. *Am J Respir Crit Care Med*. 2017;196:1040–1049.
54. Fulton CT, Cui TX, Goldsmith AM, et al. Gene expression signatures point to a male sex-specific lung mesenchymal cell PDGF receptor signaling defect in infants developing bronchopulmonary dysplasia. *Sci Rep*. 2018;8:17070.
55. Ren X, Ustiyan V, Guo M, et al. Postnatal alveologenesis depends on FOXF1 signaling in c-KIT(+) endothelial progenitor cells. *Am J Respir Crit Care Med*. 2019. Published Online June 24.
56. Ee MT, Thebaud B. The therapeutic potential of stem cells for bronchopulmonary dysplasia: "it's about time" or "not so fast" ? *Curr Pediatr Rev*. 2018;14: 227–238.
57. Augustine S, Avey MT, Harrison B, et al. Mesenchymal stromal cell therapy in bronchopulmonary dysplasia: systematic review and meta-analysis of preclinical studies. *Stem Cells Transl Med*. 2017;6:2079–2093.
58. Mobius MA, Thebaud B. Cell therapy for bronchopulmonary dysplasia: promises and perils. *Paediatr Respir Rev*. 2016;20:33–41.
59. Whitsett JA, Kalin TV, Xu Y, et al. Building and regenerating the lung cell by cell. *Physiol Rev*. 2019;99: 513–554.

CHAPTER 5

Epigenetics of Bronchopulmonary Dysplasia

CHARITHARTH VIVEK LAL, MD • NAMASIVAYAM AMBALAVANAN, MBBS, MD • VINEET BHANDARI, MBBS, MD, DM

INTRODUCTION

It has become increasingly evident that normal and disordered gene expression depends on epigenetics, including DNA methylation, histone modifications, promoter-enhancer interactions, and noncoding-RNA-mediated regulation (see Box 5.1). Cell development and responses in disease are determined by a multifaceted amalgamation of intracellular and extracellular signaling pathways. Therefore, studies of epigenetic modulation are critical for our understanding of genome regulation, transcription, and translation at the cellular level. Such an understanding is essential for elucidating mechanisms underlying complex multifactorial disorders such as bronchopulmonary dysplasia (BPD), a common morbidity in very preterm infants. The definition of BPD remains an operational one, with little functional indication of the actual lung pathologic condition and with no correlation of the underlying molecular mechanisms.[1,2] The use of newer systems biology approaches allows an understanding of the phenotypes emerging from various components and interactions in the pulmonary ecosystem.[3] The aim of this chapter is to provide an overview of the epigenetics in BPD.

GENOMICS OF BRONCHOPULMONARY DYSPLASIA

The genomics of BPD was first described by Parker et al.[4] who found a high concordance in 108 twin pairs of birth weights less than 1500 g. The first definitive study explicitly confirming and quantifying the genetic susceptibility to BPD was conducted by Bhandari et al.[5] In this multicenter retrospective study of 450 twin pairs born at ≤32 weeks of gestation, mixed effects logistic regression and latent variable probit model analyses were performed to assess the contribution of multiple covariates. Concordance rates in a subset of 252 monozygotic and dizygotic twin pairs were compared to determine the genetic contribution on prematurity-related pathologic conditions. The twin analyses concluded that BPD and some other diseases of prematurity are familial in origin. This finding was independently confirmed by Lavoie et al.,[6] who conducted a study of 318 twins and found that the susceptibility of BPD is significantly heritable. These pioneering studies have led to efforts in the identification of specific genes/single nucleotide polymorphisms (SNPs) associated with the development of BPD. Genomic variants predisposing to BPD may be SNPs, which may increase susceptibility to the disease. A total of 25 candidate genes have been studied in variable numbers of subjects, but only 3 have been independently validated (angiotensin-I-converting enzyme, *ACE*; mannose-binding lectin 2, *MBL2*; and surfactant protein B, *SP-B*). Given that the odds ratio reported for any candidate gene was less than 2.0, it is likely that any combination of the known candidate gene accounts for less than 5% of the total variance. Of the 25 candidate genes, 18 were in the inflammatory cascade (mostly interleukins or interleukin modulators) and 7 were related to apoptosis.[7] Among the more recent studies, in a Japanese cohort of infants, multivariate logistic regression showed that the polymorphism vascular endothelial growth factor (VEGF)-634C>G allele was an independent risk factor for BPD.[8] However, in a study conducted by Mahlman et al.,[9] polymorphisms in the VEGF and VEGF receptor 2 (VEGFR2) genes were not consistently associated with BPD. In a genome-wide analysis conducted by Hadchouel et al.,[10] SPOCK2 was identified as a new possible candidate susceptibility gene for BPD, but this target was not confirmed in the studies by Wang et al.[11] and Ambalavanan et al.[1]

An integrated genomic analysis was conducted by Ambalavanan et al.,[1] which identified known pathways

Updates on Neonatal Chronic Lung Disease. https://doi.org/10.1016/B978-0-323-68353-1.00005-1

BOX 5.1
Primer on Epigenetics and Metagenomics

DNA methylation: Typically represses gene transcription
Histone modifications
- Acetylation: Increases transcription activity
- Methylation: Can increase or decrease transcription of genes
- Phosphorylation: Effects not well characterized
- Ubiquitylation: Roles in transcription and DNA repair
- Sumoylation: Roles in transcription, stress response, and protein stability

Noncoding RNA (ncRNA)
- MicroRNA (miRNA): Posttranscriptional regulation of gene expression
- Small interfering RNA (siRNA): RNA silencing
- Long noncoding RNA (lncRNA): Regulates gene expression
- Small nucleolar RNA (snoRNA): Guides chemical modifications of RNA
- Small nuclear RNA (snRNA): Processing of premessenger RNA

Microbiome: Microbial genetic material in the tissue (airway in this chapter)
Exosomes: Extracellular vesicles that can carry protein and ncRNA cargo and have paracrine effects

of lung development and repair (the cell surface glycoprotein CD44, phosphorus-oxygen lyase activity) and novel molecules and pathways (adenosine deaminase, targets of microRNA or miR-219) to be involved in the genetic predisposition to BPD. Recent investigations using newer techniques such as whole exome sequencing have defined many potential target genes for further investigation.[12–14] Several other studies identifying the genetics of BPD have been published over the years, which we have reviewed in our previous publications.[15,16] Overall, it still remains to be ascertained as to how the different clinical factors and practices modulate the genomics of BPD across different populations.

DNA METHYLATION STUDIES

In addition to the role of the genome, major epigenetic mechanisms may regulate coordinated expression of genes during lung development and injury. Epigenetic regulation is subject to modification by environmental stimuli, such as oxidative stress, infection, and aging, and is thus critically important in lung diseases, pulmonary hypertension, and BPD.[17]

In a study to identify genes regulated by DNA methylation during normal and abnormal alveolar septation in mice, Cuna et al.[18] combined the analysis of gene expression by microarray with immunoprecipitation of methylated DNA followed by sequencing (MeDIP-seq). The mouse microarray gene expression data were then integrated with genome-wide DNA methylation data from human lungs (BPD vs. preterm or term lung). The authors found that changes in methylation corresponded to altered expression of a number of genes associated with lung development, suggesting that DNA methylation of these genes may regulate normal and abnormal alveolar septation. Some genes observed to be differentially methylated in mice were those involved in the *Wnt* (wingless/integrated) signaling pathway, *Angpt2* (angiopoietin 2), and *Sox9* (sex-determining region or SRY-Box 9)—all genes known to be important in lung development. Genes involved in pulmonary extracellular matrix turnover such as *Tnc* (tenascin C) and *Eln* (elastin) and genes involved with immune and antioxidant defense such as *Stat4* (signal transducer and activator of transcription 4), *Sod3* (superoxide dismutase 3), and *Prdx6* (peroxiredoxin 6) were also found to be differentially methylated. In humans, genes including detoxifying enzymes - *Gstm3* (glutathione S-transferase mu 3), transforming growth factor (TGF)-β signaling, and *Bmp7* (bone morphogenetic protein 7) were differentially methylated with reciprocal changes in expression in BPD compared with preterm or term lungs. The authors reported significant overlap in genes methylated during mouse and human lung development and with the development of BPD, thus suggesting an important role of DNA methylation in alveolar septation.[18]

Zhu et al.[19] conducted an in vivo study and found that DNA methylation and histone H3 trimethylation were present in the BPD rat model. In addition, they reported that the downregulation of Runt-related transcription factor 3 (RUNX3) may be attributed to both

DNA methyltransferase 3b (DNMT3b)-catalyzed DNA methylation and EZH2-catalyzed histone methylation. Interestingly, RUNX3 is associated with pulmonary epithelial and vascular development and is known to regulate expression at the posttranscriptional level by DNA methylation.

A study by Saugstad et al.[20] aimed to identify hyperoxia-related alterations in DNA methylation in the mouse model of BPD. Newborn mice randomized to hyperoxia or normoxia groups were assessed for genome methylation and expression profiles. The authors found the mean DNA methylation level to be higher in the hyperoxia group than in the normoxia group. The analysis of specific DNA fragments revealed hypermethylation of >1000 gene promoters in the hyperoxia group, confirming the presence of the DNA hypermethylation effect of hyperoxia. Further analysis showed significant enrichment of the TGF-β signaling pathway. The hypermethylated genes included *Tgfbr1* (transforming growth factor receptor type 1), *Creb1* (cyclic AMP response element–binding protein 1), and *Crebbp* (Creb-binding protein), which play central roles in the TGF-β signaling pathway and cell cycle regulation. Genome expression analysis in the hyperoxia group revealed complementary downregulation of genes that are crucial for cell cycle regulation (*Crebbp*, *Smad2*, and *Smad3*). These results suggested the involvement of the methylation of TGF-β pathway genes in the lung tissue response to hyperoxia exposure.

A genome-wide analysis of DNA methylation was conducted in hyperoxia-exposed Sprague-Dawley newborn rats, which identified ErbB (erythroblastic oncogene B), actin cytoskeleton, and focal adhesion signaling pathways to be epigenetically modulated by hyperoxia exposure.[21] This study pointed toward the role of aberrant DNA methylation and deregulation of the actin cytoskeleton and focal adhesion pathways of lung tissues in the pathophysiology of BPD.

Tipple et al.[22] studied miR-17∼92 cluster expression and promoter methylation in the severe BPD mouse model and found that lung miR-17∼92 cluster expression was significantly attenuated, and levels inversely correlated with DNMT expression and miR-17∼92 cluster promoter methylation.

Advances in epigenomic technology such as single-cell methylation studies and single-cell assay for transposase-accessible chromatin sequencing (ATAC-seq), are accelerating our understanding of DNA methylation in lung development and remodeling and may lead to novel treatments for chronic lung diseases such as BPD.

HISTONE MODIFICATIONS AND BRONCHOPULMONARY DYSPLASIA

Other epigenetic mechanisms, such as alteration of histones resulting in chromatin modification, may control the regulation of nongenomic information required for both lung modeling and remodeling. In a study by Cohen et al.,[23] the authors performed expression profiling on umbilical cord samples to discover molecular signatures associated with an increased risk of developing BPD. Chromatin remodeling and histone acetylation pathways appeared to be differentially regulated in umbilical cord tissues of the infants who were subsequently diagnosed with BPD in this study. Chao et al.[24] analyzed the short- and long-term effects of neonatal hyperoxia on nitric oxide synthase 3 (NOS3) and STAT3 messenger RNA (mRNA) expression and corresponding epigenetic signatures using a hyperoxia-exposed mouse model of BPD. They found that early hyperoxia exposure increased both NOS3 and STAT3 mRNA expression in pulmonary endothelial cells, with corresponding changes in histone modification patterns such as H2aZac and H3K9ac hyperacetylation at the respective gene loci. The authors speculated that these permanent changes in histone signatures at the *Nos3* and *Stat3* gene loci might partly explain the altered vascular response patterns in children with BPD.

The transcription factor peroxisome proliferator-activated receptor γ (PPARγ) is thought to contribute to lung development. One contribution of PPARγ to lung development may be its direct regulation of chromatin-modifying enzymes, such as Setd8. Joss-Moore et al.[25] hypothesized that intrauterine growth restriction (IUGR) would result in a sex-specific reduction in PPARγ, Setd8, and associated H4K20Me levels in the neonatal rat lung. Because docosahexaenoic acid (DHA) activates PPARγ, they also hypothesized that maternal DHA supplementation would normalize PPARγ, Setd8, and H4K20Me levels in the IUGR rat lung. IUGR was found to decrease PPARγ levels, with an associated decrease in Setd8 levels in both male and female rat lungs. Levels of the Setd8-dependent histone modification, H4K20Me, were reduced on the *PPARγ* gene in both male and female rat lungs, whereas only whole lung H4K20Me level was reduced in male rat lungs. Maternal DHA supplementation ameliorated these effects in the offspring. The authors concluded that IUGR decreases lung PPARγ, Setd8, and PPARγ H4K20Me independent of sex, while decreasing whole lung H4K20Me level in male rats only. These outcomes were offset by maternal DHA. Hence, these findings suggest that PPARγ is involved in regulating the epigenetics in the lung and maternal DHA supplementation in IUGR infants may be beneficial.

Histone deacetylases (HDACs) control cellular signaling and gene expression, and HDAC2 is crucial for the suppression of inflammatory gene expression. Londhe et al.[26] first found that hyperoxia exposure in newborn mice resulted in decreased HDAC1 and HDAC2 and increased p53 and p21 expression. Zhu et al.[27] had reported that attenuation of cytokine-induced neutrophil chemoattractant 1 (CINC-1)-mediated inflammation by activating HDAC may have a protective effect in a rat model of BPD. Using a similar rat model of BPD, Ni et al.[28] found that lipopolysaccharide (LPS) exposure led to a suppression of both HDAC1 and HDAC2 expression and activity, induced TGF-α expression, and disrupted alveolar morphology. Overexpression of HDAC2, but not HDAC1, suppressed LPS-induced TGF-α expression. Both the HDAC inhibitor trichostatin A and the downregulation of HDAC2 by small interfering RNA significantly increased TGF-α expression in cultured myofibroblasts. Moreover, the authors found that the preservation of HDAC activity by theophylline treatment improved alveolar development and attenuated TGF-α release. Hence, these findings indicate a therapeutic role of TGF-α attenuation in BPD by HDAC2 enhancement.

In a mechanically ventilated preterm lamb model of BPD, inhibition of histone deacetylation significantly improved alveolar formation in the lung, associated with changes in specific histone modifications.[17]

LONG NONCODING RNAS AND BRONCHOPULMONARY DYSPLASIA

In the recent years, noncoding RNAs including miR, other small RNA, and long noncoding RNA (lncRNA) have been recognized as important mediators of normal growth and disease. Using a murine lung injury model that mimicked human BPD, investigators noted that 882 lncRNAs were upregulated and 887 lncRNAs were downregulated in BPD lung tissues. This study found that the lncRNA AK033210 associated with TNC was downregulated in BPD tissues and hence might be involved in the pathogenesis of BPD.[29]

Cai et al.[30] reported that the upregulation of lncRNA metastasis-associated lung adenocarcinoma transcript 1 (MALAT1) could protect preterm infants with BPD by inhibiting cell apoptosis. In this study, the expression of MALAT1 was significantly increased in lung tissues of BPD mice (at days 14 and 29) compared with wild-type mice. Consistent with murine data, mRNA array profiling analysis in blood samples from preterm infants with BPD revealed increased MALAT1 expression levels. These data provide novel insights into MALAT1 regulation, which may be relevant to the cell fate and may shed light on BPD prevention and treatment.

MICRORNAS AND BRONCHOPULMONARY DYSPLASIA

miRs have been noted to be dysregulated in multiple disorders and are now being studied in lung biology.[31,32] Table 5.1 lists miRs currently implicated in the pathogenesis of BPD. Several miRs have been described to play a role in branching morphogenesis, a key step in early lung development.[33] The current evidence of the role of miRs in late lung development and BPD has been well summarized by Nardiello and Morty.[33] In one of the first such studies, Zhang et al.[34] identified the differential expression of miRs in the neonatal hyperoxia-exposed mouse model.

TABLE 5.1
miRNA and Their Respective Targets That Have Been Studied in the Pathogenesis of BPD.

MicroRNA Implicated in BPD	Possible Target Genes Involved in BPD Pathogenesis
miR-489[35]	Insulin like growth factor 1 (IGF-1), tenascin C (TNC)
miR-219[59]	Platelet-derived growth factor receptor α (PDGFR-α)
miR-34a[36]	Angiopoietin 1 (Ang-1)
miR-29b[37]	Transforming growth factor (TGF) β
miR-196a[38]	Heme oxygenase 1 (HO-1)
miR-150[40]	Glycoprotein nonmetastatic melanoma protein B (GPNMB)
miR-29c[41]	Neurotrophic tyrosine kinase receptor type 2 (Ntrk2)
miR-17∼92[22]	TGF-β
miR-876-3p[45]	Androgen receptor (AR)
miR-30a[53]	Delta like ligand 4 (DLL4)
miR-206	Fibronectin 1 (FN1)
miR146	Toll-like receptor 4 (TLR4), interleukin 1 receptor–associated kinase 1 (IRAK1)

BPD, bronchopulmonary dysplasia; *miR*, microRNA.

Our group has highlighted the role of miR-489 in guiding alveolar septation by modulation of its target genes insulinlike growth factor (IGF) 1 and TNC.[35] As mentioned earlier, in a large genome-wide analysis conducted on blood samples from extremely preterm infants, the pathway with lowest false discovery rate for BPD/death was the targets of miR-219.[1]

In another study, Syed et al.[36] showed that pharmacologic miR-34a inhibition may be a therapeutic option to prevent or ameliorate hyperoxia-induced lung injury in neonates. The authors found that lung miR-34a levels were significantly increased in lungs of neonatal mice exposed to hyperoxia; deletion or inhibition of miR-34a improved the pulmonary phenotype and BPD-associated pulmonary arterial hypertension in BPD mice models.

Rogers et al.[37] found that miR-29b supplementation decreased expression of matrix proteins and improved alveolarization in mice exposed to maternal inflammation and neonatal hyperoxia. Thus the above data from a prenatal LPS combined with postnatal hyperoxia mouse model suggest that miR-29b restoration may be one component of a novel therapeutic strategy to treat or prevent severe BPD in prematurely born infants. As mentioned earlier, the same group had also identified epigenetically altered miR-17∼92 cluster in the pathogenesis of severe BPD.[22]

An important factor in mitigating inflammation and oxidative stress is heme oxygenase (HO), in particular the inducible form, HO-1. This cytoprotective enzyme is highly expressed in the neonatal lung, perhaps as a defense against perinatal oxidative injury. Hayato et al.[38] found that in neonatal mice, miR-196a regulates the expression of transcriptional repressor BTB and CNC homology 1 (Bach1) and subsequently leads to higher levels of lung HO-1 mRNA than those in adults. The authors also found miR-196a to be degraded in hyperoxia, resulting in limited HO-1 induction in neonatal mice lungs. Based on this study, miR-196a appears to be a key regulator of HO-1 via Bach1 during postnatal lung development and hence represents a therapeutic target for avoidance of oxidative lung injury in neonates.

One of the miRs that is downregulated in hyperoxia is miR-150,[39] which has several angiogenic factors as targets, including glycoprotein nonmetastatic melanoma protein B (GPNMB). Narasaraju et al.[40] found that miR-150 is highly expressed in neonatal lungs and is decreased in neonatal mice exposed to hyperoxia. The study also found that mouse pups lacking miR-150, due to the upregulation of target GPNMB, were more resistant to hyperoxia-induced alveolar injury, vascular damage, and inflammation.

Abnormal lung development due to hyperoxia exposure is accompanied by significant increases in the levels of multiple miRs and corresponding decreases in the targets of these mRNA, many of which have known or suspected roles in pathways altered in the pathogenesis of BPD. One such study by Dong et al.[41] found several hyperoxia modulated genes involved in a variety of lung developmental processes, including cell cycle, cell adhesion, mobility and taxis, inflammation, and angiogenesis. In this study, miR-29 expression was prominently increased in the lungs of hyperoxia-exposed mice. The downregulation of neurotrophic tyrosine kinase receptor type 2 (Ntrk2) expression, regulated by miR-29c, was found to play a role in the pathogenesis of hyperoxia-induced BPD.

EXOSOMES AND BRONCHOPULMONARY DYSPLASIA

Exosomes are membrane-bound phospholipid vesicles (30–150 nm in diameter) actively secreted by a variety of living cells.[42] In a recent study, our group has described the important role of proteolytic exosomes in adult lung injury and in preterm BPD.[43] Exosomes are involved in cell-cell communication by shuttling various molecules, including miRs, from donor to recipient cells.[44] Our group has also recently described the role of exosomal miRs in BPD prediction and pathogenesis.[45] We found that infants with severe BPD have a higher number of exosomes in their tracheal aspirates (TAs) than gestational age–matched controls. Next, we identified that a decreased expression of miR-876-3p at birth in TAs of preterm infant predicts the future development of severe BPD. We also confirmed these findings in established newborn mice models and in vitro hyperoxia models of BPD, thus establishing the role of miR-876-3p in BPD pathogenesis. Furthermore, in vitro and in vivo studies showed that Proteobacteria and their LPS products mediate miR-876-3p expression in BPD. Gain of miR-876-3p function rescued alveolarization, establishing the cause-and-effect relationship between decreased miR-876-3p expression and BPD pathogenesis.[45] In summary, these studies establish the predictive potential and causative role of microbiota-regulated miR-876-3p in severe BPD.

SEX AND BRONCHOPULMONARY DYSPLASIA

In this section, we discuss the influence of sex on BPD. The influence of race on BPD, particularly relative protection during neonatal intensive care unit (NICU) stay but worse lung disease during infancy in black compared with white infants, has been detailed elsewhere in this book (Chapter 1, see the section Etiology and Pathogenesis of Bronchopulmonary Dysplasia). Clinical evidence suggests a major sex predilection for BPD, where male premature newborns are at higher risk and generally have greater morbidity/mortality than female newborns who are protected from the same.[46] Studies from other countries such as Japan[47] and Korea[48] also report such sex predilection, wherein male infants are more likely to develop BPD. Epigenetic mechanisms that drive the regulation of the biological processes leading to BPD are possibly influenced by sex. Epigenetic mechanisms, consisting of sex-specific reduction in PPARγ, Setd8, and associated H4K20Me levels in the neonatal rat lung, were described earlier.[25] The action of noncoding RNAs that control the regulation of information "beyond the genome"[17] required for the response to lung injury and repair will be described in the following section.

Sammour et al.[49] conducted a study to determine whether intratracheal administration of female mesenchymal stem cells to neonatal rats with experimental BPD has more beneficial reparative effects than those of male mesenchymal stem cells. Newborn Sprague-Dawley rats exposed to normoxia or hyperoxia were randomly assigned to receive male or female bone marrow derived green fluorescent protein–tagged (GFP^+) mesenchymal stem cells or placebo. Female mesenchymal stem cells were found to have greater therapeutic efficacy than male mesenchymal stem cells in reducing neonatal hyperoxia-induced lung inflammation and vascular remodeling. Furthermore, the beneficial effects of female derived cells were more pronounced in male animals. These findings establish the superior potency of female mesenchymal stem cells for lung repair in severe BPD.

Fulton et al.[50] found that mesenchymal stem cells from TAs of male infants developing BPD exhibit a pathologic gene expression profile deficient in platelet-derived growth factor receptor (PDGFR) and its downstream effectors, thereby favoring delayed lung development. In the same study, in female infants developing BPD, TA levels of proinflammatory C-C motif chemokine ligand 2 (CCL2) and profibrotic galectin-1 were higher than those in male infants developing BPD and in female infants not developing BPD.

Using male and female neonatal lung fibroblasts, Balaji et al.[51] studied the role of hyperoxia on differential Notch pathway activation. Increased Notch pathway activation was noted in male fibroblasts along with differential sex-specific modulation of key Notch pathway mediators in response to hyperoxia. There were distinct changes in expression of key fibrosis-related genes noted between male and female fibroblasts, which may contribute to the sex-specific differences seen in hyperoxia-induced fibrosis and lung development in BPD.

Lingappan et al.[52] have reported sexual dimorphism of the pulmonary transcriptome in neonatal hyperoxic lung injury. Analysis of the pulmonary transcriptome revealed differential sex-specific modulation of crucial pathways related to angiogenesis, response to hypoxia, inflammatory responses, and the p53 pathway. Analysis also revealed sex-specific differences in the modulation of crucial transcription factors. Focusing on the differential modulation of the angiogenesis pathway, the authors also showed sex-specific differential activation of *Hif-1α*-regulated genes using chromatin immunoprecipitation-quantitative polymerase chain reaction and differences in expression of crucial genes (*Vegf, VegfR2,* and prolyl hydroxylase domain 2 [Phd2]) modulating angiogenesis.[52] These studies provide insights into differential sex-specific modulation of the pulmonary transcriptome hyperoxia and highlight angiogenesis as one of the crucial pathways. Lingappan et al.[53] have also reported the role of miR-30a in the sex-specific molecular mechanisms leading to the sexual dimorphism in BPD.

Leary and colleagues[54] studied sex-based differences in mild, moderate, and severe BPD using two different strains of mice: CD1 (outbred) and C57BL/6 (inbred). In response to hyperoxia, female mice had less alveolar injury with better preservation of alveolar chord length and decreased alveolar protein leak and inflammatory cells in the bronchoalveolar lavage fluid. Gonadotropin-releasing hormone concentration was increased in female mice compared with male mice in the hyperoxia mouse model. Specific miRs (miR-146 and miR-34a) were expressed differently in male and female mice. The authors also demonstrated that in the severe BPD mouse model, administering miR-146-mimic to male mice reduced lung damage, whereas administering miR-146 inhibitor to female mice increased the resultant pulmonary injury.[54]

MICROBIOME AND BRONCHOPULMONARY DYSPLASIA

Epigenetics is influenced by the environment, and based on recent data, it is possible that the commensal microbiome may have effects on the maturation of DNA methylation signatures and the transcriptional program after birth.[55] In addition, the microbial products short-chain fatty acids butyrate and propionate are potent inhibitors of HDAC enzymes[56] and therefore may promote heterochromatin formation and increase transcriptional activity. Historically, the fetus and fetal lungs were considered sterile, but we have recently discovered that the airways of infants even as early as at birth harbor a distinct microbial signature.[57] The airways of infants with BPD show increased abundance of Proteobacteria and decreased numbers of *Lactobacillus* and infants developing severe BPD show a temporal dysbiosis, with an increase in Proteobacteria and decrease in *Lactobacillus* numbers on the way to the development of severe BPD. In addition, an early microbial dysbiosis, that is, decreased *Lactobacillus* numbers at birth, is predictive of the development of severe BPD.[57] Hence, it is very possible that this dynamic dysbiosis associated with BPD[57,58] targets microbially responsive genes through their DNA methylation status. The exact mechanisms by which the microbiome may affect epigenetic mechanisms in lung development and BPD are still unknown and need further exploration.

SUMMARY

It has been more than a decade since the definitive genetic contribution to BPD was established. Despite much effort, the identification of specific genes that contribute to the pathogenesis of BPD has remained elusive; although some genes and molecular signaling pathways have been elucidated, they still require confirmation. Regarding epigenetics, differential regulation of DNA methylation of specific genes in experimental and human BPD includes those involved in Gstm3, TGF-β, Bmp7, RUNX3, ErbB, and miR-17 ∼ 92 cluster signaling pathways. Histone modifications in NOS3, STAT3, and PPARγ were noted in rodent BPD models. Among lncRNAs, AK033210 was downregulated, whereas MALAT1 was upregulated in BPD lung tissues. miRs associated with BPD and their downstream targets have been summarized in Table 5.1. Recent studies have noted specific gene regulatory pathways to understand the sexual dimorphism in experimental and human BPD, notably PDGFR, CCL2, galectin-1, miR-30a, miR-34a, and miR-146. Epigenetic regulation is subject to modification by environmental stimuli, such as oxidative stress and infection, and hence would be critically important in a chronic remodeling disorder such as BPD.[17] The role of the microbiome regulating the BPD phenotype needs additional study, although the dysbiosis noted (increased Proteobacteria and decreased *Lactobacillus* numbers) in the airway of infants associated with the severe BPD phenotype and the interactions of the microbiome with miR release and DNA methylation are certainly intriguing.

CONCLUSIONS

Although we have presented several studies dealing with the epigenetic mechanisms associated with the development of BPD, much of the iceberg still remains hidden. It remains to be ascertained as to how different patient characteristics, clinical practices, phenotypic variations, and alterations in the host microbiome modulate epigenetic influences contributing to BPD. Sophisticated bioinformatics methodologies for integration of miRs and other epigenetic influences in the context of BPD are needed.

FUNDING

NIH K08HL141652, NIH R01 HL129907, AHA 17SDG32720009, NIH U01 HL122626, NIH U01HL133536.

REFERENCES

1. Ambalavanan N, Cotten CM, Page GP, et al. Integrated genomic analyses in bronchopulmonary dysplasia. *J Pediatr*. 2015;166(3):531−7 e13.
2. Day CL, Ryan RM. Bronchopulmonary dysplasia: new becomes old again!. *Pediatr Res*. 2017;81(1-2):210−213.
3. Sobie EA, Lee YS, Jenkins SL, Iyengar R. Systems biology–biomedical modeling. *Sci Signal*. 2011;4(190):tr2.
4. Parker RA, Lindstrom DP, Cotton RB. Evidence from twin study implies possible genetic susceptibility to bronchopulmonary dysplasia. *Semin Perinatol*. 1996;20(3):206−209.
5. Bhandari V, Bizzarro MJ, Shetty A, et al. Familial and genetic susceptibility to major neonatal morbidities in preterm twins. *Pediatrics*. 2006;117(6):1901−1906.
6. Lavoie PM, Pham C, Jang KL. Heritability of bronchopulmonary dysplasia, defined according to the consensus statement of the national institutes of health. *Pediatrics*. 2008;122(3):479−485.
7. Prosnitz A, Gruen JR, Bhandari V. In: Rimoin DL, Connor JM, Pyeritz RE, BR K, eds. *Emery and Rimoin's Principles and Practice of Medical Genetics*. Elsevier; 2013:1−22.
8. Fujioka K, Shibata A, Yokota T, et al. Association of a vascular endothelial growth factor polymorphism with the development of bronchopulmonary dysplasia in Japanese premature newborns. *Sci Rep*. 2014;4:4459.
9. Mahlman M, Huusko JM, Karjalainen MK, et al. Genes encoding vascular endothelial growth factor A (VEGF-A) and VEGF receptor 2 (VEGFR-2) and risk for bronchopulmonary dysplasia. *Neonatology*. 2015;108(1):53−59.
10. Hadchouel A, Durrmeyer X, Bouzigon E, et al. Identification of SPOCK2 as a susceptibility gene for

bronchopulmonary dysplasia. *Am J Respir Crit Care Med.* 2011;184(10):1164–1170.
11. Wang H, St Julien KR, Stevenson DK, et al. A genome-wide association study (GWAS) for bronchopulmonary dysplasia. *Pediatrics.* 2013;132(2):290–297.
12. Hamvas A, Feng R, Bi Y, et al. Exome sequencing identifies gene variants and networks associated with extreme respiratory outcomes following preterm birth. *BMC Genet.* 2018;19(1):94.
13. Carrera P, Di Resta C, Volonteri C, et al. Exome sequencing and pathway analysis for identification of genetic variability relevant for bronchopulmonary dysplasia (BPD) in preterm newborns: a pilot study. *Clin Chim Acta.* 2015;451(Pt A):39–45.
14. Li J, Yu KH, Oehlert J, et al. Exome sequencing of neonatal blood spots and the identification of genes implicated in bronchopulmonary dysplasia. *Am J Respir Crit Care Med.* 2015;192(5):589–596.
15. Lal CV, Bhandari V, Ambalavanan N. Genomics, microbiomics, proteomics, and metabolomics in bronchopulmonary dysplasia. *Semin Perinatol.* 2018;42(7):425–431.
16. Lal CV, Ambalavanan N. Genetic predisposition to bronchopulmonary dysplasia. *Semin Perinatol.* 2015;39(8): 584–591.
17. Hagood JS. Beyond the genome: epigenetic mechanisms in lung remodeling. *Physiology.* 2014;29(3):177–185.
18. Cuna A, Halloran B, Faye-Petersen O, et al. Alterations in gene expression and DNA methylation during murine and human lung alveolar septation. *Am J Respir Cell Mol Biol.* 2015;53(1):60–73.
19. Zhu Y, Fu J, Yang H, Pan Y, Yao L, Xue X. Hyperoxia-induced methylation decreases RUNX3 in a newborn rat model of bronchopulmonary dysplasia. *Respir Res.* 2015; 16:75.
20. Bik-Multanowski M, Revhaug C, Grabowska A, et al. Hyperoxia induces epigenetic changes in newborn mice lungs. *Free Radic Biol Med.* 2018;121:51–56.
21. Chen CM, Liu YC, Chen YJ, Chou HC. Genome-wide analysis of DNA methylation in hyperoxia-exposed newborn rat lung. *Lung.* 2017;195(5):661–669.
22. Robbins ME, Dakhlallah D, Marsh CB, Rogers LK, Tipple TE. Of mice and men: correlations between microRNA-17 approximately 92 cluster expression and promoter methylation in severe bronchopulmonary dysplasia. *Am J Physiol Lung Cell Mol Physiol.* 2016; 311(5):L981–L984.
23. Cohen J, Van Marter LJ, Sun Y, Allred E, Leviton A, Kohane IS. Perturbation of gene expression of the chromatin remodeling pathway in premature newborns at risk for bronchopulmonary dysplasia. *Genome Biol.* 2007; 8(10):R210.
24. Chao CM, van den Bruck R, Lork S, et al. Neonatal exposure to hyperoxia leads to persistent disturbances in pulmonary histone signatures associated with NOS3 and STAT3 in a mouse model. *Clin Epigenet.* 2018;10:37.
25. Joss-Moore LA, Wang Y, Baack ML, et al. IUGR decreases PPARgamma and SETD8 Expression in neonatal rat lung and these effects are ameliorated by maternal DHA supplementation. *Early Hum Dev.* 2010;86(12):785–791.
26. Londhe VA, Sundar IK, Lopez B, et al. Hyperoxia impairs alveolar formation and induces senescence through decreased histone deacetylase activity and up-regulation of p21 in neonatal mouse lung. *Pediatr Res.* 2011;69(5 Pt 1):371–377.
27. Zhu L, Li H, Tang J, Zhu J, Zhang Y. Hyperoxia arrests alveolar development through suppression of histone deacetylases in neonatal rats. *Pediatr Pulmonol.* 2012;47(3): 264–274.
28. Ni W, Lin N, He H, Zhu J, Zhang Y. Lipopolysaccharide induces up-regulation of TGF-alpha through HDAC2 in a rat model of bronchopulmonary dysplasia. *PLoS One.* 2014; 9(3):e91083.
29. Bao TP, Wu R, Cheng HP, Cui XW, Tian ZF. Differential expression of long non-coding RNAs in hyperoxia-induced bronchopulmonary dysplasia. *Cell Biochem Funct.* 2016;34(5):299–309.
30. Cai C, Qiu J, Qiu G, et al. Long non-coding RNA MALAT1 protects preterm infants with bronchopulmonary dysplasia by inhibiting cell apoptosis. *BMC Pulm Med.* 2017;17(1):199.
31. Stoll BJ, Hansen NI, Bell EF, et al. Neonatal outcomes of extremely preterm infants from the NICHD Neonatal Research Network. *Pediatrics.* 2010;126(3):443–456.
32. Yoder BA, Harrison M, Clark RH. Time-related changes in steroid use and bronchopulmonary dysplasia in preterm infants. *Pediatrics.* 2009;124(2):673–679.
33. Nardiello C, Morty RE. MicroRNA in late lung development and bronchopulmonary dysplasia: the need to demonstrate causality. *Mol Cell Pediatr.* 2016;3(1):19.
34. Zhang X, Peng W, Zhang S, et al. MicroRNA expression profile in hyperoxia-exposed newborn mice during the development of bronchopulmonary dysplasia. *Respir Care.* 2011;56(7):1009–1015.
35. Olave N, Lal CV, Halloran B, et al. Regulation of alveolar septation by microRNA-489. *Am J Physiol Lung Cell Mol Physiol.* 2016;310(5):L476–L487.
36. Syed M, Das P, Pawar A, et al. Hyperoxia causes miR-34a-mediated injury via angiopoietin-1 in neonatal lungs. *Nat Commun.* 2017;8(1):1173.
37. Durrani-Kolarik S, Pool CA, Gray A, et al. miR-29b supplementation decreases expression of matrix proteins and improves alveolarization in mice exposed to maternal inflammation and neonatal hyperoxia. *Am J Physiol Lung Cell Mol Physiol.* 2017;313(2):L339–L349.
38. Go H, La P, Namba F, et al. MiR-196a regulates heme oxygenase-1 by silencing Bach1 in the neonatal mouse lung. *Am J Physiol Lung Cell Mol Physiol.* 2016;311(2): L400–L411.
39. Bhaskaran M, Xi D, Wang Y, et al. Identification of microRNAs changed in the neonatal lungs in response to hyperoxia exposure. *Physiol Genom.* 2012;44(20):970–980.
40. Narasaraju T, Shukla D, More S, et al. Role of microRNA-150 and glycoprotein nonmetastatic melanoma protein B in angiogenesis during hyperoxia-induced neonatal

lung injury. *Am J Respir Cell Mol Biol.* 2015;52(2): 253–261.
41. Dong J, Carey WA, Abel S, et al. MicroRNA-mRNA interactions in a murine model of hyperoxia-induced bronchopulmonary dysplasia. *BMC Genom.* 2012;13:204.
42. Thery C, Ostrowski M, Segura E. Membrane vesicles as conveyors of immune responses. *Nat Rev Immunol.* 2009;9(8): 581–593.
43. Genschmer KR, Russell DW, Lal C, et al. Activated PMN exosomes: pathogenic entities causing matrix destruction and disease in the lung. *Cell.* 2019;176(1–2), 113–26 e15.
44. Hu G, Drescher KM, Chen XM. Exosomal miRNAs: biological properties and therapeutic potential. *Front Genet.* 2012;3:56.
45. Lal CV, Olave N, Travers C, et al. Exosomal microRNA predicts and protects against severe bronchopulmonary dysplasia in extremely premature infants. *JCI Insight.* 2018;3(5).
46. Ambalavanan N, Van Meurs KP, Perritt R, et al. Predictors of death or bronchopulmonary dysplasia in preterm infants with respiratory failure. *J Perinatol.* 2008;28(6): 420–426.
47. Ito M, Tamura M, Namba F, Neonatal Research Network of Japan. Role of sex in morbidity and mortality of very premature neonates. *Pediatr Int.* 2017;59(8):898–905.
48. Shim SY, Cho SJ, Kong KA, Park EA. Gestational age-specific sex difference in mortality and morbidities of preterm infants: a nationwide study. *Sci Rep.* 2017;7(1):6161.
49. Sammour I, Somashekar S, Huang J, et al. The effect of gender on mesenchymal stem cell (MSC) efficacy in neonatal hyperoxia-induced lung injury. *PLoS One.* 2016; 11(10):e0164269.
50. Fulton CT, Cui TX, Goldsmith AM, Bermick J, Popova AP. Gene expression signatures point to a male sex-specific lung mesenchymal cell PDGF receptor signaling defect in infants developing bronchopulmonary dysplasia. *Sci Rep.* 2018;8(1):17070.
51. Balaji S, Dong X, Li H, Zhang Y, Steen E, Lingappan K. Sex-specific differences in primary neonatal murine lung fibroblasts exposed to hyperoxia in vitro: implications for bronchopulmonary dysplasia. *Physiol Genom.* 2018; 50(11):940–946.
52. Coarfa C, Zhang Y, Maity S, et al. Sexual dimorphism of the pulmonary transcriptome in neonatal hyperoxic lung injury: identification of angiogenesis as a key pathway. *Am J Physiol Lung Cell Mol Physiol.* 2017;313(6): L991–L1005.
53. Zhang Y, Coarfa C, Dong X, et al. MicroRNA-30a as a candidate underlying sex-specific differences in neonatal hyperoxic lung injury: implications for BPD. *Am J Physiol Lung Cell Mol Physiol.* 2019;316(1):L144–L156.
54. Leary S, Das P, Ponnalagu D, Singh H, Bhandari V. Genetic strain and sex differences in a hyperoxia-induced mouse model of varying severity of bronchopulmonary dysplasia. *Am J Pathol.* 2019;189(5):999–1014.
55. Pan WH, Sommer F, Falk-Paulsen M, et al. Exposure to the gut microbiota drives distinct methylome and transcriptome changes in intestinal epithelial cells during postnatal development. *Genome Med.* 2018;10(1):27.
56. Arpaia N, Campbell C, Fan X, et al. Metabolites produced by commensal bacteria promote peripheral regulatory T-cell generation. *Nature.* 2013;504(7480):451–455.
57. Lal CV, Travers C, Aghai ZH, et al. The airway microbiome at birth. *Sci Rep.* 2016;6:31023.
58. Pammi M, Lal CV, Wagner BD, et al. Airway microbiome and development of bronchopulmonary dysplasia in preterm infants: a systematic review. *J Pediatr.* 2019;204, 126–133 e2.
59. Ambalavanan N, Cotten CM, Page GP, et al. Integrated genomic analyses in bronchopulmonary dysplasia. *J Pediatr.* 2015;166(3):531–537. e13.

CHAPTER 6

Advancing Imaging Modalities in Bronchopulmonary Dysplasia and Other Neonatal Chronic Lung Diseases

NARA S. HIGANO, PHD • JASON C. WOODS, PHD

ABBREVIATIONS

^{1}H	Hydrogen, proton
^{3}He	Helium-3
^{81}Kr	Krypton-81
^{99}Tc	Technetium-99
^{127}Xe	Xenon-127
^{129}Xe	Xenon-129
^{133}Xe	Xenon-133
Ao	Aorta
ADC	Apparent diffusion coefficient
ASD	Atrial septal defect
ASL	Arterial spin labeling (MRI)
BM	Bronchomalacia
BPD	Bronchopulmonary dysplasia
CDH	Congenital diaphragmatic hernia
CF	Cystic fibrosis
CFD	Computational fluid dynamics
CGA	Corrected gestational age
COPD	Chronic obstructive pulmonary disease
CPV	Common pulmonary vein
CT	Computed tomography
CTA	Computed tomography angiography
CTEPH	Chronic thromboembolic pulmonary hypertension
EDV	End-diastolic volume
EF	Ejection fraction
EI-d	Eccentricity index at end-diastole
EI-s	Eccentricity index at end-systole
ESV	End-systolic volume
FEV_1	Forced expiratory volume in 1 second
FRC	Functional residual capacity
FSE	Fast spin echo (MRI)
Gd	Gadolinium
GRE	Gradient echo (MRI)
HP	Hyperpolarized
IND	Investigational New Drug
IPF	Idiopathic pulmonary fibrosis
IVC	Inferior vena cava
LA	Left atrium
LINV	Left innominate vein
LM	Laryngomalacia
LPA	Left pulmonary artery
LSPV	Left superior pulmonary vein
LV	Left ventricle
LVOT	Left ventricular outflow tract
MPA	Main pulmonary artery
MRI	Magnetic resonance imaging
NICU	Neonatal intensive care unit
NSCLC	Non–small cell lung cancer
OE	Oxygen-enhanced (MRI)
PA	Pulmonary artery
PAAT	Pulmonary artery acceleration time
PAP	Pulmonary arterial pressure
PC	Phase-contrast (MRI)
PDA	Patent ductus arteriosus
PFT	Pulmonary function test
PH	Pulmonary hypertension
PMA	Postmenstrual age
PVD	Pulmonary vascular disease
qCT	Quantitative computed tomography
qMRI	Quantitative magnetic resonance imaging
RA	Right atrium
RPA	Right pulmonary artery
RV	Right ventricle
SEOP	Spin-exchange optical pumping
SGS	Subglottic stenosis
SPECT	Single-photon emission computed tomography
SV	Stroke volume
SVC	Superior vena cava
T	Tesla (magnetic field strength)

Updates on Neonatal Chronic Lung Disease. https://doi.org/10.1016/B978-0-323-68353-1.00006-3

T_1	Nuclear spin longitudinal relaxation time (MRI)
T_2*	Nuclear spin effective transverse relaxation time (MRI)
TE	Echo time (MRI)
TM	Tracheomalacia
UTE	Ultrashort echo time
V/Q	Ventilation and perfusion
VSD	Ventricular septal defect
ZTE	Zero echo time

INTRODUCTION

Imaging has been a central tool in describing structural pulmonary abnormalities related to preterm birth since the early clinical recognition of classical bronchopulmonary dysplasia (BPD) a few decades ago. Initially described by Northway et al. in the 1960s,[1] chest X-ray radiographs of preterm infants exposed to high-pressure ventilation and high oxygen concentrations demonstrated heterogeneous abnormalities, including scattered course opacities, regional cysts, and hyperinflation. Over the years since then, improvements to clinical therapies for preterm infants (described in detail in other chapters of this book) have helped to significantly reduce mortality in preterm infants. This increased rate of survival, particularly in infants born extremely preterm or with very low birth weights, has resulted in increased BPD incidence and severity,[2] with shifting clinical and radiologic characteristics of the disease. The so-called "new BPD"[3] is characterized by more diffuse disease, with regional patterns of alveolar simplification, inflammation, and fibrosis seen on both histologic examination and imaging. Patients with severe and complicated BPD often still require invasive positive-pressure ventilation, long-term oxygen support, and/or tracheostomy, leading to imaging-identified abnormalities that are often consistent with the original description of the disease. These patients have increased risks of multiple rehospitalizations, persistent respiratory symptoms, reduced long-term lung function, pulmonary hypertension (PH), and death.

There is increasing recognition that BPD is complex and multifactorial, with lung disease often comorbid with abnormalities in the major airways and pulmonary vasculature, and also that BPD-related disease phenotypes can be highly variable between individual patients. To date, diagnostic technologies have not provided us with sufficient understanding of the underlying cardiorespiratory disease, or how to treat it effectively.[4] This is precisely where new diagnostics can play a significant role in the near future.

Newer imaging techniques of the lung, airway, and cardiopulmonary systems in infants have the potential for improved understanding of BPD phenotypes and may provide a unique opportunity to better define the individual contributions and interactions of cardiorespiratory disease components in infants born extremely preterm. Serial imaging assessment and quantification offer the ability to monitor disease state, personalize medicine, and evaluate therapeutic efficacy. Cutting-edge imaging methods, such as those described here, can individually quantify parenchymal, airway, and pulmonary vascular abnormalities, holding promise for high-caliber predictions of later clinical outcomes. Although this chapter focuses primarily on BPD, many of the new imaging techniques can be applied to other chronic and congenital lung diseases likely to present in the newborn period,[5,6] such as hypoplastic disease and PH in congenital diaphragmatic hernia (CDH).

LUNG IMAGING

Chest X-ray Radiograph

Chest X-ray radiography is the most common choice for initial radiologic evaluation of acute morbidities in preterm infants, owing to its high accessibility and ease of implementation in the clinic. Chest radiography is generally safe for longitudinal imaging because of the relatively low exposure to ionizing radiation.[7] However, it lacks three-dimensional (3D) tomographic resolution and so offers limited specific structural information. Furthermore, only more severe specific abnormalities are typically apparent on radiography, resulting in marginal sensitivity in describing milder forms of lung disease (Fig. 6.1).

Even with the low sensitivity and specificity, radiography can be used to safely detect more gross structural abnormalities, such as pulmonary edema, fibrosis/scarring, lobar emphysema, and hyperinflation. Chest radiograph scoring systems (e.g., by Toce et al.[8]) have also described categories of focal or generalized hyperexpansion, emphysema, fibrous/interstitial abnormalities, cardiovascular abnormalities, and subjective severity impression, finding that radiologic scores of disease had strong correlation with clinical measures of gas exchange, respiratory distress, and growth rate.

Although X-ray radiographs themselves are relatively nonspecific due to the projection-based nature of the images, they represent an important step toward using radiographic description of parenchymal abnormalities

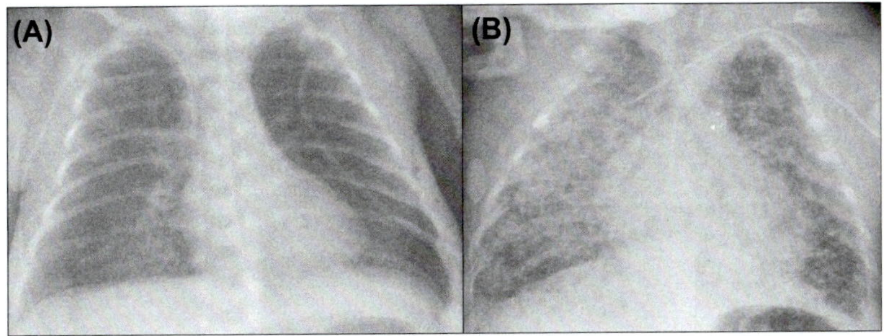

FIG. 6.1 **Chest X-ray radiograph in infants.** X-ray chest radiographs of **(A)** a 27-week corrected gestational age (CGA) preterm male infant with respiratory distress syndrome (later diagnosed with mild bronchopulmonary dysplasia [BPD]) and **(B)** a 46-week CGA preterm male infant diagnosed with severe BPD. Only more severe features of the lung disease are apparent, with marginal sensitivity to milder forms of parenchymal abnormalities. (Courtesy of Jason Woods, Ph.D., and Nara Higano, Ph.D., at Cincinnati Children's Hospital.)

to inform clinical diagnosis and evaluation. Despite this, most current definitions of BPD severity[3,9–11] only incorporate the clinically assessed need for respiratory support and forego the inclusion of radiologic findings, largely owing to the lack of sensitivity and specificity for disease and prognosis. As chest radiography is currently the most easily deployable imaging modality in the neonatal clinical setting, it currently remains the clinical gold standard but is limited by the same lack of sensitivity and specificity.

Chest X-ray Computed Tomography

Chest X-ray computed tomography (CT) offers both 3D submillimeter spatial resolution and true volumetric parenchymal tissue density; this combination yields highly sensitive detection of normal and abnormal anatomic structures (Fig. 6.2). However, chest CT is not a routine imaging clinical modality for infants and is typically employed only in the most severe cases of BPD, when higher precision is required. This is in part due to concerns over the exposure to ionizing radiation in pediatric and infant populations, which has been linked to increased risk of cancer.[7,12] There is well-justified debate over the small increased long-term risks associated with CT,[13] and radiation doses are steadily decreasing with improving technology.[14,15] It has been reported that one radiation-induced solid cancer results from every ~360 (girls) and ~1200 (boys) chest CT scans in patients under 5 years old.[7] However, pediatric chest CT scans often require sedation/anesthesia[16,17] and intubation for control of respirations and movement, which further decreases the use of CT for routine assessment in serial scanning.

While the safety risks of pediatric chest CT must be considered, significant information on lung parenchymal structure can be obtained via high-resolution CT images. Myriad chest CT protocols and nine different semiquantitative scoring systems have been utilized over the past few decades to describe parenchymal and structural abnormalities in formerly preterm patients between the ages of 35 weeks' postmenstrual age (PMA) and 33 years,[18] yet no protocol and scoring system has been broadly accepted or routinely implemented. Structural components commonly evaluated include opacities (linear and subpleural), hyperlucencies (cysts/bullae/blebs),

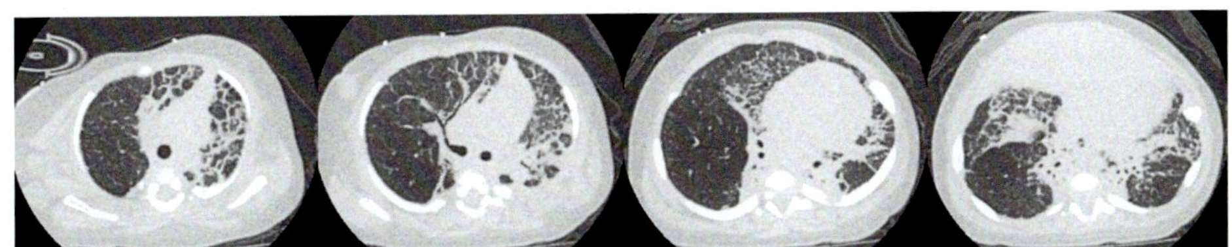

FIG. 6.2 **Chest X-ray computed tomography (CT) in an infant.** Lung CT images in an 8-month-old female infant with severe bronchopulmonary dysplasia, demonstrating clear parenchymal abnormalities. (Courtesy of Jason Woods, Ph.D., and Nara Higano, Ph.D., at Cincinnati Children's Hospital.)

emphysema, mosaic attenuation, bronchial wall thickening and collapse, consolidations/atelectasis, architectural distortion, and subjective impression.[18] All studies utilizing these scoring systems found elevated CT scores for lung disease in patients with BPD both early and later in life.[18]

Several studies found significant correlations between CT scores and pulmonary function test (PFT) parameters in older children and adults with BPD.[19,20] Two studies performed PFTs and CT imaging in pediatric patients under 2 years old at the time of discharge from the neonatal intensive care unit (NICU), linking decreases in compliance and forced residual capacity with more severe imaging findings.[21,22] Significant correlation was determined in several studies between CT scores and duration of oxygen treatment, or whether patients were discharged on oxygen.[22–24] There was some disagreement in studies' findings not only on whether CT score correlated with increased respiratory symptoms (such as wheezing, rehospitalization, or pneumonia) at a later age[22,25,26] but also on the involvement of bronchial wall thickening.[22,27,28]

Chest CT images can measure parenchymal density and so offer the possibility for quantitative and regional density analysis (quantitative CT [qCT]), unique among modalities currently used in the clinic (although cutting-edge research magnetic resonance imaging (MRI) techniques have demonstrated comparable density measurements, as described later). Stein et al.[29] demonstrated that normal lung attenuation on CT decreased rapidly with increasing lung volume and age from 0 to 2 years, with slower changes occurring between 2 and 7 years of age. Sarria et al.[30] found, using sedated chest CT, that infants and toddlers with chronic lung disease of prematurity had increased heterogeneity of lung density (as measured by standard deviation of lung attenuation on CT normalized to mean attenuation) compared with term control patients with no suspected lung issues, and in a cross-sectional CT of patients with BPD between the ages of 0 and 6 years, Spielberg et al.[31] reported decreases in lung abnormalities (opacities, lucencies, and overall heterogeneity) with age.

Multivolume CT analysis can also capture lung dynamics; for instance, specific gas volumes have been calculated via segmentation and registration of expiratory/inspiratory lung CT images, identifying regions of air trapping in adult patients with emphysema.[32–35] Similar techniques may be implemented to analyze regional alveolar simplification and gas trapping in infants with BPD.

In the infant population with CDH, the diaphragmatic surface structure has been assessed by high-resolution CT,[36] and single-photon emission CT has been used to evaluate regional lung function impairment via mapping of ventilation and perfusion, with clear disadvantages related to the use of radioactive tracers.[37] There is potential for dynamic CT to assess diaphragmatic function and evaluate surgical efficacy after repair.

Applications of qCT are more thoroughly explored in adult populations, with only limited studies in pediatrics because of concerns over ionizing radiation exposure and use of sedation/anesthesia (see earlier discussion). Interestingly, there is little emphasis in published studies regarding standardization of CT protocol details (e.g., lung volume at acquisition, slice thickness, and reconstruction kernel),[18] even though these simple parameters can significantly affect quantification and are relatively easy to standardize. As the lung imaging field moves toward more automated quantification pipelines, such standardization will be key to reliably sensitive measurements.

There is high value in quantitatively monitoring disease and density abnormalities at multiple time points. With the valuable parenchymal information provided by chest CT, recent efforts have been focused on reducing the radiation burden via low-dose CT protocols in order to increase feasibility in the pediatric and infant populations.[38–40] Although typical volumetric/spiral pediatric CT protocols have a radiation dose that is equivalent to approximately 50 chest X-ray radiographs, low-dose limited high-resolution CT protocols in pediatrics have a dose closer to approximately ~10–15 radiographs.[2] However, in limiting the radiation dose, isotropic voxel resolution is sacrificed, resulting in CT images that have an increased slice thickness. Recent developments in CT technology have generated faster X-ray tube rotation speeds, increased number of radiation detectors, and dual source CT scanners, resulting in rapid acquisition of an infant chest CT lasting a fraction of a second.[41] Such updates may reduce requirements for sedation/anesthesia and breath-hold maneuvers in the noncompliant infant population.

Despite these CT protocol upgrades, the accumulated ionizing radiation dose associated with routine or serial CT may remain prohibitive even in low-dose protocol settings, particularly in light of recent developments in MRI techniques, which can achieve CT-like visualization of parenchymal density and structure with comparable 3D resolution. Thus pulmonary imaging modalities that are both nonionizing and tomographic, such as MRI, will likely be the serial modality of choice to better understand the trajectories of BPD-related pulmonary disease.

Pulmonary Magnetic Resonance Imaging

In the recent years, the largest efforts in advanced imaging of BPD have been focused predominantly on MRI. As a nonionizing modality, MRI is ideal for both routine and longitudinal imaging in pediatrics and neonates, and there are a multitude of rapidly developing MRI techniques that can probe various structural and functional components of pulmonary disease.[42]

However, a handful of practicalities related to cost and logistics have historically kept MRI from applications in the neonatal environment. MRI systems are more expensive than CT systems, and MRI exams tend to take longer than other imaging modalities; individual MRI acquisition sequences can last several minutes at a time, with full exam durations that can at times exceed 1 hour for multiple complementary measurements. In addition, the strong magnetic field inherent in MRI occasionally limits the medical monitoring and support equipment that can be provided to neonatal imaging subjects; this challenge can be obviated with an inventory of MR-compatible equipment in the neonatal unit. A small handful of medical institutions from around the globe have installed MRI scanners within the NICU, whereas a neonatal MRI ordered at most hospitals would currently require transportation of both the patient and the clinical monitoring team to the radiology department. Pioneering works at the Hammersmith Hospital (London, United Kingdom),[43] Cincinnati Children's Hospital (United States),[44,45] and the University of Sheffield (United Kingdom)[46] serve as models for other institutions eager to bring MRI to the NICU environment. As neonatal MRI becomes more commonplace, several emerging MRI techniques may increase our understanding and treatment of BPD.

^{1}H magnetic resonance imaging

MRI of the lung is technically challenging for various reasons, including the low proton (^{1}H) density and associated image intensity of lung parenchyma compared with soft tissues.[47] In addition, lung parenchyma has a rapid signal decay (i.e., short ^{1}H T_2* relaxation time, approximately 0.5–3 ms at typical field strengths of 1.5–3 T [48–52]) due to the many air-tissue interfaces inherent in the alveolar structure, which yields local magnetic field inhomogeneities and requires rapid data acquisition after spin excitation. ^{1}H chest MRI can be subject to image quality degradation from respiratory and cardiac motion; in the neonatal population, additional challenges include the small lung size (~100 mL), fast respiratory rate (40–70 breaths per minute), and inability to perform breathing maneuvers (e.g., breath-holds).

Despite these obstacles, preliminary studies using conventional Cartesian MRI sequences, such as a gradient echo (GRE) or fast spin echo (FSE), have seen initial successes in demonstrating regionally heterogeneous tissue in preterm infants compared to controls,[48] as well as in detecting significant differences in signal intensity between patients with and without BPD.[43,51] Indeed, conventional sequences, with relatively long echo time (TE) values compared with the normal parenchymal T_2* values, have sufficient ability to visualize soft tissue or pathologic tissue specimens with a longer T_2* (such as regions of inflammation, fibrosis, consolidations, or atelectasis), which manifest on imaging as focal and diffuse high-intensity regions. As there is high contrast on conventional MR images between lung parenchyma and soft tissues, such techniques have also been used in the infant population with CDH to study the potential for catch-up growth in infants with pulmonary hypoplasia, via comparison of ipsilateral and contralateral lung volume changes between prenatal and postnatal imaging.[52] However, due to the relatively long TE compared with the parenchymal T_2* value, conventional sequences perform poorly in visualizing lung tissues with normal or simplified alveoli. As the MR signal from these normal or simplified tissues decays before being acquired, they are represented on conventional MRI with low image intensity that inaccurately represents actual tissue density and lacks much structural information.

Recent developments in 3D radial ultrashort echo time (UTE) MRI acquisitions[53–55] have in large part addressed the technical obstacles that have historically kept pulmonary MRI from high clinical utility. Radial acquisition strategies are inherently robust to cardiorespiratory and bulk motion, and with TE values much shorter than parenchymal T_2* values (in the order of $<100\ \mu s$), UTE images provide image intensities in the lung that, when normalized by muscle intensity, generate CT-like pulmonary tissue density[56] (Fig. 6.3). Furthermore, UTE acquisitions yield high resolution that is comparable to the resolution of CT; in some low-dose CT protocols with increased slice thickness and/or spacing, UTE MR images actually have higher 3D resolution than CT images. This opens the door to safe, nonionizing, tomographic quantification of regional lung density in patients with a variety of pulmonary morbidities, including BPD or hypoplastic

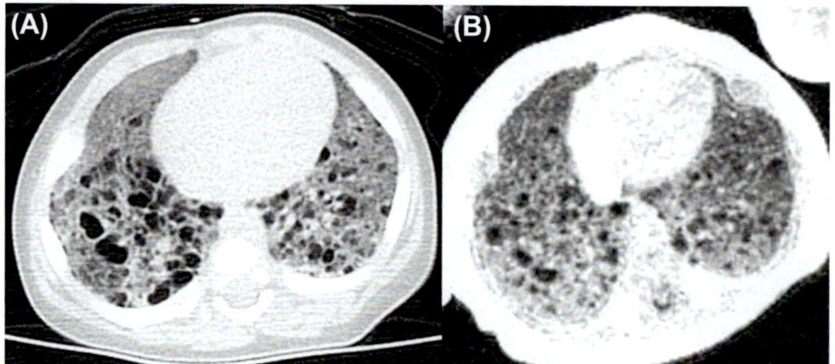

FIG. 6.3 Comparison of neonatal chest computed tomography (CT) and magnetic resonance imaging (MRI). Lung imaging in a male infant with severe bronchopulmonary dysplasia born at 26 weeks' gestation. Slice-matched images (A) from CT at 50 weeks' corrected gestational age (CGA) and (B) from ultrashort echo time (UTE) MRI at 39 weeks' CGA. The cystic and high-density nature of the parenchymal lung disease persists between these two time points. UTE MRI provides comparable tomographic information to that of CT, without requiring ionizing radiation or sedation/anesthesia. (Courtesy of Jason Woods, Ph.D., and Nara Higano, Ph.D., at Cincinnati Children's Hospital.)

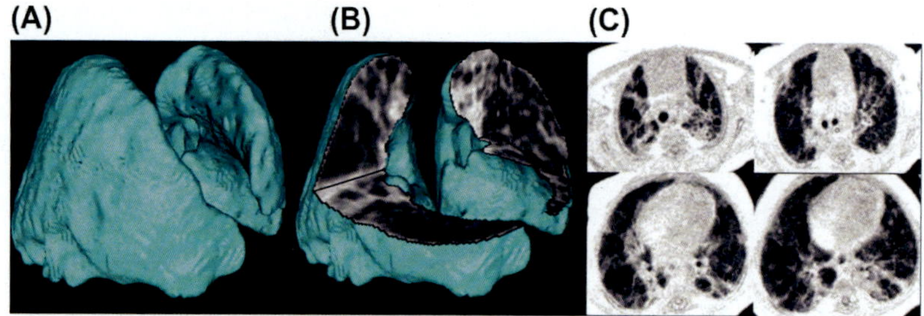

FIG. 6.4 Neonatal lung images and volume surfaces from ultrashort echo time (UTE) magnetic resonance imaging (MRI). Anatomic lung volume rendering of a neonatal patient with severe bronchopulmonary dysplasia **(A)**, with cutout **(B)**, generated from high-resolution pulmonary ultrashort echo time (UTE) MRI (axial image slices, **C**). (Courtesy of Jason Woods, Ph.D., and Nara Higano, Ph.D., at Cincinnati Children's Hospital.)

disease (e.g., CDH).[57,58] Advanced postprocessing methods that were once limited to high-resolution CT (e.g., anatomic lung/airway volume renderings or quantitative measures of lung volume and regional density) can now be achieved with nonionizing UTE MRI (Fig. 6.4).[59–61]

In a few recent studies, the BPD CT scoring system developed by Ochiai et al.[23] was modified for structural MRI acquisitions. Early investigations with conventional Cartesian MRI sequences (e.g., GRE and FSE) demonstrated that infants diagnosed with BPD had higher MRI scores than both preterm infants without BPD and term infants without BPD.[51] More recently, UTE and GRE MRI scores of patients with and without BPD near 40 weeks' PMA were integrated with standard clinical parameters (e.g., gestational age at birth, birth weight, sex, race, multiparity of pregnancy, antenatal steroids, postnatal steroids, highest level of respiratory support in the NICU) as inputs in a general linear model to predict respiratory outcomes.[62] This work demonstrated that MRI scores of parenchymal structure abnormalities describe disease severity and predicted short-term clinical outcomes (such as duration of respiratory support and level of respiratory support at discharge from NICU) more accurately than any individual standard clinical measure. As UTE images can provide measurements akin to volumetric density,[56] future work may focus on quantitative MRI analysis similar to current qCT methods. Quantitative lung density distributions from voxel intensity histograms (e.g., percentage of whole-lung volume representing lucencies or opacities) may complement or replace radiologic scoring systems in an attempt to quantify lung disease with more objective and automated processes.

Radial UTE MRI inherently captures the center of MR k-space (i.e., raw data not yet Fourier-transformed) at every acquisition every few milliseconds. It has been phenomenologically observed that the magnitude and phase of the center point in k-space are modulated by motion, which means that UTE MRI raw data can provide a self-gating waveform that tracks both bulk and respiratory motion.[63,64] This waveform can be used to distinguish between periods of quiescence and periods of bulk motion[63]; data acquired during periods of bulk motion can be retrospectively discarded and data acquired during tidal quiet-breathing can be respiratory-binned, resulting in respiratory-gated image reconstruction at various stages of the respiratory cycle that is virtually free of motion artifact. These high-resolution 3D cine-like MR images may be used to investigate various parameters of the dynamic lung, such as tidal volumes and regional ventilation via density changes. In the CDH population, this UTE technique has been used to explore the efficacy of primary and nonprimary diaphragmatic repair in seven postoperative infants.[65] Furthermore, the ability to retrospectively track and discard bulk motion from a UTE scan obviates the need for sedation/anesthesia in this difficult and often noncompliant infant population.

Radial zero echo time (ZTE) MRI has emerged in the recent years as an alternative acquisition technique to UTE MRI, achieving an extremely short TE that is milliseconds shorter than the parenchymal T_2* and $\sim 10^1-10^2$ μs shorter than the TE values achievable with UTE.[66,67] ZTE MRI offers a practical advantage over nearly all other MRI sequences—virtually silent acquisition, an important feature with noncompliant infants whose restfulness may be disturbed by typical MRI acoustics. However, ZTE acquisitions inherently miss a circle (two dimensional) or sphere (3D) data from the center of k-space at every excitation, due to the acquisition dead time of radio-frequency excitation pulsing, transmit-receive switching, and digital filtering.[68] This gap can be algebraically reconstructed, with decreasing reliability as the gap size increases (i.e., higher excitation bandwidths),[68] but the inherent gap means that ZTE MRI is not sensitive to the motion-modulated variation of the k-space center that is necessary for the retrospective respiratory gating and motion-discarding explored with neonatal UTE techniques. With conventional hearing protection used at MRI (earplugs and sound-blocking ear muffs), there are few acoustical safety concerns related to MRI in neonates.[69]

Hyperpolarized noble gas magnetic resonance imaging

As an alternative approach to direct imaging of lung parenchymal tissue, imaging of an inhaled hyperpolarized (HP) noble gas contrast agent (^{3}He or ^{129}Xe) can be performed. The field of pulmonary HP gas MRI has slowly developed for the past few decades, with rapid bursts in progress over the recent years in pediatrics. While gaseous nuclei are generally "invisible" on MRI due to the low nuclear spin density and polarization at thermal (Boltzmann) equilibrium ($\sim 10^{-6}$), the nuclear spins of ^{3}He or ^{129}Xe can be made "visible" on MRI by increasing nuclear spin polarization via a process known as spin-exchange optical pumping (SEOP). In SEOP, angular momentum is first transferred from circularly polarized laser light to the electronic spins of an alkali metal buffer gas and then transferred via collisions to the nuclear spins of ^{3}He or ^{129}Xe gas. This technique yields an HP noble gas nuclear polarization ($\sim 10^{-1}$) that far exceeds the Boltzmann polarization and provides high-signal maps of regional ventilation and gas exchange.[70] The investigation of noble gas polarization is a thriving field on its own and can be reviewed extensively elsewhere.[70,71]

HP gas MRI has been demonstrated in vivo in both healthy subjects and patients with a variety of respiratory conditions, including chronic obstructive pulmonary disease (COPD),[72,73] idiopathic pulmonary fibrosis (IPF),[74] asthma,[75,76] cystic fibrosis (CF),[77–79] and CDH (Fig. 6.5).[80] Importantly, the safety profile of HP ^{3}He and ^{129}Xe has been well established in healthy and diseased adult[81,82] and pediatric subjects,[83–85] down to the age of 4 years, and the feasibility of ^{3}He MRI has been demonstrated in infant patients under 1 year old.[86] HP gas MRI can be separated into three acquisition strategies: ventilation, diffusion, and dissolved phase. Each of these categories provide unique regional information about the structure and function of the lung.

The most straightforward HP gas MRI method is ventilation imaging, in which static spin-density maps are generated to highlight airspaces that are ventilated during inhalation; bright and dark areas indicate the presence and absence of inhaled gas, respectively. A normal lung typically demonstrates a homogenous ventilation patterning, whereas a diseased lung will present with heterogeneous ventilation defects, indicating regional function impairment and airway obstruction. In a ^{3}He MRI study of adults (18–30 years old) with a history of repaired CDH, Spoel et al.[80] demonstrated clear ventilation defects in the ipsilateral lung in six of nine patients, demonstrating persistent presence into

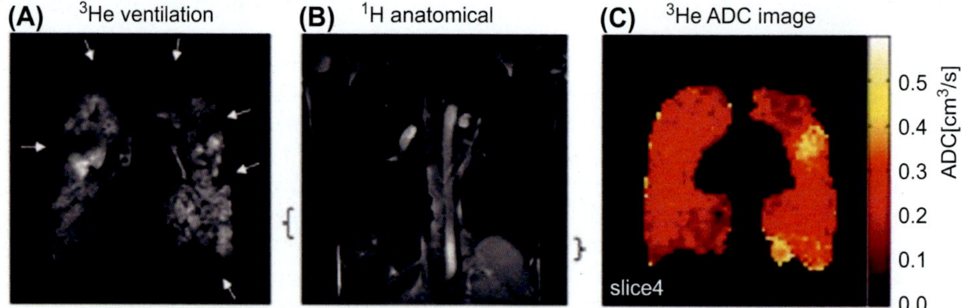

FIG. 6.5 Hyperpolarized (HP) ^{3}He ventilation and diffusion in an adult with a history of congenital diaphragmatic hernia repair. (A) HP ^{3}He ventilation magnetic resonance imaging (MRI), **(B)** spatially matched anatomic ^{1}H MRI, and **(C)** apparent diffusion coefficient (ADC) map from HP ^{3}He diffusion MRI in an 18-year-old adult with a history of congenital diaphragmatic repair in infancy. Anatomic ^{1}H images were acquired after a 1-L inhalation of air to match the inflation level during ^{3}He imaging. Ventilation defects are shown with arrows (A). Regional increases in ADC (C, a surrogate for alveolar airspace size) are apparent in the ipsilateral lung compared with the contralateral lung. (Adapted from Spoel M, Marshall H, IJsselstijn H, et al. Pulmonary ventilation and micro-structural findings in congenital diaphragmatic hernia. *Pediatr Pulmonol.* 2016; 51(5):517–524. https://doi.org/10.1002/ppul.23325.)

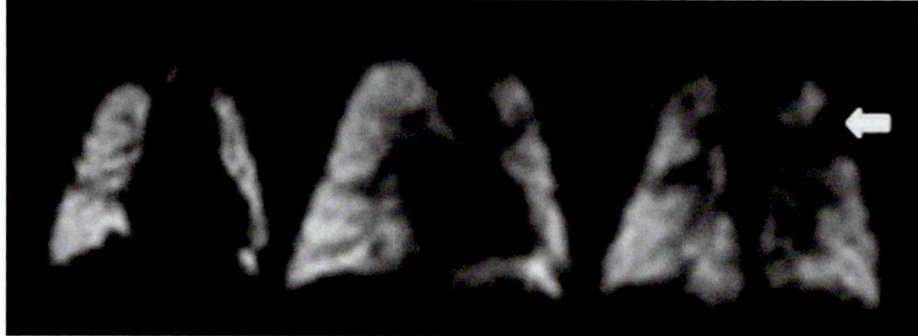

FIG. 6.6 Hyperpolarized ^{3}He lung ventilation in an infant. Coronal magnetic resonance images of hyperpolarized ^{3}He ventilation in 2-month-old preterm infant. Multiple ventilation defects are evident, with the largest highlighted (*arrow*). (From Altes TA, Meyer CH, Mata JF, Froh DK, Paget-Brown A, Gerald Teague W, Fain SB, de Lange EE, Ruppert K, Botfield MC, Johnson MA, Mugler JP third. Hyperpolarized helium-3 magnetic resonance lung imaging of non-sedated infants and young children: a proof-of-concept study. *Clin Imaging*. 2017 Sep–Oct; 45:105–110.)

adulthood of pulmonary abnormalities related to hypoplastic lung disease and repair in infancy. A few studies have implemented ^{129}Xe ventilation MRI in pediatric patients with CF and noted a correlation between the amount of regional ventilation defects and global lung function measurements (forced expiratory volume in 1 second, FEV_1)[77,78]; notably, ventilation defect as measured by MRI was more sensitive than FEV_1 in the detection of mild CF.[78] ^{3}He ventilation MRI was demonstrated in a proof-of-concept study in nonsedated infants with and without pulmonary morbidities (CF, asthma, BPD).[86] Images from a 2-month-old patient with BPD indicate the presence of focal ventilatory defects (Fig. 6.6). Further exploration of regional ventilation deficiencies and air trapping, particularly when combined with structural and morphologic information available through CT or UTE MRI as demonstrated with older pediatric and adult patients with CF,[87] will likely illuminate pulmonary structure-function relationships in infants with BPD and potentially evaluate treatment efficacy.

Alveolar microstructure and size can be probed with HP gas diffusion MRI.[88] The atoms of inhaled HP gas diffuse in the alveolar airspaces via Brownian motion, with diffusion restricted by acinar wall structures in millisecond timescales. Using diffusion-sensitizing magnetic field gradients, the apparent diffusion coefficient (ADC) of the diffusing gas atoms can be measured as a surrogate for general alveolar airspace size.[89,90] Early results from one ^{3}He diffusion MRI study indicate that children with former BPD in infancy (mean age, ~10 years) had increases in both mean and heterogeneous focal ADC values compared with age-matched controls, indicative of impaired development of alveolar structure.[91] In a separate study, Narayanan et al. reported similar alveolar sizes and numbers from ^{3}He diffusion MRI in children (ages 10–14 years) with and without former mild and moderate BPD in infancy, potentially indicative of catch-up alveolarization in the less severe BPD population.[92] The HP ^{3}He MRI study from Spoel et al.[80] (see earlier discussion) demonstrated significantly higher ADC values in the ipsilateral lung compared with the contralateral lung in eight of nine adult patients with a history of CDH, indicating that abnormalities in alveolar microstructure related to infant lung hypoplasia can persist throughout childhood and into adulthood. In addition, explanted infant lungs from one infant with filamin A deficiency (a rare genetic mutation associated with diffuse lung disease, obtained after lung transplant, 11 months old) demonstrated greater ADC values and spatial heterogeneity when compared with results from seven infant lungs with no suspected pulmonary morbidities (obtained post mortem, 0–16 months old), indicating enlarged alveolar airspaces in the diseased case, which was confirmed via quantitative histologic examination.[93,94] If longitudinally implemented in vivo, starting in the neonatal period, HP gas diffusion MRI has the potential for spatially quantifying the degree of alveolar simplification, as well as short- and long-term alveolar development and response to treatment in individual patients.

HP dissolved-phase MRI exploits the slight solubility of ^{129}Xe in tissue and blood to measure gas exchange, red blood cell uptake, and perfusion dynamics. MR signal from ^{129}Xe nuclei present in airspace, a combined interstitial barrier tissue and blood plasma environment, and red blood cell compartments can be individually distinguished to generate quantitative maps of ventilation and gas transfer, which can be binned to spatially characterize normal and abnormal physiology. ^{129}Xe dissolved-phase MRI has been implemented in patients with a variety of pulmonary conditions, including COPD, IPF, non–small cell lung cancer after radiation therapy, pulmonary arterial hypertension, and chronic thromboembolic PH.[95] Fig. 6.7 demonstrates the increased xenon signal from the barrier and decreased signal from the red blood cells in four adult patients with IPF compared with a healthy control, providing a regional assessment of thickened interstitium and impaired gas exchange in diseases with an inflammatory and/or fibrotic component.[74] As a noninvasive method for quantifying regions of interstitial thickening related to inflammation and/or fibrosis, dissolved-phase ^{129}Xe MRI may be an alternative to invasive biopsy in infants as a modality for serially monitoring of therapeutic response to treatments.

Clinical implementation of HP gas MRI techniques has been inhibited over the recent decades for a few reasons, not the least of which is the access to polarizer technology (originally limited to a few institutions with high-level polarizer expertise) and the increasing scarcity and cost of ^{3}He due to complex supply issues and international geopolitics.[96] In addition, noble gases are currently regulated in the United States as drugs, which has prolonged the timeline to clinical application. In the recent years a ^{129}Xe polarizer device has become commercially available from Polarean (Research Triangle Park, NC, USA). Notably, the field of HP gas MRI has begun to invest in imaging acquisition and analysis techniques more specific to the less scarce ^{129}Xe, which has the potential for FDA approval within a small handful of years.

In an effort to increase accessibility of HP ^{129}Xe MRI, a ^{129}Xe MRI Clinical Trials Consortium[97] was established in 2015 and currently consists of eight clinical research centers throughout North America and the United Kingdom, each of which has established the on-site technology to perform in vivo ^{129}Xe MRI and also has obtained an independent Investigational New Drug, or equivalent. The Consortium aims to facilitate collaborative clinical ^{129}Xe MRI research, to test novel approaches for biomarkers and imaging-guided interventions, and to offer a platform for sharing MRI sequences and image analysis algorithms.[97] While the Consortium has recently been investigating lung conditions in older children and adults (COPD, IPF, CF, and asthma), interest is high in applying HP gas MRI techniques to the preterm infant for biomarker identification and tracking response to treatments.

Oxygen-enhanced magnetic resonance imaging

Oxygen (O_2) is paramagnetic and when inhaled has a concentration-dependent effect on the T_1 relaxation time in parenchymal tissues. Therefore T_1 mapping via oxygen-enhanced (OE) MRI can be performed using GRE or UTE sequences at various concentrations of inhaled O_2 to quantify regional ventilation and perfusion.[98] One study reported good differentiation between OE MRI ventilation measures in control

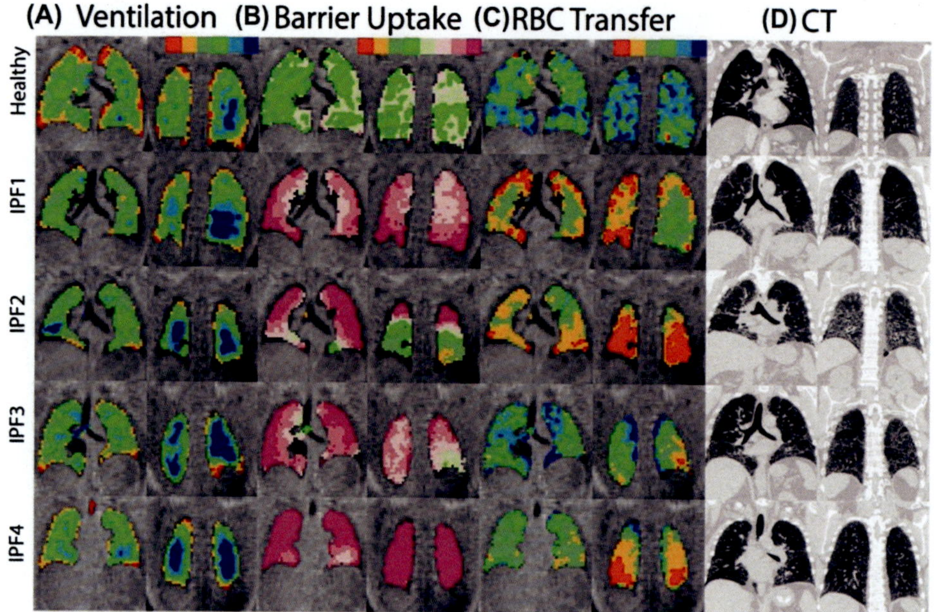

FIG. 6.7 **Hyperpolarized ^{129}Xe regional gas transfer in adults.** Coronal (central and posterior) lung maps from hyperpolarized ^{129}Xe dissolved-phase magnetic resonance imaging (MRI) in four adult patients with idiopathic pulmonary fibrosis (IPF) and one healthy control. **(A)** Ventilation maps (i.e., signal from xenon in pulmonary airspaces), where blue indicates high signal and red indicates low signal (i.e., ventilation defects). **(B)** Barrier uptake maps (i.e., signal from xenon in the barrier and plasma), where pink indicates high signal (thickened interstitium) and red indicates low signal. **(C)** Red blood cell (RBC) maps (i.e., signal from xenon in RBCs), where blue indicates high signal and red indicates low signal. **(D)** Slice-matched coronal chest computed tomographic (CT) images. When applied in infants with bronchopulmonary dysplasia, ^{129}Xe dissolved-phase MRI may provide a regional assessment of thickened interstitium and impaired gas exchange in inflammatory and/or fibrotic lung disease. (From Wang JM, Robertson SH, Wang Z, He M, Virgincar RS, Schrank GM, Smigla RM, O'Riordan TG, Sundy J, Ebner L, Rackley CR, McAdams P, Driehuys B. Using hyperpolarized 129Xe MRI to quantify regional gas transfer in idiopathic pulmonary fibrosis. *Thorax*. 2018 Jan; 73(1):21–28.)

subjects and both subjects with asthma and CF, with significant correlation to FEV_1 in diseased subjects and excellent repeatability after repeat acquisitions.[99]

OE MRI is appealing because it does not require hyperpolarizing equipment or expertise; medical oxygen is readily available in the clinical setting. However, these acquisitions typically last ~5–10 min, so application of this technique to neonates may be challenging, as a change in oxygen concentration for several minutes at a time may introduce risk to neonatal patients with severe respiratory issues.

Pulmonary Ultrasonography

Ultrasonography has played a generally small role in respiratory imaging, as the large volumes of air in a normal lung prevent ultrasonic wave transmission. Pulmonary ultrasonography performs well in detecting the presence of pleural fluid, in addition to distinguishing between a subpleural mass and lung collapse.[2] However, a study by Pieper et al.[100] reported the potential for false-positive results, with pneumonia being mistakenly identified in one infant ultrasonographic examination as a BPD-related structural abnormality; consequently, it has been noted that ultrasonography is not a reliable replacement for other pulmonary imaging modalities.[41]

Pulmonary Nuclear Medicine Scintigraphy

Radionuclide imaging (i.e., nuclear medicine scintigraphy) can generate regional, low-resolution maps of ventilation and perfusion (V/Q) using radioactive gases (e.g., ^{81}Kr, ^{127}Xe, or ^{133}Xe) or a radioactive aerosol (e.g., ^{99}Tc).[2,101,102] Pulmonary scintigraphy is a relatively straightforward modality to implement for obtaining regional lung function in infants who are unable to undergo PFTs. Of course, the method has obvious disadvantages related to the use of radioactive tracers in the infant population, requirement for sedation/anesthesia, and historically low sensitivity and/or specificity to regional impairment. As such, V/Q scintigraphy studies in infants with BPD have been limited[103–105] but have shown association between low regional perfusion and PH in BPD.[106]

PULMONARY VASCULAR IMAGING

As described in detail in other chapters, more severe cases of PH in BPD (in addition to CDH) can involve pulmonary vasculature injury and elevated pulmonary vascular resistance, yielding impaired right ventricular (RV) function, poor cardiac output, and increased pulmonary edema.[107] The incidence of PH has been reported as approximately 20%–40%[108,109] and is associated with a significant increase in morbidity and mortality among infants diagnosed with BPD.[106,110] Detection, diagnosis, and serial monitoring of PH in infants can be challenging because the symptoms are often subtle or may be attributed to lung disease alone.[107] Imaging-based biomarkers of cardiovascular abnormalities may provide important insight into the application and efficacy of PH-targeted therapies in infants with chronic lung disease, leading to improved clinical outcomes.

Echocardiography

Echocardiography is the clinical recommendation for initial noninvasive screening and management guidance for PH in infants with BPD, particularly for those patients who require prolonged ventilator support or have respiratory support needs that are incommensurate with their severity of lung disease.[107] The goal of echocardiography includes evaluating the severity of RV function impairment, evidence of pulmonary vascular resistance, and intracardiac and extracardiac shunts (such as atrial septal defect [ASD], ventricular septal defect [VSD], and patent ductus arteriosus [PDA]).[107,111] Quantitative morphologic echocardiographic biomarkers for PH include left ventricular (LV) eccentricity index at end-systole and end-diastole (EI-s and EI-d, respectively). Functional echocardiographic data is also quantified with various hemodynamic measures, such as RV systolic pressure, systolic pulmonary arterial pressure (PAP), and pulmonary artery acceleration time (PAAT) (Fig. 6.8). Qualitative evaluations include septal wall flattening, RV flattening, right atrial dilation, and RV dilation.[112]

Echocardiography utilizes Doppler ultrasonography and so is a very safe imaging modality for pediatric applications. The association between echocardiographic results and PH diagnosis has been supported in large trials of adults and older pediatric patients,[113] but this association has been less extensively explored in infants, in part because typical pulmonary characteristics of BPD (such as hyperinflation, alveolar simplification, and cysts) can impair the ability for echocardiography to accurately quantify biomarkers of PH, such as systolic PAP.[107] In a retrospective study of 25 children under 2 years old with a BPD diagnosis, Mourani et al.[114] found that echocardiography correctly detected presence or absence of PH in 79% of cases and accurately assessed severity of PH in only 46% of cases, when compared with results from cardiac catheterization (the standard method for assessing abnormalities in cardiopulmonary circulation; see later discussion). The study also demonstrated that systolic PAP could only be estimated in 61% of studies, with poor correlation between echocardiography and cardiac catheterization.[114]

Data from a prospective study of 221 preterm infants from two academic centers suggest that echocardiographic evidence of pulmonary vascular disease (PVD) at 7 days of life is a strong risk factor (in combination with other perinatal factors) for late respiratory disease during early childhood.[115] Late development or progression of PH in preterm infants in early childhood can be severe and carries a risk of mortality. Additionally, Levy et al.[116] report that preterm infants demonstrated lower PAAT on echocardiograms at 12 months old compared with age-matched term infants and that preterm infants with BPD had lower PAAT values than preterm infants without BPD, indicating that pulmonary vascular abnormalities related to prematurity can persist through early childhood. As such, clinical echocardiography adds value to identify PH in some infants with BPD but may lack a strong degree of reliability in evaluating disease severity; even so, echocardiography will likely remain the first line of routine and serial clinical screening of PH in infants with BPD due to ease and relative noninvasive nature of the test.

Cardiac Catheterization

Cardiac catheterization is the standard modality for further evaluation of PVD and contributing factors in those patients with BPD in whom echocardiographic results were nondiagnostic, and also who have persistent cardiorespiratory symptoms even after optimal management of pulmonary and airway disease or who have recurrent pulmonary edema.[107] The goal of cardiac catheterization is to describe disease severity via LV diastolic dysfunction, anatomic shunts, pulmonary vein stenosis, systemic/pulmonary collateral vessels, and anatomic cardiac lesions.[107,114]

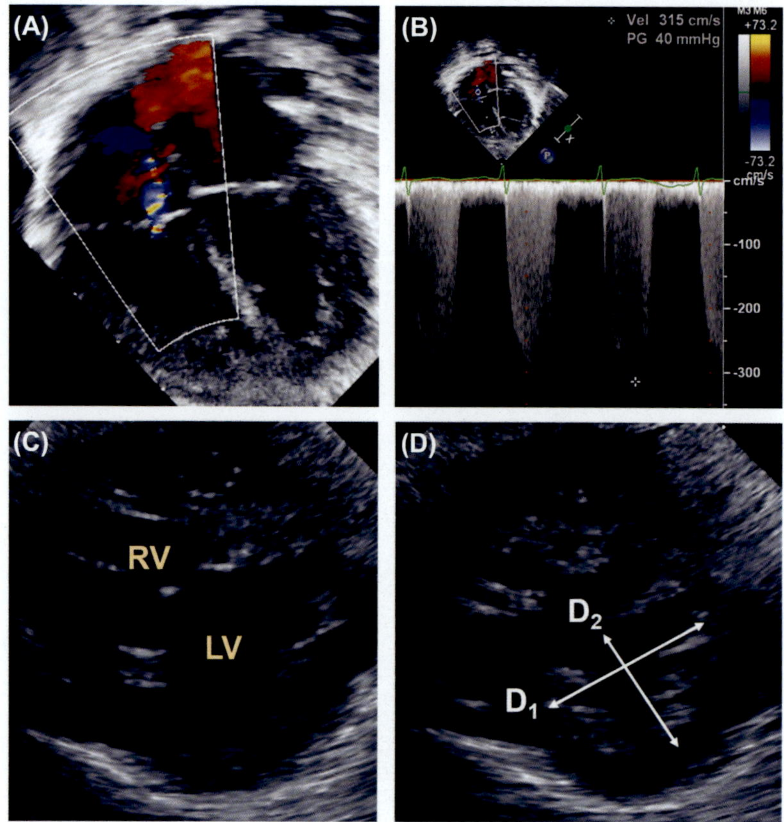

FIG. 6.8 **Infant echocardiography.** Echocardiogram from an infant diagnosed with bronchopulmonary dysplasia and moderate right ventricular hypertension. **(A,B)** An apical four-chamber view with color Doppler demonstrates tricuspid regurgitation. A parasternal short-axis view of the right ventricle (RV) and left ventricle (LV) demonstrates interventricular septal flattening in **(C)** diastole and **(D)** systole. LV eccentricity index (the ratio between major LV diameter D_1 and minor LV diameter D_2) acts as a surrogate echocardiographic biomarker for pulmonary hypertension. (Courtesy of Paul Critser, MD, at Cincinnati Children's Hospital.)

Cardiac catheterization is ordered more sparingly than echocardiography due to its invasive nature and requirement for anesthesia, and thus the procedure is typically only utilized in cases that require additional management guidance.[114] As noninvasive imaging modalities (i.e., tomographic and/or dynamic CT and MRI; see later discussion) continue to be tailored for the neonatal population, the clinical utility of cardiac catheterization for routine diagnosis of PH will likely decrease in infants with BPD.

Computed Tomography

Computed tomography angiography (CTA) can provide high-resolution tomographic visualization and reformatting of cardiac and pulmonary vascular structures (Fig. 6.9). A common contrast CT measurement of the pulmonary vasculature linked to PH is the ratio of the transverse diameters of the main pulmonary artery to ascending aorta (PA:Ao), where a ratio near 1.0 is considered normal in adults.[117,118] This parameter has been used effectively in adult patients with severe COPD, in whom an elevated PA:Ao ratio on CT outperformed echocardiographic results in the diagnosis of PH.[119] This ratio has also been linked to PH in children; a PA:Ao ratio near 1.1 is considered normal in children at 0–24 months old,[118] whereas an elevated ratio of 1.3 had a 97% positive predictive value of PH diagnosis in pediatric patients.[120] As with echocardiography, measurement of LV EI on tomographic imaging is reflective of RV dimensions and function and so is considered an indirect indicator of PH.[121] Other pulmonary vasculature findings from CT can include pulmonary vein

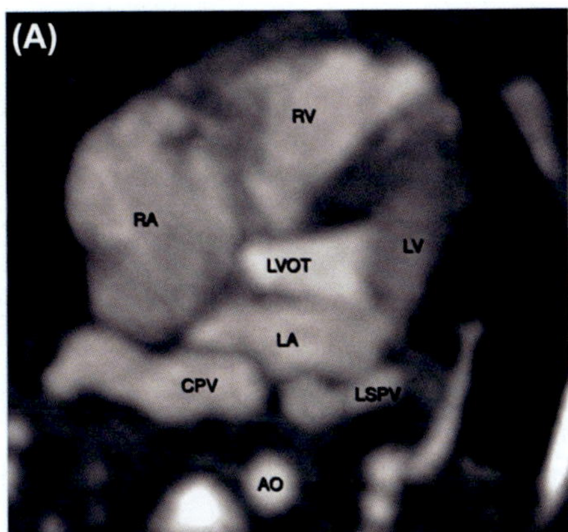

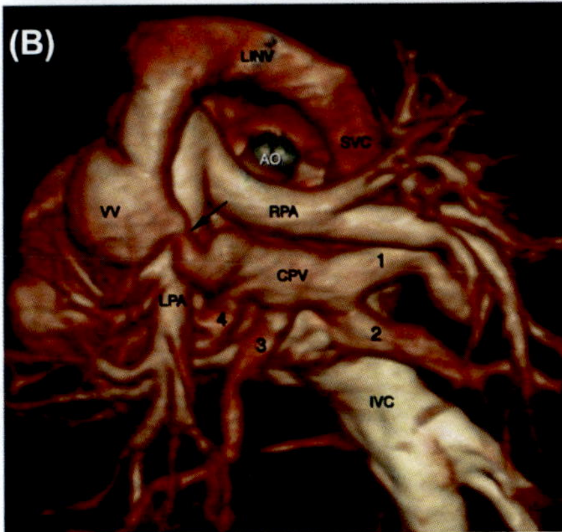

FIG. 6.9 **Neonatal cardiac computed tomography (CT).** CT angiography (CTA) in a 16-day-old male who presented with dyspnea. **(A)** An axial CTA slice demonstrates a small left ventricle (LV) and left atrium (LA), in addition to a large right atrium (RA) and right ventricle (RV). There are no observed pulmonary veins draining into the LA. **(B)** In the same patient, a posterior oblique view of a blood-volume rendering from CTA demonstrates cardiovascular anatomy and arrangement. 1–4, pulmonary veins; *AO*, aorta; *CPV*, common pulmonary vein; *IVC*, inferior vena cava; *LINV*, left innominate vein; *LPA*, left pulmonary artery; *LSPV*, left superior pulmonary vein; *LVOT*, left ventricular outflow tract; *RPA*, right pulmonary artery, *SVC*, superior vena cava; *VV*, vertical vein. (From Siripornpitak S, Pornkul R, Khowsathit P, Layangool T, Promphan W, Pongpanich B. Cardiac CT angiography in children with congenital heart disease. *Eur J Radiol*. 2013 Jul; 82(7):1067–82.)

stenosis, systemic to pulmonary collaterals, ASD, VSD, and PDA.[106]

CTA is used sparingly in the neonatal population due to concerns over exposure to ionizing radiation (see the section Lung Imaging). Additionally, CT-based assessment of the circulatory system is highly dependent on imaging contrast agent, and although severe adverse reactions to intravenous contrast materials are uncommon in children,[122] imaging contrast use in young pediatric patients is limited. Few studies exist on CT-based measurements of cardiopulmonary circulation in the BPD population. As such, CT assessment of pulmonary vasculature abnormalities in infants with BPD may remain limited to those patients with more severe disease who require additional management guidance or to those for whom other imaging tests are nondiagnostic.

Cardiac Magnetic Resonance Imaging

Cardiac MRI is routinely used in adults and older pediatric patients to reproducibly and noninvasively evaluate cardiovascular structure, function, and flow with high spatial and/or temporal resolution and without using ionizing radiation.[123] Morphologic assessment of cardiovascular structures can be achieved with cardiac gated "black-blood" MRI,[120] with parameters similar to those obtained via CT (such as PA:Ao and LV EI). Measurements such as biventricular volume and mass can be found from cine MRI, with functional parameters similar to those obtained via echocardiography, such as end-diastolic volume, end-systolic volume, ejection fraction, and stroke volume for both ventricles.[123] Dynamic septal flattening/motion is evident in the short-axis view; this finding indicates a pressure difference between ventricles and has been correlated with the severity of PH in adults.[125] Pulmonary artery blood flow measurements can be obtained via phase-contrast MRI, which has been correlated with vessel pressure and resistance obtained from invasive cardiac catheterization in adults with suspected PH.[126] Intravenous gadolinium (Gd) contrast is useful for imaging pulmonary vasculature and perfusion; however, as Gd is a highly toxic heavy metal, there is concern regarding adverse effects of prolonged deposition or retention in the pediatric population.[127] Alternatively, regional perfusion can be measured via arterial spin labeling (ASL) MRI, which uses magnetically labeled flowing blood as an endogenous contrast material.[128] As ASL MRI obviates the need for intravenous contrast or radioactive tracers, it is highly suitable for use in pediatrics. One study of 33 pediatric patients with CF and 5 healthy volunteers (13 ± 5 years old) demonstrated correlation between pulmonary perfusion from ASL MRI and PFT (FEV_1).[129] Although ASL MRI has been used in infants to study cerebral blood flow,[130] the technique has not to date been implemented for pulmonary applications in the neonatal population.

As neonatal MRI in general has become more feasible (see the section Lung Imaging), cardiac applications in the neonatal and pediatric populations are now emerging; Fig. 6.10 demonstrates interventricular septal flattening and increased LV EI-s in a term-aged infant with severe BPD and PH. Tkach et al.[121] studied the pulmonary blood flow and RV remodeling of infants with BPD using cardiac MRI, finding that the discrepancy between blood flow in right and left pulmonary arteries was significantly increased in infants with BPD compared with control infants, particularly in infants with BPD who later died. This study additionally found elevated EI-s values in patients with BPD compared with controls, suggesting the presence of increased PAP. Tkach et al.[131] also applied similar techniques in a second study on nine infants with CDH and six infants with no suspected cardiopulmonary function abnormalities, finding that cardiac MRI methods can detect changes in pulmonary hemodynamics.

Future work may elucidate the predictive relationship between hemodynamic MRI measures of PH in early life and later clinical outcomes in infants with BPD. Indeed, Critser et al. also implemented cardiac MRI in the neonatal BPD population, finding that MRI biomarkers of PH (EI-s and PA:Ao), were associated with clinical outcomes such as hospital length of stay and use of PH therapies during hospitalization and at discharge.[132] As cardiac MRI provides PH-related measurements similar to those from other imaging modalities, but with the advantages of being potentially more sensitive or specific, MRI has the potential to provide an accurate and sensitive assessment of cardiovascular circulatory abnormalities in infants with BPD.

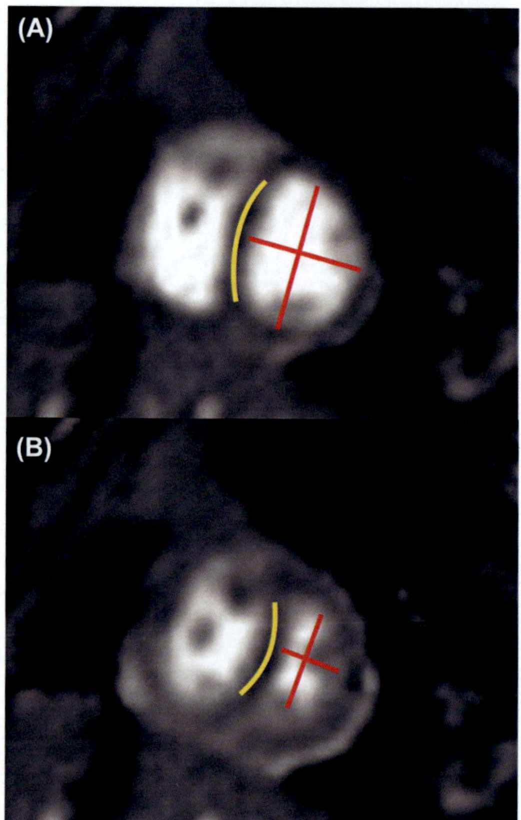

FIG. 6.10 Neonatal cardiac magnetic resonance imaging (MRI). Short-axis view from cine cardiac MRI at **(A)** diastole and **(B)** systole in a term-aged male infant with severe bronchopulmonary dysplasia and pulmonary hypertension, demonstrating interventricular septal flattening and an increased eccentricity index at systole of the left ventricle (LV), suggestive of increased pressure in the pulmonary circulatory system. Red lines, LV major and minor diameters; yellow lines, septal curvature. (Courtesy of Jason Woods, Ph.D., and Nara Higano, Ph.D., at Cincinnati Children's Hospital.)

IMAGING OF THE MAJOR AIRWAYS

Bronchoscopy

Bronchoscopy is the current clinical standard for diagnosing and assessing the severity of airway comorbidities of BPD and other respiratory conditions in pediatric patients and provides a real-time visual examination throughout the respiratory cycle of abnormalities in airway structure and dynamics (Fig. 6.11), such as subglottic stenosis, laryngomalacia, tracheomalacia (TM), and bronchomalacia, or tracheal obstruction from innominate artery compression.

However, bronchoscopy in infants and children has various disadvantages, including the requirement for sedation/anesthesia and the invasiveness of the procedure, which increase patient risks and may alter the airflow structure and dynamics under investigation; for example, the airway anatomy may be modified due to stenting during a rigid bronchoscopy.[133] There are also inconsistences between flexible and rigid bronchoscopic techniques,[134] and poor agreement has been demonstrated between readers on the presence and severity of pediatric TM.[135] Furthermore, scoring of collapse on bronchoscopy is visually assessed, with a lack of quantitative assessment or established reference baseline; the absence of quantification is due in part to measurement artifacts from the varying depths of view that are difficult to correct.[136]

Bronchoscopy is useful in assessing severe airway abnormalities in those patients with BPD who present with clear symptoms of airway morbidities, but its use in longitudinal and cross-sectional studies is largely prohibitive.

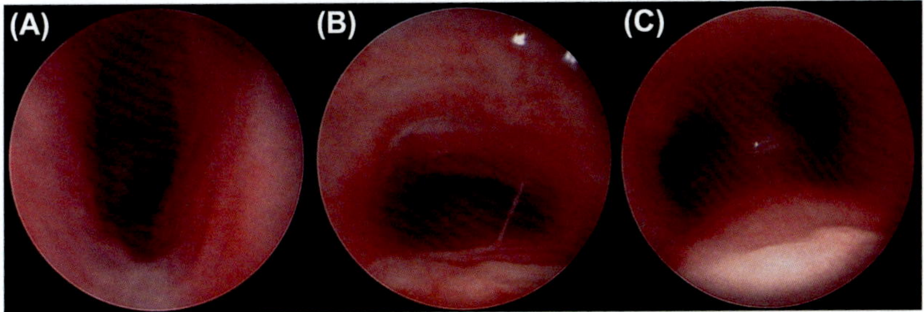

FIG. 6.11 **Bronchoscopy in an infant.** Bronchoscopic views in infants with BPD: **(A)** subglottic stenosis, **(B)** moderate malacia of the mid-trachea, and **(C)** mild malacia of the distal trachea. (Courtesy of Erik Hysinger, MD, at Cincinnati Children's Hospital.)

Airway Computed Tomography

CT can be used to visualize both static and dynamic airway abnormalities in infants with BPD with high spatial resolution; Fig. 6.12 shows axial images from cine CT in a 5-month-old female infant at end-inspiratory and end-expiratory phases, demonstrating dynamic excessive collapse of the posterior tracheal wall (TM).[137]

The limitations of CT as a tool for airway evaluation in infants are numerous. As with chest CT in children and infants, exposure to ionizing radiation and sedation/anesthesia is a concern when using airway CT in pediatrics (see the Lung Imaging section). Additionally, the trachealis can be affected by sedation/anesthesia and infant CT can require endotracheal intubation, both of which may interfere with assessment of airway malacia. The temporal resolution of dynamic CT scans is limited by gantry rotation; most airway CT protocols require breath-hold maneuvers at end-expiration or end-inspiration, such that the resultant images are not representative of the airway under natural breathing conditions. One study of infants with diagnosed TM found that CT detected known TM at a rate of 42.9%, with positive CT findings specifying the severity and segment of malacia only 36.4% and 54.5% of the time, respectively.[133] In contrast, Goo et al. reported that sensitivity, specificity, and accuracy of free-breathing cine CT diagnosis of TM were 96.3%, 97.2%, and 97.1%, respectively[137]; this study implemented sedation in children under 6 years old.

Evaluation of the airway via CT has seen initial successes in correlating imaging biomarkers with later outcomes. Sarria et al. found significant differences between infants and toddlers with chronic lung disease of infancy and age-matched term controls using CT-based measurements of airway size and airway generation. Increased size of the first and second airway generations in preterm patients correlated with

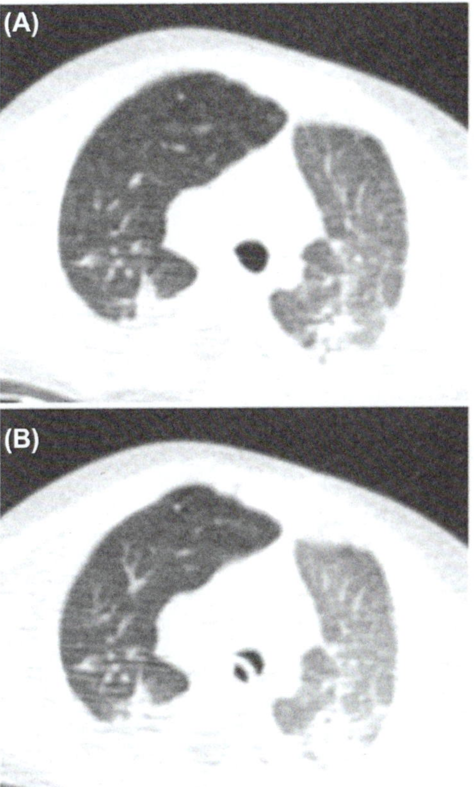

FIG. 6.12 **Cine computed tomography (CT) of the infant airway.** Axial image slices from cine airway CT in a 5-month-old female infant diagnosed with tracheomalacia on bronchoscopy. Comparison between the **(A)** inspiratory phase and **(B)** expiratory phase images demonstrates dynamic excessive collapse of the posterior tracheal wall, with cross-sectional area changes that exceed 60%. (From Goo HW. Free-breathing cine CT for the diagnosis of tracheomalacia in young children. *Pediatr Radiol*. 2013 Aug; 43(8):922–8.)

increased duration of mechanical ventilation in the neonatal period.[30]

The airway does not always share orientation with imaging axes, and so from an image analysis perspective, airway measurements taken from misaligned image slices have limited accuracy and utility. For this reason, 3D volumetric reconstructions from high-resolution CT are of high interest because they can provide virtual bronchoscopic views of abnormal airway anatomy.[138] This CT airway technique has not yet been explored rigorously in infants with BPD, in large part due to the higher exposure to ionizing radiation, but recent advancements in MRI techniques have begun to explore 3D airway modeling applications.

Airway Magnetic Resonance Imaging

As a nonionizing and tomographic modality, MRI is an alternative to CT for assessing central airway abnormalities in the young pediatric population. There have been prior successes in using conventional MRI techniques (typically using Cartesian-based sequences) to assess the dynamic airway, but these studies have often been limited to adults or older, compliant pediatric populations in whom breathing maneuvers can be coached and achieved.[139,140] Exploration of conventional MRI methods has been limited in part due to the lack of spatiotemporal resolution necessary to visualize the small airway anatomy of a rapidly breathing infant, and in the young pediatric population, sedation/anesthesia is often required.[133]

Recent developments in radial MRI acquisitions[141,142] (i.e., UTE; see the Lung Imaging section) have addressed many of the concerns regarding the use of MRI in assessing the pediatric airway. 3D UTE MRI provides submillimeter spatial resolutions comparable to that achieved with CT and provides 3D isotropic voxels.[53,56,143] Further, UTE MRI in the nonsedated neonate allows for retrospective respiratory gating during tidal free-breathing, due to the radial k-space acquisition scheme,[63] providing a continuous view of the breathing cycle and obviating the need for breath-hold maneuvers often required by CT or traditional MRI protocols. As such, airway abnormalities in infants with BPD can be evaluated in their "natural state" via UTE MRI, without the need for invasive procedures, ionizing radiation, or sedation/anesthesia.[141,144]

3D modeling of airway surfaces from high-resolution imaging, such as UTE MRI (Fig. 6.13B), can provide accurate measurement of airway geometry in infants and allows for alignment of geometric measurements with the airway axis.[145,146] A study from Bates et al.[141] highlighted a novel technique using tracheal surfaces at end-expiration and end-inspiration from retrospectively respiratory-gated UTE MRI in neonates with various respiratory diagnoses, including 17 BPD patients; this work addresses the misalignment between airway and imaging axes by drawing a centerline along the airway. From this method, regional geometric parameters (e.g., cross-sectional area or ratio between minimum and maximum diameters) can be extracted

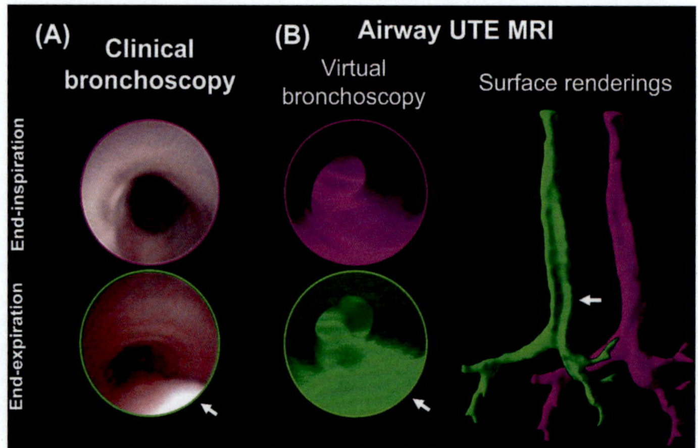

FIG. 6.13 **Neonatal airway surfaces and virtual bronchoscopy from ultrashort echo time (UTE) magnetic resonance imaging (MRI).** A male infant with severe bronchopulmonary dysplasia underwent (A) bronchoscopy and (B) UTE MRI of the airway near term age. (B) Airway surface renderings and virtual bronchoscopy from noninvasive, nonsedated UTE MRI demonstrated severe tracheomalacia in the middle and lower trachea, which matched closely with bronchoscopic findings. (Courtesy of Jason Woods, Ph.D., and Nara Higano, Ph.D., at Cincinnati Children's Hospital.)

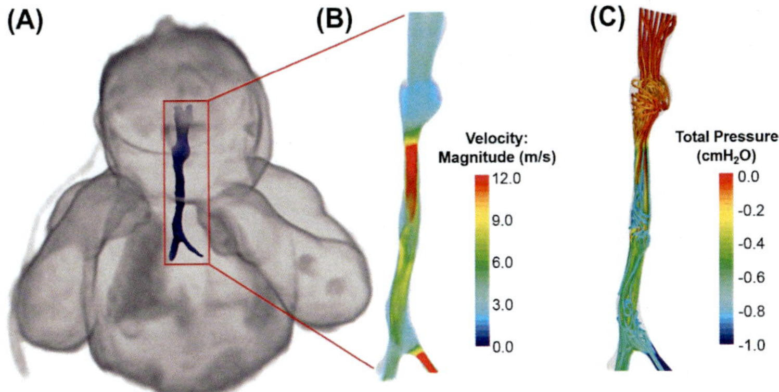

FIG. 6.14 **Computational fluid dynamics from ultrashort echo time magnetic resonance imaging (MRI) of the neonatal airway.** A nonsedated female infant with severe bronchopulmonary dysplasia underwent ultrashort echo time (UTE) MRI of the chest and airway near term age. **(A)** A three-dimensional model of the body volume (gray) and airway (dark blue, from oropharynx to main stem bronchi). **(B)** The interior of the airway is colored by the airflow velocity field during peak inhalation. **(C)** Streamlines following the path of the airflow inside the airway are colored by the total pressure of the air during peak inhalation. A high-velocity jet forms in the larynx (B, red) and extends through the upper trachea. The shape and curvature of this patient's trachea cause this velocity jet to extend further along the trachea than in the normal anatomy, increasing the inspiratory pressure loss (C) and the patient's work of breathing. (Courtesy of Alister Bates, Ph.D., and Chamindu Gunatilaka, BS, at Cincinnati Children's Hospital.)

along the length of the airway, both in static and dynamic conditions. Preliminary validation in infants is encouraging; comparison between UTE MRI and clinical bronchoscopy for the regional diagnosis of TM has demonstrated strong agreement.[142] Although the resolution of UTE MR images is still slightly below that of CT images (for example, 0.7 mm compared with 0.3 mm), UTE MRI has similar potential as CT for generating noninvasive virtual bronchoscopy, but without ionizing radiation (Fig. 6.13). This overcomes obstacles in current diagnostic methods and may serve as the foundation for management guidance and serial assessment of response to pharmacologic therapy in infants with BPD and comorbid airway issues.

With the recent progress in high-resolution imaging techniques that are safe and feasible in infants with BPD, and with continued increases in computational power, computational fluid dynamics (CFD) simulations pose an exciting opportunity for exploring the relationship between respiratory aerodynamics and airway anatomy, in addition to the effects of abnormal aerodynamics on therapeutic response and later clinical outcomes in preterm infants. CFD simulations have been used in previous studies of adult patients with goiters[147,148] and transplanted trachea,[149,150] providing functional information about the airway, including work of breathing and regional pressures and forces, as well as assessment of the deposition of therapeutic particles to tailor drug delivery within the airways.[151] Requirements of CFD simulations include high-resolution imaging and, in dynamic conditions, temporal resolution of airway wall motion.[152,153] As shown in Fig. 6.14, recent developments in imaging and quantifying the dynamic neonatal airway via nonionizing UTE MRI are a key step forward in using CFD applications to measure respiratory effort and energy expenditure of dynamic airway collapse in infants with BPD.

Airway Ultrasonography

Ultrasonography is a nonionizing, rapid, and repeatable imaging modality that is well tolerated by the majority of patient populations and is also portable, cheap, and readily available in nearly all institutions. As technical advancements to ultrasound technology have improved image quality and resolution over the past few decades, exploration of the use of ultrasound imaging for therapeutic and diagnostic airway imaging has increased.[154,155]

Airway ultrasonographic studies in the pediatric population (Fig. 6.15) have been somewhat limited, however, and have disagreed somewhat on the modality's utility in children. One case report from Dalesio et al.[154] used airway ultrasonography in three pediatric patients in an operating room setting to demonstrate real-time imaging assessment of airway interventions. In a larger study, echocardiograms for 30 pediatric

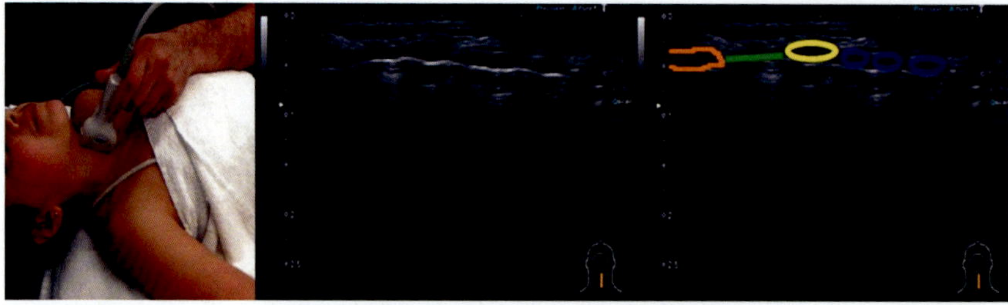

FIG. 6.15 **Pediatric airway ultrasonography.** Pediatric ultrasonography with a midline longitudinal view visualizes the structures of the larynx and upper trachea (ordered cranial to caudal): thyroid cartilage (orange), cricothyroid membrane (green), cricoid cartilage (yellow), and tracheal rings (blue). Visualization of deeper structures is limited by air in the airways (a continuous bright line deep to the larynx and upper trachea structures). (From Stafrace S. Essential ultrasound techniques of the pediatric airway. *Paediatr Anaesth*. 2016 Feb; 26(2):122–31.)

patients with diagnosed TM did not add new information about the airway malacia or compression beyond that available through bronchoscopy, and so did not provide any additional management guidance.[133] Although ultrasonography may have many logistic advantages over rapidly developing tomographic airway imaging modalities, ultrasonography may be limited to settings that require real-time visualization for management guidance rather than playing an independent role in defining airway pathologic conditions.

CONCLUSIONS

Advanced imaging techniques may soon play a pivotal role in refining the understanding and treatment of cardiorespiratory disease related to preterm birth, in addition to other neonatal chronic lung diseases. As more sophisticated technology is introduced to quantitatively assess lung, airway, and cardiac abnormalities in this patient population, there are exciting opportunities for defining and identifying individual patient phenotypes related to preterm birth.

Novel imaging techniques may provide safe and effective imaging of cardiopulmonary structure and function to increase our understanding of lung disease of prematurity and its treatment. Although current clinical modalities such as chest X-ray radiograph, bronchoscopy, and echocardiography will likely remain the initial radiologic assessment of parenchymal, pulmonary vascular, and airway abnormalities in patients with BPD, respectively, recent advancements in other modalities may provide an opportunity for quantitative imaging to help define BPD lung disease and assess clinical progress.

In particular, pulmonary MRI is experiencing rapid progress in the research setting, with high potential for clinical translation (particularly for UTE and HP gas MRI) in the near future. Various other modalities, such as ultrasonography and scintigraphy of the lungs and ultrasonography of the airway, will likely continue to play more limited roles in routine clinical imaging of preterm infants due to lack of high sensitivity, specificity, and/or safety. Cardiorespiratory applications of CT are enticing due to high-resolution visualization of anatomic structures, but safety concerns regarding sedation/anesthesia and intubation persist. Although low-dose CT protocols have reduced the exposure to ionizing radiation, new methods in quantitative, nonsedated free-breathing ^{1}H UTE MRI can provide comparable structural information of the lung parenchyma and major airways, and cutting-edge HP gas MRI can generate spatial information on regional lung microstructure, function, and gas-exchange abnormalities that are not available through any other modality. As these research MRI techniques mature, they are likely to become more readily implementable in the NICU setting, with institutional hardware and software upgrades. While some methods have been explored more thoroughly than others in the BPD population, existing data suggest that pulmonary MRI holds great promise in understanding lung disease in infants who are born extremely preterm.

With the continued development of advanced imaging techniques specific to the neonatal population, we are now poised to understand the structural and functional cardiorespiratory abnormalities of preterm birth and other neonatal chronic lung diseases at a more in-depth level than previously possible. New imaging methods allow for serial description of disease trajectory and enhanced differentiation between the individual contributions of lung, airway, and pulmonary vascular morbidities. Advanced cardiorespiratory imaging may soon significantly inform management guidance and individualized treatment strategies for neonatal patients born preterm or with chronic lung disease.

REFERENCES

1. Northway WHJ, Rosan RC, Porter DY. Pulmonary disease following respirator therapy of hyaline-membrane disease. Bronchopulmonary dysplasia. *N Engl J Med*. 1967; 276(7):357–368. https://doi.org/10.1056/NEJM196702162760701.
2. Rossi UG, Owens CM. The radiology of chronic lung disease in children. *Arch Dis Child*. 2005;90(6):601–607. https://doi.org/10.1136/adc.2004.051383.
3. Jobe AH. The new bronchopulmonary dysplasia. *Curr Opin Pediatr*. 2011;23(2):167–172. https://doi.org/10.1097/MOP.0b013e3283423e6b.
4. Pryhuber GS. Renewed promise of nonionizing radiation imaging for chronic lung disease in preterm infants. *Am J Respir Crit Care Med*. 2018;198(10):1248–1249. https://doi.org/10.1164/rccm.201805-0963ED.
5. Liang T, Vargas SO, Lee EY. Childhood interstitial (diffuse) lung disease: pattern recognition approach to diagnosis in infants. *Am J Roentgenol.*. 2019:1–10 https://doi.org/10.2214/AJR.18.20696.
6. Sood S, Rissmiller J, Hryhorczuk A. Pediatric chest: a review of the must-know diagnoses. *Appl Radiol*. 2018; 47(4):4–14.
7. Miglioretti DL, Johnson E, Williams A, et al. The use of computed tomography in pediatrics and the associated radiation exposure and estimated cancer risk. *JAMA Pediatr*. 2013;167(8):700–707. https://doi.org/10.1001/jamapediatrics.2013.311.
8. Toce SS, Farrell PM, Leavitt LA, Samuels DP, Edwards DK. Clinical and roentgenographic scoring systems for assessing bronchopulmonary dysplasia. *Am J Dis Child*. 1984; 138(6):581–585.
9. Stoll BJ, Hansen NI, Bell EF, et al. Neonatal outcomes of extremely preterm infants from the NICHD Neonatal Research Network. *Pediatrics*. 2010;126(3):443–456. https://doi.org/10.1542/peds.2009-2959.
10. Morrow LA, Wagner BD, Ingram DA, et al. Antenatal determinants of bronchopulmonary dysplasia and late respiratory disease in preterm infants. *Am J Respir Crit Care Med*. 2017;196(3):364–374. https://doi.org/10.1164/rccm.201612-2414OC.
11. Higgins RD, Jobe AH, Koso-Thomas M, et al. Bronchopulmonary dysplasia: executive summary of a workshop. *J Pediatr*. 2018;197:300–308. https://doi.org/10.1016/j.jpeds.2018.01.043.
12. Pearce MS, Salotti JA, Little MP, et al. Radiation exposure from CT scans in childhood and subsequent risk of leukaemia and brain tumours: a retrospective cohort study. *Lancet*. 2012;380(9840):499–505. https://doi.org/10.1016/S0140-6736(12)60815-0.
13. Berrington de Gonzalez A, Journy N, Lee C, et al. No association between radiation dose from pediatric CT scans and risk of subsequent hodgkin lymphoma. *Cancer Epidemiol Biomark Prev*. 2017;26(5):804–806. https://doi.org/10.1158/1055-9965.EPI-16-1011.
14. Singh S, Kalra MK, Moore MA, et al. Dose reduction and compliance with pediatric CT protocols adapted to patient size, clinical indication, and number of prior studies. *Radiology*. 2009;252(1):200–208. https://doi.org/10.1148/radiol.2521081554.
15. Yu H, Zhao S, Hoffman EA, Wang G. Ultra-low dose lung CT perfusion regularized by a previous scan. *Acad Radiol*. 2009;16(3):363–373. https://doi.org/10.1016/j.acra.2008.09.003.
16. Cravero JP, Beach ML, Blike GT, Gallagher SM, Hertzog JH. The incidence and nature of adverse events during pediatric sedation/anesthesia with propofol for procedures outside the operating room: a report from the Pediatric Sedation Research Consortium. *Anesth Analg*. 2009;108(3):795–804. https://doi.org/10.1213/ane.0b013e31818fc334.
17. Mahmoud M, Ishman SL, McConnell K, et al. Upper airway reflexes are preserved during dexmedetomidine sedation in children with down syndrome and obstructive sleep apnea. *J Clin Sleep Med*. 2017;13(5):721–727. https://doi.org/10.5664/jcsm.6592.
18. van Mastrigt E, Logie K, Ciet P, et al. Lung CT imaging in patients with bronchopulmonary dysplasia: a systematic review. *Pediatr Pulmonol*. 2016;51(9):975–986. https://doi.org/10.1002/ppul.23446.
19. Aquino SL, Schechter MS, Chiles C, Ablin DS, Chipps B, Webb WR. High-resolution inspiratory and expiratory CT in older children and adults with bronchopulmonary dysplasia. *Am J Roentgenol*. 1999;173(4):963–967. https://doi.org/10.2214/ajr.173.4.10511158.
20. Wong P, Murray C, Louw J, French N, Chambers D. Adult bronchopulmonary dysplasia: computed tomography pulmonary findings. *J Med Imaging Radiat Oncol*. 2011;55(4):373–378. https://doi.org/10.1111/j.1754-9485.2011.02285.x.
21. de Mello RR, Dutra MVP, Ramos JR, Daltro P, Boechat M, de Andrade Lopes JM. Lung mechanics and high-resolution computed tomography of the chest in very low birth weight premature infants. *Sao Paulo Med J*. 2003;121(4):167–172.
22. Mahut B, De Blic J, Emond S, et al. Chest computed tomography findings in bronchopulmonary dysplasia and correlation with lung function. *Arch Dis Child Fetal Neonatal Ed*. 2007;92(6):F459–F464. https://doi.org/10.1136/adc.2006.111765.
23. Ochiai M, Hikino S, Yabuuchi H, et al. A new scoring system for computed tomography of the chest for assessing the clinical status of bronchopulmonary dysplasia. *J Pediatr*. 2008;152(1). https://doi.org/10.1016/j.jpeds.2007.05.043, 90-95, 95.e1-3.
24. Aukland SM, Rosendahl K, Owens CM, Fosse KR, Eide GE, Halvorsen T. Neonatal bronchopulmonary dysplasia predicts abnormal pulmonary HRCT scans in long-term survivors of extreme preterm birth. *Thorax*. 2009;64(5):405–410. https://doi.org/10.1136/thx.2008.103739.
25. Boechat MCB, Mello RR de, Silva KS da, et al. A computed tomography scoring system to assess pulmonary disease among premature infants. *Sao Paulo Med J*. 2010; 128(6):328–335.

26. Shin S-M, Kim WS, Cheon J-E, et al. Bronchopulmonary dysplasia: new high resolution computed tomography scoring system and correlation between the high resolution computed tomography score and clinical severity. *Korean J Radiol.* 2013;14(2):350–360. https://doi.org/10.3348/kjr.2013.14.2.350.
27. Tonson la Tour A, Spadola L, Sayegh Y, et al. Chest CT in bronchopulmonary dysplasia: clinical and radiological correlations. *Pediatr Pulmonol.* 2013;48(7):693–698. https://doi.org/10.1002/ppul.22714.
28. Brostrom EB, Thunqvist P, Adenfelt G, Borling E, Katz-Salamon M. Obstructive lung disease in children with mild to severe BPD. *Respir Med.* 2010;104(3):362–370. https://doi.org/10.1016/j.rmed.2009.10.008.
29. Stein JM, Walkup LL, Brody AS, Fleck RJ, Woods JC. Quantitative CT characterization of pediatric lung development using routine clinical imaging. *Pediatr Radiol.* 2016;46(13):1804–1812. https://doi.org/10.1007/s00247-016-3686-8.
30. Sarria EE, Mattiello R, Rao L, et al. Quantitative assessment of chronic lung disease of infancy using computed tomography. *Eur Respir J.* 2012;39(4):992–999. https://doi.org/10.1183/09031936.00064811.
31. Spielberg DR, Walkup LL, Stein JM, et al. Quantitative CT scans of lung parenchymal pathology in premature infants ages 0-6 years. *Pediatr Pulmonol.* 2018;53(3):316–323. https://doi.org/10.1002/ppul.23921.
32. Galban CJ, Han MK, Boes JL, et al. Computed tomography-based biomarker provides unique signature for diagnosis of COPD phenotypes and disease progression. *Nat Med.* 2012;18(11):1711–1715. https://doi.org/10.1038/nm.2971.
33. Pennati F, Salito C, Baroni G, Woods J, Aliverti A. Comparison between multivolume CT-based surrogates of regional ventilation in healthy subjects. *Acad Radiol.* 2014;21(10):1268–1275. https://doi.org/10.1016/j.acra.2014.05.022.
34. Salito C, Barazzetti L, Woods JC, Aliverti A. Heterogeneity of specific gas volume changes: a new tool to plan lung volume reduction in COPD. *Chest.* 2014;146(6):1554–1565. https://doi.org/10.1378/chest.13-2855.
35. Pennati F, Salito C, Roach D, Clancy JP, Woods J, Aliverti A. Regional ventilation in infants quantified by multi-volume high resolution computed tomography (HRCT) and multi-volume proton magnetic resonance imaging (MRI). *Eur Respir J.* 2015;46(suppl 59):OA2949. https://doi.org/10.1183/13993003.congress-2015.OA2949.
36. Schneider A, Koob M, Sananes N, Senger B, Hemmerle J, Becmeur F. Computed tomographic study of the pediatric diaphragmatic growth: application to the treatment of congenital diaphragmatic hernia. *Eur J Pediatr Surg.* 2017;27(2):177–180. https://doi.org/10.1055/s-0036-1582242.
37. Bjorkman KC, Kjellberg M, Bergstrom SE, et al. Postoperative regional distribution of pulmonary ventilation and perfusion in infants with congenital diaphragmatic hernia. *J Pediatr Surg.* 2011;46(11):2047–2053. https://doi.org/10.1016/j.jpedsurg.2011.06.042.
38. Li X, Samei E, Segars WP, Sturgeon GM, Colsher JG, Frush DP. Patient-specific radiation dose and cancer risk for pediatric chest CT. *Radiology.* 2011;259(3):862–874. https://doi.org/10.1148/radiol.11101900.
39. Macdougall RD, Strauss KJ, Lee EY. Managing radiation dose from thoracic multidetector computed tomography in pediatric patients: background, current issues, and recommendations. *Radiol Clin N Am.* 2013;51(4):743–760. https://doi.org/10.1016/j.rcl.2013.04.007.
40. Kim J-E, Newman B. Evaluation of a radiation dose reduction strategy for pediatric chest CT. *AJR Am J Roentgenol.* 2010;194(5):1188–1193. https://doi.org/10.2214/AJR.09.3726.
41. Semple T, Akhtar MR, Owens CM. Imaging bronchopulmonary dysplasia-A multimodality update. *Front Med.* 2017;4:88. https://doi.org/10.3389/fmed.2017.00088.
42. Walkup LL, Higano NS, Woods JC. *Structural and Functional Pulmonary Magnetic Resonance Imaging in Pediatrics—From the Neonate to the Young Adult.* Academic Radiology; 2018.
43. Adams EW, Harrison MC, Counsell SJ, et al. Increased lung water and tissue damage in bronchopulmonary dysplasia. *J Pediatr.* 2004;145(4):503–507. https://doi.org/10.1016/j.jpeds.2004.06.028.
44. Tkach JA, Merhar SL, Kline-Fath BM, et al. MRI in the neonatal ICU: initial experience using a small-footprint 1.5-T system. *AJR Am J Roentgenol.* 2014;202(1):W95–W105. https://doi.org/10.2214/AJR.13.10613.
45. Merhar SL, Tkach JA, Woods JC, et al. Neonatal imaging using an on-site small footprint MR scanner. *Pediatr Radiol.* 2017;47(8):1001–1011. https://doi.org/10.1007/s00247-017-3855-4.
46. Griffiths PD, Jarvis D, Armstrong L, Connolly DJA, Bayliss P, Cook J, Hart AR, Pilling E, Williams T, Paley MNJ. Initial experience of an investigational 3T MR scanner designed for use on neonatal wards. *Eur Radiol.* 2018 Oct;28(10):4438–4446. https://doi.org/10.1007/s00330-018-5357-7. Epub 2018 Apr 30.
47. Hatabu H, Alsop DC, Listerud J, Bonnet M, Gefter WB. T2* and proton density measurement of normal human lung parenchyma using submillisecond echo time gradient echo magnetic resonance imaging. *Eur J Radiol.* 1999;29(3):245–252.
48. Adams EW, Counsell SJ, Hajnal JV, et al. Magnetic resonance imaging of lung water content and distribution in term and preterm infants. *Am J Respir Crit Care Med.* 2002;166(3):397–402. https://doi.org/10.1164/rccm.2104116.
49. Stock KW, Chen Q, Hatabu H, Edelman RR. Magnetic resonance T2* measurements of the normal human lung in vivo with ultra-short echo times. *Magn Reson Imaging.* 1999;17(7):997–1000.
50. Yu J, Xue Y, Song HK. Comparison of lung T2* during free-breathing at 1.5 T and 3.0 T with ultrashort echo time imaging. *Magn Reson Med.* 2011;66(1):248–254. https://doi.org/10.1002/mrm.22829.

51. Walkup LL, Tkach JA, Higano NS, et al. Quantitative magnetic resonance imaging of bronchopulmonary dysplasia in the neonatal intensive care unit environment. *Am J Respir Crit Care Med.* 2015;192(10):1215–1222. https://doi.org/10.1164/rccm.201503-0552OC.
52. Schopper MA, Walkup LL, Tkach JA, et al. Evaluation of neonatal lung volume growth by pulmonary magnetic resonance imaging in patients with congenital diaphragmatic hernia. *J Pediatr.* 2017;188. https://doi.org/10.1016/j.jpeds.2017.06.002, 96-102.e1.
53. Johnson KM, Fain SB, Schiebler ML, Nagle S. Optimized 3D ultrashort echo time pulmonary MRI. *Magn Reson Med.* 2013;70(5):1241–1250. https://doi.org/10.1002/mrm.24570.
54. Lederlin M, Cremillieux Y. Three-dimensional assessment of lung tissue density using a clinical ultrashort echo time at 3 tesla: a feasibility study in healthy subjects. *J Magn Reson Imaging.* 2014;40(4):839–847. https://doi.org/10.1002/jmri.24429.
55. Dournes G, Grodzki D, Macey J, et al. Quiet submillimeter MR imaging of the lung is feasible with a PETRA sequence at 1.5 T. *Radiology.* 2015;276(1):258–265. https://doi.org/10.1148/radiol.15141655.
56. Higano NS, Fleck RJ, Spielberg DR, et al. Quantification of neonatal lung parenchymal density via ultrashort echo time MRI with comparison to CT. *J Magn Reson Imaging.* 2017;46(4):992–1000. https://doi.org/10.1002/jmri.25643.
57. Adaikalam SA, Higano NS, Tkach JA, et al. Neonatal lung growth in congenital diaphragmatic hernia: evaluation of lung density and mass by pulmonary MRI. *Pediatr Res.* 2019. https://doi.org/10.1038/s41390-019-0480-y.
58. Higano NS, Fleck RJ, Schapiro AH, House M, Kingma PS, Woods JC. Lung density and disease severity of neonatal bronchopulmonary dysplasia: objective quantification via ultrashort echo-time MRI and comparison to reader scoring. In: *Proceedings of the American Thoracic Society.* 2019:A4005.
59. Yoder LM, Higano NS, Schapiro AH, et al. Elevated lung volumes in neonates with bronchopulmonary dysplasia measured via MRI. *Pediatr Pulmonol.* 2019;54(8): 1311–1318. https://doi.org/10.1002/ppul.24378.
60. Salito C, Aliverti A, Gierada DS, et al. Quantification of trapped gas with CT and 3 He MR imaging in a porcine model of isolated airway obstruction. *Radiology.* 2009; 253(2):380–389. https://doi.org/10.1148/radiol.2532081941.
61. Pennati F, Quirk JD, Yablonskiy DA, Castro M, Aliverti A, Woods JC. Assessment of regional lung function with multivolume (1)H MR imaging in health and obstructive lung disease: comparison with (3)He MR imaging. *Radiology.* 2014;273(2):580–590. https://doi.org/10.1148/radiol.14132470.
62. Higano NS, Spielberg DR, Fleck RJ, et al. Neonatal pulmonary magnetic resonance imaging of bronchopulmonary dysplasia predicts short-term clinical outcomes. *Am J Respir Crit Care Med.* 2018;198(10):1302–1311. https://doi.org/10.1164/rccm.201711-2287OC.
63. Higano NS, Hahn AD, Tkach JA, et al. Retrospective respiratory self-gating and removal of bulk motion in pulmonary UTE MRI of neonates and adults. *Magn Reson Med.* 2017;77(3):1284–1295. https://doi.org/10.1002/mrm.26212.
64. Tibiletti M, Paul J, Bianchi A, et al. Multistage three-dimensional UTE lung imaging by image-based self-gating. *Magn Reson Med.* 2016;75(3):1324–1332. https://doi.org/10.1002/mrm.25673.
65. Hite C, Higano NS, Tkach JA, et al. Effect of post-natal surgical repair methods on diaphragmatic movement in infants with congenital diaphragmatic hernia. In: *Proceedings of the American Thoracic Society.* Vol. 197. 2018: A3657.
66. Gibiino F, Sacolick L, Menini A, Landini L, Wiesinger F. Free-breathing, zero-TE MR lung imaging. *Magn Reson Mater Physics, Biol Med.* 2015;28(3):207–215. https://doi.org/10.1007/s10334-014-0459-y.
67. Bae K, Jeon KN, Hwang MJ, et al. Comparison of lung imaging using three-dimensional ultrashort echo time and zero echo time sequences: preliminary study. *Eur Radiol.* 2018. https://doi.org/10.1007/s00330-018-5889-x.
68. Weiger M, Brunner DO, Tabbert M, Pavan M, Schmid T, Pruessmann KP. Exploring the bandwidth limits of ZTE imaging: spatial response, out-of-band signals, and noise propagation. *Magn Reson Med.* 2015;74(5):1236–1247. https://doi.org/10.1002/mrm.25509.
69. Tkach JA, Li Y, Pratt RG, et al. Characterization of acoustic noise in a neonatal intensive care unit MRI system. *Pediatr Radiol.* 2014;44(8):1011–1019. https://doi.org/10.1007/s00247-014-2909-0.
70. Walker TG, Happer W. Spin-exchange optical pumping of noble-gas nuclei. *Rev Mod Phys.* 1997;69(2):629–642. https://doi.org/10.1103/RevModPhys.69.629.
71. Goodson BM. Nuclear magnetic resonance of laser-polarized noble gases in molecules, materials, and organisms. *J Magn Reson.* 2002;155(2):157–216. https://doi.org/10.1006/jmre.2001.2341.
72. Saam BT, Yablonskiy DA, Kodibagkar VD, et al. MR imaging of diffusion of (3)He gas in healthy and diseased lungs. *Magn Reson Med.* 2000;44(2):174–179.
73. Ruppert K, Qing K, Patrie JT, Altes TA, Mugler 3rd JP. Using hyperpolarized xenon-129 MRI to quantify early-stage lung disease in smokers. *Acad Radiol.* 2018. https://doi.org/10.1016/j.acra.2018.11.005.
74. Wang JM, Robertson SH, Wang Z, et al. Using hyperpolarized (129)Xe MRI to quantify regional gas transfer in idiopathic pulmonary fibrosis. *Thorax.* 2018;73(1): 21–28. https://doi.org/10.1136/thoraxjnl-2017-210070.
75. Cadman RV, Lemanske RFJ, Evans MD, et al. Pulmonary 3He magnetic resonance imaging of childhood asthma. *J Allergy Clin Immunol.* 2013;131(2):365–369. https://doi.org/10.1016/j.jaci.2012.10.032.
76. Thomen RP, Sheshadri A, Quirk JD, et al. Regional ventilation changes in severe asthma after bronchial thermoplasty with (3)He MR imaging and CT. *Radiology.* 2015; 274(1):250–259. https://doi.org/10.1148/radiol.14140080.

77. Koumellis P, van Beek EJR, Woodhouse N, et al. Quantitative analysis of regional airways obstruction using dynamic hyperpolarized 3He MRI-preliminary results in children with cystic fibrosis. *J Magn Reson Imaging*. 2005;22(3):420–426. https://doi.org/10.1002/jmri.20402.
78. Thomen RP, Walkup LL, Roach DJ, Cleveland ZI, Clancy JP, Woods JC. Hyperpolarized (129)Xe for investigation of mild cystic fibrosis lung disease in pediatric patients. *J Cyst Fibros*. 2017;16(2):275–282. https://doi.org/10.1016/j.jcf.2016.07.008.
79. Santyr G, Kanhere N, Morgado F, Rayment JH, Ratjen F, Couch MJ. Hyperpolarized gas magnetic resonance imaging of pediatric cystic fibrosis lung disease. *Acad Radiol*. 2018. https://doi.org/10.1016/j.acra.2018.04.024.
80. Spoel M, Marshall H, IJsselstijn H, et al. Pulmonary ventilation and micro-structural findings in congenital diaphragmatic hernia. *Pediatr Pulmonol*. 2016;51(5):517–524. https://doi.org/10.1002/ppul.23325.
81. Driehuys B, Martinez-Jimenez S, Cleveland ZI, et al. Chronic obstructive pulmonary disease: safety and tolerability of hyperpolarized 129Xe MR imaging in healthy volunteers and patients. *Radiology*. 2012;262(1):279–289. https://doi.org/10.1148/radiol.11102172.
82. Lutey B a, Lefrak SS, Woods JC, et al. Hyperpolarized 3He MR imaging: physiologic monitoring observations and safety considerations in 100 consecutive subjects. *Radiology*. 2008;248(2):655–661. https://doi.org/10.1148/radiol.2482071838.
83. Walkup LL, Thomen RP, Akinyi TG, et al. Feasibility, tolerability and safety of pediatric hyperpolarized (129) Xe magnetic resonance imaging in healthy volunteers and children with cystic fibrosis. *Pediatr Radiol*. 2016;46(12):1651–1662. https://doi.org/10.1007/s00247-016-3672-1.
84. Narayanan M, Owers-Bradley J, Beardsmore CS, et al. Alveolarization continues during childhood and adolescence: new evidence from helium-3 magnetic resonance. *Am J Respir Crit Care Med*. 2012;185(2):186–191. https://doi.org/10.1164/rccm.201107-1348OC.
85. Altes TA, Mata J, de Lange EE, Brookeman JR, Mugler 3rd JP. Assessment of lung development using hyperpolarized helium-3 diffusion MR imaging. *J Magn Reson Imaging*. 2006;24(6):1277–1283. https://doi.org/10.1002/jmri.20723.
86. Altes TA, Meyer CH, Mata JF, et al. Hyperpolarized helium-3 magnetic resonance lung imaging of non-sedated infants and young children: a proof-of-concept study. *Clin Imaging*. 2017;45:105–110. https://doi.org/10.1016/j.clinimag.2017.04.004.
87. Thomen R, Walkup L, Roach D, et al. Investigation of structure-function relationships in cystic fibrosis lung disease using hyperpolarized xenon and ultra-short echo MRI. In: *Proceedings of the American Thoracic Society*. Vol. 197. 2018:A6386.
88. Woods JC, Conradi MS. (3)He diffusion MRI in human lungs. *J Magn Reson*. 2018;292:90–98. https://doi.org/10.1016/j.jmr.2018.04.007.
89. Woods JC, Yablonskiy DA, Choong CK, et al. Long-range diffusion of hyperpolarized 3He in explanted normal and emphysematous human lungs via magnetization tagging. *J Appl Physiol*. 2005;99(5):1992–1997. https://doi.org/10.1152/japplphysiol.00185.2005.
90. Thomen RP, Quirk JD, Roach D, et al. Direct comparison of (129) Xe diffusion measurements with quantitative histology in human lungs. *Magn Reson Med*. 2017;77(1):265–272. https://doi.org/10.1002/mrm.26120.
91. Altes TA, Mata J, Froh DK, Paget-Brown A, de Lange EE, Mugler JP. Abnormalities of lung structure in children with bronchopulmonary dysplasia as assessed by diffusion hyperpolarized helium-3 MRI. In: *Proceedings of the International Society for Magnetic Resonance in Medicine*. 2006.
92. Narayanan M, Beardsmore CS, Owers-Bradley J, et al. Catch-up alveolarization in ex-preterm children: evidence from (3)He magnetic resonance. *Am J Respir Crit Care Med*. 2013;187(10):1104–1109. https://doi.org/10.1164/rccm.201210-1850OC.
93. Higano N, Thomen R, Quirk J, et al. Hyperpolarized 3He gas MRI in infant lungs: investigating alveolar-airspace size with restricted gas diffusion. In: *Proceedings of the International Society for Magnetic Resonance in Medicine*. 2017:A2663.
94. Pratt R, Giaquinto R, Ireland C, et al. A novel switched frequency 3He/1H high-pass birdcage coil for imaging at 1.5 tesla. *Concepts Magn Reson B Magn Reson Eng*. 2015;45(4):174–182. https://doi.org/10.1002/cmr.b.21309.
95. Wang Z, He M, Bier E, et al. *Hyperpolarized (129) Xe gas transfer MRI: the transition from 1.5T to 3T*. Magn Reson Med; July 2018. https://doi.org/10.1002/mrm.27377.
96. Woods JC. Mine the moon for 3He MRI? Not yet. *J Appl Physiol*. 2013;114(6):705–706. https://doi.org/10.1152/japplphysiol.00035.2013.
97. Woods J. The 129Xe MRI Clinical Trials Consortium: a route for multi-site trials. In: *International Workshop on Pulmonary Imaging*. 2017.
98. Kruger SJ, Fain SB, Johnson KM, Cadman RV, Nagle SK. Oxygen-enhanced 3D radial ultrashort echo time magnetic resonance imaging in the healthy human lung. *NMR Biomed*. 2014;27(12):1535–1541. https://doi.org/10.1002/nbm.3158.
99. Zha W, Kruger SJ, Johnson KM, et al. Pulmonary ventilation imaging in asthma and cystic fibrosis using oxygen-enhanced 3D radial ultrashort echo time MRI. *J Magn Reson Imaging*. 2018;47(5):1287–1297. https://doi.org/10.1002/jmri.25877.
100. Pieper CH, Smith J, Brand EJ. The value of ultrasound examination of the lungs in predicting bronchopulmonary dysplasia. *Pediatr Radiol*. 2004;34(3):227–231. https://doi.org/10.1007/s00247-003-1102-7.
101. Sanchez-Crespo A, Rohdin M, Carlsson C, et al. A technique for lung ventilation-perfusion SPECT in neonates and infants. *Nucl Med Commun*. 2008;29(2):173–177. https://doi.org/10.1097/MNM.0b013e3282f25905.

102. Kjellberg M, Bjorkman K, Rohdin M, Sanchez-Crespo A, Jonsson B. Bronchopulmonary dysplasia: clinical grading in relation to ventilation/perfusion mismatch measured by single photon emission computed tomography. *Pediatr Pulmonol.* 2013;48(12):1206–1213. https://doi.org/10.1002/ppul.22751.
103. Moylan FM, Shannon DC. Preferential distribution of lobar emphysema and atelectasis in bronchopulmonary dysplasia. *Pediatrics.* 1979;63(1):130–134.
104. Soler C, Figueras J, Roca I, Perez JM, Jimenez R. Pulmonary perfusion scintigraphy in the evaluation of the severity of bronchopulmonary dysplasia. *Pediatr Radiol.* 1997;27(1):32–35. https://doi.org/10.1007/s002470050058.
105. Murray C, Pilling DW, Shaw NJ. Persistent acquired lobar overinflation complicating bronchopulmonary dysplasia. *Eur J Pediatr.* 2000;159(1–2):14–17.
106. del Cerro MJ, Sabate Rotes A, Carton A, et al. Pulmonary hypertension in bronchopulmonary dysplasia: clinical findings, cardiovascular anomalies and outcomes. *Pediatr Pulmonol.* 2014;49(1):49–59. https://doi.org/10.1002/ppul.22797.
107. Abman SH, Hansmann G, Archer SL, et al. Pediatric pulmonary hypertension: guidelines from the American heart association and American thoracic society. *Circulation.* 2015;132(21):2037–2099. https://doi.org/10.1161/CIR.0000000000000329.
108. Bhat R, Salas AA, Foster C, Carlo WA, Ambalavanan N. Prospective analysis of pulmonary hypertension in extremely low birth weight infants. *Pediatrics.* 2012;129(3):e682–e689. https://doi.org/10.1542/peds.2011-1827.
109. Slaughter JL, Pakrashi T, Jones DE, South AP, Shah TA. Echocardiographic detection of pulmonary hypertension in extremely low birth weight infants with bronchopulmonary dysplasia requiring prolonged positive pressure ventilation. *J Perinatol.* 2011;31(10):635–640. https://doi.org/10.1038/jp.2010.213.
110. Subhedar NV, Shaw NJ. Changes in pulmonary arterial pressure in preterm infants with chronic lung disease. *Arch Dis Child Fetal Neonatal Ed.* 2000;82(3):F243–F247.
111. McGoon M, Gutterman D, Steen V, et al. Screening, early detection, and diagnosis of pulmonary arterial hypertension: ACCP evidence-based clinical practice guidelines. *Chest.* 2004;126(1 Suppl):14S–34S. https://doi.org/10.1378/chest.126.1_suppl.14S.
112. Carlton EF, Sontag MK, Younoszai A, et al. Reliability of echocardiographic indicators of pulmonary vascular disease in preterm infants at risk for bronchopulmonary dysplasia. *J Pediatr.* 2017;186:29–33. https://doi.org/10.1016/j.jpeds.2017.03.027.
113. Arcasoy SM, Christie JD, Ferrari VA, et al. Echocardiographic assessment of pulmonary hypertension in patients with advanced lung disease. *Am J Respir Crit Care Med.* 2003;167(5):735–740. https://doi.org/10.1164/rccm.200210-1130OC.
114. Mourani PM, Sontag MK, Younoszai A, Ivy DD, Abman SH. Clinical utility of echocardiography for the diagnosis and management of pulmonary vascular disease in young children with chronic lung disease. *Pediatrics.* 2008;121(2):317–325. https://doi.org/10.1542/peds.2007-1583.
115. Mourani PM, Mandell EW, Meier M, et al. Early pulmonary vascular disease in preterm infants is associated with late respiratory outcomes in childhood. *Am J Respir Crit Care Med.* 2018. https://doi.org/10.1164/rccm.201803-0428OC.
116. Levy PT, Patel MD, Choudhry S, Hamvas A, Singh GK. Evidence of echocardiographic markers of pulmonary vascular disease in asymptomatic infants born preterm at one year of age. *J Pediatr.* 2018;197:48–56. https://doi.org/10.1016/j.jpeds.2018.02.006. e2.
117. Siripornpitak S, Pornkul R, Khowsathit P, Layangool T, Promphan W, Pongpanich B. Cardiac CT angiography in children with congenital heart disease. *Eur J Radiol.* 2013;82(7):1067–1082. https://doi.org/10.1016/j.ejrad.2011.11.042.
118. Compton GL, Florence J, MacDonald C, Yoo S-J, Humpl T, Manson D. Main pulmonary artery-to-ascending aorta diameter ratio in healthy children on MDCT. *AJR Am J Roentgenol.* 2015;205(6):1322–1325. https://doi.org/10.2214/AJR.15.14301.
119. Iyer AS, Wells JM, Vishin S, Bhatt SP, Wille KM, Dransfield MT. CT scan-measured pulmonary artery to aorta ratio and echocardiography for detecting pulmonary hypertension in severe COPD. *Chest.* 2014;145(4):824–832. https://doi.org/10.1378/chest.13-1422.
120. Caro-Domínguez P, Compton G, Humpl T, Manson DE. Pulmonary arterial hypertension in children: diagnosis using ratio of main pulmonary artery to ascending aorta diameter as determined by multi-detector computed tomography. *Pediatr Radiol.* 2016;46(10):1378–1383. https://doi.org/10.1007/s00247-016-3636-5.
121. Tkach J, Taylor M, Moore R, et al. MRI measures of pulmonary arterial blood flow and RV remodeling in BPD. *Proc Am Thorac Soc.* 2017;195:A7202.
122. Callahan MJ, Poznauskis L, Zurakowski D, Taylor GA. Nonionic iodinated intravenous contrast material-related reactions: incidence in large urban children's hospital–retrospective analysis of data in 12,494 patients. *Radiology.* 2009;250(3):674–681. https://doi.org/10.1148/radiol.2503071577.
123. Swift AJ, Wild JM, Nagle SK, et al. Quantitative magnetic resonance imaging of pulmonary hypertension: a practical approach to the current state of the art. *J Thorac Imaging.* 2014;29(2):68–79. https://doi.org/10.1097/RTI.0000000000000079.
124. Song HK, Wright AC, Wolf RL, Wehrli FW. Multislice double inversion pulse sequence for efficient black-blood MRI. *Magn Reson Med.* 2002;47(3):616–620.
125. Dellegrottaglie S, Sanz J, Poon M, et al. Pulmonary hypertension: accuracy of detection with left ventricular septal-to-free wall curvature ratio measured at cardiac MR.

Radiology. 2007;243(1):63–69. https://doi.org/10.1148/radiol.2431060067.

126. Sanz J, Kuschnir P, Rius T, et al. Pulmonary arterial hypertension: noninvasive detection with phase-contrast MR imaging. *Radiology*. 2007;243(1):70–79. https://doi.org/10.1148/radiol.2431060477.
127. Blumfield E, Moore MM, Drake MK, et al. Survey of gadolinium-based contrast agent utilization among the members of the society for pediatric radiology: a quality and safety committee report. *Pediatr Radiol*. 2017;47(6):665–673. https://doi.org/10.1007/s00247-017-3807-z.
128. Hopkins SR, Prisk GK. Lung perfusion measured using magnetic resonance imaging: new tools for physiological insights into the pulmonary circulation. *J Magn Reson Imaging*. 2010;32(6):1287–1301. https://doi.org/10.1002/jmri.22378.
129. Schraml C, Schwenzer NF, Martirosian P, et al. Noninvasive pulmonary perfusion assessment in young patients with cystic fibrosis using an arterial spin labeling MR technique at 1.5 T. *Magma*. 2012;25(2):155–162. https://doi.org/10.1007/s10334-011-0271-x.
130. Mabray P, Thewamit R, Whitehead MT, et al. Increased cerebral blood flow on arterial spin labeling magnetic resonance imaging can localize to seizure focus in newborns: a report of 3 cases. *Epilepsia*. 2018;59(5):e63–e67. https://doi.org/10.1111/epi.14060.
131. Tkach J, Taylor M, Moore R, et al. Quantitative MRI measures of pulmonary arterial blood flow and morphology in congenital diaphragmatic hernia. In: *Proceedings of the American Thoracic Society*. Vol. 195. 2017:A7201.
132. Critser PJ, Higano NS, Tkach JA, Olson ES, Spielberg DR, Kingma PS, Fleck RJ, Lang SM, Moore RA, Taylor MD, Woods JC. Cardiac MRI evaluation of neonatal bronchopulmonary dysplasia associated pulmonary hypertension. *Am J Respir Crit Care Med*. 2019 Sep 20. https://doi.org/10.1164/rccm.201904-0826OC [Epub ahead of print].
133. Deacon JWF, Widger J, Soma MA. Paediatric tracheomalacia - a review of clinical features and comparison of diagnostic imaging techniques. *Int J Pediatr Otorhinolaryngol*. 2017;98:75–81. https://doi.org/10.1016/j.ijporl.2017.04.027.
134. Wood RE, Postma D. Endoscopy of the airway in infants and children. *J Pediatr*. 1988;112(1):1–6. https://doi.org/10.1016/S0022-3476(88)80109-4.
135. Burg G, Hysinger E, Hossain M, Wood R. Evaluation of agreement on presence and severity of tracheobronchomalacia in pediatric patients by dynamic flexible bronchoscopy. In: *Proceedings of the American Thoracic Society*. Vol. 197. 2018:A3660.
136. Masters IB, Eastburn MM, Wootton R, et al. A new method for objective identification and measurement of airway lumen in paediatric flexible videobronchoscopy. *Thorax*. 2005;60(8):652–658. https://doi.org/10.1136/thx.2004.034421.
137. Goo HW. Free-breathing cine CT for the diagnosis of tracheomalacia in young children. *Pediatr Radiol*. 2013;43(8):922–928. https://doi.org/10.1007/s00247-013-2637-x.
138. Dunham ME, Wolf RN. Visualizing the pediatric airway: three-dimensional modeling of endoscopic images. *Ann Otol Rhinol Laryngol*. 1996;105(1):12–17. https://doi.org/10.1177/000348949610500103.
139. Ciet P, Wielopolski P, Manniesing R, et al. Spirometer-controlled cine magnetic resonance imaging used to diagnose tracheobronchomalacia in paediatric patients. *Eur Respir J*. 2014;43(1):115–124. https://doi.org/10.1183/09031936.00104512.
140. Malik TH, Bruce IA, Kaushik V, Willatt DJ, Wright NB, Rothera MP. The role of magnetic resonance imaging in the assessment of suspected extrinsic tracheobronchial compression due to vascular anomalies. *Arch Dis Child*. 2006;91(1):52–55. https://doi.org/10.1136/adc.2004.070250.
141. Bates A, Higano N, Hysinger E, et al. Quantitative assessment of regional dynamic airway collapse in neonates via retrospectively respiratory-gated 1 H ultrashort echo time MRI. *J Magn Reson Imaging*. 2018. https://doi.org/10.1002/jmri.26296 [Epub ahead of print].
142. Hysinger E, Bates A, Higano N, et al. Quantitative assessment of tracheomalacia using ultra-short echo time MRI. San Diego, CA. In: *Proceedings of the American Thoracic Society*. Vol. 197. 2018:A4466.
143. Hahn AD, Higano NS, Walkup LL, et al. Pulmonary MRI of neonates in the intensive care unit using 3D ultrashort echo time and a small footprint MRI system. *J Magn Reson Imaging*. 2017;45(2):463–471. https://doi.org/10.1002/jmri.25394.
144. Higano NS, Bates AJ, Tkach JA, et al. Pre- and post-operative visualization of neonatal esophageal atresia/tracheoesophageal fistula via magnetic resonance imaging. *J Pediatr Surg Case Rep*. 2018;29:5–8. https://doi.org/10.1016/j.epsc.2017.10.001.
145. Theilmann RJ, Smales E, DeYoung PN, Malhotra A, Darquenne CJ. Dynamic movement of upper airway structures during sleep and apnea in obstructive sleep apnea subjects (OSA). In: *A30. Upper Airway Dynamics: Insights from Human and Animal Studies*. A1245. doi: 10.1164/ajrccm-conference.2018.197.1_MeetingAbstracts.A1245.
146. Bates AJ, Schuh A, McConnell K, et al. A novel method to generate dynamic boundary conditions for airway CFD by mapping upper airway movement with non-rigid registration of dynamic and static MRI. *Int J Numer Method Biomed Eng*; 2018. http://doi.wiley.com/10.1002/cnm.3144.
147. Bates AJ, Comerford A, Cetto R, Schroter RC, Tolley NS, Doorly DJ. Power loss mechanisms in pathological tracheas. *J Biomech*. 2016;49(11):2187–2192. https://doi.org/10.1016/j.jbiomech.2015.11.033.
148. Bates AJ, Cetto R, Doorly DJ, Schroter RC, Tolley NS, Comerford A. The effects of curvature and constriction on airflow and energy loss in pathological tracheas. *Respir Physiol Neurobiol*. 2016;234:69–78. https://doi.org/10.1016/j.resp.2016.09.002.
149. Jahani N, Choi S, Choi J, Iyer K, Hoffman EA, Lin C-L. Assessment of regional ventilation and deformation

using 4D-CT imaging for healthy human lungs during tidal breathing. *J Appl Physiol*. 2015;119(10): 1064–1074. https://doi.org/10.1152/japplphysiol.00339.2015.

150. Hamilton NJ, Kanani M, Roebuck DJ, et al. Tissue-engineered tracheal replacement in a child: a 4-year follow-up study. *Am J Transplant*. 2015;15(10): 2750–2757. https://doi.org/10.1111/ajt.13318.
151. Bates AJ, Doorly DJ, Cetto R, et al. Dynamics of airflow in a short inhalation. *J R Soc Interface*. 2014;12(102). https://doi.org/10.1098/rsif.2014.0880.
152. Bates AJ, Schuh A, Amine-Eddine G, et al. Assessing the relationship between movement and airflow in the upper airway using computational fluid dynamics with motion determined from magnetic resonance imaging. *Clin Biomech*. 2017;0(0). https://doi.org/10.1016/j.clinbiomech.2017.10.011.
153. Miyawaki S, Hoffman EA, Lin CL. Effect of static vs. dynamic imaging on particle transport in CT-based numerical models of human central airways. *J Aerosol Sci*. 2016; 100:129–139. https://doi.org/10.1016/j.jaerosci.2016.07.006.
154. Dalesio NM, Kattail D, Ishman SL, Greenberg RS. Ultrasound use in the pediatric airway: the time has come. *AA Case Rep*. 2014;2(3):23–26. https://doi.org/10.1097/ACC.0b013e3182a070d2.
155. Stafrace S, Engelhardt T, Teoh WH, Kristensen MS. Essential ultrasound techniques of the pediatric airway. *Paediatr Anaesth*. 2016;26(2):122–131. https://doi.org/10.1111/pan.12787.

CHAPTER 7

Pulmonary Function Tests in Bronchopulmonary Dysplasia: Why, What, and How

CINDY T. MCEVOY, MD, MCR • JUDY L. ASCHNER, MD

INTRODUCTION

Bronchopulmonary dysplasia (BPD) is the most common form of chronic lung disease in infancy.[1] As described in 1967 by Northway et al.,[2] BPD occurred in modestly premature infants with surfactant deficiency who were exposed to ventilator-induced volutrauma and high oxygen concentrations. Today, BPD occurs primarily in extremely premature infants (23–28 weeks of gestation) born during the late canalicular/early saccular stage of lung development.[3] In contrast to the inflammation, fibrosis, and scarring that characterized "classic BPD" as described by Northway, BPD today is conceptualized as a disruption and impairment of lung development ("new BPD").[4] Importantly, a diagnosis of BPD carries the risk of lifelong altered pulmonary function test (PFT) results, with significant clinical and functional respiratory abnormalities that can persist into adolescence and adulthood.[5]

With the changing epidemiology and pathology of BPD and with more former premature infants reaching adulthood, the life-course trajectory of PFTs in former preterm infants with BPD is an important area for study. The natural history of PFTs in infants with the "new BPD" may not be significantly different than the natural history of those with "classic BPD." Both groups of individuals manifest with persistent respiratory symptoms and reduced lung function. PFTs show expiratory flow limitation at school age, which may improve with bronchodilator treatment[6] and has been documented into adulthood.[7,8] There is concern that BPD will predispose to chronic obstructive pulmonary disease (COPD) because infants are beginning life with reduced lung function, and longitudinal cohorts indicate that individuals track along their predetermined PFT percentiles throughout life.[9] This emphasizes the important need for increased focus on the primary prevention of BPD to optimize lung function and normalize PFT parameters as early as possible.

Pathologic datasets from newborns and infants with BPD are limited and histologic examination of lung tissue from patients with the "new BPD" is fortunately rare. Therefore PFTs play a crucial role in documenting and quantifying the natural history and trajectory of pulmonary function alterations in BPD. In this chapter, we will summarize the current knowledge of the life course of BPD by emphasizing recent and key articles notating its natural history in terms of PFTs from the newborn period through adulthood and building the case for a continued focus on its primary prevention to reset pulmonary function trajectories.

OVERVIEW: THE IMPORTANCE OF EARLY LIFE LUNG FUNCTION/PULMONARY FUNCTION TRAJECTORIES

There are convincing data from a number of longitudinal cohorts primarily born at term that an individual will continue to track along a pulmonary function trajectory that is established very early in life. For example, the Tucson Children's Respiratory Study[9] enrolled 169 nonselected infants at birth and performed PFTs at 2–3 months of age before any respiratory illness occurred and then at least once at ages 11, 16, and 22 years. This study demonstrated that those infants who were in the lowest quartile for the initial infant PFT had persistently diminished PFT results through 22 years of age.[9] In addition, it is being increasingly recognized that the origins of some COPD phenotypes, particularly the nonsmoking-related phenotype, occur very early. Until recently, the hallmark of COPD (now the third most

Updates on Neonatal Chronic Lung Disease. https://doi.org/10.1016/B978-0-323-68353-1.00007-5

common cause of death in the United States) was considered to be a rapid age-related decline in pulmonary function in adulthood.[10] However, recent studies[11] show that 50% of individuals who develop COPD have a normal decrease in pulmonary function as adults but develop COPD because they never reached a normal maximum pulmonary function in early adulthood.

There are many factors that can impact the placement of an individual on a PFT trajectory. However, preterm delivery is the most common cause of altered lung development and BPD is a complication of extreme prematurity. An infant born preterm with suboptimal lung function, particularly if BPD develops, is at risk for not attaining an optimal lung function as a young adult and therefore developing symptomatic respiratory disease as he/she ages (Fig. 7.1). This emphasizes the importance of (1) primary prevention of BPD (and of preterm birth) to optimize lung development; (2) longitudinal PFTs in this at-risk population to follow their trajectory, which may even worsen over time; and (3) the application of PFTs to quantify early interventions targeted to primary and secondary prevention.

NATURAL HISTORY OF PULMONARY FUNCTION TESTING MEASUREMENTS IN BRONCHOPULMONARY DYSPLASIA

It is unclear when BPD begins, but there is increasing evidence that its origins occur in utero[4] due to factors such as chorioamnionitis, preeclampsia, preexisting hypertensive disorders, gestational diabetes, maternal obesity, and smoking among other factors that are associated with an increased risk for BPD.[12] For instance, a prospective, longitudinal study of 587 preterm infants 500–1250 g demonstrated that maternal smoking during pregnancy and maternal hypertension were each associated with a significant twofold increase in the odds of developing BPD after preterm birth.[12,13] Therefore detailed assessment of neonatal pulmonary function after a premature delivery can be important to understand the evolution of disease and to identify potential windows of vulnerability and intervention. In

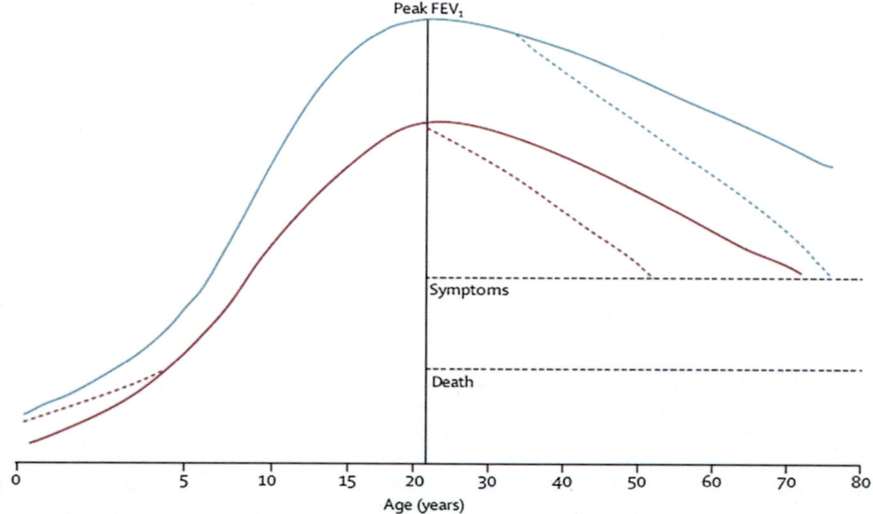

FIG. 7.1 Early origins of adult lung disease. In healthy children, continuous growth of the lungs and thorax throughout childhood results in maximum lung function at around 22 years of age (*solid blue line*). Subsequently, despite gradual age-related changes, considerable reserves are maintained into old age unless there is an accelerated rate of decline (*dashed blue line*) because of, for example, the effects of smoking. If a child is born with suboptimum lung function due to intrauterine insults (*red solid line*), or has impaired airway lung and airway growth during the first 5 years of life (*dashed red line*) because of early postnatal insults, lung function might remain diminished throughout childhood. Failure to achieve optimal lung function as a young adult means that even in the absence of any further insults, such individuals will be prone to develop symptomatic respiratory disease as they age. Onset of such symptoms can occur much earlier in the presence of any additional risk factors for accelerated lung aging (*red dashed line*). FEV_1, forced expiratory volume in 1 s. (Reprinted with permission from Elsevier publications Stocks J, Hislop A, Sonnappa S. Early lung development: lifelong effect on respiratory health and disease. *Lancet Respir Med.* 2013;1(9):728–742.)

preterm infants, lung development that would normally occur in utero happens postnatally under altered mechanical and environmental conditions. These include active tidal breathing with strain and stretch of immature intrathoracic structures, and a state of relative hyperoxia, even with room air.[14] Lung development is also affected by conditions precipitating premature delivery, often including inflammatory and infectious processes.[15]

Premature delivery not only impacts normal alveolarization and pulmonary vascularization but also affects respiratory mechanical processes.[16] Neonatal pulmonary mechanics or PFTs have been useful to reproducibly quantify the newborn's response to a variety of antenatal and postnatal exposures, therapies, or conditions (including preterm birth itself). These PFT results correlate with clinical outcomes. PFTs have given useful insights into normal and aberrant lung development in preterm infants and have strengthened the physiologic basis (or lack thereof) for therapies used for the prevention and treatment of respiratory distress syndrome (RDS) and evolving BPD. Antenatal steroids and surfactant, which have been shown in randomized controlled trials (RCTs) to significantly decrease the incidence of death and RDS, have been shown to significantly improve measurements of neonatal PFTs.[17–21] Therapies unproven in large RCTs, such as inhaled nitric oxide (iNO) for BPD prevention, are not associated with improvements in neonatal PFT results.[22] International guidelines are published regarding specific methodologies, acceptance criteria, and standardized equipment for performing PFTs in neonates and young infants.[23,24]

Neonatal PFTs can be challenging because the patient is often not cooperative, but they can be accomplished noninvasively during quiet sleep and do not require sedation. Published studies examining the mechanical properties of the newborn respiratory system have primarily applied passive and dynamic techniques to measure respiratory compliance (Crs) and resistance (Rrs).[16,19] Lung volumes have been measured by gas washout methods, helium dilution, or body plethysmography.[25] Table 7.1 summarizes PFTs that have

TABLE 7.1
Pulmonary Function Tests That Have Been Used to Monitor the Natural History of BPD.

NEONATES (UP TO 44 WEEKS OF PMA)				
Measurement	**Technique**	**What it tells us**	**Units of measure**	**Is sedation needed?**
Crs = passive respiratory system compliance	Single breath or multiple breath occlusion	Respiratory system mechanics (stiffness of lungs) Assess effectiveness of medications, i.e., prenatal and postnatal steroids, surfactant, and others Decreased in BPD	mL/cm H_2O and mL/cm H_2O/kg	No
Rrs = passive respiratory system resistance	Single breath or multiple breath occlusion	Respiratory system mechanics (flow in airways/airspaces) Assess effectiveness of medication as aforementioned Increased in BPD	cm H_2O/mL/s	No
Cdyn = dynamic compliance	Least mean square analysis and others; uses a pneumotachograph	Dynamic respiratory system mechanics (stiffness of lungs) Assess effectiveness of medications as aforementioned Decreased in BPD	mL/cm H_2O mL/cm H_2O/kg	No

Continued

TABLE 7.1
Pulmonary Function Tests That Have Been Used to Monitor the Natural History of BPD.—cont'd

Measurement	Technique	What it tells us	Units of measure	Is sedation needed?
NEONATES (UP TO 44 WEEKS OF PMA)				
FRC = functional residual capacity	Nitrogen washout, helium dilution, SF_6	Volume in the lungs at the end of a normal expiration; assesses effectiveness of medications as aforementioned Decreased in "new BPD"	mL and mL/kg	No
Z_{rs} = impedance of respiratory system	Forced oscillation technique	Describes the resistance, compliance, and inertance, as well as resonance frequency, of the respiratory system		No
LCI = lung clearance index/mixing efficiency	Multiple breath washout	Measure of lung homogeneity		No
INFANTS (FROM 44 WEEKS OF PMA TO 2 YEARS OF AGE)				
As aforementioned can measure Crs, Rrs, Cdyn, FRC, Z_{rs}[a], and LCI[a]	As aforementioned in neonatal tests	As aforementioned	As aforementioned	Yes
FEFs = forced expiratory flows (FEF_{75}, FEF_{50}, FEF_{25-75}, VmaxFRC)	Raised volume RTC technique; tidal breathing RTC (also called VmaxFRC)	Expiratory flow during forced expiration; decreased in BPD	mL/s	Yes
FVC= forced vital capacity $FEV_{0.5}$ = forced expiratory volume in 0.5 s	Raised volume RTC and tidal breathing RTC	Volume change between full inspiration and complete expiration Volume change in first 0.5 s. $FEV_{0.5}$ decreased in BPD	mL	Yes
FRCp = functional residual capacity	Plethysmography	Volume in the lungs at the end of a normal expiration; assesses effectiveness of medications as aforementioned Decreased in "new BPD"	mL	Yes
D_{LCO} = diffusing capacity of lung for carbon monoxide V_A = alveolar volume	Single breath hold	Used to assess lung growth and parenchymal lung disease D_{LCO} decreased in BPD; V_A normal in BPD	mLCO/min/mm Hg mL	Yes
Children/Adolescents/Adults				
FEFs = forced expiratory flows (FEF_{25-75}, FEF_{75}, FEF_{50})	Spirometry	Expiratory flow during forced expiration Decreased in BPD	mL/s	No
FVC = forced vital capacity FEV_1 = forced expiratory volume in 1 s	Spirometry	FVC as aforementioned FEV_1, volume change in first 1 s of expiration Decreased in BPD	mL or L	No

TABLE 7.1
Pulmonary Function Tests That Have Been Used to Monitor the Natural History of BPD.—cont'd

NEONATES (UP TO 44 WEEKS OF PMA)				
Measurement	**Technique**	**What it tells us**	**Units of measure**	**Is sedation needed?**
FRC, RV = residual volume, TLC = total lung capacity, and other volumes	Spirometry	FRC as aforementioned RV/TLC increased with air trapping	mL or L	No
DLCO = diffusing capacity of lung for carbon monoxide	Single breath hold	DLCO as above	mLCO/min/mm Hg	No

Other techniques have been used in neonates but may require sedation.
This list is not comprehensive/inclusive. Peak oxygen consumption has also been measured during exercise tolerance in children and adults.
BPD, bronchopulmonary dysplasia; *PMA*, postmenstrual age; *RTC*, rapid thoracic compression; *SF*$_6$, sulfur hexafluoride.
[a] Studies are underway evaluating the ability to measure Z_{rs} and LCI in infants without sedation.

been used to monitor the natural history of BPD from the neonatal stage through adulthood.

Neonatal Studies

PFTs have been used to examine the effects of pharmacologic agents on the premature lung, including those of antenatal steroids,[17–20] surfactant,[21,26] and postnatal steroids.[27] Similar to results in animal models, studies have demonstrated a significant increase in Crs and functional residual capacity (FRC) after a timely single course of antenatal steroids,[17] thereby supporting accelerated lung maturation with antenatal steroid treatment (Fig. 7.2). These PFT improvements correlated with improved clinical outcomes with less surfactant use and less supplemental oxygen need. Neonatal PFTs have been used to quantify the duration of the clinical effect of a single course of antenatal steroids[18] and to quantify the effects of a single rescue course of antenatal steroids versus placebo given to women undelivered more than 14 days after their first course of antenatal steroids.[19] This study demonstrated a significantly increased Crs in the preterm infants (n = 113) whose mothers received the rescue course of antenatal steroids and provided a physiologic basis for a large RCT[28] showing improved clinical respiratory outcomes after a rescue course of antenatal steroids. Another study[29] documented a significant increase in Crs after a single course of antenatal steroids in late-preterm infants delivered between 34 and 34$^6/_7$ weeks. This study[29] is consistent with the findings of an RCT[30] of a single course of antenatal steroids versus placebo in over 2800 pregnant women who delivered infants between 34 and <37 weeks of gestation, which found significantly decreased neonatal composite outcome in those who received the course of antenatal steroids. The use of neonatal PFTs may allow the quantification of response to medications such as antenatal steroids in low- and middle-income countries[31] and the

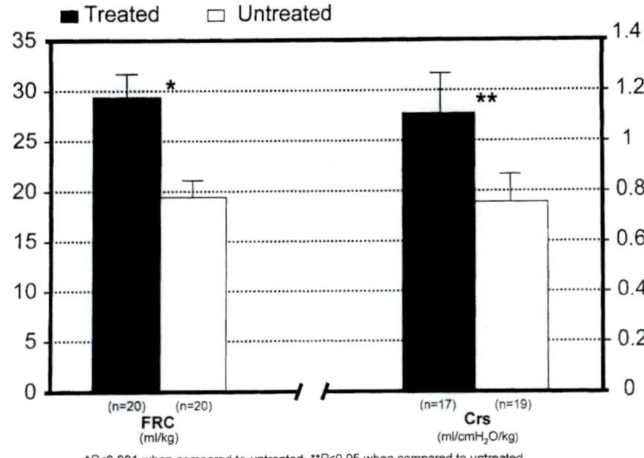

FIG. 7.2 Measurements of functional residual capacity (FRC) in mL/kg in 40 preterm infants (20 treated vs. 20 untreated infants) and of respiratory compliance (Crs) in mL/cm H_2O/kg in 36 preterm infants (mean ± standard error of mean). FRC and respiratory compliance values were significantly increased in the betamethasone-treated group compared with the untreated group. (Reprinted with permission from John Wiley & Sons publications McEvoy C, Bowling S, Williamson K, Stewart M, Durand M. Functional residual capacity and passive compliance measurements after antenatal steroid therapy in preterm infants. *Pediatr Pulmonol*. 2001;31(6):425–430.)

identification of BPD phenotypes responsive to bronchodilators.[32] Clinical studies examined the effect of surfactant in preterm newborns with RDS and demonstrated an increase in FRC before an increase in Crs.[16,21]

Preterm delivery is the most common cause of abnormal lung development, with BPD in the extremely preterm infant at one end of the spectrum. Studies have shown that even "healthy" preterm infants have a lower Crs and higher Rrs than healthy term infants.[33,34] Preterm infants with BPD have lower FRC values than preterm infants without BPD.[35,36] Infants with BPD studied at 34–36 weeks had significantly lower Crs and FRC and higher Rrs than matched, healthy late-preterm infants studied at comparable postmenstrual ages.[37,38] A longitudinal study demonstrated that the Crs was 50% of predicted during the acute phase of BPD and was associated with abnormal Rrs values. These values normalized over the first 2 years of life but significant airway dysfunction persisted in many infants.[39] This illustrates the importance of defining the trajectory of the "healthy" premature lung for an appropriate comparison or control for infants at risk for or diagnosed with BPD.[39] Representative PFT studies in neonates and infants are presented in Table 7.2.

Infants

Infant PFTs are more challenging than neonatal PFTs because both the patients are not cooperative and the techniques applied to this age group require sedation, with normative values established during sleep induced with chloral hydrate, a drug no longer available in the United States. However, the period of lung growth during the first 2 years of life is the most rapid and therefore may be the most relevant to the investigations of the natural history of PFTs in BPD. Infant PFTs have primarily been the measurement of forced expiratory flows (FEFs) and volumes with the raised or tidal volume rapid thoracic compression technique and of FRC with the plethysmograph[23] (Table 7.1).

Extremely preterm infants are born before the onset of alveolar formation leading to failed septation and a reduced number of alveoli. To understand the growth of the preterm lung, a term reference lung is needed. Studies of infants with healthy term lungs show their lungs grow in concordance with somatic growth and their lung volume or forced vital capacity (FVC) increases faster than their airway flows.[40,41] Lung growth can occur by two possible mechanisms: by increasing the number of alveoli and by increasing the size of

TABLE 7.2
Representative PFT Studies in Neonates and Infants Reporting Response to Therapies and Elucidating Natural History of BPD.

TREATMENT STUDIES (ANTENATAL STEROIDS, SURFACTANT, BRONCHODILATORS, EFFECTS OF PEEP, POSTNATAL STEROIDS)					
Study/year	**Aim**	**Study design**	**Study groups**	**Methods**	**Conclusion/outcome**
Go (2018)[29]	Study changes in Crs in late preterm infants after one course of ASs	Case control	25 Preterm infants $34^{0}/_{7}$–$34^{6}/_{7}$ weeks treated with ASs versus 25 matched untreated infants	SBOT	Crs was significantly increased in these late-preterm infants after AS use
Morrow (2015)[32]	Quantify changes in Rrs in preterm infants with evolving BPD	Descriptive	40 Preterm infants with evolving BPD	SBOT	50% Of preterm infants with evolving BPD had a ≥10% decrease in Rrs in response to a bronchodilator
McEvoy (2001)[17]	Document changes in Crs and FRC after single course of ASs	Case control	20 Preterm infants treated with ASs versus 20 preterm untreated infants	SBOT; nitrogen washout	A single course of ASs within 7 days of delivery significantly increases Crs and FRC
		Case control		SBOT	

McEvoy (2008)[18]	To compare PFT results in infants born at different intervals after AS therapy		28 Preterm infants born within 7 days of AS therapy versus 28 preterm infants born >7 days after AS therapy		Infants born >7 days after AS therapy had a significant ↓ in Crs because of the dissipation of the beneficial effects of surfactant induced by ASs
McEvoy (2010)[19]	To evaluate whether a "rescue" course of ASs improves PFT results in preterm infants	RCT	56 Infants randomized to rescue AS course versus 57 randomized to placebo	SBOT; nitrogen washout	Preterm infants who received a rescue course of ASs had improved Crs and less oxygen need
Hjalmarson (2011)[20]	To evaluate if AS-induced lung changes persist	Case control	22 Infants treated with ASs but born at term versus 50 term infants untreated with ASs	SBOT; nitrogen washout; gas mixing efficiency	No signs of a permanent effect of ASs on lung function
Dinger (2002)[26]	To understand mechanisms of improved oxygenation after surfactant use	Descriptive	90 Preterm infants with severe RDS studied before and serially after surfactant use	SBOT; SF_6 washout	↑ In FRC within 1 h of treatment, with ↑ in Crs 3–24 h after treatment depending on the type of surfactant used
Dinger (2001)[21]	Effect of PEEP levels on lung mechanics	Descriptive	20 Infants at 24–32 weeks of gestation and 72 h after surfactant use	SBOT; SF_6 washout	↑ In FRC with ↑ PEEP, but ↓ Crs with increasing PEEP
Durand (2002)[27]	Compare 7 days of low-dose versus high-dose postnatal steroids on pulmonary function	RCT	24 Preterm infants randomized to low-dose and 23 to high-dose dexamethasone	Cdyn	Similar ↑ in Cdyn with both doses by day 7 of treatment, no difference in BPD
STUDIES IN NEONATES AND INFANTS WITH BPD					
Shepherd (2018)[50]	Investigate potential severe BPD phenotypes with infant PFTs	Prospective cohort	110 Infants with severe BPD studied at a median age of 52 weeks PMA	RVRTC	The current diagnosis of severe BPD includes patients with obstructive, mixed, and restrictive phenotypes
Kavvadia (1998)[35]	Compare FRC in preterm infants with BPD with that in preterm infants without BPD	Case control	16 Infants with BPD at 28 days and 8 infants without BPD had FRC done at 14 and 28 days	Helium dilution	Decreased FRC in patients with BPD compared to those without BPD
Kavvadia (2000)[36]	Predictive value of FRC, Crs, and Rrs	Descriptive	100 Consecutive VLBW infants	SBOT; helium dilution	Decreased FRC (<19 mL/kg) best

Continued

TABLE 7.2
Representative PFT Studies in Neonates and Infants Reporting Response to Therapies and Elucidating Natural History of BPD.—cont'd

TREATMENT STUDIES (ANTENATAL STEROIDS, SURFACTANT, BRONCHODILATORS, EFFECTS OF PEEP, POSTNATAL STEROIDS)					
Study/year	**Aim**	**Study design**	**Study groups**	**Methods**	**Conclusion/outcome**
	on day 2 of life in 100 VLBW infants		ventilated within 6 h of life and studied on day 2		predictor of BPD at 28 days in patients <28 weeks of gestation
McEvoy (2014)[37]	Compare PFT results at 34 −36 weeks in BPD with healthy patients born at 34 −36 weeks	Case control	20 Patients with BPD and 20 matched healthy infants	SBOT; nitrogen washout	Infants with BPD have significantly ↓FRC and ↓Crs compared with healthy infants studied at the same PMA
Hjalmarson (2005)[38]	Compare PFT results of BPD and healthy preterm infants, all studied at term	Case control	50 Infants with BPD and 19 healthy preterm controls	SBOT; nitrogen washout; gas mixing efficiency	Infants with severe BPD had lower FRC, less efficient gas mixing, and ↑ specific conductance than those with mild, moderate BPD or healthy preterm infants
Baraldi (1997)[39]	Follow PFT results through 2 years in infants with BPD	Longitudinal cohort	24 Patients with BPD	SBOT; nitrogen Washout; VmaxFRC	Pulmonary mechanics improve over first 2 years but low FEFs persist
Fakhoury (2010)[47]	Describe PFTs in infants with BPD in the first 3 years of life	Longitudinal cohort	44 Patients with BPD	TVRTC	Persistent low partial expiratory flows through 24 months of age
Filbrun (2011)[48]	Assess longitudinal changes in PFT results over first 3 years of life in relation to somatic growth	Longitudinal cohort	18 Patients with BPD studied at a mean of 59 and 91 weeks of age	RVRTC	Children with BPD have significant and persistent airflow obstruction. Those with above average somatic growth had greater lung growth.
Thunqvist (2014)[49]	PFTs at 6 and 18 months in relation to BPD severity	Longitudinal cohort	55 Infants with BPD studied at 6 and 18 months	SBOT; FRC by plethysmography; TVRTC; RVRTC	Initial low Crs and high Rrs improved over time but FEFs remained low indicating impaired expiratory flows
Balinotti (2010)[43]	Compare DLCO and V_A in patients with BPD with those in term controls	Case control	39 Infants with BPD and 61 term infants studied at about 12 months of age	DLCO with single breath hold	Infants with BPD had ↓DLCO but normal V_A compared to term controls, consistent with ↓alveolarization
STUDIES IN HEALTHY PRETERM OR TERM NEONATES AND INFANTS (NEEDED AS REFERENCE GROUP OR CONTROL GROUP AS BPD IS STUDIED)					
		Case control		VA and DLCO	

Assaf (2015)[44]	Measure D_{LCO} and V_A in healthy preterm infants and term controls		48 Healthy preterm and 88 healthy term infants studied at 3–33 months of PMA		Prematurity without BPD did not impair lung parenchymal development
Hjalmarson (2002)[34]	Compare PFT results in healthy preterm and term infants	Case control	32 Healthy preterm and 53 healthy term infants studied at the same PMA	SBOT; nitrogen washout; gas mixing efficiency	Preterm infants show signs of dysfunction of terminal respiratory units
McEvoy (2013)[33]	Compare PFT results in healthy LPIs at term PMA with PFT results in healthy term infants	Case control	31 Healthy LPIs and 30 healthy term infants studied at 40 weeks of PMA	SBOT; nitrogen washout	Healthy LPIs have ↓Crs, altered flow volume loops, and ↑Rrs compared with term infants
Balinotti (2009)[42]	To measure the ratio of D_{LCO} to V_A in healthy term infants	Observational	50 Healthy infants between 3 and 23 months of age	D_{LCO} and V_A	Lung growth in this age occurs mostly by addition of alveoli rather than by expansion of current alveoli
Jones (2000)[41]	Establish reference values for FEFs for term infants	Observational/ normative	155 Healthy infants between 3 and 149 weeks of age	RVRTC	FEFs increase with increasing length
Friedrich (2007)[40]	Compare longitudinal FEFs in healthy preterm infants with those in healthy term infants	Prospective cohort	26 Preterm (average GA of 32.7 weeks) and 24 term infants studied in year 1 and 2 of life	RVRTC	Healthy preterm infants have persistently lower FEFs than term infants suggesting no catch up growth in airway function

This list of studies is not inclusive.

ASs, antenatal steroids; *BPD*, bronchopulmonary dysplasia; *CO*, carbon monoxide; *Cdyn*, dynamic respiratory compliance; *Crs*, passive respiratory system compliance; *D_{LCO}*, diffusing capacity of lung for carbon monoxide; *FEFs*, forced expiratory flows; *FRC*, functional residual capacity; *GA*, gestational age; *LPIs*, late-preterm infants; *PEEP*, positive end-expiratory pressure; *PFT*, pulmonary function test; *PMA*, postmenstrual age; *RCT*, randomized controlled trial; *RDS*, respiratory distress syndrome; *Rrs*, passive respiratory system resistance; *RVRTC*, raised volume rapid thoracic compression; *SBOT*, single breath occlusion technique; *SF_6*, sulfur hexafluoride; *TVRTC*, tidal volume rapid thoracic compression; *V_A*, alveolar volume; *VLBW*, very low-birth-weight.

existing alveoli. Studies measuring alveolar volumes and gas diffusion in healthy term infants between 3 and 23 months of age[42] have shown that the ratio of diffusing capacity of lung for carbon monoxide (DLCO) and alveolar volume (V_A) is linear. This indicates that lung growth increases primarily by the addition of new alveoli rather than by the expansion of existing alveoli and that DLCO/V_A is constant through the first 2 years of life. Infants with BPD have a normal V_A but have a lower DLCO for the same than term control infants (Fig. 7.3A and B), supporting the premise that in BPD there are fewer (but larger) alveoli.[43] Interestingly, Assaf et al.[44] compared former preterm infants born at an average of 31.7 weeks' gestation without BPD with term infants and found that in the absence of extreme prematurity without BPD, prematurity itself did not impair lung parenchymal development in terms of V_A and DLCO. A study using aerosol-derived airway morphometry demonstrated that the number of alveoli remained constant from 6 years of age and above.[45]

In infants with BPD, there are fewer and larger alveoli and less tethering of the airways through the elastic components in alveolar walls,[14] which can affect both gas transfer and elastic recoil. Infants with BPD have lower FEFs than the reference values from healthy term controls.[46–49] Shepherd et al.[50] studied infants with severe BPD (median gestational age at birth of 25 weeks, median birth weight of 707 g) at a mean postmenstrual age of 52 weeks who were still in the neonatal intensive care unit. They demonstrated distinct phenotypes of PFTs within the global definition of BPD, with 51% having obstructive, 40% with mixed, and 9% with restrictive phenotypes. Targeting specific phenotypes of BPD would increase the likelihood of success of future intervention trials. Infants with BPD who wheeze have lower FEFs than infants with BPD who do not wheeze.[51] Infants with BPD studied at 6 and 12 months of age have decreased FEFs that remain subnormal and may worsen over time.[52] Studies have shown that healthy preterm infants (with minimal oxygen and ventilation need) have decreased FEFs compared with normal term infants and their FEFs do not appear to catch up over time[40] (Table 7.2).

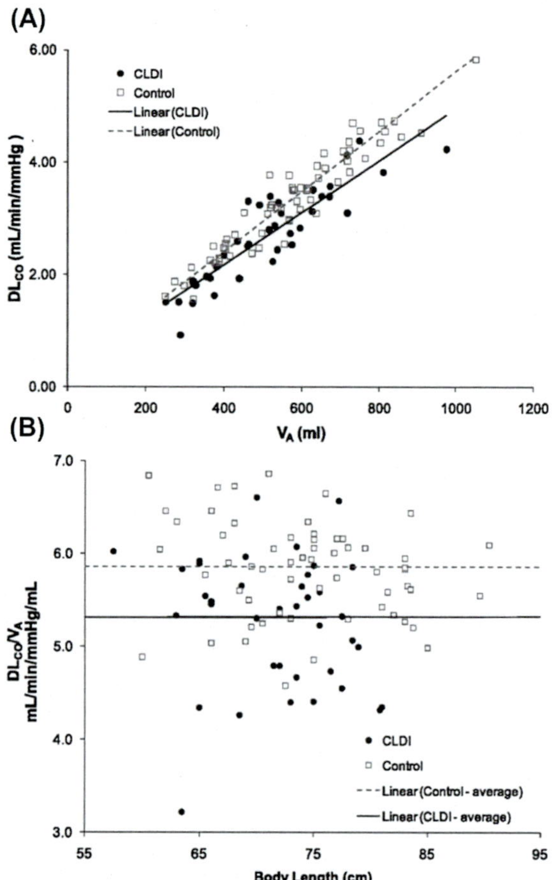

FIG. 7.3 **(A)** Diffusing capacity of lung for carbon monoxide, DLCO, versus alveolar volume, V_A. Individual data for subjects with chronic lung disease of infancy (CLDI) (*solid circles*) and control subjects (*open squares*), as well as the linear regressions for each group are presented. DLCO was significantly lower for subjects with CLDI than control subjects when adjusted for alveolar volume by analysis of covariance ($P = .0004$). **(B)** Ratio of pulmonary diffusing capacity to alveolar volume, DLCO/V_A, was not related to body length. Individual data for subjects with CLDI (*solid circles*) and control subjects (*open squares*) are presented, as well as the average data for each group. DLCO/V_A was significantly lower for subjects with CLDI than control subjects ($P = .0004$). (Reprinted with permission from the American Thoracic Society. Copyright © 2015 American Thoracic Society. Balinotti JE, Chakr VC, Tiller C, et al. Growth of lung parenchyma in infants and toddlers with chronic lung disease of infancy. *Am J Respir Crit Care Med*. 2010; 181(10): 1093–97.Official Journal of the American Thoracic Society.)

Children and Adolescents

Studies evaluating the effect of BPD on school-aged children have in general documented measurements of airflow obstruction with decreased FEFs and forced expiratory volume at 1 s (FEV_1) compared to term controls.[53–55] Measurements of residual volume/total lung capacity were suggestive of air trapping and diffusing capacity was decreased.[55] Baraldi et al.[56] demonstrated that structural abnormalities in the small airways of children with BPD accounts for at least part of their manifested airflow obstruction. These investigators compared children with BPD to children with asthma with a similar degree of airflow obstruction and found those with BPD had lower levels of exhaled NO and were less responsive to β-agonists, supporting a structural abnormality. Vrijilandt et al.[57] applied forced oscillometry in 3- to 5-year-old children with a history of BPD and found higher resonant frequency and lower mean reactance than children without BPD, suggesting those with BPD had decreased peripheral airway patency.

Follow-up of extremely preterm infants from the EPICURE study at 11 years of age demonstrated that 56% of the children had significantly decreased FEFs and 27% had a positive bronchodilator response, with reductions in lung function being more severe in the infants with a prior BPD diagnosis.[58] A subset of these patients were further tested showing lung function abnormalities in 78% of the extremely preterm children with evidence of airway obstruction, ventilation inhomogeneity, gas trapping, and airway hyperresponsiveness.[59]

Several investigators[60,61] demonstrated that as children, former very low-birth-weight (VLBW) infants with BPD have decreased lung function compared with former VLBW infants without BPD, whereas other investigators reported no differences in lung function or diffusing capacity in VLBW infants with and without BPD.[62] Simpson et al.[63] performed longitudinal studies between 4 and 12 years of age in preterm children with and without BPD and in term controls and demonstrated that those with and without BPD had declines in spirometry *z* scores compared with controls. FEV_1 decreased by a rate of at least 0.1 *z* score per year in those with BPD.[63] Doyle et al.[54] reported a decline in lung function measured at 8 and 18 years of age in BPD survivors. Doyle et al.[64] compared changes in spirometry from 8 to 18 years of age in preterm survivors born in the surfactant era with those in controls and demonstrated that the preterm group had significant decreases in airflow at both ages with mean differences in *z* scores for FEV_1; at 8 years, −1.02, 95% confidence interval (CI), −1.21 to −0.82 and at 18 years, −0.92, 95% CI, −1.14 to −0.71. This airflow obstruction increased over time if the preterm infants had BPD or were smokers at 18 years of age.[64] This same group also compared expiratory flow data at 8 years of age from preterm infants born in three different epochs, 1991–92, 1997, and 2005,[65] and demonstrated that despite increases in the use of less invasive ventilation after birth, airflows at 8 years of age were worse in the 2005 epoch than the two earlier ones.[65] These data again likely speaks to the importance of primary prevention and in utero/perinatal origins of infant lung disease. Hospital readmissions in the first 2 years of life and FEV_1 and FVC in patients between 8 and 15 years of age have been shown to be significantly associated with initial BPD severity.[66]

Adults

In general, studies of BPD survivors in adulthood have utilized case control or prospective cohort study designs and have consistently reported significantly lower FEFs and FEV_1 than term controls. Several studies have demonstrated significantly decreased FEFs in adult survivors of BPD compared with adults who were preterm without BPD,[7,8] whereas other studies have not demonstrated this difference.[67] A regional cohort study[68] reported respiratory outcomes of 26 extremely preterm survivors (≤28 weeks of gestational age or ≤1000 g of birth weight) at 25 years of age compared to matched term-born subjects. Lung function was in the normal range in the majority of the extremely preterm survivors and few subjects reported respiratory symptoms, but methacholine responsiveness was more pronounced in the extremely preterm survivors than in the term-born young adults.[68]

The Padova BPD study[69] reported a longitudinal assessment of lung function in 17 survivors of moderate to severe BPD (born between 1991 and 1993) from birth to adulthood. These patients had Crs measurements done through 24 months of age and then FEFs at 2, 9, 15, 20, and 24 years of age. These patients demonstrated significant airway obstruction early in life, which tracked into adulthood with an FEV_1 at 24 years of age with a *z* score of −2.14 (i.e., 64% of predicted) demonstrating these survivors of BPD failed to achieve optimal lung function in early adulthood.[69] There was a significant correlation between Crs in the first days of life and subsequent measurements of forced flows and a significant correlation between forced flows at 2 years of age and subsequent flows. Therefore the assessment of neonatal/early infant lung function in preterm infants may help identify those at greatest risk for the development of ongoing lung disease and COPD as an adult.[69]

EVOLUTION OF EXERCISE TOLERANCE THROUGH ADULTHOOD

A meta-analysis[70] of 20 studies (685 preterm and 680 control subjects) showed that children and adults born preterm with or without BPD have a significantly lower oxygen uptake at maximal exercise than term-born controls, although the effect size was small. Some individual studies have not shown differences in exercise capacity between children born preterm and those born full term. In adults with a history of extreme prematurity, Clemm et al.[71] found only a minor reduction in exercise capacity that was primarily related to self-reported physical activity.

A study[72] performed ventilatory and sensory measurements before and during exercise in three groups of 18- to 31-year–old adults: 20 former premature adults without BPD, 15 former premature adults with BPD, and 20 full-term controls. The adults born very preterm with and without BPD demonstrated severe dyspnea and leg discomfort, which was associated with critical constraints on tidal volume expansion and reduced exercise tolerance. This occurred despite differences in expiratory flow limitation in patients with and without BPD, emphasizing the potential limitations of spirometry alone in the assessment of very preterm survivors. Continued research is needed to fully elucidate exercise capacity limitations in patients with BPD as they age.

NEED FOR PRIMARY PREVENTION OF BRONCHOPULMONARY DYSPLASIA IN VIEW OF PULMONARY FUNCTION TEST TRAJECTORIES

There are extremely preterm infants who do not develop BPD, supporting the premise that primary prevention of BPD is attainable. To accomplish this goal, interventions would likely have to occur prenatally or within a short period after birth[73] and many barriers must be overcome. These include the refinement of BPD risk and diagnosis by phenotype/endotypes, use of PFT phenotyping in patient recruitment, inclusion of BPD severity classifications in outcome measures, and improving the sensitivity and accuracy of the diagnosis of BPD as a modifiable outcome in future trials. Moreover, increased understanding of the molecular causal pathways that underlie the pathogenesis of BPD is required to design strategies to prevent BPD.

The recognition and refinement of BPD phenotypes, with increased focus on antenatal factors such as maternal smoking during pregnancy, intrauterine growth retardation, and placental dysfunction (which are major risk factors for BPD[12]), is underway. Vitamin C supplementation to pregnant smokers has been shown to improve infant PFT results and decrease wheeze through 1 year of age in term infants,[74,75] as well as could modify the development of BPD in preterm infants born to smokers. An increasingly recognized phenotype is BPD associated with pulmonary hypertension (PH). A longitudinal study[76] demonstrated echocardiogram-derived risk factors at 7 days of age were associated with the development of both BPD and PH.

The Challenge of Defining a "Healthy Lung" in the Premature Infant

To define the abnormal trajectory of a premature lung evolving to BPD, we must define "normal" lung growth, development, and function in the "healthy" preterm infant who does not progress to BPD. This is challenging given that premature infants are born at various junctures of the late canalicular/saccular stage of lung development and are exposed to a wide range of pre- and postnatal circumstances contributing to lung injury and repair. It also necessitates a new paradigm with increased focus and research on the evolution of lung health in the well infant delivered at term, a group largely unstudied, particularly in infancy.

BPD-related research has focused on the cause, risk factors, and interventions for this poorly defined and evolving disease. Several studies[77,78] have documented the clinical pulmonary evolution in extremely preterm infants and offer insight into possible postnatal windows for BPD prevention. A study of 1340 extremely preterm infants described three patterns of pulmonary disease over the first 2 weeks of life: 20% of infants had consistently low oxygen requirements and 17% of these infants developed BPD, nearly 38% had low initial oxygen needs that increased in week 2 of life and 51% developed BPD, and 43% of the infants had initial and consistently high oxygen needs and 76% developed BPD.[77] Future studies examining risk factors and exposures, particularly antenatal, and collecting robust functional and molecular biomarkers associated with the different phenotypes of premature infants and their pulmonary dysfunction are crucial to the primary prevention of BPD (Box 7.1).

BOX 7.1
Barriers to Primary Prevention Research and Clinical Trials in Bronchopulmonary Dysplasia

A. BARRIERS RELATED TO THE TARGETED PATIENT POPULATION

- Vulnerable (immature, developing) population of very premature infants.
- Need to balance risk/benefit of preventative strategies or interventions—some premature babies that would never get the disease will be exposed to an experimental therapy that could have side effects or cause harm.
- Institutional Review Board consent and ethical issues of dealing with children and vulnerable populations, including possible harm with no guarantee of benefit in a high-risk population.
- Bronchopulmonary dysplasia (BPD) is a rare disease necessitating multi-institutional collaborations:
  - De-regionalization of neonatal care
  - Need to organize academic centers into "consortiums" with the capacity to collect data and enroll patients in intervention trials for rapid scientific discovery
- Pharmaceutical companies are reluctant to study the neonatal population, given the limited numbers of patients and inherent risks of studying a critically ill pediatric population with high mortality and a long statute of limitations.
  - Best Pharmaceutical for Children Act: limitations in studying drug therapies in neonatal population.[79]

B. BARRIERS RELATED TO SCIENTIFIC KNOWLEDGE GAPS

- Limited understanding of normal lung growth and repair mechanisms; few tissue repositories for anatomic studies of lungs of babies who die from BPD or premature babies who recover from BPD and die of other causes.
- Poorly understood pathophysiology—multiple pathways to BPD.
- Unclear timing for primary prevention—does BPD start in utero, at delivery?
- Need for more information on how various BPD phenotypes evolve/mature over time
  - Limited BPD model systems: rodents may not be an ideal model for studying BPD prevention.
  - Long-standing primate model in San Antonio no longer funded.
  - History of novel, promising therapies in rodent studies that have not been translated to early phase clinical trials.
- Lack of validated early biomarkers that predict later disease onset.
- No good surrogates for important long-term respiratory outcomes.
  - Relatively poor correlation between a diagnosis of BPD and childhood respiratory disease.

C. SYSTEMATIC CLINICAL AND BUREAUCRATIC BARRIERS

- Poor phenotyping/definition of BPD: definition provides no information about pathophysiology, disease progression, or variability in lung pathology.
- Failure to examine severity of disease; some interventions (i.e., inhaled nitric oxide) may reduce disease severity but not incidence, as currently defined by O_2 use at 36 weeks.
- Failure to identify subpopulations with distinct mechanisms of disease.
- Clinical trials of combination therapies are hard to design and interpret but may be what is needed given the various mechanistic pathways and phenotypes.
- Double standard for the evidence: high bar for new therapies but not for established approaches, which may cause harm.
- Need for redesign of the clinical research machine plagued with inefficiencies and bureaucratic barriers.

Modified from McEvoy CT, Jain L, Schmidt B, Abman S, Bancalari E, Aschner JL. Bronchopulmonarydysplasia: NHLBI workshop on the primary prevention of chronic lung diseases. Ann Am Thorac Soc. *2014; 11 Suppl 3:S146–S153.*

FUTURE GOALS AND RESEARCH PRIORITIES FOR BRONCHOPULMONARY DYSPLASIA PREVENTION

BPD is categorized as a rare disease because there are an estimated 10,000–15,000 new cases per year in the United States. However, the significance of BPD spans the individual's lifetime, which at an estimated 65 years places the estimated prevalence of BPD at 1 million.[80]

Although adults with persistent symptoms of wheeze, breathlessness, and reduced exercise tolerance may have bronchial asthma, it is important to consider preterm birth as a potential cause; a medical history of prematurity is not consistently and specifically elicited by many internists and adult pulmonologists. Future progress will require longitudinal studies of PFTs, will ideally employ the same sensitive and specific PFT throughout the life span that does not require sedation, and will be performed in large populations of well-phenotyped individuals born preterm (with and without BPD) and healthy term controls to follow the progression of PFTs in the context of lung injury, developmental disruption, environmental exposures, and natural aging. There needs to be a particular focus during early adulthood on the maximum PFTs performed and whether there is an accelerated decline in PFT measurements with aging. Multifaceted physiologic and quantitative assessments are needed to define specific phenotypes to facilitate targeted biologic and genetic interventions that may need to begin very early to accomplish primary prevention of BPD.

The holy grail is the prevention of prematurity, which has proven elusive. Aside from prematurity prevention, perinatal interventions represent a unique opportunity in BPD prevention, as longitudinal studies show that small improvements in neonatal PFT results translate into large improvements in childhood and adult respiratory health.

FUNDING SOURCES

NHLBI R01 HL105447; NHLBI R01 HL129060 to CTM, UH3OD023320 to JLA.

Conflict of Interest

The authors have no conflicts of interest or affiliations with the companies that have direct financial interests in the subject matter of this article.

REFERENCES

1. Baraldi E, Carraro S, Filippone M. Bronchopulmonary dysplasia: definitions and long-term respiratory outcome. *Early Hum Dev*. 2009;85(Suppl 10):S1–S3.
2. Northway Jr WH, Rosan RC, Porter DY. Pulmonary disease following respirator therapy of hyaline-membrane disease. Bronchopulmonary dysplasia. *N Engl J Med*. 1967;276(7):357–368.
3. Jobe AH, Bancalari E. Bronchopulmonary dysplasia. *Am J Respir Crit Care Med*. 2001;163(7):1723–1729.
4. McEvoy CT, Jain L, Schmidt B, Abman S, Bancalari E, Aschner JL. Bronchopulmonary dysplasia: NHLBI workshop on the primary prevention of chronic lung diseases. *Ann Am Thorac Soc*. 2014;11(Suppl 3):S146–S153.
5. Stocks J, Hislop A, Sonnappa S. Early lung development: lifelong effect on respiratory health and disease. *Lancet Respir Med*. 2013;1(9):728–742.
6. Vom HM, Prenzel F, Uhlig HH, Robel-Tillig E. Pulmonary outcome in former preterm, very low birth weight children with bronchopulmonary dysplasia: a case-control follow-up at school age. *J Pediatr*. 2014;164(1):40–45.
7. Gough A, Linden M, Spence D, Patterson CC, Halliday HL, McGarvey LP. Impaired lung function and health status in adult survivors of bronchopulmonary dysplasia. *Eur Respir J*. 2014;43(3):808–816.
8. Gibson AM, Reddington C, McBride L, Callanan C, Robertson C, Doyle LW. Lung function in adult survivors of very low birth weight, with and without bronchopulmonary dysplasia. *Pediatr Pulmonol*. 2014;50(10):987–994.
9. Stern DA, Morgan WJ, Wright AL, Guerra S, Martinez FD. Poor airway function in early infancy and lung function by age 22 years: a non-selective longitudinal cohort study. *Lancet*. 2007;370(9589):758–764.
10. Martinez FD. Early-life origins of chronic obstructive pulmonary disease. *N Engl J Med*. 2016;375(9):871–878.
11. Lange P, Celli B, Agusti A, et al. Lung-function trajectories leading to chronic obstructive pulmonary disease. *N Engl J Med*. 2015;373(2):111–122.
12. Taglauer E, Abman SH, Keller RL. Recent advances in antenatal factors predisposing to bronchopulmonary dysplasia. *Semin Perinatol*. 2018;42(7):413–424.
13. Morrow LA, Wagner BD, Ingram DA, et al. Antenatal determinants of bronchopulmonary dysplasia and late respiratory disease in preterm infants. *Am J Respir Crit Care Med*. 2017;196(3):364–374.
14. Colin AA, McEvoy C, Castile RG. Respiratory morbidity and lung function in preterm infants of 32 to 36 weeks' gestational age. *Pediatrics*. 2010;126(1):115–128.
15. Kallapur SG, Kramer BW, Nitsos I, et al. Pulmonary and systemic inflammatory responses to intra-amniotic IL-1alpha in fetal sheep. *Am J Physiol Lung Cell Mol Physiol*. 2011;301(3):L285–L295.
16. Gappa M, Pillow JJ, Allen J, Mayer O, Stocks J. Lung function tests in neonates and infants with chronic lung disease: lung and chest-wall mechanics. *Pediatr Pulmonol*. 2006;41(4):291–317.
17. McEvoy C, Bowling S, Williamson K, Stewart M, Durand M. Functional residual capacity and passive compliance measurements after antenatal steroid therapy in preterm infants. *Pediatr Pulmonol*. 2001;31(6):425–430.
18. McEvoy C, Schilling D, Spitale P, Peters D, O'Malley J, Durand M. Decreased respiratory compliance in infants less than or equal to 32 weeks' gestation, delivered more than 7 days after antenatal steroid therapy. *Pediatrics*. 2008;121(5):e1032–e1038.
19. McEvoy C, Schilling D, Peters D, et al. Respiratory compliance in preterm infants after a single rescue course of antenatal steroids: a randomized controlled trial. *Am J Obstet Gynecol*. 2010;202(6):544–549.
20. Hjalmarson O, Sandberg KL. Effect of antenatal corticosteroid treatment on lung function in full-term newborn infants. *Neonatology*. 2011;100(1):32–36.
21. Dinger J, Topfer A, Schaller P, Schwarze R. Effect of positive end expiratory pressure on functional residual capacity and compliance in surfactant-treated preterm infants. *J Perinat Med*. 2001;29(2):137–143.
22. Di Fiore JM, Hibbs AM, Zadell AE, et al. The effect of inhaled nitric oxide on pulmonary function in preterm infants. *J Perinatol*. 2007;27(12):766–771.

23. Beydon N, Davis SD, Lombardi E, et al. An official American Thoracic Society/European Respiratory Society statement: pulmonary function testing in preschool children. *Am J Respir Crit Care Med*. 2007;175(12):1304–1345.
24. Rosenfeld M, Allen J, Arets BH, et al. An official American Thoracic Society workshop report: optimal lung function tests for monitoring cystic fibrosis, bronchopulmonary dysplasia, and recurrent wheezing in children less than 6 years of age. *Ann Am Thorac Soc*. 2013;10(2):S1–S11.
25. Wanger J, Clausen JL, Coates A, et al. Standardisation of the measurement of lung volumes. *Eur Respir J*. 2005; 26(3):511–522.
26. Dinger J, Topfer A, Schaller P, Schwarze R. Functional residual capacity and compliance of the respiratory system after surfactant treatment in premature infants with severe respiratory distress syndrome. *Eur J Pediatr*. 2002;161(9): 485–490.
27. Durand M, Mendoza ME, Tantivit P, Kugelman A, McEvoy C. A randomized trial of moderately early low-dose dexamethasone therapy in very low birth weight infants: dynamic pulmonary mechanics, oxygenation, and ventilation. *Pediatrics*. 2002;109(2):262–268.
28. Garite TJ, Kurtzman J, Maurel K, Clark R. Impact of a 'rescue course' of antenatal corticosteroids: a multicenter randomized placebo-controlled trial. *Am J Obstet Gynecol*. 2009;200(3):248–249.
29. Go M, Schilling D, Nguyen T, Durand M, McEvoy CT. Respiratory compliance in late preterm infants (34(0/7)-34(6/7) weeks) after antenatal steroid therapy. *J Pediatr*. 2018; 201:21–26.
30. Gyamfi-Bannerman C, Thom EA, Blackwell SC, et al. Antenatal betamethasone for women at risk for late preterm delivery. *N Engl J Med*. 2016;374(14):1311–1320.
31. Althabe F, Belizan JM, McClure EM, et al. A population-based, multifaceted strategy to implement antenatal corticosteroid treatment versus standard care for the reduction of neonatal mortality due to preterm birth in low-income and middle-income countries: the ACT cluster-randomised trial. *Lancet*. 2015;385(9968):629–639.
32. Morrow DK, Schilling D, McEvoy CT. Response to bronchodilators in very preterm infants with evolving bronchopulmonary dysplasia. *Res Rep Neonatol*. 2015;5: 113–117.
33. McEvoy C, Venigalla S, Schilling D, Clay N, Spitale P, Nguyen T. Respiratory function in healthy late preterm infants delivered at 33-36 weeks of gestation. *J Pediatr*. 2013; 162(3):464–469.
34. Hjalmarson O, Sandberg K. Abnormal lung function in healthy preterm infants. *Am J Respir Crit Care Med*. 2002; 165(1):83–87.
35. Kavvadia V, Greenough A, Dimitriou G, Itakura Y. Lung volume measurements in infants with and without chronic lung disease. *Eur J Pediatr*. 1998;157(4):336–339.
36. Kavvadia V, Greenough A, Dimitriou G. Early prediction of chronic oxygen dependency by lung function test results. *Pediatr Pulmonol*. 2000;29(1):19–26.
37. McEvoy C, Schilling D. *Pulmonary function in extremely low birth weight infants with bronchopulmonary dysplasia before hospital discharge. E-PAS 3540.6*. 2014.
38. Hjalmarson O, Sandberg KL. Lung function at term reflects severity of bronchopulmonary dysplasia. *J Pediatr*. 2005; 146(1):86–90.
39. Baraldi E, Filippone M, Trevisanuto D, Zanardo V, Zacchello F. Pulmonary function until two years of life in infants with bronchopulmonary dysplasia. *Am J Respir Crit Care Med*. 1997;155(1):149–155.
40. Friedrich L, Pitrez PM, Stein RT, Goldani M, Tepper R, Jones MH. Growth rate of lung function in healthy preterm infants. *Am J Respir Crit Care Med*. 2007;176(12): 1269–1273.
41. Jones M, Castile R, Davis S, et al. Forced expiratory flows and volumes in infants. Normative data and lung growth. *Am J Respir Crit Care Med*. 2000;161(2 Pt 1): 353–359.
42. Balinotti JE, Tiller CJ, Llapur CJ, et al. Growth of the lung parenchyma early in life. *Am J Respir Crit Care Med*. 2009; 179(2):134–137.
43. Balinotti JE, Chakr VC, Tiller C, et al. Growth of lung parenchyma in infants and toddlers with chronic lung disease of infancy. *Am J Respir Crit Care Med*. 2010;181(10): 1093–1097.
44. Assaf SJ, Chang DV, Tiller CJ, et al. Lung parenchymal development in premature infants without bronchopulmonary dysplasia. *Pediatr Pulmonol*. 2015;50(12): 1313–1319.
45. Zeman KL, Bennett WD. Growth of the small airways and alveoli from childhood to the adult lung measured by aerosol-derived airway morphometry. *J Appl Physiol*. 2006;100(3):965–971.
46. Lum S, Hulskamp G, Merkus P, Baraldi E, Hofhuis W, Stocks J. Lung function tests in neonates and infants with chronic lung disease: forced expiratory maneuvers. *Pediatr Pulmonol*. 2006;41(3):199–214.
47. Fakhoury KF, Sellers C, Smith EO, Rama JA, Fan LL. Serial measurements of lung function in a cohort of young children with bronchopulmonary dysplasia. *Pediatrics*. 2010; 125(6):e1441–e1447.
48. Filbrun AG, Popova AP, Linn MJ, McIntosh NA, Hershenson MB. Longitudinal measures of lung function in infants with bronchopulmonary dysplasia. *Pediatr Pulmonol*. 2011;46(4):369–375.
49. Thunqvist P, Gustafsson P, Norman M, Wickman M, Hallberg J. Lung function at 6 and 18 months after preterm birth in relation to severity of bronchopulmonary dysplasia. *Pediatr Pulmonol*. 2014;50(10):978–986.
50. Shepherd EG, Clouse BJ, Hasenstab KA, et al. Infant pulmonary function testing and phenotypes in severe bronchopulmonary dysplasia. *Pediatrics*. 2018;141(5): e20173350.
51. Robin B, Kim YJ, Huth J, et al. Pulmonary function in bronchopulmonary dysplasia. *Pediatr Pulmonol*. 2004; 37(3):236–242.

52. Hofhuis W, Huysman MW, Van Der Wiel EC, et al. Worsening of V'maxFRC in infants with chronic lung disease in the first year of life: a more favorable outcome after high-frequency oscillation ventilation. *Am J Respir Crit Care Med.* 2002;166(12 Pt 1):1539–1543.
53. Doyle LW. Respiratory function at age 8-9 years in extremely low birthweight/very preterm children born in Victoria in 1991-1992. *Pediatr Pulmonol.* 2006;41(6):570–576.
54. Doyle LW, Faber B, Callanan C, Freezer N, Ford GW, Davis NM. Bronchopulmonary dysplasia in very low birth weight subjects and lung function in late adolescence. *Pediatrics.* 2006;118(1):108–113.
55. Korhonen P, Laitinen J, Hyodynmaa E, Tammela O. Respiratory outcome in school-aged, very-low-birth-weight children in the surfactant era. *Acta Paediatr.* 2004;93(3):316–321.
56. Baraldi E, Bonetto G, Zacchello F, Filippone M. Low exhaled nitric oxide in school-age children with bronchopulmonary dysplasia and airflow limitation. *Am J Respir Crit Care Med.* 2005;171(1):68–72.
57. Vrijilandt EJ, Boezen HM, Gerritsen J, Stremmelaar EF, Duiverman EJ. Respiratory health in prematurely born preschool children with and without bronchopulmonary dysplasia. *J Pediatr.* 2007;150(3):256–261.
58. Fawke J, Lum S, Kirkby J, et al. Lung function and respiratory symptoms at 11 years in children born extremely preterm: the EPICure study. *Am J Respir Crit Care Med.* 2010;182(2):237–245.
59. Lum S, Kirkby J, Welsh L, Marlow N, Hennessy E, Stocks J. Nature and severity of lung function abnormalities in extremely pre-term children at 11 years of age. *Eur Respir J.* 2011;37(5):1199–1207.
60. Doyle LW, Ford GW, Olinsky A, Knoches AM, Callanan C. Bronchopulmonary dysplasia and very low birthweight: lung function at 11 years of age. *J Paediatr Child Health.* 1996;32(4):339–343.
61. Ronkainen E, Dunder T, Peltoniemi O, et al. New BPD predicts lung function at school age: follow-up study and meta-analysis. *Pediatr Pulmonol.* 2015;50(11):1090–1098.
62. Cazzato S, Ridolfi L, Bernardi F, Faldella G, Bertelli L. Lung function outcome at school age in very low birth weight children. *Pediatr Pulmonol.* 2013;48(8):830–837.
63. Simpson SJ, Turkovic L, Wilson AC, et al. Lung function trajectories throughout childhood in survivors of very preterm birth: a longitudinal cohort study. *Lancet Child Adolesc Health.* 2018;2(5):350–359.
64. Doyle LW, Adams AM, Robertson C, et al. Increasing airway obstruction from 8 to 18 years in extremely preterm/low-birthweight survivors born in the surfactant era. *Thorax.* 2017;72(8):712–719.
65. Doyle LW, Carse E, Adams AM, Ranganathan S, Opie G, Cheong JLY. Ventilation in extremely preterm infants and respiratory function at 8 years. *N Engl J Med.* 2017;377(4):329–337.
66. Landry JS, Chan T, Lands L, Menzies D. Long-term impact of bronchopulmonary dysplasia on pulmonary function. *Can Respir J.* 2011;18(5):265–270.
67. Vrijlandt EJ, Gerritsen J, Boezen HM, Grevink RG, Duiverman EJ. Lung function and exercise capacity in young adults born prematurely. *Am J Respir Crit Care Med.* 2006;173(8):890–896.
68. Vollsaeter M, Clemm HH, Satrell E, et al. Adult respiratory outcomes of extreme preterm birth - a regional cohort study. *Ann Am Thorac Soc.* 2015;12(3):313–322.
69. Moschino L, Stocchero M, Filippone M, Carraro S, Baraldi E. Longitudinal assessment of lung function in survivors of bronchopulmonary dysplasia from birth to adulthood. The Padova BPD study. *Am J Respir Crit Care Med.* 2018;198(1):134–137.
70. Edwards MO, Kotecha SJ, Lowe J, et al. Effect of preterm birth on exercise capacity: a systematic review and meta-analysis. *Pediatr Pulmonol.* 2015;50(3):293–301.
71. Clemm HH, Vollsaeter M, Roksund OD, Eide GE, Markestad T, Halvorsen T. Exercise capacity after extremely preterm birth. Development from adolescence to adulthood. *Ann Am Thorac Soc.* 2014;11(4):537–545.
72. Lovering AT, Elliott JE, Laurie SS, et al. Ventilatory and sensory responses in adult survivors of preterm birth and bronchopulmonary dysplasia with reduced exercise capacity. *Ann Am Thorac Soc.* 2014;11(10):1528–1537.
73. Higgins RD, Jobe AH, Koso-Thomas M, et al. Bronchopulmonary dysplasia: executive summary of a workshop. *J Pediatr.* 2018;197:300–308.
74. McEvoy CT, Schilling D, Clay N, et al. Vitamin C supplementation for pregnant smoking women and pulmonary function in their newborn infants: a randomized clinical trial. *JAMA.* 2014;311(20):2074–2082.
75. McEvoy CT, Shorey-Kendrick LE, Milner K, et al. Oral vitamin C (500 mg/day) to pregnant smokers improves infant airway function at 3 Months (VCSIP): a randomized trial. *Am J Respir Crit Care Med.* 2018. https://doi.org/10.1164/rccm.201805-1011OC [Epub ahead of print].
76. Mourani PM, Sontag MK, Younoszai A, et al. Early pulmonary vascular disease in preterm infants at risk for bronchopulmonary dysplasia. *Am J Respir Crit Care Med.* 2015;191(1):87–95.
77. Laughon M, Allred EN, Bose C, et al. Patterns of respiratory disease during the first 2 postnatal weeks in extremely premature infants. *Pediatrics.* 2009;123(4):1124–1131.
78. Rojas MA, Gonzalez A, Bancalari E, Claure N, Poole C, Silva-Neto G. Changing trends in the epidemiology and pathogenesis of neonatal chronic lung disease. *J Pediatr.* 1995;126(4):605–610.
79. Davis JM, Connor EM, Wood AJ. The need for rigorous evidence on medication use in preterm infants: is it time for a neonatal rule? *JAMA.* 2012;308:1435–1436.
80. Bhandari A, McGrath-Morrow S. Long-term pulmonary outcomes of patients with bronchopulmonary dysplasia. *Semin Perinatol.* 2013;37(2):132–137.

Pulmonary Hypertension and Cardiac Changes in BPD: Etiology, Detection, and Management

DOUGLAS BUSH, MD • ERICA W. MANDELL, MD • STEVEN H. ABMAN, MD • CHRISTOPHER D. BAKER, MD

INTRODUCTION

Pulmonary hypertension (PH) is frequently identified in neonates and infants in the neonatal intensive care unit (NICU) and has diverse underlying etiologies, including failure in transition to extrauterine life resulting in persistent pulmonary hypertension of the newborn (PPHN); congenital heart disease (CHD) both with and without intracardiac shunts; pulmonary vein stenosis or capillary hemangiomatosis; developmental lung diseases such as omphalocele and other conditions associated with lung hypoplasia; conditions thought to be due to single-gene mutations such as FOXF1 (alveolar capillary dysplasia), TBX4 and other genes[1]; congenital diaphragmatic hernia (CDH); bronchopulmonary dysplasia (BPD); and others (Table 8.1). Despite major advances in our understanding of disease pathophysiology and the growing availability of PH-specific drug therapies, PH continues to contribute to high, and perhaps increasing, morbidity and mortality in infants and children. As recently summarized by the Pediatric Task Force of the World Symposium on PH in 2018, PH associated with preterm infants, especially in the setting of BPD, has become recognized as one of the most common causes of PH throughout childhood.[2] As such, PH remains a frequent and significant challenge to neonatologists and related consultants.

Novel insights into the structural growth and maturation of the lung circulation during development as well as sustained abnormalities of lung vascular growth and function in response to perinatal injury have broadened the concept of "pulmonary vascular disease (PVD)" beyond the clinical problem of PH alone (Fig. 8.1).[3] High pulmonary artery pressure (PAP) due to altered regulation of vascular tone and structural remodeling of the vascular wall have been long recognized as key components of PH.[4] Additionally, recent studies have highlighted the importance of decreased lung vascular growth due to altered vasculogenic or angiogenic mechanisms as further contributors to PH.[5] Early disruption of vascular growth may slow growth of the distal lung microvasculature and decrease lung surface area for gas exchange and injury to the developing pulmonary vascular endothelium may further impair alveolar growth through disruption of paracrine or "angiocrine" signaling between endothelium and epithelium. Abnormal lung vascular growth may not only increase susceptibility for PH and contribute to the severity of BPD in preterm infants, but such changes persist into late childhood and early adulthood.[6–8] Thus, our understanding of the lung circulation now includes greater awareness of several distinct phenotypes of PVD associated with prematurity, including problems during the perinatal transition ("early PH"), the development of sustained or chronic PH later in the clinical course ("late PH"), and finally, sustained PVD that is characterized by exercise intolerance, higher risk for PH later in life, and cardiovascular (CV) problems during adulthood.[6]

In this chapter, we present our current understanding of BPD-associated PH and its clinical management. We first discuss mechanisms that contribute to early PH in preterm infants, highlighting distinct features of PPHN physiology in preterm infants and the potential role of early PVD by echocardiography as a clinical biomarker of the risk for subsequent PH and BPD severity in preterm infants. We then present diagnostic approaches and challenges in assessing PH in BPD infants; clinical strategies for treatment; and finally, a brief

Updates on Neonatal Chronic Lung Disease. https://doi.org/10.1016/B978-0-323-68353-1.00008-7

TABLE 8.1
Developmental Lung Disorders Associated With Pulmonary Hypertension.

Clinical Disorder	Associated Gene Mutation
Bronchopulmonary dysplasia	
Congenital diaphragmatic hernia	
Down syndrome	Trisomy 21
Alveolar capillary dysplasia with "misalignment of veins"	FOXF1 (Forkhead boxFl)
Lung hypoplasia, acinar dysplasia	
Abdominal wall defects	
Giant omphalocele	
Gastroschisis	
Prune-belly syndrome	
Small patella syndrome	TBX4 (T-box 4)
Childhood interstitial lung disorders	
Surfactant protein abnormalities	
	SFTPB (surfactant protein B)
	SFTPC (surfactant protein C)
	ABCA3 (ATP binding cassette subfamily A member 3)
	TTF-1 (Thyroid transcription factor-I) NKX2.1 (NK2 homeobox 1)
Pulmonary interstitial glycogenosis	
Pulmonary alveolar proteinosis	CSF2RA (colony stimulating factor 2 receptor alpha)
Pulmonary lymphangiectasia	
Filamin A mutations	FLXA (Filamin A)

Adapted from Rosenzweig, EB., et al., Paediatric pulmonary arterial hypertension: updates on definition, classification, diagnostics and management. *Eur Respir J*. 2018 and Abman, S.H., et al., Pediatric pulmonary hypertension: guidelines from the American heart association and American thoracic society. *Circulation*. 2015;132(21) 2037–2099.

discussion of the late manifestations of PH or PVD after NICU discharge.

PULMONARY HYPERTENSION: DEFINITIONS

The definition of PH has recently been updated and is now defined as a mean pulmonary arterial pressure (mPAP) $\geq$ 20 mmHg for both pediatric and adult diagnoses.[2] PH is further differentiated into pulmonary arterial hypertension (PAH) if pulmonary vascular resistance (PVR) is elevated in the setting of a normal pulmonary artery occlusion pressure (PAOP) and pulmonary hypertensive venous disease if PAOP is elevated.[2,9] The World Health Organization (WHO) characterizes PH into five main groups.[2] Group I is characterized by PAH with five of seven subgroups relevant to infant disease including PH associated with CHD, with overt pulmonary veno-occlusive or capillary disease (PVOD/PCH), with PPHN (early PH), with identified genetic causes or that are idiopathic. Group II is PH secondary to left-sided heart disease and can frequently be identified in neonates with left ventricular (LV) outflow tract obstructions causing postcapillary hypertension (e.g., coarctation of the aorta). Group III is PH due to lung disease and/or hypoxia and includes developmental lung diseases such as BPD and pulmonary hypoplasia, such as that associated with CDH and interstitial lung diseases including surfactant protein abnormalities (Table 8.1). Group IV is pulmonary artery obstruction such as chronic thromboembolic PH, a rare etiology of PH in children. Finally, Group V is PH with unclear or multifactorial mechanisms, which includes various hematologic, systemic, and metabolic disorders that do not easily fit into other classification groups.[9] Appropriate classification of PH, related to etiology, is critical as this allows for appropriate targeting of therapeutic intervention.

Physiologically defining PH in the first few months after term or preterm birth presents several unique challenges due to the dynamic nature of the transition of the lung circulation during this time period.[2,9] Elevated PAP represents normal physiology in utero and is not uncommon to detect by echocardiogram in term and preterm infants during the early postnatal period. There is clearly, however, a need to more accurately define pathologic PH in this time window. PPHN is defined by the presence of extrapulmonary right-to-left shunting across the foramen ovale or patent ductus arteriosus (PDA), which leads to hypoxemia. Similar to term and near-term neonates, PPHN physiology can also contribute to hypoxemia in preterm infants shortly after

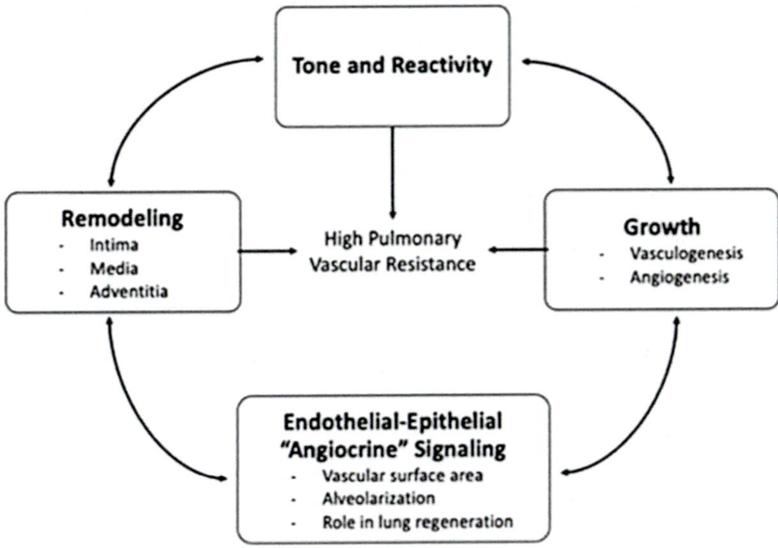

FIG. 8.1 Components of neonatal pulmonary vascular disease. (With permission from S.H. Abman.)

birth.[2,9,10] A clearly defined level of estimated PAP to define PH in this setting is lacking. As such, PPHN is currently defined physiologically by hypoxemia due to the demonstration of predominant right-to-left shunt, as best defined by echocardiography, and not by oxygenation alone. Many infants, especially preterm infants, can have evidence of delayed transition of the lung circulation due to the failure of pulmonary vasodilation at birth. This delayed transition can be associated with variable degrees of postnatal lung parenchymal disease, lung hypoplasia including that from mid-trimester onset oligohydramnios, in utero abnormalities of pulmonary blood flow (e.g., premature closure of the ductus arteriosus), and other diseases. These infants may also have evidence of pulmonary venous hypertension due to left heart dysfunction.[11] Cardiopulmonary interactions during the acute transitional period after birth often contribute to the degree of hypoxemia related to shunt and must be accounted for during the diagnostic evaluation. Assessment of oxygenation including oxygenation index (OI) reflects the severity of overall cardiopulmonary disease but is not specific for PPHN physiology in term or preterm neonates. Furthermore, it does not accurately differentiate between the severity of parenchymal lung disease and the degree of shunt as the primary cause of hypoxemic respiratory failure. As a result, many sick neonates, for example with severe surfactant deficiency or respiratory distress syndrome (RDS), will have markedly elevated OI in the absence of PPHN physiology. Therefore, OI and other assessments of inadequate oxygenation have no diagnostic role for PH in sick neonates. Nevertheless, hypoxia is an indicator of potential PH and responsiveness to increased oxygenation and hyperventilation can be useful as markers for predicting reversibility of PH with pulmonary vasodilator therapy, especially if hypoxemia is due to extrapulmonary shunt.

There remains a need for developing a better understanding of the different patterns of change in PAP during the dynamic period after birth in preterm and term infants and related physiologic implications. Although in the past, neonatologists often thought that premature infants lacked the vessel muscularization to present with PPHN due to vasoconstriction, several studies clearly demonstrate that this is incorrect. Several case series over the past 3 decades have clearly shown that inhaled NO can induce marked increases in oxygenation in selected preterm infants with echo-confirmed PPHN physiology.[9] More recently, a study of serial changes in the estimated levels of PH by echocardiography described several different patterns of transition in preterm infants and demonstrated striking changes in delayed pulmonary vascular transition that were associated with the degree of prematurity (Fig. 8.2).[12] Importantly, preterm infants with delayed pulmonary vascular transition had the highest risk for the subsequent development of BPD and late death.

The association of PH in established BPD fits into the WHO Group III classification. In 2001, an NICHD/NHLBI workgroup defined BPD, the chronic lung disease of prematurity, as an oxygen requirement or greater respiratory support for at least 28 days.[13]

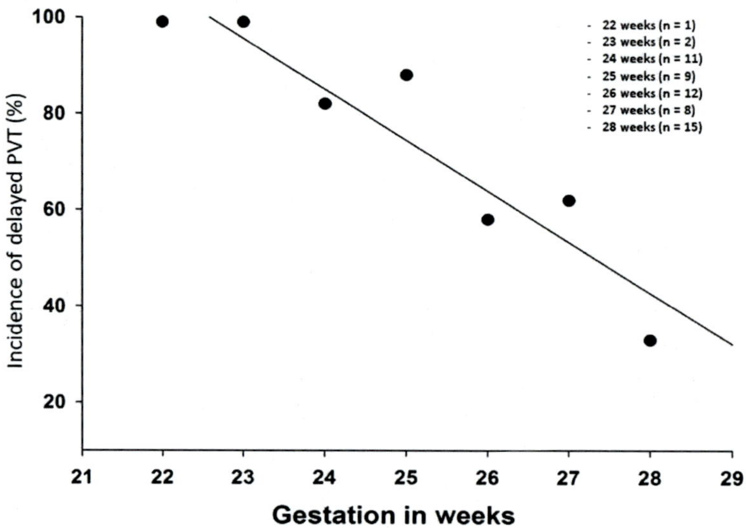

FIG. 8.2 Association of delayed pulmonary vascular transition (PVT) with gestational age (Mirza H., et al. Natural history of postnatal cardiopulmonary adaptation in infants born extremely preterm and risk for death or bronchopulmonary dysplasia. *J Pediatr*. 2018;198:187-193 e1.)

BPD severity is then determined by the level of respiratory support at 36 weeks postconceptual age: no oxygen therapy for mild BPD, $FiO_2 < 0.30$ for moderate BPD, and $FiO_2 \geq 0.30$ or positive pressure dependence for severe BPD.[13] Using this definition, a recent metaanalysis identified a prevalence of PH in 6% of neonates with mild BPD, 12% with moderate BPD, and 39% in severe BPD.[14] This same report identified a high cumulative mortality rate of 16% among infants with both BPD and PH, increasing to 40% in studies that followed children through the first 2 years of life.[14] BPD is therefore a significant risk factor for the development of late PH. Furthermore, with relatively stable rates of BPD (approximately 40%) in infants born at less than 28 weeks gestation, PH continues to have a significant impact on morbidity and mortality in this population.[15,16] Managing PH in preterm infants requires early screening of those at risk and an understanding of their complex cardiopulmonary physiology in order to appropriately intervene.

PATHOBIOLOGY OF PH IN BRONCHOPULMONARY DYSPLASIA

Impaired pulmonary vascular development secondary to genetic predisposition, antenatal complications of pregnancy, premature delivery, as well as perinatal and postnatal insults contributes to the development of BPD (Table 8.2).[17] Many of these insults impair

TABLE 8.2
Risk Factors for the Development of BPD.

Prenatal Risk Factors	Intrauterine Growth Restriction Mid-trimester oligohydramnios Lack of antenatal corticosteroids Maternal chorioamnionitis Maternal tobacco exposure Maternal drug use Gestational diabetes Maternal hypertension and preeclampsia Genetic factors Male gender
Risk factors at birth	Premature birth Low birth weight Lower level of neonatal intensive care at birth hospital Lower APGAR scores Perinatal asphyxia
Postnatal risk factors	Hyperoxia Hypoxia Inflammation Infection Ventilator-induced lung injury Patent ductus arteriosus Atrial septal defect Gastroesophageal reflux

Adapted from Higgins RD., et al., Bronchopulmonary dysplasia: executive summary of a workshop. *J Pediatr*. 2018;197 300–308.

vascular growth secondary to their modulating effects on vascular endothelial growth factor (VEGF) activity.[18] VEGF has been identified as a critical growth factor in pulmonary vascular development and subsequent alveolarization. In preclinical models, impairments in VEGF signaling have been shown to cause the hypoplastic vascular and alveolar phenotype seen in BPD.[19,20] A reduced vascular surface area limits the capacitance of the pulmonary capillary bed and leads to early vascular recruitment and full distension of the vasculature with increased cardiac output and pulmonary vascular blood flow.[21,22] Ohm's law implies that increased pulmonary blood flow directly results in increased PAP if resistance does not decrease (as pressure = flow x resistance). Therefore, a reduced vascular surface area, particularly when coupled with hemodynamically significant left-to-right intracardiac shunt lesions (PDA, atrial septal defect (ASD), ventricular septal defect (VSD)), increases the risk of developing PH.[23] Such pulmonary overcirculation can contribute to further endothelial injury and dysfunction, which can impair endothelial-mediated suppression of quiescent smooth muscle cells leading to medial thickening, pulmonary arterial smooth muscle remodeling, and increased PVR.[4,24] This concept is further supported by recent studies in which the persistence of an ASD in preterm infants accelerated the development of PH in BPD.[25,26] Vascular resistance is further challenged in the presence of significant pulmonary disease resulting in hypoxia and hypercarbia (Fig. 8.3).

Early respiratory challenges in ventilator management of the critically ill premature neonate increase the risk of ventilator-induced lung injury due to volutrauma, atelectasis, regional hypoxemia, hyperoxia, infection, and aspiration. Each of these factors contributes to disrupted lung development, regional vasoconstriction, and increased PVR.[27,28] Airways disease, mucus plugging, and inflammation cause regional hyperinflation, prolonged time constants, retained carbon dioxide, and acidosis in mechanically ventilated neonates.[29] Regional hyperinflation can compress intraalveolar pulmonary capillaries and increase mechanical stress and resistance within the pulmonary circulation. Adjacent atelectatic lung regions also experience hypoxic pulmonary vasoconstriction. These early insults, especially if sustained over prolonged periods, contribute to the development of PH in children with BPD.[27,28]

RISK FACTORS FOR DEVELOPING PH IN NEONATES WITH BPD

Given the substantial morbidity, mortality, and considerable expense in evaluating and treating infants with PH,[30] it is important to have a high index of suspicion

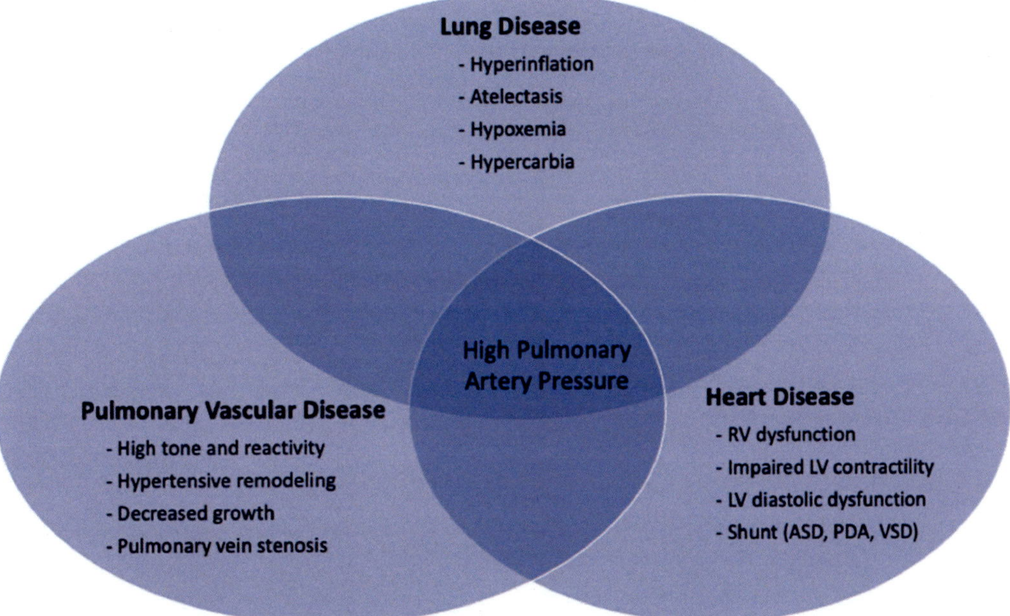

FIG. 8.3 The role of heart-lung-pulmonary vascular interactions in the physiology of pulmonary hypertension in bronchopulmonary dysplasia. *ASD*, atrial septal defect; *LV*, left ventricular; *PDA*, patent ductus arteriosus; *VSD*, ventricular septal defect.

and to implement strategic screening practices. Both antenatal and postnatal risk factors for the development of PH in infants with BPD have been identified and warrant consideration (Fig. 8.4). Fetal growth restriction is a major risk factor for progression to PH, particularly in those with birth weight below the 25th percentile.[31,32] Placental insufficiency due to maternal vascular underperfusion in the clinical setting of preeclampsia, chronic hypertension, and chorioamnionitis were significant in utero risk factors for the development of PH in infants with BPD[33] although some of these remain controversial.[14] Further, an antiangiogenic state may contribute to impaired lung development as suggested by reduced levels of cord blood proangiogenic factors[34] and increased levels of maternal antiangiogenic factors[35,36] suggesting a pathomechanism for reduced fetal vascular development and a possible therapeutic target (Fig. 8.5).[37] A recent metaanalysis concluded that a gestational age (GA) of less than 28 weeks at birth, low birth weight, oligohydramnios, and other antenatal factors are strongly associated with a diagnosis of BPD-associated PH.[14] In the postnatal period, PH has a strong association with necrotizing enterocolitis (NEC) as well as a weak association with the presence of a PDA and the need for its ligation.[14,32] Thus, the most premature and smallest infants are at significant risk for developing PH and those experiencing inflammatory insults, such as NEC, are at even greater risk. Additional comorbidities associated with PH in infants with BPD include retinopathy of prematurity, intraventricular hemorrhage, LV dysfunction, and the presence of an ASD.[14,38,39] Recently, LV dysfunction has been reported as a potential contributor to the development of PH in children with severe BPD.[39,40] An ASD with left-to-right shunt may be a previously underappreciated risk factor warranting additional consideration and study.[25,38]

SCREENING AND EVALUATION

While the gold standard for diagnosing PH remains a right heart catheterization and direct measurement of pulmonary hemodynamics, this is not always practical or possible in neonates with BPD. Echocardiography is a well-established, noninvasive tool for screening neonates with BPD for PH.[41,42] Importantly, echocardiographic screening in preterm infants as early as day 7 of life can predict late PH (as defined by PH at 36 weeks GA) offering opportunity for earlier therapeutic interventions.[43] Early echocardiogram screening and evaluation of preterm infants with BPD for PH has been recommended in the 2015 American Heart Association and American Thoracic Society pediatric PH guidelines and by the Pediatric Pulmonary Hypertension Network

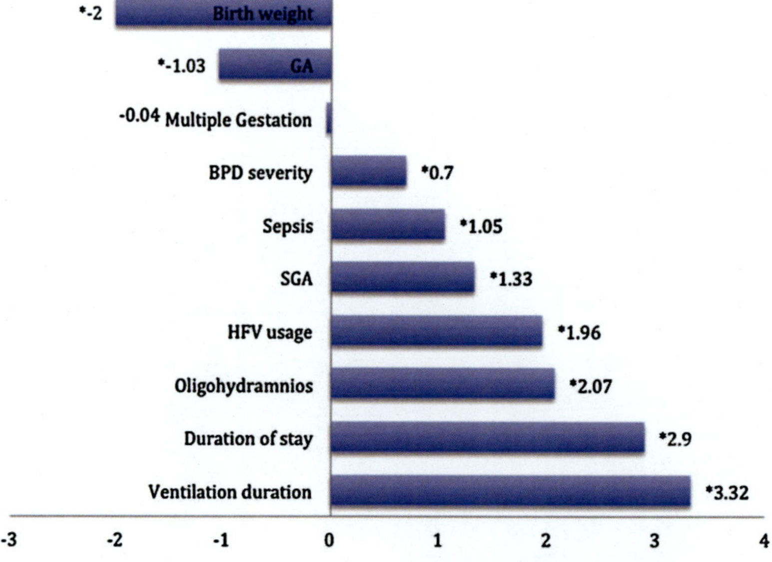

FIG. 8.4 Risk factors for BPD-Associated pulmonary hypertension. *BPD*, bronchopulmonary dysplasia; *GA*, gestational age; *HFV*, high-frequency ventilation; *SGA*, small for gestational age (From Nagiub M., et al. Risk factors for development of pulmonary hypertension in infants with bronchopulmonary dysplasia: systematic review and meta-analysis. *Paediatr Respir Rev*. 2017;23:27–32.)

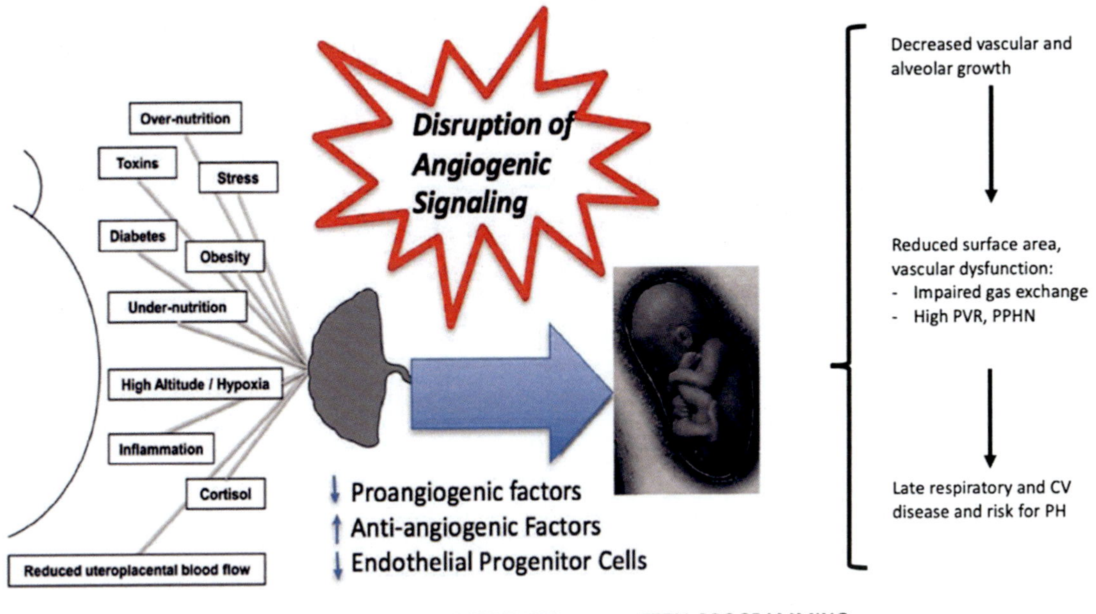

FIG. 8.5 Antenatal vascular origins of bronchopulmonary dysplasia. *CV*, cardiovascular; *PH*, pulmonary hypertension; *PPHN*, persistent pulmonary hypertension of the newborn; *PVR*, pulmonary vascular resistance. (Adapted from Mandell EW., Abman SH. Fetal vascular origins of bronchopulmonary dysplasia. *J Pediatr*. 2017;185:7-10 e1.)

(PPHNet).[9,43,44] Among other recommendations, these guidelines suggest early echocardiographic screening of preterm infants with severe respiratory distress requiring high levels of respiratory support, especially those with more extreme prematurity (<26 weeks) and those with a slow rate of clinical improvement of underlying cardiopulmonary disease. Additionally, per consensus recommendation, infants with established BPD as diagnosed at 36 weeks gestation by NIH criteria should be screened for PH with echocardiography, especially in those with severe BPD due to the high prevalence of PH (up to 50%) in this subgroup (Fig. 8.6).[9,44] This is important because a diagnosis of PH affects clinical management in the NICU and long-term follow-up after NICU discharge (see below). For example, the presence of echocardiographic evidence of PH would suggest the need to target higher oxygen saturations, to avoid even brief exposure to intermittent hypoxia and to follow clinical course more closely after NICU discharge. Infants with BPD and PH are at greater risk for recurrent respiratory readmissions, acute exacerbations, and severe PH during acute viral illness or other stresses.

The role of cardiac catheterization in infants with BPD and suspected or identified PH is uncertain, but is generally considered for infants with severe levels of PH by echocardiogram, poor responsiveness to aggressive respiratory support, sustained PH despite PH-targeted drug therapy or consideration for systemic prostanoid therapy (see below), concern for or identification of pulmonary vein stenosis by echocardiogram, uncertain physiologic role of PDA, ASD, or VSD in contributing to PH, and recurrent or persistent pulmonary edema that may worsen with PH therapy.

In addition to echocardiography, brain natriuretic peptide (BNP) or its prohormone, N-terminal probrain natriuretic peptide (NT-proBNP) may be helpful biomarkers for use in trending PH progression or the response to therapy in children with established BPD and PH.[45–48] NT-proBNP is secreted by cardiomyocytes in response to increased stretch and may serve as a useful biomarker for monitoring PVD in pediatric PAH.[49] The European Pediatric Pulmonary Vascular Disease Network and PPHNet have recommended the use of BNP or NT-proBNP as biomarkers for monitoring PH disease in children with PH associated with chronic lung diseases of prematurity, although cutoff values have not been suggested.[44,50] Levels can be assessed at the time of initial diagnosis of PH and can be used to monitor response to therapies or to suggest acute

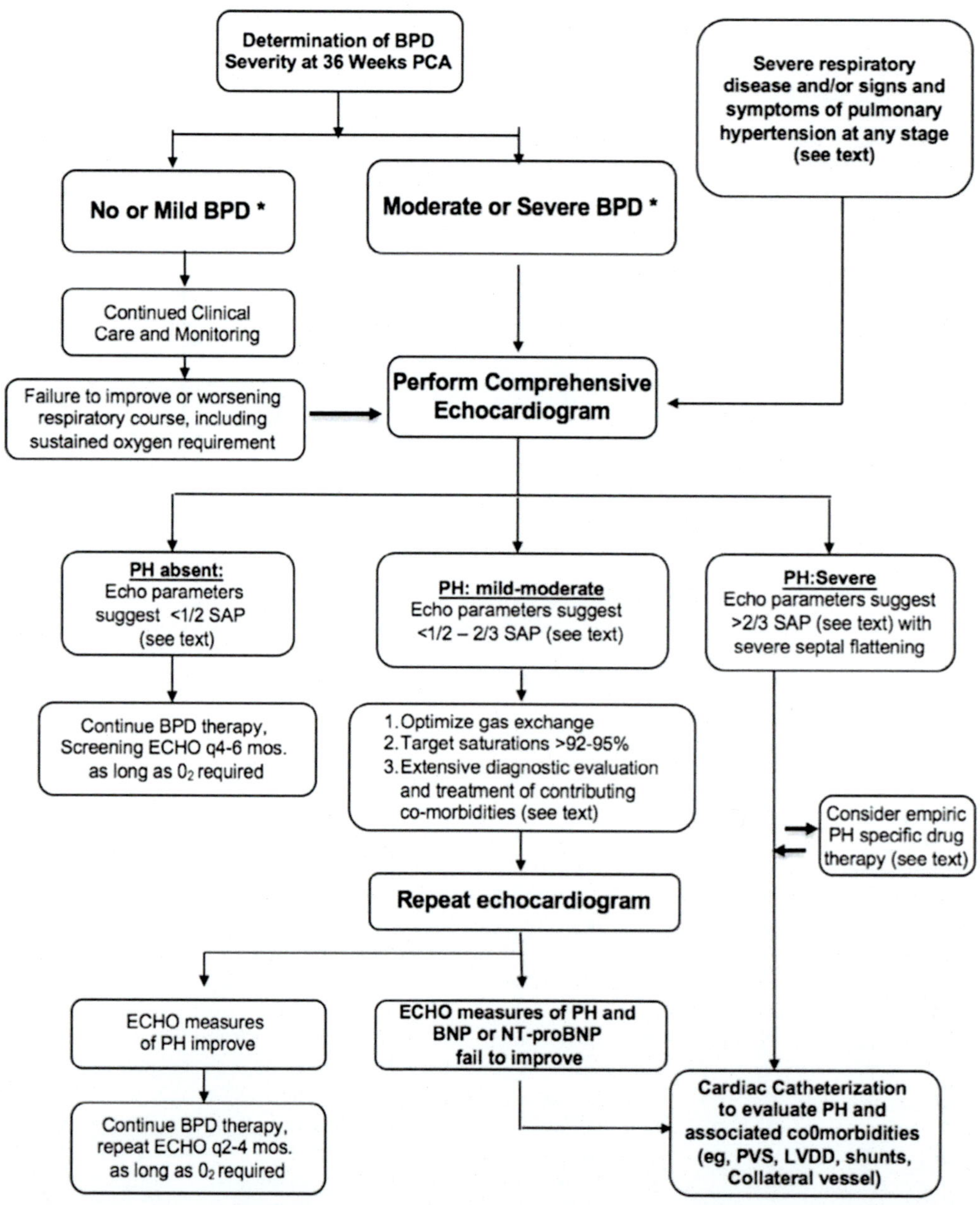

FIG. 8.6 Algorithm for diagnostic approach to evaluation of BPD-Associated PH. *BPD*, bronchopulmonary dysplasia; *PCA*, postconceptual age; *PH*, pulmonary hypertension. (From Krishnan U., et al. Evaluation and management of pulmonary hypertension in children with bronchopulmonary dysplasia. *J Pediatr*. 2017;188:24-34 e1.)

clinical decompensations when other tools, such as echocardiogram, are not readily available. Importantly, BNP and NT-proBNP are not specific for the diagnosis of PH since they may also be altered by other causes of myocardial stress.[49] However, changes in these levels along with serial echocardiograms may aid clinicians in deciding when to alter clinical strategies or adjust PH-targeted medications in preterm infants. Although novel biomarkers for identifying preterm infants at risk for developing PH in the NICU have been reported, these have yet to be sufficiently validated for clinical use. Recently, an unbiased, aptamer-based approach identified 18 such proteins, including several involved in angiogenesis.[51] These important studies may suggest molecular pathways involved in disease pathogenesis and may provide opportunity for therapeutic intervention.

MANAGEMENT

A recent interdisciplinary work group has put forth a review of management strategies for infants with severe BPD[29] and a consensus guideline has been published by the PPHNet[44] both of which are relevant to the discussion below. It is important to recognize that children with BPD and PH may benefit more from treatment of underlying respiratory disease than from pulmonary arterial vasodilator therapy.[9] Targeting appropriate respiratory support for the evolving lung disease or hypoxemia is critical to reducing the risk of progressive PH and right ventricular dysfunction. Given the prior discussion on the pathophysiology of PH in children with BPD, one should consider interventions that target hemodynamically significant intracardiac shunts, appropriate ventilatory and oxygenation strategies, those that reduce the degree of pulmonary arterial vasoconstriction, and those that reduce the risk or burden of ongoing respiratory insults (such as aspiration).

Closure of ASD and PDA in Infants with BPD and PH: Cardiac catheterization can be utilized in select infants with BPD, although with some risk, to understand the hemodynamic contribution of ASD or PDA shunts to the diagnosis of PH and differentiate between high pulmonary blood flow and high PVR. In the setting of high PVR, closure should be delayed; if high mPAP is due to high flow, these lesions can often be test-occluded during the study and then closed within the same procedure if necessary.

Ventilation and Oxygenation Strategies in BPD: The BPD Collaborative recently summarized the challenges of and strategies for mechanical ventilation in infants with BPD, especially with severe PH.[29] Briefly, the heterogeneous nature of lung disease in evolving or established BPD, as reflected by marked regional variation of time constants, mandates a different approach to ventilator management that is distinct from the traditional "lung protective strategies" for early ventilator management of preterm infants (see Chapter 18 Management of severe BPD requiring chronic medical support). After the early stages of respiratory distress in preterm infants, sustained ventilator dependence often reflects the need to transition ventilator approaches to better match the strikingly different lung physiology observed in established chronic lung disease.[29] Often, this requires a combination of larger tidal volumes, longer inspiratory times, and slower rates to enhance gas distribution throughout the lung, avoid atelectasis, reduce dead space ventilation, and reduce the level of supplemental oxygen needed to maintain adequate oxygenation (Fig. 8.7). These strategies can be challenging to implement and often run contrary to ventilator strategies utilized for RDS.

Further, sustaining optimal lung volumes (e.g., functional residual capacity (FRC)) and avoiding atelectasis requires a multifaceted approach necessitating higher positive end expiratory pressure (PEEP; >6–8 cmH_2O) and larger tidal volumes (Vt; 8–12 mL/kg) than those used for RDS. If high peak pressures are observed, a prolongation of inspiratory time (Ti) can be considered to improve mean airway pressure (MAP) while reducing peak pressures required to obtain the targeted Vt. Prone positioning allows for improved postural drainage of secretions in the posterior lung fields, reduces atelectasis, improves respiratory system resistance, improves ventilation-to-perfusion (V/Q) matching, and may reduce PVR in doing so.[23,52] Targeting a higher PEEP improves the recruitment of atelectatic lung regions, may reduce airways resistance, and optimizes chest wall compliance by improving ventilation around FRC and improving the mechanics of the diaphragm in relation to the thoracic cage.[53] However, excessively high PEEP may reduce right ventricle (RV) preload and increase PVR in extraalveolar vessels. The impact of PEEP on pulmonary blood flow must be taken into consideration in managing the child with PH.[54]

The long time constant, or time it takes a lung region to exhale 2/3 of its volume, requires a prolonged exhalation time for appropriate ventilation. This typically means a reduction in the mechanical ventilator set respiratory rate. Minute ventilation should be accommodated through increases in Vt (~8–12 mL/kg) once acute respiratory insults are no longer active. Increased Vt with an elongated Ti allows for improved distribution of gas through heterogeneous lung regions and may improve recruitment by reducing atelectasis.

In the acutely ill neonate, agitation can contribute to patient-ventilator asynchrony, tachypnea, and impaired exhalation time which may exacerbate hyperinflation and further increase PVR. Temporary use of agents for sedation, analgesia, and even neuromuscular blockade may be required in those with life-threatening PH crises or those who remain unstable after ventilatory support

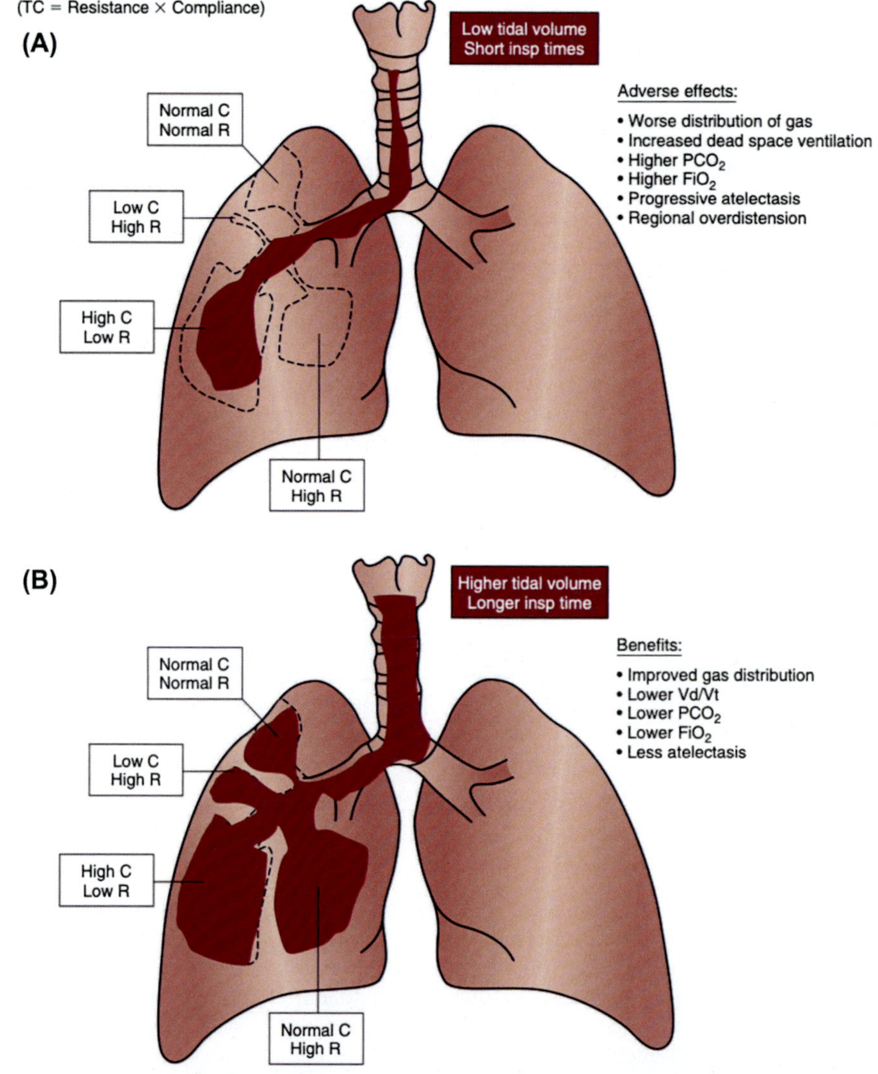

FIG. 8.7 Heterogeneity of lung disease in established BPD: role of variable time constants. BPD, bronchopulmonary dysplasia. (From Abman SH, Nelin L. Management of severe BPD. In, *The Newborn Lung: Neoanatology Questions and Controversies*, 2nd ed, Bancalari E (ed), Philadelphia: Elsevier, 2012.)

has been optimized. Overall success of long-term respiratory support is often defined by reduced distress, enhanced interactions with mother and staff, resolution of cyanotic spells, reduced need for sedatives, and greater tolerance of handling and developmental therapies, rather than by strict blood gas criteria alone.

Promoting Pulmonary Arterial Vasodilation

Targeted ventilator strategies (as discussed above) can improve the acid-base status of the neonate with PH due to severe BPD. In addition to hypoxic pulmonary vasoconstriction, acidosis has long been recognized as a potent pulmonary vasoconstrictor and can lead to marked increases in PVR. Elevated partial pressure of arterial carbon dioxide can contribute to pulmonary vasoconstriction, but is much less potent when pH is maintained at or close to a normal physiologic pH.[55,56] As such, we recommend targeting a normal pH (7.40).[57] Small increases in supplemental oxygen may be required and can assist in pulmonary arterial vasodilation. Targeting SPO2 90%–95% may be associated with less risk of developing PH.[58] However, its use

TABLE 8.3
Pharmacotherapy of Pulmonary Hypertension in BPD

Names	Dose/Titration	Side Effects	Comments
Sildenafil (phosphodiesterase-5 inhibitor)	PO: 1 mg/kg q 6–8 h; start with low dose (0.3–0.5 mg/kg/dose) and increase gradually to 1 mg/kg/dose as tolerated; slower as outpatient. Maximal dose of 10 mg q 8 h per EMA guidelines for infants. Intravenous: 0.25–0.5 mg/kg/dose q 6–8 h.	Hypotension, GER, irritability (headache), bronchospasm, nasal stuffiness, fever, rarely priapism.	Monitor for adverse effects, lower the dose, or switch to alternate therapy if not tolerated.
Bosentan (endothelin receptor antagonist)	1 mg/kg PO q 12 h as starting dose; may increase to 2 mg/kg BID in 2–4 wk, if tolerated and liver enzymes stable.	Liver dysfunction especially during viral infections, VQ mismatch, hypotension, anemia (edema and airway issues rare in infants).	Monitor LFTs monthly (earlier with respiratory infections); monitor CBC quarterly. Teratogenicity precautions for caregivers.
Inhaled iloprost	2.5–5 mcg every 2–4 h. Can be given as continuous inhalation during mechanical ventilation. Can titrate dose from 1 to 5 mcg and frequency from every 4 h to continuous.	Bronchospasm, hypotension, ventilator tube crystallization and clogging, pulmonary hemorrhage, prostanoid side effects (GI disturbances), may be teratogenic to caregivers.	Need close monitoring for clogged tubing, may need further dilution. May need bronchodilators or inhaled steroid pretreatment with bronchospasm.
Inhaled epoprostenol (Flolan)	10–50 ng/kg/min. Given as continuous inhalation during mechanical ventilation with titration from 10 to 50 ng/kg/min monitoring for hypotension and improved oxygenation.	Bronchospasm, hypotension, ventilator tube crystallization and clogging, pulmonary hemorrhage (especially with anticoagulation/ECMO), prostanoid side effects (GI disturbances),	Need close monitoring for accurate dose delivery, clogged tubing, may need further dilution.
Intravenous epoprostenol (Flolan)	Start at 1–2 ng/kg/min, titrate up slowly every 4–6 h to 20 ng/kg/min; need to increase dose at regular intervals because of tachyphylaxis. Further increases guided by clinical targets and avoiding adverse effects.	Hypotension, VQ mismatch, GI disturbances. Needs dedicated line, very short half-life with high risk for rebound PH with brief interruption of therapy; line-related complications include infection, clogging, breaks in line, thrombosis, arrhythmia.	Monitor closely if added to other rinone; careful attention to line care is essential.
Treprostinil (Remodulin) IV or subcutaneous	Start at 2 ng/kg/min and titrate every 4–6 h up to 20 ng/kg/min, then slowly increase dose as tolerated (dose often 1.5–2 times greater than equivalent epoprostenol dose, if switching medications).	SQ: Local site pain; IV: similar risks as with epoprostenol, but treprostinil has a longer half-life, which reduces risk for severe PH with interruption of infusion	Site pain managed with local and systemic measures
	0.15–0.5 mcg/kg/min—lower dosage range	Arrhythmogenic; systemic hypotension and high risk	May need to add a pressor, such as vasopressin, to

Continued

TABLE 8.3
Pharmacotherapy of Pulmonary Hypertension in BPD—cont'd

Names	Dose/Titration	Side Effects	Comments
Milrinone IV (Phosphodiesterase-3 inhibitor)	when used with other vasodilators.	for decreased myocardial perfusion; caution with renal dysfunction.	mitigate effects of decrease in systemic pressures.

BID, twice a day; CBC, complete blood count; EMA, European Medicines Agency; GER, gastroesophageal reflux; GI, gastrointestinal; IV, intravenous; LFT, liver function test; PO, oral; SC, subcutaneous; SR, sustained release; VQ, ventilation-perfusion.
From Krishnan U., et al. Evaluation and management of pulmonary hypertension in children with bronchopulmonary dysplasia. *J Pediatr*. 2017; 188:24-34 e1 and McIntyre CM., et al. Safety of epoprostenol and treprostinil in children less than 12 months of age. *Pulm Circ*. 2013;3(4): 862–869.

should be balanced with the potential toxic effects on lung tissue, the molecular[59] and genetic[60] mechanisms of which are still under investigation.[61] Intermittent hypoxia likely contributes to the pathogenesis of PH in BPD and can exacerbate existing PH. Interventions that reduce the frequency of alveolar hypoxia through lung recruitment maneuvers, augmented mobilization of airway secretions, and appropriate ventilatory support should reduce the need for a high fraction of inspired oxygen (FiO_2).[29]

In neonates with severe PH and BPD, it can be challenging to differentiate signs of respiratory distress due to lung disease from the contribution of PH. Currently available PH-targeted drugs are generally used for pulmonary vasodilator effects but should not be used without prior rigorous assessment and management of underlying respiratory disease and cardiac performance. With prolonged vasoconstriction and increased PAP, pulmonary arterial remodeling can occur, leading to thickening of the medial layer of muscular arteries and neomuscularization of small vessels.[28] For those neonates with PAH with evidence of significantly elevated PVR and RV dysfunction unrelated to left heart disease, initiation of pulmonary artery vasodilator therapy should be considered. However, much of the evidence for their use is based on clinical experience, case series, retrospective database studies, and related observations, without large-scale, multicenter randomized clinical trials (MRCTs). Therapies and dosages are summarized in Table 8.3.[44]

Except for inhaled nitric oxide (iNO), which is approved for term and near-term infants with acute respiratory failure often associated with PH, FDA-approved medications for the treatment of PH due to lung disease (WHO Group III) is lacking. However, the FDA has recently approved bosentan, a nonselective endothelin receptor antagonist (ERA) for use in children with PAH (WHO Group I) weighing more than 4 kg.[62] Some studies have suggested ERA therapy may be beneficial in neonates with PPHN,[63] but a recent Cochrane review of the literature does not fully support its use for neonatal early PH.[64] Lack of efficacy may be due to delayed absorption of bosentan during treatment initiation in the critically ill neonate.[65] ERA use as a therapy for PH in infants with BPD is likely only to be beneficial when true reactive pulmonary arterial disease is recognized (response to vasodilator challenge during cardiac catheterization) and caution should be utilized when prescribing. Alternative ERAs are available for use in the adult population; however, there are limited studies supporting their use in infants with PH. Bosentan causes a liver transaminitis in a small percentage of treated adult patients. This side effect appears to occur less frequently in children but liver function tests (LFTs) should be monitored.

Low-dose sildenafil, a phosphodiesterase 5 (PDE5) inhibitor, has long been used off-label for BPD infants with PH in the NICU and with long-term follow-up.[66] A recent meta-analysis suggested sildenafil may be efficacious in treating PH in premature neonates and may improve echocardiographic markers of PAH.[67] Similarly, a Cochrane review found that sildenafil may have a role in reducing mortality and improving oxygenation in these infants.[68]

Inhaled pulmonary vasodilator therapy, in particular iNO, is well tolerated, has a limited side effect profile, and has proven efficacious for near-term and term neonates with PPHN.[69] However, its use remains controversial in those with PH secondary to BPD. Confusion persists among neonatologists regarding its use in preterm infants for the prevention of BPD versus its use for PH-specific therapy. Whereas MRCT data do not support generalized use of early iNO therapy for the prevention of BPD, there have been no MRCTs that have examined its effects on PH in the critically ill newborn or in infants with established BPD. While improved pulmonary hemodynamics and gas exchange have been demonstrated when iNO is utilized acutely during cardiac catheterization of BPD infants with PH, questions regarding its long-term efficacy and considerable cost remain barriers to use.[70] Current guidelines support the transient use of iNO at a dose between 10 and 20 ppm during acute PH crises along with addressing underlying etiologies of the acute crisis (e.g., respiratory infection, gastroesophageal reflux (GER), aspiration, or agitation) and slowly weaning after stabilization.[44] Inhaled prostacyclin analogues (e.g., Iloprost or epoprostenol) have demonstrated efficacy for neonates with PPHN[71,72] and PH secondary to BPD.[73,74] However, its use as an acute or chronic therapy for children with PH secondary to BPD has not been thoroughly evaluated. Additionally, inhaled prostacyclin analogues may have adverse systemic hemodynamic effects including hypotension and flushing.

Parenteral prostacyclin therapy can improve RV function in children with severe PH.[75] However, there are few studies specifically evaluating use in children with PH secondary to BPD. Despite this, intravenous prostacyclin may be considered in infants with severe PH acknowledging that the therapy poses significant challenges, including systemic side effects and maintenance of a central line. Subcutaneous treprostinil may be efficacious in the treatment of severe PH in infants with chronic lung disease[76] and may have an improved side effect profile as compared to intravenous use.[77,78] Importantly, prostacyclin analogues are not currently FDA approved for use in the pediatric population.

In infants with PH refractory to prostacyclin therapy or those that appear to worsen while on prostacyclin therapy, it may be valuable to further evaluate the etiology of PH. When acutely reducing PVR, significant increases in pulmonary arterial flow may lead to pulmonary edema or capillary leak and a clinical worsening in the child's respiratory status if the etiology of PH is postcapillary. A cardiac catheterization in patients in this scenario should be considered in order to assess those suspected with left heart dysfunction (LV diastolic dysfunction) or pulmonary vein stenosis.[9]

Limiting Ongoing or New Insults to the Lung: Prevention of additional insult to lung injury is paramount to the successful treatment of PH in BPD. Strategies to reduce exposure to hyperoxia, lung derecruitment, aspiration, and infections require close monitoring. Frequent aggressive airway clearance is critical to reducing airways resistance. Given the potent toxicity of oxygen free radicals on lung tissue, recent guidelines for the management of PH in BPD have recommended targeting oxyhemoglobin saturations (SpO_2) between 92% and 95%.[44] The maintenance of hemoglobin levels between 10 and 12 g/dL can have a more significant impact on oxygen delivery to tissues as long as cardiac output remains adequate.[79] Strategies to reduce the need for high concentrations of supplemental oxygen should be targeted, including the mechanical ventilation strategies described above and aggressive airway clearance to reduce V/Q mismatch.

GER is frequently identified in prematurely born neonates, but its impact on lung disease remains controversial.[80–82] GER with aspiration may be more challenging in the BPD infant with PH, in particular for those on PH targeted therapy such as PDE5 inhibitors (sildenafil or tadalafil) and ERAs (bosentan or ambrisentan) which can reduce lower esophageal sphincter tone.[83] Reducing the acid content of refluxate through acid-suppression medications may allow for gastric bacterial overgrowth, aspiration of which may lead to additional respiratory infections.[84] As such, initiation of antiacid therapies is limited to those with associated esophagitis. Pepsin, a proteolytic enzyme produced in the first portion of the duodenum, can be aspirated in infants with GER and may contribute to additional lung injury, although causality has not been established.[85–87] As such, in those with significant aspiration concerns, we recommend initiation of nasojejunal tube feeds with consideration for gastric fundoplication. However, additional research is warranted to support this recommendation.

In addition to reducing the potential for gastrointestinal flora infections in the lung, it is important to evaluate for airway infections with acute changes in secretion viscosity, volume, or odor. Early and aggressive antimicrobial therapy coupled with frequent and aggressive airway clearance can reduce the impact of tracheitis or pneumonitis on the developing lung.[29] Routine infant immunizations should be administered as well as palivizumab for RSV prophylaxis when indicated.

For BPD infants with PH that have progressed to chronic respiratory failure with a prolonged need for mechanical ventilation, a tracheostomy tube should be considered.[88] Tracheostomy tubes are shorter than endotracheal tubes and can reduce resistance to the circuit, improving the work the patient requires for ventilation. Further, a tracheostomy is more secure, reducing the need for urgent reintubation and associated trauma. Most importantly, a tracheostomy provides the opportunity for weaning sedation, interaction between the infant and family members or therapists, and the potential for improved neurocognitive, physical, and social development.[29]

SHORT- AND LONG-TERM MANAGEMENT

Current recommendations for acute management of children with BPD and PH support a multidisciplinary approach including neonatologists, pulmonologists, cardiologists, intensivists, and PH specialists.[44] When clinically stable, infants with BPD and PH should be followed by serial echocardiograms and BNP (or NT-ProBNP) at 3–4 month intervals.[29] In time, lung growth may lead to improved PVD and medications can be reduced, discontinued, or the child allowed to "grow out of" the dose.[44] Ongoing inpatient multidisciplinary evaluation may help manage acute worsening of PH which can be secondary to ongoing or new airways disease (e.g., asthma, tracheomalacia, aspiration), cardiac disease including LV dysfunction, pulmonary venous disease, or new infectious insults.

When the patient with BPD and PH has been successfully treated and discharge is being planned, a similar pattern of outpatient specialists is recommended with the pediatrician and neurodevelopmental specialists taking the place of the intensivists. If PH and lung disease have stabilized, rehabilitation and neurocognitive development become the more pressing challenge as recent work has suggested that children with BPD and PH are more likely to have long-term growth and neurodevelopmental challenges at 3 years of life than those with BPD alone.[89] Given the association of severe BPD and significant respiratory support, in particular those with PH, these children may be more likely to have quadriparesis compared with infants without PH who required only supplemental oxygen at 36 weeks post conceptional age.[90] With physical therapy, infants with PH and BPD may require slight increases in FiO_2 during exercise given the effect of exercise on cardiac output and PAP. It is important to acknowledge the importance of physical rehabilitation. As such, brief adjustments to respiratory support can improve duration or tolerance of physical activity. Currently, there are no studies evaluating the CV effects of physical therapy on the infant with BPD and PVD. However, we recommend returning the FiO_2 or level of respiratory support to baseline levels after cessation of activity.

There is a growing body of literature reporting late outcomes of children and adult survivors with severe BPD. In particular, BPD appears to increase the risk of having elevated PAP in school-aged children and adults born before 29 weeks gestation.[6,91] Adults with a history of preterm birth may not be identified as having PH during routine resting evaluations, but may develop increased PAP during exercise suggesting a previously unrecognized maladaptation to increased cardiac output in these patients.[92] Further, a similar study identified an abnormal ventilatory efficiency (minute ventilation/VCO2) with a low minute ventilation during exercise in adults previously born premature.[93] Advances in postnatal care in NICUs including the use of noninvasive respiratory support (e.g., CPAP) have failed to result in improved lung function in children after extremely preterm birth.[91,94]

With the potential for ongoing cardiopulmonary challenges, children with BPD and PH warrant follow-up with appropriate subspecialists at regular intervals, particularly if PH persists. Currently, there are no prospective studies reporting frequency or duration of follow-up. Nevertheless, we recommend frequent follow-up for those with active or challenging disease, in particular for those on ERA therapy necessitating frequent liver function evaluation. For those with stable disease, we recommend follow-up with a PH provider every 3–4 months until disease improves or resolves. With time, growth, and stability, the PH provider can reduce the frequency of follow-up visits. Serial echocardiograms suggesting resolved disease while off of therapies can eventually lead to a further reduction in office visit frequency and may permit eventual discharge from PH Clinic.

CONCLUSIONS

To date, treating PH in children with BPD remains challenging and outcomes too often can be poor. However, with careful physiologic phenotyping of BPD infants to define heart-lung interactions, characterization of disease severity and underlying factors contributing to PH, and an individualized approach to clinical care by an interdisciplinary team, long-term outcomes look promising. Further prospective studies evaluating large populations from multiple institutions are required to more thoroughly and accurately understand this condition and to optimize therapy.[9,44]

DISCLOSURE STATEMENT

The authors do not have anything to disclose.

REFERENCES

1. Kerstjens-Frederikse WS, Bongers BM, Roofthooft MT, et al. TBX4 mutations (small patella syndrome) are associated with childhood-onset pulmonary arterial hypertension. *J Med Genet*. 2013;50(8):500–506.
2. Rosenzweig EB, Abman SH, Adatia I, et al. Paediatric pulmonary arterial hypertension: updates on definition, classification, diagnostics and management. *Eur Respir J*. 2018; 53(1):1801916.

3. Mourani PM, Abman SH. Pulmonary hypertension and vascular abnormalities in bronchopulmonary dysplasia. *Clin Perinatol.* 2015;42(4):839–855.
4. Rabinovitch M. Molecular pathogenesis of pulmonary arterial hypertension. *J Clin Investig.* 2012;122(12):4306–4313.
5. Baker CD, Abman SH. Impaired pulmonary vascular development in bronchopulmonary dysplasia. *Neonatology.* 2015;107(4):344–351.
6. Goss KN, Beshish AG, et al. Early pulmonary vascular disease in young adults born preterm. *Am J Respir Crit Care Med.* 2018;**198**(12):1549–1558.
7. Maron BA, Abman SH. Translational advances in the field of pulmonary hypertension. Focusing on developmental origins and disease inception for the prevention of pulmonary hypertension. *Am J Respir Crit Care Med.* 2017;195(3): 292–301.
8. Abman SH, Lovering AT, Maron BA. Pulmonary vascular disease across the life span: a call for bridging pediatric and adult cardiopulmonary research and care. *Am J Respir Crit Care Med.* 2018;**198**(12):1471–1473.
9. Abman SH, Hansmann G, Archer SL, et al. Pediatric pulmonary hypertension: guidelines from the American heart association and American thoracic society. *Circulation.* 2015;132(21):2037–2099.
10. Chandrasekharan P, Kozielski R, Kumar VH, et al. Early use of inhaled nitric oxide in preterm infants: is there a rationale for selective approach? *Am J Perinatol.* 2017;34(5): 428–440.
11. Giesinger RE, More K, Odame J, Jain A, Jankov RP, McNamara PJ. Controversies in the identification and management of acute pulmonary hypertension in preterm neonates. *Pediatr Res.* 2017;82(6):901–914.
12. Mirza H, Garcia JA, Crawford E. Natural history of postnatal cardiopulmonary adaptation in infants born extremely preterm and risk for death or bronchopulmonary dysplasia. *J Pediatr.* 2018;198, 187-193 e1.
13. Jobe AH, Bancalari E. Bronchopulmonary dysplasia. *Am J Respir Crit Care Med.* 2001;163(7):1723–1729.
14. Arjaans S, Zwart EAH, Ploegstra MJ. Identification of gaps in the current knowledge on pulmonary hypertension in extremely preterm infants: a systematic review and meta-analysis. *Paediatr Perinat Epidemiol.* 2018;32(3):258–267.
15. Lapcharoensap W, Gage SC, Kan P. Hospital variation and risk factors for bronchopulmonary dysplasia in a population-based cohort. *JAMA Pediatr.* 2015;169(2): e143676.
16. Stoll BJ, Hansen NI, Bell EF. Trends in care practices, morbidity, and mortality of extremely preterm neonates, 1993–2012. *JAMA.* 2015;314(10):1039–1051.
17. Higgins RD, Jobe AH, Koso-Thomas M. Bronchopulmonary dysplasia: executive summary of a workshop. *J Pediatr.* 2018;197:300–308.
18. Stenmark KR, Abman SH. Lung vascular development: implications for the pathogenesis of bronchopulmonary dysplasia. *Annu Rev Physiol.* 2005;67:623–661.
19. Jakkula M, Le Cras TD, Gebb S. Inhibition of angiogenesis decreases alveolarization in the developing rat lung. *Am J Physiol Lung Cell Mol Physiol.* 2000;279(3):L600–L607.
20. Abman SH. Bronchopulmonary dysplasia: "a vascular hypothesis". *Am J Respir Crit Care Med.* 2001;164(10 Pt 1):1755–1756.
21. Caskey S, Gough A, Rowan S. Structural and functional lung impairment in adult survivors of bronchopulmonary dysplasia. *Ann Am Thorac Soc.* 2016;13(8):1262–1270.
22. MacLean JE, DeHaan K, Fuhr D. Altered breathing mechanics and ventilatory response during exercise in children born extremely preterm. *Thorax.* 2016;71(11): 1012–1019.
23. Vyas-Read S, Kanaan U, Shankar P. Early characteristics of infants with pulmonary hypertension in a referral neonatal intensive care unit. *BMC Pediatr.* 2017;17(1):163.
24. Abe K, Shinoda M, Tanaka M. Haemodynamic unloading reverses occlusive vascular lesions in severe pulmonary hypertension. *Cardiovasc Res.* 2016;111(1):16–25.
25. Choi EK, Jung YH, Kim HS. The impact of atrial left-to-right shunt on pulmonary hypertension in preterm infants with moderate or severe bronchopulmonary dysplasia. *Pediatr Neonatol.* 2015;56(5):317–323.
26. Vyas-Read S, Guglani L, Shankar P, Travers C, Kanaan U. Atrial septal defects accelerate pulmonary hypertension diagnoses in premature infants. *Front Pediatr.* 2018;6:342.
27. Gorenflo M, Vogel M, Obladen M. Pulmonary vascular changes in bronchopulmonary dysplasia: a clinicopathologic correlation in short- and long-term survivors. *Pediatr Pathol.* 1991;11(6):851–866.
28. Bush A, Busst CM, Knight WB, Hislop AA, Busst SG, Shinebourne EA. Changes in pulmonary circulation in severe bronchopulmonary dysplasia. *Arch Dis Child.* 1990; 65(7):739–745.
29. Abman SH, Collaco JM, Shepherd EG, et al. Interdisciplinary care of children with severe bronchopulmonary dysplasia. *J Pediatr.* 2017;181:12–28 e1.
30. Alvarez-Fuente M, Arruza L, Muro M, et al. The economic impact of prematurity and bronchopulmonary dysplasia. *Eur J Pediatr.* 2017;176(12):1587–1593.
31. Check J, Gotteiner N, Liu X, et al. Fetal growth restriction and pulmonary hypertension in premature infants with bronchopulmonary dysplasia. *J Perinatol.* 2013;33(7): 553–557.
32. Nagiub M, Kanaan U, Simon D, Guglani L. Risk factors for development of pulmonary hypertension in infants with bronchopulmonary dysplasia: systematic review and meta-analysis. *Paediatr Respir Rev.* 2017;23:27–32.
33. Mestan KK, Check J, Minturn L, et al. Placental pathologic changes of maternal vascular underperfusion in bronchopulmonary dysplasia and pulmonary hypertension. *Placenta.* 2014;35(8):570–574.
34. Mestan KK, Gotteiner N, Porta N, Grobman W, Su EJ, Ernst LM. Cord blood biomarkers of placental maternal vascular underperfusion predict bronchopulmonary dysplasia-associated pulmonary hypertension. *J Pediatr.* 2017;185:33–41.
35. Maynard SE, Min JY, Merchan J, et al. Excess placental soluble fms-like tyrosine kinase 1 (sFlt1) may contribute to endothelial dysfunction, hypertension, and proteinuria in preeclampsia. *J Clin Investig.* 2003;111(5):649–658.

36. Allen RE, Rogozinska E, Cleverly K, Aquilina J, Thangaratinam S. Abnormal blood biomarkers in early pregnancy are associated with preeclampsia: a meta-analysis. *Eur J Obstet Gynecol Reprod Biol*. 2014;182:194–201.
37. Wallace B, Peisl A, Seedorf G, et al. Anti-sFlt-1 therapy preserves lung alveolar and vascular growth in antenatal models of bronchopulmonary dysplasia. *Am J Respir Crit Care Med*. 2018;197(6):776–787.
38. Weismann CG, Asnes JD, Bazzy-Asaad A, Tolomeo C, Ehrenkranz RA, Bizzarro MJ. Pulmonary hypertension in preterm infants: results of a prospective screening program. *J Perinatol*. 2017;37(5):572–577.
39. Sehgal A, Malikiwi A, Paul E, Tan K, Menahem S. A new look at bronchopulmonary dysplasia: postcapillary pathophysiology and cardiac dysfunction. *Pulm Circ*. 2016;6(4): 508–515.
40. Mourani PM, Ivy DD, Rosenberg AA, Fagan TE, Abman SH. Left ventricular diastolic dysfunction in bronchopulmonary dysplasia. *J Pediatr*. 2008;152(2):291–293.
41. Ehrmann DE, Mourani PM, Abman SH, et al. Echocardiographic measurements of right ventricular mechanics in infants with bronchopulmonary dysplasia at 36 weeks postmenstrual age. *J Pediatr*. 2018;203:210–217 e1.
42. Carlton EF, Sontag MK, Younoszai A, et al. Reliability of echocardiographic indicators of pulmonary vascular disease in preterm infants at risk for bronchopulmonary dysplasia. *J Pediatr*. 2017;186:29–33.
43. Mourani PM, Sontag MK, Younoszai A, et al. Early pulmonary vascular disease in preterm infants at risk for bronchopulmonary dysplasia. *Am J Respir Crit Care Med*. 2015;191(1):87–95.
44. Krishnan U, Feinstein JA, Adatia I, et al. Evaluation and management of pulmonary hypertension in children with bronchopulmonary dysplasia. *J Pediatr*. 2017;188, 24-34 e1.
45. Cuna A, Kandasamy J, Sims B. B-type natriuretic peptide and mortality in extremely low birth weight infants with pulmonary hypertension: a retrospective cohort analysis. *BMC Pediatr*. 2014;14:68.
46. Konig K, Guy KJ, Nold-Petry CA, et al. BNP, troponin I, and YKL-40 as screening markers in extremely preterm infants at risk for pulmonary hypertension associated with bronchopulmonary dysplasia. *Am J Physiol Lung Cell Mol Physiol*. 2016;311(6):L1076–L1081.
47. Amdani SM, Mian MUM, Thomas RL, Ross RD. NT-pro BNP-A marker for worsening respiratory status and mortality in infants and young children with pulmonary hypertension. *Congenit Heart Dis*. 2018;13(4):499–505.
48. Montgomery AM, Bazzy-Asaad A, Asnes JD, Bizzarro MJ, Ehrenkranz RA, Weismann CG. Biochemical screening for pulmonary hypertension in preterm infants with bronchopulmonary dysplasia. *Neonatology*. 2016;109(3): 190–194.
49. Takatsuki S, Wagner BD, Ivy DD. B-type natriuretic peptide and amino-terminal pro-B-type natriuretic peptide in pediatric patients with pulmonary arterial hypertension. *Congenit Heart Dis*. 2012;7(3):259–267.
50. Hilgendorff A, Apitz C, Bonnet D, Hansmann G. Pulmonary hypertension associated with acute or chronic lung diseases in the preterm and term neonate and infant. The European paediatric pulmonary vascular disease network, endorsed by ISHLT and DGPK. *Heart*. 2016;102(Suppl 2): ii49–56.
51. Wagner BD, , et alBabinec AE, Carpenter C. Proteomic profiles associated with early echocardiogram evidence of pulmonary vascular disease in preterm infants. *Am J Respir Crit Care Med*. 2018;197(3):394–397.
52. Yin T, Yuh YS, Liaw JJ, Chen YY, Wang KW. Semi-prone position can influence variability in respiratory rate of premature infants using nasal CPAP. *J Pediatr Nurs*. 2016;31(2): e167–e174.
53. Thome U, Topfer A, Schaller P, Pohlandt F. The effect of positive endexpiratory pressure, peak inspiratory pressure, and inspiratory time on functional residual capacity in mechanically ventilated preterm infants. *Eur J Pediatr*. 1998; 157(10):831–837.
54. Ross PA, Khemani RG, Rubin SS, Bhalla AK, Newth CJ. Elevated positive end-expiratory pressure decreases cardiac index in a rhesus monkey model. *Front Pediatr*. 2014;2: 134.
55. Rudolph AM, Yuan S. Response of the pulmonary vasculature to hypoxia and H+ ion concentration changes. *J Clin Investig*. 1966;45(3):399–411.
56. Ketabchi F, Egemnazarov B, Schermuly RT, et al. Effects of hypercapnia with and without acidosis on hypoxic pulmonary vasoconstriction. *Am J Physiol Lung Cell Mol Physiol*. 2009;297(5):L977–L983.
57. Gordon JB, Halla TR, Fike CD, Madden JA, et al. Mediators of alkalosis-induced relaxation in pulmonary arteries from normoxic and chronically hypoxic piglets. *Am J Physiol*. 1999;276(1 Pt 1):L155–L163.
58. Laliberte C, Hanna Y, Ben Fadel N, et al. Target oxygen saturation and development of pulmonary hypertension and increased pulmonary vascular resistance in preterm infants. *Pediatr Pulmonol*. 2019;54(1):73–81.
59. Menon RT, Shrestha AK, Barrios R, Shivanna B, et al. Hyperoxia disrupts extracellular signal-regulated kinases 1/2-induced angiogenesis in the developing lungs. *Int J Mol Sci*. 2018;19(5).
60. Bik-Multanowski M, Revhaug C, Grabowska A, et al. Hyperoxia induces epigenetic changes in newborn mice lungs. *Free Radic Biol Med*. 2018;121:51–56.
61. Deneke SM, Fanburg BL. Normobaric oxygen toxicity of the lung. *N Engl J Med*. 1980;303(2):76–86.
62. *Tracleer (bosentan)*. San Francisco, CA: Actelion Pharmaceuticals US; 2017.
63. Maneenil G, Thatrimontrichai A, Janjindamai W, Dissaneevate S. Effect of bosentan therapy in persistent pulmonary hypertension of the newborn. *Pediatr Neonatol*. 2018;59(1):58–64.
64. More K, Athalye-Jape GK, Rao SC, Patole SK. Endothelin receptor antagonists for persistent pulmonary hypertension in term and late preterm infants. *Cochrane Database Syst Rev*. 2016;(8):CD010531.

65. Steinhorn RH, Fineman J, Kusic-Pajic A, et al. Bosentan as adjunctive therapy for persistent pulmonary hypertension of the newborn: results of the randomized multicenter placebo-controlled exploratory trial. *J Pediatr*. 2016;177: 90–96 e3.
66. Mourani PM, Sontag MK, Ivy DD, Abman SH. Effects of long-term sildenafil treatment for pulmonary hypertension in infants with chronic lung disease. *J Pediatr*. 2009; 154(3), 379-384, 384 e1-2.
67. Tan K, Krishnamurthy MB, O'Heney JL, Paul E, Sehgal A. Sildenafil therapy in bronchopulmonary dysplasia-associated pulmonary hypertension: a retrospective study of efficacy and safety. *Eur J Pediatr*. 2015;174(8):1109–1115.
68. Kelly LE, Ohlsson A, Shah PS. Sildenafil for pulmonary hypertension in neonates. *Cochrane Database Syst Rev*. 2017;8: CD005494.
69. Kinsella JP, Steinhorn RH, Krishnan US, et al. Recommendations for the use of inhaled nitric oxide therapy in premature newborns with severe pulmonary hypertension. *J Pediatr*. 2016;170:312–314.
70. Mourani PM, Ivy DD, Gao D, Abman SH. Pulmonary vascular effects of inhaled nitric oxide and oxygen tension in bronchopulmonary dysplasia. *Am J Respir Crit Care Med*. 2004;170(9):1006–1013.
71. Kahveci H, Yilmaz O, Avsar UZ, et al. Oral sildenafil and inhaled iloprost in the treatment of pulmonary hypertension of the newborn. *Pediatr Pulmonol*. 2014;49(12): 1205–1213.
72. Ehlen M, Wiebe B. Iloprost in persistent pulmonary hypertension of the newborn. *Cardiol Young*. 2003;13(4): 361–363.
73. Piastra M, De Luca D, De Carolis MP, et al. Nebulized iloprost and noninvasive respiratory support for impending hypoxaemic respiratory failure in formerly preterm infants: a case series. *Pediatr Pulmonol*. 2012;47(8):757–762.
74. Brown AT, Gillespie JV, Miquel-Verges F, et al. Inhaled epoprostenol therapy for pulmonary hypertension: improves oxygenation index more consistently in neonates than in older children. *Pulm Circ*. 2012;2(1):61–66.
75. Hopper RK, Wang Y, DeMatteo V, et al. Right ventricular function mirrors clinical improvement with use of prostacyclin analogues in pediatric pulmonary hypertension. *Pulm Circ*. 2018;8(2), 2045894018759247.
76. Ferdman DJ, Rosenzweig EB, Zuckerman WA,, Krishnan U. Subcutaneous treprostinil for pulmonary hypertension in chronic lung disease of infancy. *Pediatrics*. 2014;134(1): e274–e278.
77. McIntyre CM, Hanna BD, Rintoul N, Ramsey EZ. Safety of epoprostenol and treprostinil in children less than 12 months of age. *Pulm Circ*. 2013;3(4):862–869.
78. Carpentier E, Mur S, Aubry E, et al. Safety and tolerability of subcutaneous treprostinil in newborns with congenital diaphragmatic hernia and life-threatening pulmonary hypertension. *J Pediatr Surg*. 2017;52(9):1480–1483.
79. Lumb A. *Nunn's Applied Respiratory Physiology*. 8th ed. Elsevier; 2017.
80. Akinola E, Rosenkrantz TS, Pappagallo M, McKay K, Hussain N. Gastroesophageal reflux in infants < 32 weeks gestational age at birth: lack of relationship to chronic lung disease. *Am J Perinatol*. 2004;21(2):57–62.
81. Jensen EA, Munson DA, Zhang H, Blinman TA, Kirpalani H. Anti-gastroesophageal reflux surgery in infants with severe bronchopulmonary dysplasia. *Pediatr Pulmonol*. 2015;50(6):584–587.
82. Nobile S, Noviello C, Cobellis G, Carnielli VP. Are infants with bronchopulmonary dysplasia prone to gastroesophageal reflux? A prospective observational study with esophageal pH-impedance monitoring. *J Pediatr*. 2015;167(2): 279–285 e1.
83. Kim HS, Conklin JL, Park H. The effect of sildenafil on segmental oesophageal motility and gastro-oesophageal reflux. *Aliment Pharmacol Ther*. 2006;24(7):1029–1036.
84. Rosen R, Amirault J, Liu H, et al. Changes in gastric and lung microflora with acid suppression: acid suppression and bacterial growth. *JAMA Pediatr*. 2014;168(10): 932–937.
85. Garland JS, Alex CP, Johnston N, Yan JC, Werlin SL. Association between tracheal pepsin, a reliable marker of gastric aspiration, and head of bed elevation among ventilated neonates. *J Neonatal Perinat Med*. 2014;7(3): 185–192.
86. Gopalareddy V, He Z, Soundar S, et al. Assessment of the prevalence of microaspiration by gastric pepsin in the airway of ventilated children. *Acta Paediatr*. 2008;97(1): 55–60.
87. Farhath S, He Z, Nakhla T, et al. Pepsin, a marker of gastric contents, is increased in tracheal aspirates from preterm infants who develop bronchopulmonary dysplasia. *Pediatrics*. 2008;121(2):e253–e259.
88. Gien J, Abman SH, Baker CD. Interdisciplinary care for ventilator-dependent infants with chronic lung disease. *J Pediatr*. 2014;165(6):1274–1275.
89. Nakanishi H, Uchiyama A, Kusuda S. Impact of pulmonary hypertension on neurodevelopmental outcome in preterm infants with bronchopulmonary dysplasia: a cohort study. *J Perinatol*. 2016;36(10):890–896.
90. Newman JB, Debastos AG, Batton D, Raz S. Neonatal respiratory dysfunction and neuropsychological performance at the preschool age: a study of very preterm infants with bronchopulmonary dysplasia. *Neuropsychology*. 2011; 25(5):666–678.
91. Zivanovic S, Pushparajah K, Calvert S, et al. Pulmonary artery pressures in school-age children born prematurely. *J Pediatr*. 2017;191:42–49 e3.
92. Laurie SS, Elliott JE, Beasley KM, et al. Exaggerated increase in pulmonary artery pressure during exercise in adults born preterm. *Am J Respir Crit Care Med*. 2018;197(6):821–823.
93. Lovering AT, Elliott JE, Laurie SS, et al. Ventilatory and sensory responses in adult survivors of preterm birth and bronchopulmonary dysplasia with reduced exercise capacity. *Ann Am Thorac Soc*. 2014;11(10):1528–1537.
94. Doyle LW, Carse E, Adams AM, et al. Ventilation in extremely preterm infants and respiratory function at 8 years. *N Engl J Med*. 2017;377(4):329–337.
95. Mandell EW, Abman SH. Fetal vascular origins of bronchopulmonary dysplasia. *J Pediatr*. 2017;185, 7-10 e1.

CHAPTER 9

The Inflammation Superhighway: Tolls, Signals, and Pathways to Bronchopulmonary Dysplasia

JOHN IBRAHIM, MD • STAVROS GARANTZIOTIS, MD • RASHMIN C. SAVANI, MBCHB

INTRODUCTION

Inflammation is a key contributor to the development and severity of a wide variety of diseases, including atherosclerosis, liver and kidney failure, diabetes, cancer, and neurodegeneration.[1] Similarly, inflammation is a key component in the pathogenesis of neonatal disorders such as bronchopulmonary dysplasia (BPD),[2] hypoxic ischemic encephalopathy (HIE),[3–5] necrotizing enterocolitis (NEC),[6,7] retinopathy of prematurity (ROP),[8] and sepsis.[9,10] Indeed, preterm birth is also driven by both infectious and sterile inflammation.[11] Recently, our understanding of the common mechanisms and specific modulators of inflammation has increased dramatically and has raised the possibility of developing novel therapeutic approaches to limit the effects of inflammation in these conditions without the complications of glucocorticoids that are the current mainstay of anti-inflammatory approaches in medicine.

BPD is a devastating chronic lung disease seen largely in preterm infants with respiratory failure.[12,13] It affects approximately 15,000 infants per year and inflicts lifelong disease-specific and social burdens to affected neonates and their families, as well as substantial healthcare costs.[14,15] BPD has a multifactorial pathogenesis, but ultimately is a disease of inflammation and dysregulated lung development.[16] Lung development occurs in a finely orchestrated series of molecularly distinct yet overlapping phases that include embryonic, pseudoglandular, canalicular, saccular, and alveolar stages.[17] A number of influences, both *in utero* and postnatal, can accelerate or retard the timeline for lung development. Thus, antenatal stresses, such as chorioamnionitis and placental insufficiency, stimulate the expression of cytokines and glucocorticoids that accelerate lung development. Indeed, antenatal administration of glucocorticoids to women in preterm labor is a mainstay of accelerating lung surfactant maturation in the fetus. Congenital diaphragmatic hernia, on the other hand, inhibits the normal growth of the lung, resulting in both alveolar and vascular defects with severe consequences after birth. With preterm birth, the newborn is exposed to a higher ambient oxygen than in the in utero environment, resulting in hyperoxia-induced injury even if they are maintained in 21% oxygen, and may eventually need intubation and invasive mechanical ventilation. Together with a propensity for systemic and pulmonary infection, this results in lung injury that establishes an inflammatory cascade that has profound extended effects on lung development that now has to be completed *ex utero*. Combined with an inability to provide nutrition that matches that from the placenta and exposure to other medications such as postnatal glucocorticoids, lung development is dysregulated and results in an arrest of normal alveolar and vascular development that we recognize as BPD.[2,16]

THE DIFFERENCES BETWEEN INNATE AND ADAPTIVE IMMUNE RESPONSES

Exposure to an environment with an abundance of microorganisms and noxious substances bombards the host with invading bacteria, viruses, and toxins. This has required the evolution of both innate and adaptive immune systems to combat these attacks. The innate immune system is evolutionarily ancient and provides defense to nonvertebrate and vertebrate animals, whereas the adaptive immune system is only found in vertebrate animals. These two systems are distinct in their characteristics (Table 9.1). Innate immune responses are antigen independent and not antigen specific. They achieve an immediate and maximum

Updates on Neonatal Chronic Lung Disease. https://doi.org/10.1016/B978-0-323-68353-1.00009-9

TABLE 9.1
Innate and Adaptive Immune Responses.

Innate Immunity	Adaptive or Specific Immunity
Evolutionarily ancient	Evolutionarily more recent
Found in invertebrates and vertebrates	Found only in vertebrates
Response is antigen independent	Antigen dependent
Not antigen specific	Antigen specific
Immediate maximal response	Lag time between exposure and maximal response
No immunologic memory	Exposure results in immunologic memory

response that lacks immunologic memory. In contrast, adaptive immune responses are antigen dependent and antigen specific, have a lag time between exposure and maximum response, and the exposure results in long-lasting immunologic memory. Indeed, immunization against various mostly viral diseases is based on these properties of adaptive immunity and has been successful in the eradication or effective containment of diseases such as smallpox and polio that previously affected large numbers of people.

NONIMMUNE DEFENSES OF THE INNATE IMMUNE SYSTEM

A number of nonimmune defense systems consisting of physical, chemical, cellular, and microbiological components contribute to preventing microorganism entry. First, the stratum corneum of the epithelium resists bacterial invasion because of its low water content, acidic environment, and antimicrobial lipids that are present.[18] Physical barriers also exist in the epithelia of respiratory, gastrointestinal, and genitourinary tracts with mucus layers that prevent exposure of the epithelium to organisms[19] and epithelial tight junctions that prevent microorganism penetration.[20] Next, mechanical forces such as ciliary beat movement of mucus in the upper airways, the airway mucus itself with appropriate regulation of salt and hydration,[21] and tears and saliva are also multifunctional barriers to invading organisms.[22]

A number of chemical factors in saliva, tears, stomach, gastrointestinal and genitourinary tracts, and the lungs also serve as antimicrobial defenses. These include lysozyme, lactoferrin, uric acid, leukoprotease inhibitor, secretory phospholipase A2, defensins, cathelicidins, and collectins.[23] In addition, nitric oxide is produced in both upper and lower respiratory tracts and has antimicrobial properties.[24] In the lung, we will focus particular attention to defensins, cathelicidins, and collectins.

DEFENSINS AND CATHELICIDINS

Defensins and cathelicidins, produced mainly by inflammatory and epithelial cells, are amphipathic peptides of less than 100 amino acids that disrupt microbial membranes.[25] They not only directly kill pathogens but also play important roles in modulating immune responses. Initially called "alarmins" because of their ability to stimulate inflammatory responses, defensins and cathelicidins can also have anti-inflammatory properties.[26] There are two main classes of defensins in humans, namely alpha (α) and beta (ß) defensins.[27] They have a distinct three-dimensional structure with a characteristic triple strand beta sheet and six cysteines that participate in disulfide bonds. While the specific amino acid sequences of defensins vary, clusters of positively charged residues are present and the cysteine framework is conserved.[28] α-defensins are synthesized as preproproteins that are enzymatically cleaved by metalloproteinases and stored together with glycosaminoglycans in intracellular granules until secreted. β-defensins are simpler and lack the large propeptide of α-defensins. Triggers for defensin release include exposure to bacteria, phagocytosis or cholinergic stimuli, and the principal mechanism of antimicrobial activity is the permeabilization of membranes.[29] The only human cathelicidin, hCAP18/LL-37, is molecularly distinct from defensins and contains a signal peptide, an intermediate domain and an antimicrobial domain. Proteolytic cleavage results in the release of the antimicrobial domain (LL-37) which has similar activities to those of the defensins.[30]

These antimicrobial peptides have the ability to kill bacteria, viruses, fungi, and protozoa, as well as inhibit the actions of toxins. Other activities of defensins include the stimulation of chemotaxis by binding to chemokine receptors such as CCR6, whereas the cathelicidin LL-37 uses the formyl peptide receptor-like 1 (FPRL1). These peptides can also interfere with LPS-stimulated, Toll-Like Receptor 4 (TLR4)-mediated responses in cultured macrophages.[31] In a counter system, bacteria have developed mechanisms to protect themselves from these peptides with changes in cell membrane constituents that make their cell surfaces less able to be bound by these peptides.[27]

COLLECTINS

Collagen-containing C-type lectins (collectins) are soluble pattern recognition receptors (PRRs) that have multiple properties that include binding of pathogen- and danger-associated molecular patterns (PAMPs/DAMPs), competing with organisms for TLR binding, direct stimulation of TLRs and other receptors to induce intracellular signaling, opsonization, and phagocytosis of invading organisms and apoptotic cells, as well as stimulation of growth factor expression and inflammatory cell chemotaxis.[32] Members of the collectin family include C1q that activates the classical complement pathway,[33,34] mannose binding lectin (MBL) that can activate complement independently from the classical or alternative pathways,[35] and the pulmonary collectins Surfactant Protein A (SP-A) and SP-D.[36–38] (Fig. 9.1) The basic structure of collectins includes a cysteine rich N-terminal noncollagenous domain, a collagen-like domain, an α-helical, coiled-coil neck domain, and a carbohydrate recognition domain (CRD).

SP-A and SP-D are large, hydrophilic proteins that were first described in pulmonary surfactant but are widely expressed in extrapulmonary tissues, including the female reproductive, urinary, and gastrointestinal tracts, the eye, nose, central nervous system, coronary arteries, and the skin.[39,40] In the lung, SP-A associates with phosphatidylcholine of surfactant and promotes surfactant turnover and homeostasis, whereas SP-D binds to phosphatidylinositol.

The structures of SP-A and SP-D are complex, forming large multimeric complexes by assembly of individual polypeptides (Fig. 9.1). Thus, three 35 kDa SP-A polypeptide chains bind via disulfide bonds to generate a 105 kDa subunit. Six of these subunits associate to create an 18 chain 630 kDa molecule that forms a bouquet-shaped structure. Similarly, four homotrimers of 43 kDa SP-D polypeptide chains are bound at their N-terminus to generate a 520 kDa cruciform-shaped SP-D. Further oligomerization can occur with up to 96 individual chains.[41]

The CRDs of both proteins mediate binding to viruses, bacteria, yeast, and fungi that results in opsonization and presentation to inflammatory cells. In addition, these proteins also interact with inflammatory

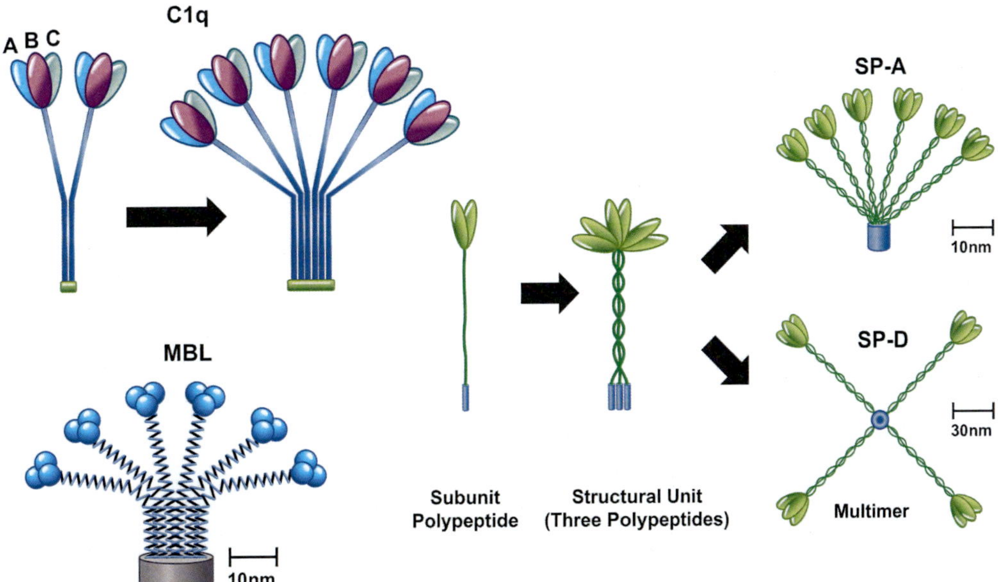

FIG. 9.1 **The Collectins.** Collagen-containing C-type lectins (collectins) are soluble pattern recognition receptors that have multiple functions, including binding of PAMPs and DAMPs, toll-like receptor (TLR) binding with direct stimulation of growth factor expression and chemotaxis, as well as opsonization and phagocytosis of invading organisms and apoptotic cells. Members include C1q, mannose binding lectin (MBL), and Surfactant Proteins A (SP-A) and D (SP-D). Collectins have subunit polypeptides that have a cysteine-rich N-terminal noncollagenous domain, a collagen-like domain, an α-helical coiled coil neck domain, and a carbohydrate recognition domain. Three polypeptides form trimers and then higher-order multimers to create structures that are able to interact with pathogens and TLRs. *DAMP*, danger-associated molecular pattern; *PAMP*, pathogen-associated molecular pattern.

cells to compete with invading organisms' binding to TLRs, in particular TLR2 and TLR4, stimulation of chemotaxis, phagocytosis, and killing of invading organisms.[41] Interestingly, Gardai et al.[42] showed that SPA acts as a dual function surveillance molecule to enhance or suppress cytokine production depending on the binding orientation of the CRD of SPA. SPA maintains normal lung homeostasis by binding to SIRPα (signal inhibitory regulatory protein) that blocks proinflammatory signaling by activating SHP-1, a phosphatase that in turn dephosphorylates p38. However, upon recognition of PAMPs on foreign organisms, the collagenous tail of SPA binds to calreticulin/CD91 and elicits the phosphorylation of p38 and downstream activation of the NFκB proinflammatory signal pathway[42] (Fig. 9.2). Our own studies of SP-A demonstrated that SP-A binding to TLR2 activates Jnk and Erk and stimulates production of TGFß that acts to recruit macrophages to the site[43] (Fig. 9.3).

The multimeric organization of SP-D confers anti-inflammatory properties to this protein. Two cysteine residues at the N-terminus (amino acids 15 and 20) are responsible for the formation of the large SP-D multimer.[44] Our studies showed that S-nitrosylation of SP-D (SNO-SP-D) results in the disruption of the SP-D multimer and promotes an inflammatory signal via calreticulin/CD91 and p38 MAP kinase and macrophage chemotaxis.[45] Further, acute, noninfectious injury with intratracheal bleomycin is associated with increased SNO-SP-D and a loss of the multimeric nature of native SP-D. Taken together with the fact that mutation of the two cysteine residues prevents the formation of multimeric SP-D[44] and that expression of this mutant SP-D in *Spd*$^{-/-}$ mice does not rescue the inflammatory phenotype of the knockout (KO) mice[46] establishes the contribution of the two cysteine residues and multimeric SP-D to the anti-inflammatory state of the quiescent lung.

The expression of SP-A and SP-D are developmentally regulated and both proteins show dramatically increased expression during late gestation.[47–51] Therefore, infants born prematurely will have a developmental deficiency of these proteins, have a greater propensity for inflammation, and be less able to defend

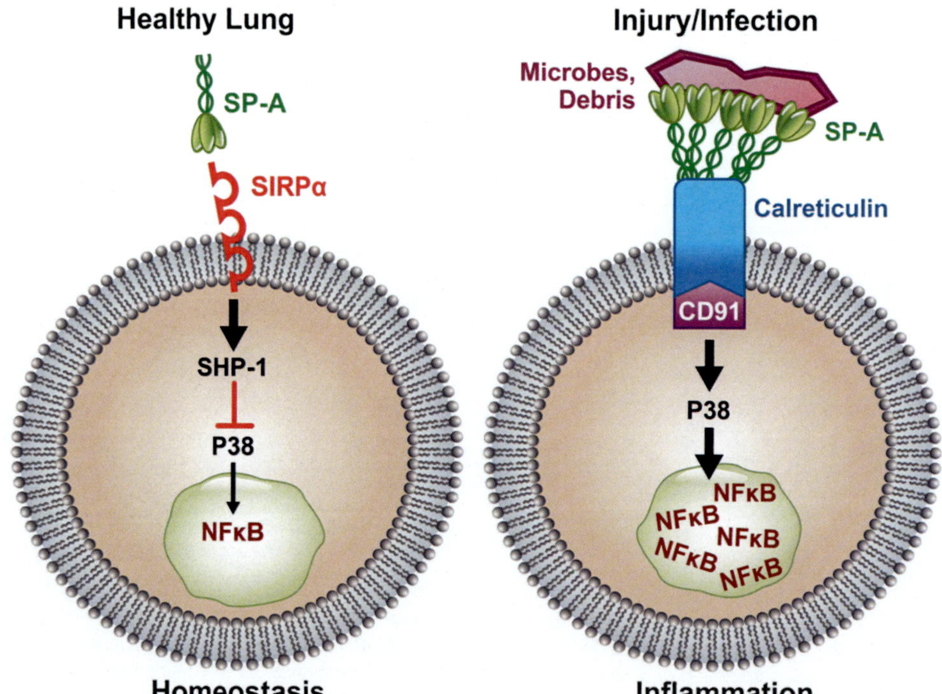

FIG. 9.2 Dual function of SP-A in inhibition or activation of NFκB. During normal homeostasis, SP-A binds SIRP-α using its carbohydrate recognition domain. This binding activates the phosphatase SHP-1, which in turn dephosphorylates p38 and blocks the activation of NFκB. In the presence of microbial invasion or accumulation of debris, the carbohydrate recognition domain of SP-A binds this foreign material and the tail of SP-A binds to calreticulin/CD91. This binding results in phosphorylation of p38 and activation of NFκB.

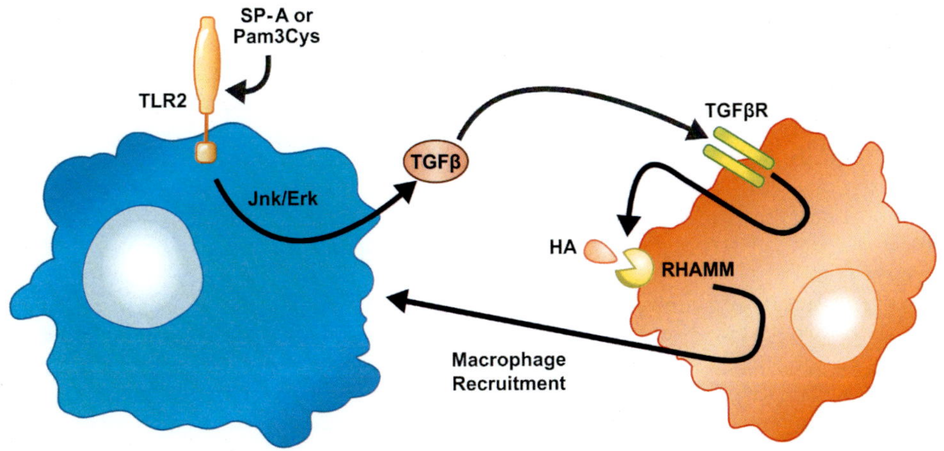

FIG. 9.3 **SP-A stimulation of TLR2 results in Jnk/Erk-mediated TGFß production which recruits macrophages using the hyaluronan receptor RHAMM.** Stimulation of TLR2, either by SP-A or by the TLR2-specific ligand Pam3Cys, activates Jnk and Erk and leads to the expression and activation of TGFß. Chemotactic gradients of this growth factor recruit macrophages to the site and require the hyaluronan receptor RHAMM.

themselves from infectious challenges.[52] Exogenous surfactant preparations are lipid extracts of either lung tissue or lavage, and therefore do not contain SP-A and SP-D which are hydrophilic proteins. Addition of SP-A to exogenous surfactant, however, is problematic and results in the stimulation of an inflammatory response.[53] Interestingly, Mendelson described a role for SP-A in the fetal lung as a hormonal signal for the initiation of parturition.[54] SP-A stimulated NFκB activation and IL1ß production in fetal macrophages that then migrated to the uterine wall and initiated labor.[54] In support of these observations, SP-A and SP-D double KO mice and TLR2 KO mice have delayed parturition.[55]

ENDOGENOUS DANGER SIGNALS

The notion that the innate immune system can respond to self-derived mediators as "danger signals" was originally proposed by Matzinger in 1994.[56] DAMPs are both cytosolic and extracellular matrix (ECM) molecules that undergo changes and/or are released in response to tissue injury and promote innate immune responses.[57–59] These danger signals are sensed by PRRs predominantly in immune cells and activate signaling pathways that result in the elaboration of inflammatory mediators that alter the responses in target tissues and result in an inflammatory response and fibrotic consequence.[60–62] A number of endogenous danger signals have been characterized and the major ones will be summarized here. It should be noted that these DAMPs have been identified in humans and in preclinical models of ventilator-induced lung injury.[63]

Recently, the concept of nanoparticle-associated molecular patterns (NAMPs) has been proposed. A number of nanoparticles, including nanosilica, carbon nanotubes, and titanium dioxide, activate the NLRP3 inflammasome and stimulate IL1ß production in a wide variety of organs, including the lung.[64] In addition, nanosilica can have effects on the developing fetus causing placental dysfunction and intrauterine growth restriction.[65]

HMGB1: HMGB1 was one of the first endogenous danger signals to be characterized. Its expression is increased by gram-negative bacterial (LPS) challenge mediated by interaction with TLR4/myeloid differentiation factor 2 (MD2), but this is a response measured in days after challenge and associated with mortality.[66–68] Notably, sterile injury is also associated with elevated serum concentrations of HMGB1 in a wide variety of injury models, including sepsis, hemorrhagic shock, and liver injury.[69] In preclinical models, blockade of HMGB1 ameliorates these changes and protects animals from the effects of injury. Binding of HMGB1 to TLR4/MD2 on immune cells stimulates the production of cytokines and chemokines that promote inflammation via NFκB activation.[70] A number of other receptors for HMGB1 have also been described and include RAGE, integrins, TLR2, and IL1R.[67] A tetrapeptide (P5779, sequence FSSE), a specific inhibitor of HMGB1 that disrupts the HMGB1/TLR4/MD2 complex, ameliorates preclinical models of sepsis and liver injury.[71]

Interestingly, concentrations of HMGB1 are elevated in the tracheal aspirates of preterm infants destined to develop death or BPD at 36 weeks PMA.[72] In mice, lung HMGB1 mRNA and protein increase with exposure to hyperoxia in the neonatal period,[73] and antibody blockade of HMGB1 improves neutrophil infiltration, expression of IL1ß, and decreased alveolarization seen with neonatal hyperoxia exposure.[74] These studies suggest that HMGB1 acts as a danger signal in the development of BPD.

Monosodium urate crystals: Hyperuricemia, a disorder of purine metabolism, results in elevated monosodium urate crystal deposition in tissues and inflammatory arthritis that is debilitating.[75,76] Although not a neonatal disease, it is important to note that these crystals activate the NLRP3 inflammasome to produce IL1ß that promotes the acute inflammatory flare-ups that are common in this disease. Decreased purine synthesis by allopurinol is the mainstay of therapy for this disorder, but gout provides a classic example of crystal-based danger signals.

Soluble biglycan: Biglycan, a member of the small leucine-rich proteoglycans (SLRPs) family, is either bound to the ECM or is released as soluble biglycan in the blood and in synovial fluid where it can be used as a biomarker for disease.[77–79] This soluble form, generated by the action of proteinases on the ECM-bound biglycan, acts as an endogenous danger signal.[80] It interacts with TLR2 and TLR4 in macrophages, dendritic cells (DCs), and chondrocytes to activate several intracellular signaling pathways, including mitogen-activated protein kinase (MAPK) p38, extracellular signal-regulated kinase (Erk), as well as NFκB and activation of the NLRP3 inflammasome pathway leading to the production of TNFα, C-C motif and C-X-C motif ligands and IL1ß to stimulate an inflammatory response.[81,82]

Biglycan regulation of the expression of IL1ß is complex. Soluble biglycan can interact with TLR2 and TLR4 either individually or both together, resulting in different outcomes.[77] Thus, the interaction of biglycan with both TLR2 and TLR4, using MyD88 and requiring NADPH oxidase (NOX) 1 and NOX4, results in the production of IL1ß.[83] Biglycan interaction with TLR4/MyD88/TRIF results in increased expression of NOX2, whereas the interaction of biglycan with TLR2 stimulates the expression of Heat Shock Protein 70 (HSP70) which activates the NOX2.[83] This oxidase negatively regulates the expression of IL1ß, thereby providing tight control of the activation of the principal activator of the innate immune pathway.[83] To our knowledge, only one study of biglycan in neonatal hyperoxia has been reported in rats, demonstrating that its expression increases with chronic postnatal exposure to hyperoxia.[84]

Hyaluronan: Hyaluronan (hyaluronic acid, HA) is a polymer of repeating disaccharide units of glucuronic acid and N-acetyl glucosamine, and an important mediator of sterile inflammation.[85,86] HA regulation of inflammation is molecular size dependent.[87] High molecular weight (HMW) HA inhibits a number of inflammatory cell properties, including chemotaxis,[43,88] phagocytosis,[89] elastase release,[90] and respiratory burst activity.[89] Conversely, low molecular weight or oligomeric HA (LMW HA) promotes proinflammatory properties, including the stimulation of IL1ß expression, suggesting that it is able to activate the NLRP3 inflammasome.[91,92] Increased lung HA occurs in sarcoidosis,[93] occupational disorders,[94] ARDS,[95] and after acute lung injury, as well as in rodent models such as intratracheal bleomycin instillation.[96–98] Further, the increased recovery of HA temporally correlates with an influx of inflammatory cells.[99]

There are three mammalian HA synthases, HAS1, 2, and HAS3. Although HAS3 produces HA of a smaller molecular size compared to the other two synthases, all essentially produce HMW HA, and the generation of LMW HA occurs either through the actions of hyaluronidases or by oxidative and nitrative fragmentation of HMW HA.[100–102] Of note, preterm infants destined to develop BPD have increased superoxide and peroxynitrite early in their postnatal course.[103,104] LMW HA acts as an endogenous danger signal that interacts with HA receptors and TLRs to activate the innate immune system.[100,105–108] Interestingly, we and others have demonstrated that HA fragments are able to activate the NLRP3 inflammasome.[91,92]

HA interacts with specific cell-associated receptors, including CD44 and Receptor for HA-Mediated Motility (RHAMM, CD168). Both of these receptors have been implicated in acute lung injury.[85] Expression of CD44, an ubiquitously expressed type 1 transmembrane HA receptor, is increased after bleomycin injury.[109,110] Bleomycin-induced lung injury in CD44 KO mice is associated with unrelenting inflammation and HA accumulation, suggesting that CD44 is necessary for the resolution of inflammation.[111] RHAMM expression is more restricted and occurs largely in response to injury in a wide variety of cells.[86,108,112,113] RHAMM expression has been reported on the cell surface, in the cytoplasm and in the nucleus, with functions related to cell locomotion, proliferation, and mitosis.[113–115] After intratracheal bleomycin-induced acute lung injury, RHAMM expression is increased in macrophages responding to injury.[116,117] Interestingly, antibody blockade of RHAMM *in vivo* decreases the accumulation of macrophages into the bleomycin-injured lung, and RHAMM KO mice have decreased inflammation and fibrosis compared to wild-type controls.[118]

Interestingly, HA content in the lung decreases with increasing gestation,[119] is decreased by antenatal betamethasone administration,[120] and the presence of HMW HA in early gestation fetal skin is associated with scarless wound healing.[121] However, when wounds are made large enough, expression of HA receptors is noted in association with wound fibrosis.[122] This suggests that, in the quiescent state, HMW HA is anti-inflammatory and antifibrotic, and that HA receptor expression is necessary for the fibrotic phenotype.

Since HA has never been shown to directly bind to TLRs, it has been proposed that LMW HA uses HA receptors as a complex with TLRs to allow signaling to activate the NLRP3 inflammasome. A number of studies support this proposal. Gallo's group demonstrated that both TLR4 and CD44 are involved in HA stimulated MIP2 expression.[123] Importantly, CD44 coimmunoprecipitated with TLR4 and MD2.[123] In further studies, they have proposed that CD44 participates in internalization of medium chain HA which is degraded in lysosomes to activate NLRP3 intracellularly.[92]

Importantly, we have previously demonstrated that an RHAMM-derived peptide is able to inhibit macrophage accumulation and fibrosis after intratracheal bleomycin in rodents,[116] demonstrating that HA is upstream of and critical for the inflammatory response to lung injury. These data also suggest that these peptides are likely inhibiting inflammasome activation. The ability of these and more advanced peptides in blocking the activation of the TLR-NFκB-NLRP3 inflammasome pathway are currently being evaluated and hold promise of the ability to prevent BPD or to significantly ameliorate its adverse effects on inflammation and lung structure.

Of note, the HA and HA receptor system has also been implicated in other aspects of innate immunity. For example, in bronchial epithelial cells, HMW HA binds to and holds inactive tissue kallikrein, a distal lung bronchoconstrictor. With infectious or other challenges, HMW HA is fragmented, kallikrein is released, and the resulting LMW HA stimulates increased ciliary beat frequency using RHAMM as the receptor.[124–126] This mechanism serves two purposes, distal bronchoconstriction to limit the invasion to the lower respiratory tract and increased mucociliary clearance of the upper airway.

SENSORS OF PAMPS AND DAMPS

Toll-Like Receptors

The best characterized PRRs are the TLRs, which are named after Toll, a protein identified in *Drosophilia* that was initially identified as important for dorsoventral body patterning, but was also found to interact with fungi and activate NFκB.[127] There are 11 known human TLRs with varying ligand specificities.[128] (Fig. 9.4) Most prominently, lipopolysaccharide (LPS) of gram-negative organisms interacts with TLR4, whereas peptidoglycan (PGN) of gram-positive organisms and zymosan of yeast cell walls interact with TLR2. Activation of each TLR results in intracellular signaling that activates growth factor and cytokine production, including IL1ß, TGFß, and TNFα.

The cell surface TLRs include TLR 1, 2, 4, 5, 6, 10, and 11, whereas TLR 3, 7, 8, and 9 are endosomal[61] (Fig. 9.4). The cell surface TLRs have a large extracellular portion that interacts with PAMPs and DAMPs, a transmembrane domain and cytoplasmic tail that contains a domain bearing homology to the IL1 receptor family. This domain is called the Toll/IL1 receptor (TIR) domain and is present in all TLRs except TLR3. The TIRs interact with adaptors of which myeloid differentiation primary response gene 88 (MyD88) is used by all TLRs except TLR3 and signals the activation of NFκB and the production of inflammatory cytokines and growth factors. Thus, the interaction of bacterial, fungal, and viral components with TLRs initiates a robust elaboration of cytokines and growth factors, as well as inducible nitric oxide synthase (iNOS), leading to shock, surfactant deficiency, respiratory distress, and a systemic inflammatory response.[129]

Inflammasomes and IL1ß as Master Regulators of the Innate Immune System

IL1ß is a master inflammatory cytokine that has been implicated in the pathogenesis of a wide variety of diseases such as atherosclerosis, type 1 diabetes, gout, as well as many autoinflammatory disorders including familial cold inflammatory syndrome (FCAS), Muckle-Wells syndrome (MWS), chronic infantile neurologic cutaneous and articular syndrome/neonatal onset multisystem inflammatory disease (CINCA/NOMID).[130–132] The IL1ß-mediated autoinflammatory diseases differ from the classic autoimmune diseases in that there is no role for adaptive immunity in their induction.

IL1ß has a complex activation system (Fig. 9.5). Stimulation of TLRs by PAMPs and DAMPs signals via the adaptor molecule MyD88 to activate NFκB that then mediates a transcriptional increase in the expression of pro-IL1ß.[133] A family of exclusively intracellular proteins called nucleotide-binding oligomerization domain (NOD)-like receptors, or NLRs, also bind to DAMPs.[134] One such NLR, NLRP3, forms a protein complex with the adaptor molecule ASC and procaspase1 to

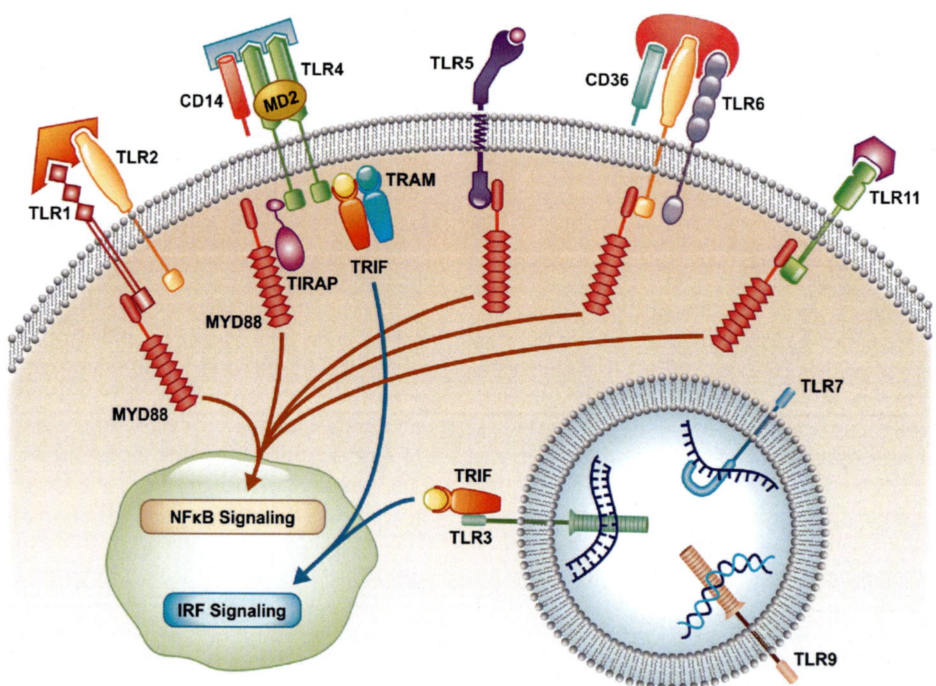

FIG. 9.4 The toll-like receptors. TLRs are pattern recognition receptors that are located either on the cell surface or intracellular. Of the 11 human TLRs, TLR1, TLR2, TLR4, TLR5, TLR6, TLR10, and TLR11 are cell surface receptors and TLR3, TLR7, 8, and 9 are intracellular. Each TLR has its own specific ligands. Thus, TLR1 binds to triacyl-lipoprotein, TLR2 to peptidoglycan (gram positive organisms) and zymosan (fungi), TLR3 to viral double stranded RNA or poly I:C, TLR4 to lipopolysaccharide (gram-negative organisms), TLR5 to bacterial flagellin, TLR6 to mycoplasma diacyl lipopeptides, TLR7 and 8 to viral single-stranded RNA, TLR9 to unmethylated CpG DNA, and TLR11 to *Toxoplasma gondii* profilin-like peptide. The ligand for TLR10 is currently unknown. Each cell surface TLR interacts with MyD88 and activates specific transcription factors, in particular NFκB. TLR4 and intracellular TLRs also activate an alternate pathway involving interferon regulatory factor (IRF) 3.

form the NLRP3 inflammasome.[135,136] Activation of the purinergic receptor P2X7 by extracellular ATP promotes the formation of the NLRP3 inflammasome.[137,138] Formation of this complex cleaves procaspase1 to caspase1 (p20), which in turn proteolytically cleaves pro-IL1ß to produce mature IL1ß. A number of mechanisms have been proposed for the release of IL1ß from cells. Rubartelli proposed autophagy as a route of IL-1ß release. LPS treatment of macrophages stimulated the recruitment of IL-1ß to autophagosomes. When autophagy was inhibited, the sequestered IL1ß was released, but when it was activated, IL-1ß was degraded in the autophagosomes.[139,140] Other reports support release of IL1ß via exosomes,[141] by pyroptosis where the cell dies and releases IL1ß[140] and by an increase in the permeability of cells independent of the activation of NLRP3[142] with extracellular release of pro-IL1ß undergoing further proteolytic cleavage by a variety of proteases.[143] Released IL1ß interacts with its receptor, IL1R, to signal inflammatory pathways. Importantly, IL1 receptor antagonist (IL1ra) is a circulating glycosylated protein that prevents the binding of IL1ß to its receptor.[144] Recombinant IL1ra (rIL1ra, Kineret; Anakinra) is not glycosylated and is used in humans for rheumatic and monogenic disorders that have excess IL1ß production.[145]

A number of studies have shown an association between increased IL1ß and the development of BPD. Yoon et al.[146,147] evaluated the relationship between amniotic fluid cytokines and the risk of BPD. After adjusting for gestational age at birth, elevated levels of amniotic fluid IL-1ß, IL-6, and IL-8, but not TNF-α, were associated with increased risk of developing BPD.[146,147] Koksal et al.[148] showed that elevated

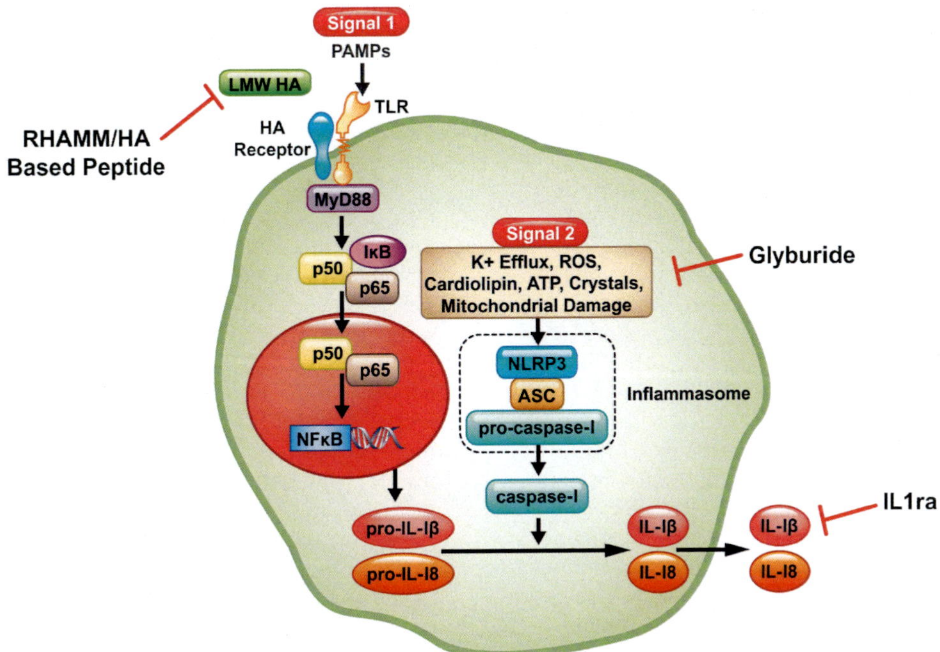

FIG. 9.5 **The TLR-NFκB-NLRP3 inflammasome pathway and inhibitors of IL1ß expression or activity.** The production of IL1ß is tightly controlled and requires two signals. The first signal involves stimulation of TLRs by pathogens or endogenous danger signals such as hyaluronan (HA) and results in the activation of NFκB and transcription of pro-IL1ß and pro-IL18. The second signal, activated by a number of signals including potassium efflux, reactive oxygen species (ROS), ATP, and crystals, results in the formation of the NLRP3 inflammasome, a complex of NLRP3, ASC, and pro-caspase 1. Activation of this complex results in the enzymatic cleavage of procaspase-1 to the active caspase-1, which in turn converts pro-IL1ß and pro-IL18 to their mature forms. Glyburide blocks the formation of the NLRP3 inflammasome and recombinant IL1ra blocks the interaction of IL1β with its receptor. We believe that novel peptides derived from the hyaluronan receptor RHAMM can block TLR signaling to activate this system.

concentrations of IL-1ß, TNF-α, and IL-6 and low concentrations of IL10 in both blood and tracheal aspirates (TA) at 24 hours after birth were associated with the development of BPD. Ambalavanan et al.[149] evaluated 25 cytokines in over 1000 extremely low birth weight infants at 4 hours and on 3,7,14, and 21 days of life. Elevated blood content of IL1ß and other cytokines were associated with death or BPD. Some studies have suggested that an elevated IL1ß:IL1ra ratio is associated with the development of BPD. Rindfleisch et al.[150] demonstrated a high correlation between IL1ß concentration and IL1ß activity that was increased 60-fold on day five of life, while concentrations of IL1ra remained unchanged during the first month of life. Kakkera et al.[151] showed that, compared to infants that did not develop BPD, tracheal aspirate IL1ß as well neutrophil content were significantly increased on days 3 and 5 in the infants that progressed to BPD. While IL1ra concentrations also rose during that time, the IL1ß:IL1ra ratio was significantly increased on days 5 and 7 in the BPD group. Our own studies confirm that an elevated IL1ß:IL1ra ratio at days 1–3 of life is significantly associated with death or BPD at 36 weeks postmenstrual age (PMA).[152]

Elegant mouse studies by Bry et al. showed that, even in the absence of injury, conditional expression of mature IL1ß in lung epithelial cells in the perinatal and postnatal periods was associated with inflammation, downstream cytokine elaboration, decreased vascular endothelial growth factor (VEGF), abnormal α-smooth muscle actin and elastin deposition, and disrupted alveolar septation.[153] These studies establish that excess lung IL1ß alone can recapitulate all the features of BPD, making this cytokine an ideal target for therapeutic blockade. Indeed, Johnson et al. showed that rIL1ra treatment of neonatal rats exposed to 60%

O_2 resulted in decreased inflammation, improved alveolarization, and partially restored vessel density.[154] Nold et al.[155] injected pregnant dams with LPS to induce perinatal inflammation that precipitated BPD and then exposed the rearing pups to a second hit with hyperoxia at either 65% or 85% oxygen. Pups were then treated with rIL-1ra daily or a vehicle for up to 28 days. Hyperoxia exposure was associated with large increases in IL1ß and inflammation. Treatment with rIL1ra decreased inflammation and cytokine elaboration, but its effect was partial and dependent on the oxygen concentration. Using the same model, Rudloff et al.[156] tested an increased dose of rIL1ra, but showed no additional benefit for the ability to decrease inflammation and the changes associated with the development of BPD. Our studies using rIL1ra in mice exposed to postnatal hyperoxia showed substantial improvements in cytokine and growth factor elaboration, inflammation, and alveolar septation.[152] Additionally, in our studies, blockade of the formation of the NLRP3 inflammasome by glyburide[157] also blocked IL1ß protein expression and inflammation, and improved alveolarization.[152] Taken together with studies that demonstrated that LPS exposure of cultured fetal lungs inhibits airway branching which can be reversed by antibody blockade of IL1ß or in fetal lungs from *Il1ß*$^{-/-}$ mice,[158] these studies suggest that rIL1ra might be a useful therapeutic intervention to prevent or limit the severity of BPD, but that *in utero* infection or inflammation might decrease its effectiveness.

CELLS INVOLVED IN INNATE IMMUNITY

A number of investigators have reported the association of an inflammatory influx with subsequent development of BPD in preterm infants with lung disease. Elastase activity and neutrophil counts in tracheal aspirates of intubated preterm infants in the first week of life are higher in infants that subsequently develop BPD.[6] These infants not only have higher neutrophil counts, but their tracheal aspirates also have increased chemoattractive properties and increased concentrations of neutrophil chemoattractants such as IL-8.[7] Neutrophil and macrophage accumulation commences early in the first week of life and counts remain elevated in infants that develop BPD.[8,9] Interestingly, increased concentrations of IL-8 precede the influx of neutrophils in tracheal aspirates of infants that develop BPD.[10] Inflammation results in the elaboration of proinflammatory and profibrotic growth factors, an imbalance of the proteolytic activity in the lung, and increased vascular permeability.[4,5] A number of cell types are involved in the innate immune response, including neutrophils, macrophages, DCs, natural killer (NK) cells, and most recently, innate lymphoid cells (ILCs).

Neutrophils: The classical view of neutrophils was that they represented the initial cellular response to pathogens, were designed to provide immediate counterattack to rid the host of the invasion, and then underwent apoptosis. However, more recent studies suggest a more nuanced set of functions for neutrophils, including proreparative functions and the ability to move out of affected tissues.[159] Neutrophils are recruited from the circulation in response to both PAMPs and DAMPs. Resident cells such as DCs and resident macrophages sense these signals and create the local ATP and chemokine gradients, as well as adhesion molecule expression to promote neutrophil recruitment.[160] Interestingly, initial neutrophil adhesion is mediated by CD44 and endothelial HA when PAMPs are driving the response, but by macrophage antigen 1 (MAC1) and intercellular adhesion molecule (ICAM) in the face of sterile injury.[161] Neutrophils contain a multitude of damaging molecules, including metalloproteinases, reactive oxygen and nitrogen species, the production of neutrophil extracellular traps (NETs) and antimicrobial peptides, that are sequestered in phagolysosomes within neutrophil granules, and that can cause tissue injury.[162,163] On the other hand, more recent evidence provides insight into several key protective roles that neutrophils play in the response to injury. Phagocytosis and clearance of necrotic cells and enzymatic degradation of DAMPs limit the continuation of the initial stimulus that initiated inflammation.[164,165] Some of the secreted products of infiltrating neutrophils are proreparative, such as VEGF that promotes angiogenesis.[166] Further, extracellular membrane vesicles released from neutrophils exposes phosphatidylserine and Annexin A1 on the surface which are anti-inflammatory signals for macrophages and DCs.[167,168]

There is evidence for neutrophil apoptosis in the target tissue that triggers engulfment by macrophages and the secretion of transforming growth factor beta (TGFß), an anti-inflammatory growth factor.[169] However, recent studies using intravital microscopy and tracking of neutrophils and macrophages have questioned this dogma and have demonstrated that neutrophils are able to migrate back into the blood, a process called reverse transmigration.[170] The mechanisms regulating this reverse migration remain to be resolved.

Macrophages: Both alveolar macrophages and DCs are derived from a common progenitor population and are sentinel cells that serve to maintain quiescence in the lung.[171] These immediate response cells remove pathogens and apoptotic cells by phagocytosis, bind invading organisms to present them to immune cells, and activate the adaptive immune system.[172] The generation of alveolar macrophages is dependent on granulocyte monocyte colony stimulating factor (GM-CSF) that also regulates surfactant turnover. Thus, patients with mutations in the GM-CSF receptor have increased susceptibility to infection and develop alveolar proteinosis.[173] Alveolar macrophages produce anti-inflammatory molecules such as TGFß, IL10 receptor, and SIRPα, a receptor that engages the CRD of SP-A to inhibit NFκB activation.[174]

With lung injury or infection, monocyte-derived macrophages are recruited from the bone marrow and circulation to form an inflammatory influx at the site of injury. Interaction of these cells with PAMPs and DAMPs using PRRs such as TLRs induces the activation of the TLR-NFκB-NLRP3 inflammasome pathway and phenotypic changes in the macrophages.[175] Macrophage phenotype is controlled by a variety of factors, including the gut and lung microbiome as well as the lung microenvironment. Initially, two major macrophage phenotypes were described. Classically activated macrophages, called M1 macrophages, are proinflammatory, involved in killing organisms and produce cytokines, growth factors, and iNOS. Alternatively activated macrophages, called M2 macrophages, are reparative cells that promote tissue repair.[176] However, this simple construct has been challenged with the discovery of M2 macrophage subtypes, some of which respond to proinflammatory signals such as LPS and IL6.[177]

Resolution of inflammation is an important part of the inflammatory process and disturbance of these pathways results in pathologic inflammation and tissue damage.[178] Several mechanisms exist to switch off an inflammatory response. First, the orderly removal of dead cells, a process called efferocytosis, is orchestrated by communication mediated by products released by dead cells with macrophages that seek out, recognize, and then phagocytose the dead cells.[179] Second, as noted above, the activation of NOX2 by TLR signaling also serves to inhibit the synthesis of IL1ß and dampen the inflammatory process.[83] Interestingly, CD44 KO mice given intratracheal bleomycin have unrelenting inflammation, suggesting that this HA receptor plays a role in the resolution of inflammation, although the mechanisms by which it has these effects have not been fully elucidated.[111]

Dendritic Cells: DCs induce and maintain tolerance in the homeostatic state but are also critical for the ability of the innate immune system to perform surveillance against invading organisms and activate the adaptive immune system.[180–183] Immature DC have a high capacity to take up antigens via receptor-mediated endocytosis and micropinocytosis. As such, they act as surveillance cells that can clear nonself antigens as well as dead cells. This action does not mature these cells and induces T-cell apoptosis or anergy rather than differentiation, a property that forms the basis of immune tolerance in the unchallenged state.[184] Interaction of immature DC with PAMPs and DAMPs results in multiple changes in gene expression that define the process of maturation.[185] Mature DC migrate through the lymphatics to lymph nodes and act as antigen-presenting cells that interact with naïve T-cells to generate T-helper (Th) cells such as Th1, Th2, and Th17 cells, as well as cytotoxic T cells and B cells to mount a complete adaptive immune response to invasion.[186]

Distinct subsets of DC have been described.[187] Plasmacytoid DC (pDC) express TLR7 and TLR9, respond to viral infections, and produce interferon gamma (IFNγ) that activates a robust Th1 response.[188,189] Myeloid or conventional DC (cDC) express lectins, TLRs, and NLRs and interaction with bacteria or fungi results in the expression of IL1ß, IL12, and IL23 which stimulate Th2, Th17, Th22, and prime $CD4^+$ T-cells.[190,191]

Very few studies have examined DCs in BPD. De Paepe et al. used DC-specific immunostaining of autopsy sections of the lungs of preterm infants that had respiratory failure compared to controls.[192] While DCs were present in controls, a dramatic increase in DC numbers was noted in infants that had either been ventilated or whose mothers had a history of chorioamnionitis.[192] Interestingly, rhinovirus infection or poly I:C treatment of hyperoxia-exposed neonatal mice was associated with increased accumulation of $CD103^+$ DC in the lung and increased airway hyperresponsiveness, suggesting that the development of BPD increases the DC response and potentially worsens the outcome.[193]

Natural Killer Cells: NK cells are cytotoxic T cells that possess innate properties in that they mediate cell killing, but do not require prior antigen exposure. Although NK cells express a wide array of markers, two in particular, CD27 and CD11b (MAC1), define the maturation of these cells from double negative, to $CD27^+$ $CD11b^-$, to double positive, to $CD27^-$ $CD11b^+$.[194] NK cells are directly cytotoxic, lysing "non-self" cells such as cancer cells or cells that are infected. The mechanism of cytotoxicity requires the recognition of the target cell, formation of the immunologic synapse with the target cell, and killing of the cell.[195] This killing is achieved by two mechanisms.

First, INFγ produced by the NK cells activates death receptors such as TNF-Related Apoptosis-Inducing Ligand Receptor (TRAIL-R) and Fas (CD95) on the target cell. These bind to their ligands TRAIL and Fas ligand (FasL) on NK cells which initiates an apoptotic pathway in the target cell leading to death.[196] The second and more prominent mechanism of killing by NK cells is the formation of lytic granules in the NK cells and their delivery to the target cell by fusion of the membranes at the immunologic synapse. The lytic granules contain perforin that creates a pore in the cell membrane and granzyme B which enzymatically activates the apoptotic pathway in the target cell.[197] NK cells also produce a wide array of Th1-type cytokines that serve to attract other cells such as lymphocytes and macrophages to the site to assist in the defense of the host.[198] Of note, using flow cytometry of whole blood samples, Ballabh et al. showed that CD4+ lymphocytes were decreased in the first 2 weeks of life in infants destined to develop BPD and that infants with respiratory distress syndrome have higher NK cell content.[199] Interestingly, Pelkonen et al. have reported that decreased CD4+ lymphocytes remain decreased in school-aged children that were born preterm.[200]

Innate Lymphoid Cells: ILCs are self-renewing lymphocytes that reside in tissues rather than circulate in the blood. They lack the normal repertoire of antigens displayed by T and B lymphocytes, but produce cytokines, stimulate adaptive immune responses, and regulate inflammation.[201] Three types of ILCs have been described. ILC1s react to viruses and tumors, ILC2s respond to parasites and allergens, and ILC3s attack bacteria and fungi. ILCs respond to inducer cytokines and act immediately, mirroring the innate and not the adaptive immune response.

In a manner similar to that seen in NK cells, ILC1s produce INFγ and are a first-line defense against viruses and certain types of bacteria including Toxoplasma. ILC2s produce Th2-like cytokines including IL4 and IL13 in response to helminth infections and allergens. ILC3s develop after birth and are largely found at mucosal sites where they respond to bacterial challenge. With tissue injury, ILC1s are geared to remove microbes, dead cells, and debris, ILC2s undertake remodeling and repair of the damaged tissue, and ILC3s produce IL22 as a protective cytokine.[202]

In the lung, while the actual frequency of ILC2s is low, this ILC is the most predominant, representing 30% of all ILCs in the lung.[203,204] Allergic disorders are associated with a substantial increase in the ILC2 content, which is dependent on GATA3 stimulated by IL25, IL33, and thymic stromal lymphopoietin (TSLP).[205] Interestingly, ILC2s are increased in an IL33-dependent manner during mouse alveolarization in the first 7 days of life.[206,207]

ILC3s have been reported in the lung and are activated by IL23 and IL1ß. Increased ILC3s are noted both in bacterial infections of the lung, but also during asthmatic disorders, where IL22 is protective and IL17 worsens the condition.[208,209]

GUT AND LUNG MICROBIOTA AND INNATE IMMUNITY

Long considered to be a sterile environment, non-culture-based techniques to evaluate lung microbial presence have revealed the existence of a microbiota of both the upper and lower respiratory tracts.[210] In comparison to the gut (10^{11} CFU/g colonic luminal content), the lung microbiota is of low density (2.2×10^3 bacterial genomes/cm^2), and studies of the role of the lung microbiome are in their infancy.[211] However, there has been a shift from the notion that any bacteria found in the lung are pathogenic to the current thinking that the lung microbiota are essential for normal homeostasis. An airway microbiome has been described for infants at birth.[212] The balance of immigration and elimination of bacteria determines the nature of the lung microbiota.[211] Thus, inhalation, microaspiration, and mucosal dispersion allow bacteria into the lung, whereas cough, mucociliary clearance, and immune responses serve to eliminate lung bacteria.[213] Given the changes in pH, humidity, temperature, and oxygen and carbon dioxide contents, the composition of the lung microbiota changes by location with greater diversity in the upper versus the lower respiratory tract.[211] The mode of delivery and feeding influence the acquisition of the lung microbiota with vaginal birth and breastfeeding being associated with a health-promoting microbiota that includes *Bifidobacterium* spp. and *Lactobacillus* spp.[213] Breast milk itself has a microbiota and also delivers maternal antibodies that are protective to the baby.[214,215] A number of other factors influence the composition of the microbiota, including the composition of other bacteria in the microenvironment, exposure to antibiotics and smoke, vaccination, season, and day-care attendance.[211]

The microbiota of the gut and the lung appear to influence both structural development and physiologic function of the lung. Thus, germ-free mice have smaller lungs[216] and fewer alveoli.[217]

A number of mechanisms of a gut-lung microbiota cross-talk have been proposed.[218] The direct transfer of bacteria or bacterial fragments can occur through reflux as well as by penetration of the organisms into the blood and lymphatic system. The lymphatic invasion of bacteria or their fragments can also elicit an adaptive immune response with T and B cells. The nutritional activity of gut microbes changes the metabolic products that are released and may be metabolized or influence host cells in the gut and the lung.[219]

With respect to neonates, a number of studies have demonstrated the presence of a lung microbiome soon after birth that evolves over time and with environmental influences.[220] The major phyla of the neonatal airway microbiota are Firmicutes and Proteobacteria with *Staphylococcus* and *Ureaplasma* being the principal genera found. There appears to be a greater turnover of microbes and lower *Lactobacilli* in patients with BPD.[220] However, there is great variability in the reported literature and there is an urgent need for the standardization of methodologies for sampling and analysis in this vulnerable population that are currently lacking.

SUMMARY

A number of non-immune and immune mechanisms contribute to the innate immune response in the preterm infant that influences the development of BPD. While the adaptive immune system is immature in preterm infants, the innate immune system is robust and contributes greatly to the development of an inflammatory response after preterm birth and exposure to ventilation, oxygenation, and environmental factors, including microorganisms. This evolutionarily conserved system has multiple complex features that together orchestrate the immune response. Thus, antimicrobial peptides, pathogen-related and endogenous danger signals such as hyaluronan and biglycan, sensors of these signals such as collectins, TLRs, and NLRs, and effector cells such as neutrophils and macrophages represent the immune recognition and activation systems that regulate the immune response. Critically, the elaboration of IL1ß is a principal activator of the innate immune system and contributes greatly to the pathogenesis of BPD. Further studies to elucidate how endogenous danger signals are generated and the full repertoire of receptors involved in the activation of this pathway will likely reveal new therapeutic targets. In particular, it will be important to determine the role that exposure to oxygen, mechanical ventilation, and infection play in this biology. Thus far, a number of therapeutic approaches, including IL1ra, glyburide, and RHAMM-derived peptides, hold promise for the ability to block the activation of the innate immune system to either prevent or reduce the severity of BPD. Much remains to be studied with respect to the influence of the gut and lung microbiota on innate and adaptive immunity and to the development of BPD. The future will likely reveal even more complexity and interrelated functions of these systems. However, this new knowledge will allow the development of even more sophisticated approaches to prevent or ameliorate the disastrous consequences of BPD on patients, their families, and society in general.

ACKNOWLEDGMENTS

The authors are mindful that this review is not intended to be all encompassing and any omission of work that would be relevant to the topic of this review is not intentional. RCS is a cofounder of Eravon Therapeutics, Inc. that is focused on RHAMM-HA-based therapeutics. There are no conflicts of interest. Funding for the studies described that were conducted in the Savani laboratory was from NIH R01 awards HL62868, HL62472, and HL093535, and U01 award HL075900. Additional funding was obtained from the William Buchanan Chair in Pediatrics and Children's Hospital Foundation Dallas grant (#137).

REFERENCES

1. Hunter P. The inflammation theory of disease. The growing realization that chronic inflammation is crucial in many diseases opens new avenues for treatment. *EMBO Rep*. 2012;13(11):968–970.
2. Savani RC. Modulators of inflammation in bronchopulmonary dysplasia. *Semin Perinatol*. 2018;42(7):459–470.
3. Disdier C, Chen X, Kim JE, Threlkeld SW, Stonestreet BS. Anti-cytokine therapy to attenuate ischemic-reperfusion associated brain injury in the perinatal period. *Brain Sci*. 2018;8(6).
4. Li B, Concepcion K, Meng X, Zhang L. Brain-immune interactions in perinatal hypoxic-ischemic brain injury. *Prog Neurobiol*. 2017;159:50–68.
5. Lai JCY, Rocha-Ferreira E, Ek CJ, Wang X, Hagberg H, Mallard C. Immune responses in perinatal brain injury. *Brain Behav Immun*. 2017;63:210–223.
6. Neu J. Multiomics-based strategies for taming intestinal inflammation in the neonate. *Curr Opin Clin Nutr Metab Care*. 2019;22(3):217–222.
7. Mihi B, Good M. Impact of toll-like receptor 4 signaling in necrotizing enterocolitis: the state of the science. *Clin Perinatol*. 2019;46(1):145–157.
8. Rivera JC, Holm M, Austeng D, et al. Retinopathy of prematurity: inflammation, choroidal degeneration, and novel promising therapeutic strategies. *J Neuroinflammation*. 2017;14(1):165.

9. Skirecki T, Cavaillon JM. Inner sensors of endotoxin - implications for sepsis research and therapy. *FEMS Microbiol Rev.* 2019;43(3):239–256.
10. Cuenca AG, Wynn JL, Moldawer LL, Levy O. Role of innate immunity in neonatal infection. *Am J Perinatol.* 2013;30(2):105–112.
11. Brien ME, Baker B, Duval C, Gaudreault V, Jones RL, Girard S. Alarmins at the maternal-fetal interface: involvement of inflammation in placental dysfunction and pregnancy complications (1). *Can J Physiol Pharmacol.* 2019;97(3):206–212.
12. Sahni M, Mowes AK. *Bronchopulmonary Dysplasia*. Treasure Island (FL): StatPearls; 2019.
13. Jobe AH. The new bronchopulmonary dysplasia. *Curr Opin Pediatr.* 2011;23(2):167–172.
14. Tracy MK, Berkelhamer SK. Bronchopulmonary dysplasia and pulmonary outcomes of prematurity. *Pediatr Ann.* 2019;48(4):e148–e153.
15. Reiterer F, Scheuchenegger A, Resch B, Maurer-Fellbaum U, Avian A, Urlesberger B. Bronchopulmonary dysplasia in very preterm infants: outcome up to preschool age, in a single center of Austria. *Pediatr Int.* 2019;61(4):381–387.
16. Chess PR, D'Angio CT, Pryhuber GS, Maniscalco WM. Pathogenesis of bronchopulmonary dysplasia. *Semin Perinatol.* 2006;30(4):171–178.
17. Warburton D, Schwarz M, Tefft D, Flores-Delgado G, Anderson KD, Cardoso WV. The molecular basis of lung morphogenesis. *Mech Dev.* 2000;92(1):55–81.
18. Elias PM. The skin barrier as an innate immune element. *Semin Immunopathol.* 2007;29(1):3–14.
19. Schenk M, Mueller C. The mucosal immune system at the gastrointestinal barrier. *Best Pract Res Clin Gastroenterol.* 2008;22(3):391–409.
20. Karczewski J, Troost FJ, Konings I, et al. Regulation of human epithelial tight junction proteins by Lactobacillus plantarum in vivo and protective effects on the epithelial barrier. *Am J Physiol Gastrointest Liver Physiol.* 2010; 298(6):G851–G859.
21. Knowles MR, Boucher RC. Mucus clearance as a primary innate defense mechanism for mammalian airways. *J Clin Investig.* 2002;109(5):571–577.
22. Nieuw Amerongen AV, Veerman EC. Current therapies for xerostomia and salivary gland hypofunction associated with cancer therapies. *Support Care Cancer.* 2003; 11(4):226–231.
23. Waterer GW. Airway defense mechanisms. *Clin Chest Med.* 2012;33(2):199–209.
24. Bogdan C, Rollinghoff M, Diefenbach A. Reactive oxygen and reactive nitrogen intermediates in innate and specific immunity. *Curr Opin Immunol.* 2000;12(1):64–76.
25. Tecle T, Tripathi S, Hartshorn KL. Review: defensins and cathelicidins in lung immunity. *Innate Immun.* 2010; 16(3):151–159.
26. Doss M, White MR, Tecle T, Hartshorn KL. Human defensins and LL-37 in mucosal immunity. *J Leukoc Biol.* 2010; 87(1):79–92.
27. Ganz T. Defensins: antimicrobial peptides of innate immunity. *Nat Rev Immunol.* 2003;3(9):710–720.
28. Yount NY, Weaver DC, Lee EY, et al. Unifying structural signature of eukaryotic alpha-helical host defense peptides. *Proc Natl Acad Sci USA.* 2019;116(14): 6944–6953.
29. Ganz T. Antimicrobial polypeptides. *J Leukoc Biol.* 2004; 75(1):34–38.
30. van der Does AM, Hiemstra PS, Mookherjee N. Antimicrobial host defence peptides: immunomodulatory functions and translational prospects. *Adv Exp Med Biol.* 2019; 1117:149–171.
31. Lee EY, Lee MW, Wong GCL. Modulation of toll-like receptor signaling by antimicrobial peptides. *Semin Cell Dev Biol.* 2019;88:173–184.
32. Cummings RD, McEver RP. C-type lectins. In: Varki A, Cummings RD, Esko JD, et al., eds. *Essentials of Glycobiology*. NY: Cold Spring Harbor; 2015:435–452.
33. Reid KBM. Complement component C1q: historical perspective of a functionally versatile, and structurally unusual, serum protein. *Front Immunol.* 2018;9:764.
34. Galindo-Sevilla N, Reyes-Arroyo F, Mancilla-Ramirez J. The role of complement in preterm birth and prematurity. *J Perinat Med.* 2019;47(8):793–803.
35. Dos Santos Silva PM, de Oliveira WF, Albuquerque PBS, Dos Santos Correia MT, Coelho L. Insights into anti-pathogenic activities of mannose lectins. *Int J Biol Macromol.* 2019;140:234–244.
36. Casals C, Campanero-Rhodes MA, Garcia-Fojeda B, Solis D. The role of collectins and galectins in lung innate immune defense. *Front Immunol.* 2018;9:1998.
37. Chroneos ZC, Sever-Chroneos Z, Shepherd VL. Pulmonary surfactant: an immunological perspective. *Cell Physiol Biochem.* 2010;25(1):13–26.
38. Crouch E, Hartshorn K, Ofek I. Collectins and pulmonary innate immunity. *Immunol Rev.* 2000;173:52–65.
39. Waters P, Vaid M, Kishore U, Madan T. Lung surfactant proteins A and D as pattern recognition proteins. *Adv Exp Med Biol.* 2009;653:74–97.
40. Ujma S, Horsnell WG, Katz AA, Clark HW, Schafer G. Non-pulmonary immune functions of surfactant proteins a and D. *J Innate Immun.* 2017;9(1):3–11.
41. Kishore U, Greenhough TJ, Waters P, et al. Surfactant proteins SP-A and SP-D: structure, function and receptors. *Mol Immunol.* 2006;43(9):1293–1315.
42. Gardai SJ, Xiao YQ, Dickinson M, et al. By binding SIRPa or Calreticulin/CD91, lung collectins act as dual function surveillance moleculaes to suppress or enhance inflammation. *Cell.* 2003;115:13–23.
43. Foley JP, Lam D, Jiang H, et al. Toll-like receptor 2 (TLR2), transforming growth factor-beta, hyaluronan (HA), and receptor for HA-mediated motility (RHAMM) are required for surfactant protein A-stimulated macrophage chemotaxis. *J Biol Chem.* 2012;287(44):37406–37419.
44. Brown-Augsburger P, Chang D, Rust K, Crouch EC. Biosynthesis of surfactant protein D. Contributions of conserved NH2-terminal cysteine residues and collagen

helix formation to assembly and secretion. *J Biol Chem.* 1996;271(31):18912–18919.
45. Guo CJ, Atochina-Vasserman EN, Abramova E, et al. S-nitrosylation of surfactant protein-D controls inflammatory function. *PLoS Biol.* 2008;6(11):e266.
46. Zhang L, Ikegami M, Crouch EC, Korfhagen TR, Whitsett JA. Activity of pulmonary Surfactant Protein-D (SP-D) in vivo is dependent on oligomeric structure. *J Biol Chem.* 2001;276(22):19214–19219.
47. Mendelson CR, Boggaram V. Hormonal and developmental regulation of pulmonary surfactant synthesis in fetal lung. *Baillieres Clin Endocrinol Metab.* 1990;4(2): 351–378.
48. Wong CJ, Akiyama J, Allen L, Hawgood S. Localization and developmental expression of surfactant proteins D and A in the respiratory tract of the mouse. *Pediatr Res.* 1996;39(6):930–937.
49. Crouch E, Rust K, Marienchek W, Parghi D, Chang D, Persson A. Developmental expression of pulmonary surfactant protein D (SP-D). *Am J Respir Cell Mol Biol.* 1991; 5(1):13–18.
50. Khoor A, Gray ME, Hull WM, Whitsett JA, Stahlman MT. Developmental expression of SP-A and SP-A mRNA in the proximal and distal respiratory epithelium in the human fetus and newborn. *J Histochem Cytochem.* 1993; 41(9):1311–1319.
51. Boggaram V. Regulation of lung surfactant protein gene expression. *Front Biosci.* 2003;8:d751–764.
52. Awasthi S, Coalson JJ, Yoder BA, Crouch E, King RJ. Deficiencies in lung surfactant proteins A and D are associated with lung infection in very premature neonatal baboons. *Am J Respir Crit Care Med.* 2001;163(2):389–397.
53. Kramer BW, Jobe AH, Bachurski CJ, Ikegami M. Surfactant protein A recruits neutrophils into the lungs of ventilated preterm lambs. *Am J Respir Crit Care Med.* 2001; 163(1):158–165.
54. Condon JC, Jeyasuria P, Faust JM, Mendelson CR. Surfactant protein secreted by the maturing mouse fetal lung acts as a hormone that signals the initiation of parturition. *Proc Natl Acad Sci USA.* 2004;101(14):4978–4983.
55. Montalbano AP, Hawgood S, Mendelson CR. Mice deficient in surfactant protein A (SP-A) and SP-D or in TLR2 manifest delayed parturition and decreased expression of inflammatory and contractile genes. *Endocrinology.* 2013;154(1):483–498.
56. Matzinger P. Tolerance, danger, and the extended family. *Annu Rev Immunol.* 1994;12:991–1045.
57. Taylor KR, Gallo RL. Glycosaminoglycans and their proteoglycans: host-associated molecular patterns for initiation and modulation of inflammation. *FASEB J.* 2006; 20(1):9–22.
58. Timmermans K, Kox M, Scheffer GJ, Pickkers P. Danger in the intensive care unit: damps in critically ill patients. *Shock.* 2016;45(2):108–116.
59. Schaefer L. Complexity of danger: the diverse nature of damage-associated molecular patterns. *J Biol Chem.* 2014;289(51):35237–35245.
60. Karampitsakos T, Woolard T, Bouros D, Tzouvelekis A. Toll-like receptors in the pathogenesis of pulmonary fibrosis. *Eur J Pharmacol.* 2017;808:35–43.
61. Zhang X, Mosser DM. Macrophage activation by endogenous danger signals. *J Pathol.* 2008;214(2):161–178.
62. Anders HJ, Schaefer L. Beyond tissue injury-damage-associated molecular patterns, toll-like receptors, and inflammasomes also drive regeneration and fibrosis. *J Am Soc Nephrol.* 2014;25(7):1387–1400.
63. Kuipers MT, van der Poll T, Schultz MJ, Wieland CW. Bench-to-bedside review: damage-associated molecular patterns in the onset of ventilator-induced lung injury. *Crit Care.* 2011;15(6):235.
64. Shirasuna K, Karasawa T, Takahashi M. Exogenous nanoparticles and endogenous crystalline molecules as danger signals for the NLRP3 inflammasomes. *J Cell Physiol.* 2019;234(5):5436–5450.
65. Shirasuna K, Usui F, Karasawa T, et al. Nanosilica-induced placental inflammation and pregnancy complications: different roles of the inflammasome components NLRP3 and ASC. *Nanotoxicology.* 2015; 9(5):554–567.
66. Yang H, Wang H, Ju Z, et al. MD-2 is required for disulfide HMGB1-dependent TLR4 signaling. *J Exp Med.* 2015;212(1):5–14.
67. Yang H, Wang H, Chavan SS, Andersson U. High mobility group box protein 1 (HMGB1): the prototypical endogenous danger molecule. *Mol Med.* 2015; 21(Suppl 1):S6–S12.
68. Vijayakumar EC, Bhatt LK, Prabhavalkar KS. High mobility group box-1 (HMGB1): a potential target in therapeutics. *Curr Drug Targets.* 2019;20(14): 1474–1485.
69. Wang H, Bloom O, Zhang M, et al. HMG-1 as a late mediator of endotoxin lethality in mice. *Science.* 1999; 285(5425):248–251.
70. Li J, Kokkola R, Tabibzadeh S, et al. Structural basis for the proinflammatory cytokine activity of high mobility group box 1. *Mol Med.* 2003;9(1–2):37–45.
71. Yang H, Ochani M, Li J, et al. Reversing established sepsis with antagonists of endogenous high-mobility group box 1. *Proc Natl Acad Sci USA.* 2004;101(1):296–301.
72. Aghai ZH, Saslow JG, Meniru C, et al. High-mobility group box-1 protein in tracheal aspirates from premature infants: relationship with bronchopulmonary dysplasia and steroid therapy. *J Perinatol.* 2010;30(9):610–615.
73. Feng J, Deng C, Yu JL, Guo CB, Zhao QQ. [Expression of high mobility group protein-B1 in mice with hyperoxia-induced bronchopulmonary dysplasia]. *Zhong Guo Dang Dai Er Ke Za Zhi.* 2010;12(3):219–223.
74. Yu B, Li X, Wan Q, Han W, Deng C, Guo C. High-Mobility group box-1 protein disrupts alveolar elastogenesis of hyperoxia-injured newborn lungs. *J Interferon Cytokine Res.* 2016;36(3):159–168.
75. Dalbeth N, Merriman TR, Stamp LK. Gout. *Lancet.* 2016; 388(10055):2039–2052.
76. Dalbeth N, Choi HK, Joosten LAB, et al. Gout. *Nat Rev Dis Primers.* 2019;5(1):69.

77. Roedig H, Nastase MV, Wygrecka M, Schaefer L. Breaking down chronic inflammatory diseases: the role of biglycan in promoting a switch between inflammation and autophagy. *FEBS J*. 2019;286(15):2965–2979.
78. Nastase MV, Young MF, Schaefer L. Biglycan: a multivalent proteoglycan providing structure and signals. *J Histochem Cytochem*. 2012;60(12):963–975.
79. Hsieh LT, Nastase MV, Zeng-Brouwers J, Iozzo RV, Schaefer L. Soluble biglycan as a biomarker of inflammatory renal diseases. *Int J Biochem Cell Biol*. 2014;54: 223–235.
80. Schaefer L. Small leucine-rich proteoglycans in kidney disease. *J Am Soc Nephrol*. 2011;22(7):1200–1207.
81. Babelova A, Moreth K, Tsalastra-Greul W, et al. Biglycan, a danger signal that activates the NLRP3 inflammasome via toll-like and P2X receptors. *J Biol Chem*. 2009; 284(36):24035–24048.
82. Moreth K, Frey H, Hubo M, et al. Biglycan-triggered TLR-2- and TLR-4-signaling exacerbates the pathophysiology of ischemic acute kidney injury. *Matrix Biol*. 2014;35: 143–151.
83. Hsieh LT, Frey H, Nastase MV, et al. Bimodal role of NADPH oxidases in the regulation of biglycan-triggered IL-1beta synthesis. *Matrix Biol*. 2016;49:61–81.
84. Veness-Meehan KA, Rhodes DN, Stiles AD. Temporal and spatial expression of biglycan in chronic oxygen-induced lung injury. *Am J Respir Cell Mol Biol*. 1994;11(5): 509–516.
85. Savani RC, DeLisser HM. Hyaluronan and its receptors in lung health and disease. In: Garg HG, Roughley PJ, Hales CA, eds. *Proteoglycans and Lung Disease*. New York: Marcel Dekker; 2003:73–106.
86. Jiang D, Liang J, Noble PW. Hyaluronan as an immune regulator in human diseases. *Physiol Rev*. 2011;91(1): 221–264.
87. Stern R, Asari AA, Sugahara KN. Hyaluronan fragments: an information-rich system. *Eur J Cell Biol*. 2006;85(8): 699–715.
88. Tamoto K, Nochi H, Tada M, et al. High-molecular weight hyaluronic acids inhibit chemotaxis and phagocytosis but not lysosomal enzyme release induced by receptor-mediated stimulations in Guinea pig phagocytes. *Microbiol Immunol*. 1994;38(1):73–80.
89. Suzuki Y, Yamaguchi T. Effects of hyaluronic acid on macrophage phagocytosis and active oxygen release. *Agents Actions*. 1993;38:32–37.
90. Akatsuka M, Yamamoto Y, Tobetto K, Yasui K, Ando T. Suppressive effects of hyaluronic acid on elastase release from rat peritoneal leucocytes. *J Pharm Pharmacol*. 1993; 45:110–114.
91. Østerholt HC, Dannevig I, Wyckoff MH, et al. Antioxidant protects against increases in low molecular weight hyaluronan and inflammation in asphyxiated newborn pigs resuscitated with 100% oxygen. *PLoS One*. 2012; 7(6):e38839.
92. Yamasaki K, Muto J, Taylor KR, et al. NLRP3/Cryopyrin is necessary for interleukin-1{beta} (IL-1{beta}) release in response to hyaluronan, an endogenous trigger of inflammation in response to injury. *J Biol Chem*. 2009; 284(19):12762–12771.
93. Hällgren R, Eklund A, Engstrom-Laurent A, Schmekel B. Hyaluronate in bronchoalveolar lavage fluid: a new marker in sarcoidosis reflecting pulmonary disease. *Br Med J*. 1985;290:1778–1781.
94. Bjermer L, Engstrom-Laurent A, Lundgren R, Rosenhall L, Hallgren R. Hyaluronate and type III procollagen peptide concentrations in bronchoalveolar lavage fluid as markers of disease activity in farmer's lung. *Br Med J*. 1987;295:803–806.
95. Hällgren R, Samuelsson T, Laurent TC, Modig J. Accumulation of hyaluronan (hyaluronic acid) in the lung in adult respiratory distress syndrome. *Am Rev Respir Dis*. 1989;139:682–687.
96. Bray BA, Sampson PM, Osman M, Giandomenico A, Turino GM. Early changes in lung tissue hyaluronan (hyaluronic acid) and hyaluronidase in bleomycin-induced alveolitis in hamsters. *Am Rev Respir Dis*. 1991;143: 284–288.
97. Nettelbladt O, Bergh J, Schenholm M, Tengblad A, Hallgren R. Accumulation of hyaluronic acid in the alveolar interstitial tissue in bleomycin-induced alveolitis. *Am Rev Respir Dis*. 1989;139:759–762.
98. Nettelbladt O, Hallgren R. Hyaluronan (hyaluronic acid) in bronchoalveolar fluid during the development of bleomycin-induced alveolitis in the rat. *Am Rev Respir Dis*. 1989;140:1028–1032.
99. Giri SN, Hyde DM, Nakashima JM. Analysis of bronchoalveolar lavage fluid from bleomycin-induced pulmonary fibrosis in hamsters. *Toxicol Pathol*. 1986;14(2): 149–157.
100. Moseley R, Waddington RJ, Embery G. Degradation of glycosaminoglycans by reactive oxygen species derived from stimulated polymorphonuclear leukocytes. *Biochim Biophys Acta*. 1997;1362(2–3):221–231.
101. Kennett EC, Davies MJ. Degradation of matrix glycosaminoglycans by peroxynitrite/peroxynitrous acid: evidence for a hydroxyl-radical-like mechanism. *Free Radic Biol Med*. 2007;42(8):1278–1289.
102. Soltes L, Kogan G, Stankovska M, et al. Degradation of high-molar-mass hyaluronan and characterization of fragments. *Biomacromolecules*. 2007;8(9):2697–2705.
103. Banks BA, Ischiropoulos H, McClelland M, Ballard PL, Ballard RA. Plasma 3-nitrotyrosine is elevated in premature infants who develop bronchopulmonary dysplasia. *Pediatrics*. 1998;101(5):870–874.
104. Davis JM. Role of oxidant injury in the pathogenesis of neonatal lung disease. *Acta Paediatr Suppl*. 2002; 91(437):23–25.
105. Deguine V, Menasche M, Ferrari P, Fraisse L, Pouliquen Y, Robert L. Free radical depolymerization of hyaluronan by Maillard reaction products: role in liquefaction of aging vitreous. *Int J Biol Macromol*. 1998;22(1):17–22.
106. Hrabarova E, Juranek I, Soltes L. Pro-oxidative effect of peroxynitrite regarding biological systems: a special focus on high-molar-mass hyaluronan degradation. *Gen Physiol Biophys*. 2011;30(3):223–238.

107. Li M, Rosenfeld L, Vilar RE, Cowman MK. Degradation of hyaluronan by peroxynitrite. *Arch Biochem Biophys*. 1997; 341(2):245–250.
108. Manzanares D, Monzon ME, Savani RC, Salathe M. Apical oxidative hyaluronan degradation stimulates airway ciliary beating via RHAMM and RON. *Am J Respir Cell Mol Biol*. 2007;37(2):160–168.
109. Kasper M, Bierhaus A, Whyte A, Binns RM, Schuh D, Muller M. Expression of CD44 isoforms during bleomycin- or radiation-induced pulmonary fibrosis in rats and mini-pigs. *Histochem Cell Biol*. 1996;105:221–230.
110. Teder P, Nettelbladt O, Heldin P. Characterization of the mechanism involved in bleomycin-induced increased hyaluronan production in rat lung. *Am J Respir Cell Mol Biol*. 1995;12:181–189.
111. Teder P, Vandivier RW, Jiang D, et al. Resolution of lung inflammation by CD44. *Science*. 2002;296(5565): 155–158.
112. Hall CL, Collis LA, Bo AJ, et al. Fibroblasts require protein kinase C activation to respond to hyaluronan with increased locomotion. *Matrix Biol*. 2001;20(3):183–192.
113. Savani RC, Wang C, Yang B, et al. Migration of bovine aortic smooth muscle cells after wounding injury. The role of hyaluronan and RHAMM. *J Clin Investig*. 1995; 95(3):1158–1168.
114. Hardwick C, Hoare K, Owens R, et al. Molecular cloning of a novel Hyaluronan receptor that mediates tumor cell motility. *J Cell Biol*. 1992;117(6):1343–1350.
115. Hall CL, Yang B, Yang X, et al. Overexpression of the hyaluronan receptor RHAMM is transforming and is also required for H-ras transformation. *Cell*. 1995;82(1): 19–26.
116. Savani RC, Hou G, Liu P, et al. A role for hyaluronan in macrophage accumulation and collagen deposition after bleomycin-induced lung injury. *Am J Respir Cell Mol Biol*. 2000;23(4):475–484.
117. Zaman A, Cui Z, Foley JP, et al. Expression and role of the hyaluronan receptor RHAMM in inflammation after bleomycin injury. *Am J Respir Cell Mol Biol*. 2005;33(5): 447–454.
118. Cui Z, Liao J, Cheong N, et al. The receptor for hyaluronan-mediated motility (CD168) promotes inflammation and fibrosis after acute lung injury. *Matrix Biol*. 2019;78–79:255–271.
119. Johnsson H. *Lung Hyaluronan and Lung Water in the Perinatal Period*. Uppsala: Faculty of Medicine, Uppsala University; 2001 [Dissertation].
120. Johnsson H, Eriksson L, Sedin G. Antenatal betamethasone administration decreases the lung hyaluronan concentration in preterm rabbit pups. *Pediatr Res*. 2001; 49(4):566–571.
121. Bullard KM, Longaker MT, Lorenz HP. Fetal wound healing: current biology. *World J Surg*. 2003;27(1):54–61.
122. Lovvorn HN, Cass DL, Sylvester KG, et al. Hyaluronan receptor expression increases in fetal excisional skin wounds and correlates with fibroplasia. *J Pediatr Surg*. 1998;33(7):1062–1070.
123. Taylor KR, Yamasaki K, Radek KA, et al. Recognition of hyaluronan released in sterile injury involves a unique receptor complex dependent on Toll-like receptor 4, CD44, and MD-2. *J Biol Chem*. 2007;282(25):18265–18275.
124. Forteza R, Lauredo I, Abraham WM, Conner GE. Bronchial tissue kallikrein activity is regulated by hyaluronic acid binding. *Am J Respir Cell Mol Biol*. 1999;21:666–674.
125. Lieb T, Forteza R, Salathe M. Hyaluronic acid in cultured ovine tracheal cells and its effect on ciliary beat frequency in vitro. *J Aerosol Med*. 2000;13(3):231–237.
126. Forteza R, Lieb T, Aoki T, Savani RC, Conner GE, Salathe M. Hyaluronan serves a novel role in airway mucosal host defense. *FASEB J*. 2001;15(12):2179–2186.
127. Lemaitre B, Nicolas E, Michaut L, Reichhart JM, Hoffmann JA. The dorsoventral regulatory gene cassette spatzle/Toll/cactus controls the potent antifungal response in Drosophila adults. *Cell*. 1996;86(6):973–983.
128. Becker CE, O'Neill LA. Inflammasomes in inflammatory disorders: the role of TLRs and their interactions with NLRs. *Semin Immunopathol*. 2007;29(3):239–248.
129. Gao H, Leaver SK, Burke-Gaffney A, Finney SJ. Severe sepsis and Toll-like receptors. *Semin Immunopathol*. 2008;30(1):29–40.
130. Dinarello CA, Wolff SM. The role of interleukin-1 in disease. *N Engl J Med*. 1993;328(2):106–113.
131. Church LD, Cook GP, McDermott MF. Primer: inflammasomes and interleukin 1beta in inflammatory disorders. *Nat Clin Pract Rheumatol*. 2008;4(1):34–42.
132. Goldbach-Mansky R, Dailey NJ, Canna SW, et al. Neonatal-onset multisystem inflammatory disease responsive to interleukin-1beta inhibition. *N Engl J Med*. 2006;355(6):581–592.
133. Gasse P, Mary C, Guenon I, et al. IL-1R1/MyD88 signaling and the inflammasome are essential in pulmonary inflammation and fibrosis in mice. *J Clin Investig*. 2007;117(12):3786–3799.
134. Ye Z, Ting JP. NLR, the nucleotide-binding domain leucine-rich repeat containing gene family. *Curr Opin Immunol*. 2008;20(1):3–9.
135. Mariathasan S, Monack DM. Inflammasome adaptors and sensors: intracellular regulators of infection and inflammation. *Nat Rev Immunol*. 2007;7(1):31–40.
136. Petrilli V, Dostert C, Muruve DA, Tschopp J. The inflammasome: a danger sensing complex triggering innate immunity. *Curr Opin Immunol*. 2007;19(6):615–622.
137. Mariathasan S, Weiss DS, Newton K, et al. Cryopyrin activates the inflammasome in response to toxins and ATP. *Nature*. 2006;440(7081):228–232.
138. Kolliputi N, Shaik RS, Waxman AB. The inflammasome mediates hyperoxia-induced alveolar cell permeability. *J Immunol*. 2010;184(10):5819–5826.
139. Tapia VS, Daniels MJD, Palazon-Riquelme P, et al. The three cytokines IL-1beta, IL-18, and IL-1alpha share related but distinct secretory routes. *J Biol Chem*. 2019; 294(21):8325–8335.
140. Lopez-Castejon G, Brough D. Understanding the mechanism of IL-1beta secretion. *Cytokine Growth Factor Rev*. 2011;22(4):189–195.

141. Piccioli P, Rubartelli A. The secretion of IL-1beta and options for release. *Semin Immunol*. 2013;25(6):425–429.
142. Martin-Sanchez F, Diamond C, Zeitler M, et al. Inflammasome-dependent IL-1beta release depends upon membrane permeabilisation. *Cell Death Differ*. 2016;23(7):1219–1231.
143. Joosten LA, Netea MG, Dinarello CA. Interleukin-1beta in innate inflammation, autophagy and immunity. *Semin Immunol*. 2013;25(6):416–424.
144. Hallegua DS, Weisman MH. Potential therapeutic uses of interleukin 1 receptor antagonists in human diseases. *Ann Rheum Dis*. 2002;61(11):960–967.
145. Jesus AA, Goldbach-Mansky R. IL-1 blockade in autoinflammatory syndromes. *Annu Rev Med*. 2014;65: 223–244.
146. Yoon BH, Romero R, Jun JK, et al. Amniotic fluid cytokines (interleukin-6, tumor necrosis factor-alpha, interleukin-1 beta, and interleukin-8) and the risk for the development of bronchopulmonary dysplasia. *Am J Obstet Gynecol*. 1997;177(4):825–830.
147. Yoon BH, Romero R, Kim KS, et al. A systemic fetal inflammatory response and the development of bronchopulmonary dysplasia. *Am J Obstet Gynecol*. 1999;181(4): 773–779.
148. Koksal N, Kayik B, Cetinkaya M, et al. Value of serum and bronchoalveolar fluid lavage pro- and anti-inflammatory cytokine levels for predicting bronchopulmonary dysplasia in premature infants. *Eur Cytokine Netw*. 2012; 23(2):29–35.
149. Ambalavanan N, Carlo WA, D'Angio CT, et al. Cytokines associated with bronchopulmonary dysplasia or death in extremely low birth weight infants. *Pediatrics*. 2009; 123(4):1132–1141.
150. Rindfleisch MS, Hasday JD, Taciak V, Broderick K, Viscardi RM. Potential role of interleukin-1 in the development of bronchopulmonary dysplasia. *J Interferon Cytokine Res*. 1996;16(5):365–373.
151. Kakkera DK, Siddiq MM, Parton LA. Interleukin-1 balance in the lungs of preterm infants who develop bronchopulmonary dysplasia. *Biol Neonate*. 2005;87(2): 82–90.
152. Liao J, Kapadia VS, Brown LS, et al. The NLRP3 inflammasome is critically involved in the development of bronchopulmonary dysplasia. *Nat Commun*. 2015;6:8977.
153. Bry K, Hogmalm A, Backstrom E. Mechanisms of inflammatory lung injury in the neonate: lessons from a transgenic mouse model of bronchopulmonary dysplasia. *Semin Perinatol*. 2010;34(3):211–221.
154. Johnson BH, Yi M, Masood A, et al. A critical role for the IL-1 receptor in lung injury induced in neonatal rats by 60% O_2. *Pediatr Res*. 2009;66(3):260–265.
155. Nold MF, Mangan NE, Rudloff I, et al. Interleukin-1 receptor antagonist prevents murine bronchopulmonary dysplasia induced by perinatal inflammation and hyperoxia. *Proc Natl Acad Sci USA*. 2013;110(35): 14384–14389.
156. Rudloff I, Cho SX, Bui CB, et al. Refining anti-inflammatory therapy strategies for bronchopulmonary dysplasia. *J Cell Mol Med*. 2017;21(6):1128–1138.
157. Lamkanfi M, Mueller JL, Vitari AC, et al. Glyburide inhibits the Cryopyrin/Nalp3 inflammasome. *J Cell Biol*. 2009;187(1):61–70.
158. Stouch AN, McCoy AM, Greer RM, et al. IL-1beta and inflammasome activity link inflammation to abnormal fetal airway development. *J Immunol*. 2016;196(8):3411–3420.
159. Peiseler M, Kubes P. More friend than foe: the emerging role of neutrophils in tissue repair. *J Clin Investig*. 2019; 129(7):2629–2639.
160. Soehnlein O, Steffens S, Hidalgo A, Weber C. Neutrophils as protagonists and targets in chronic inflammation. *Nat Rev Immunol*. 2017;17(4):248–261.
161. McDonald B, McAvoy EF, Lam F, et al. Interaction of CD44 and hyaluronan is the dominant mechanism for neutrophil sequestration in inflamed liver sinusoids. *J Exp Med*. 2008;205(4):915–927.
162. Potey PM, Rossi AG, Lucas CD, Dorward DA. Neutrophils in the initiation and resolution of acute pulmonary inflammation: understanding biological function and therapeutic potential. *J Pathol*. 2019;247(5):672–685.
163. Ravindran M, Khan MA, Palaniyar N. Neutrophil extracellular trap formation: physiology, pathology, and pharmacology. *Biomolecules*. 2019;9(8).
164. Henson PM. Dampening inflammation. *Nat Immunol*. 2005;6(12):1179–1181.
165. Wang J. Neutrophils in tissue injury and repair. *Cell Tissue Res*. 2018;371(3):531–539.
166. Varricchi G, Loffredo S, Galdiero MR, et al. Innate effector cells in angiogenesis and lymphangiogenesis. *Curr Opin Immunol*. 2018;53:152–160.
167. Gasser O, Schifferli JA. Activated polymorphonuclear neutrophils disseminate anti-inflammatory microparticles by ectocytosis. *Blood*. 2004;104(8):2543–2548.
168. Eken C, Gasser O, Zenhaeusern G, Oehri I, Hess C, Schifferli JA. Polymorphonuclear neutrophil-derived ectosomes interfere with the maturation of monocyte-derived dendritic cells. *J Immunol*. 2008;180(2): 817–824.
169. Huynh ML, Fadok VA, Henson PM. Phosphatidylserine-dependent ingestion of apoptotic cells promotes TGF-beta1 secretion and the resolution of inflammation. *J Clin Investig*. 2002;109(1):41–50.
170. Serhan CN, Chiang N, Van Dyke TE. Resolving inflammation: dual anti-inflammatory and pro-resolution lipid mediators. *Nat Rev Immunol*. 2008;8(5):349–361.
171. Collin M, Bigley V. Monocyte, macrophage, and dendritic cell development: the human perspective. *Microbiol Spectr*. 2016;4(5).
172. Huang X, Xiu H, Zhang S, Zhang G. The role of macrophages in the pathogenesis of ALI/ARDS. *Mediat Inflamm*. 2018;2018, 1264913.
173. Trapnell BC, Nakata K, Bonella F, et al. Pulmonary alveolar proteinosis. *Nat Rev Dis Primers*. 2019;5(1):16.

174. Allard B, Panariti A, Martin JG. Alveolar macrophages in the resolution of inflammation, tissue repair, and tolerance to infection. *Front Immunol*. 2018;9:1777.
175. Arora S, Dev K, Agarwal B, Das P, Syed MA. Macrophages: their role, activation and polarization in pulmonary diseases. *Immunobiology*. 2018;223(4–5):383–396.
176. Martinez FO, Sica A, Mantovani A, Locati M. Macrophage activation and polarization. *Front Biosci*. 2008;13:453–461.
177. Martinez FO, Gordon S. The M1 and M2 paradigm of macrophage activation: time for reassessment. *F1000Prime Rep*. 2014;6:13.
178. Robb CT, Regan KH, Dorward DA, Rossi AG. Key mechanisms governing resolution of lung inflammation. *Semin Immunopathol*. 2016;38(4):425–448.
179. McCubbrey AL, Curtis JL. Efferocytosis and lung disease. *Chest*. 2013;143(6):1750–1757.
180. Soloff AC, Barratt-Boyes SM. Enemy at the gates: dendritic cells and immunity to mucosal pathogens. *Cell Res*. 2010;20(8):872–885.
181. Banchereau J, Briere F, Caux C, et al. Immunobiology of dendritic cells. *Annu Rev Immunol*. 2000;18:767–811.
182. Merad M, Sathe P, Helft J, Miller J, Mortha A. The dendritic cell lineage: ontogeny and function of dendritic cells and their subsets in the steady state and the inflamed setting. *Annu Rev Immunol*. 2013;31:563–604.
183. Patente TA, Pelgrom LR, Everts B. Dendritic cells are what they eat: how their metabolism shapes T helper cell polarization. *Curr Opin Immunol*. 2019;58:16–23.
184. Skoberne M, Beignon AS, Larsson M, Bhardwaj N. Apoptotic cells at the crossroads of tolerance and immunity. *Curr Top Microbiol Immunol*. 2005;289:259–292.
185. Manfredi AA, Capobianco A, Bianchi ME, Rovere-Querini P. Regulation of dendritic- and T-cell fate by injury-associated endogenous signals. *Crit Rev Immunol*. 2009;29(1):69–86.
186. Lambrecht BN, Hammad H. Lung dendritic cells in respiratory viral infection and asthma: from protection to immunopathology. *Annu Rev Immunol*. 2012;30:243–270.
187. Collin M, Bigley V. Human dendritic cell subsets: an update. *Immunology*. 2018;154(1):3–20.
188. Jarrossay D, Napolitani G, Colonna M, Sallusto F, Lanzavecchia A. Specialization and complementarity in microbial molecule recognition by human myeloid and plasmacytoid dendritic cells. *Eur J Immunol*. 2001;31(11):3388–3393.
189. Lynch JP, Mazzone SB, Rogers MJ, et al. The plasmacytoid dendritic cell: at the cross-roads in asthma. *Eur Respir J*. 2014;43(1):264–275.
190. Bharadwaj AS, Bewtra AK, Agrawal DK. Dendritic cells in allergic airway inflammation. *Can J Physiol Pharmacol*. 2007;85(7):686–699.
191. Haniffa M, Collin M, Ginhoux F. Ontogeny and functional specialization of dendritic cells in human and mouse. *Adv Immunol*. 2013;120:1–49.
192. De Paepe ME, Hanley LC, Lacourse Z, Pasquariello T, Mao Q. Pulmonary dendritic cells in lungs of preterm infants: neglected participants in bronchopulmonary dysplasia? *Pediatr Dev Pathol*. 2011;14(1):20–27.
193. Cui TX, Maheshwer B, Hong JY, Goldsmith AM, Bentley JK, Popova AP. Hyperoxic exposure of immature mice increases the inflammatory response to subsequent rhinovirus infection: association with danger signals. *J Immunol*. 2016;196(11):4692–4705.
194. Abel AM, Yang C, Thakar MS, Malarkannan S. Natural killer cells: development, maturation, and clinical utilization. *Front Immunol*. 2018;9:1869.
195. Hesker PR, Krupnick AS. The role of natural killer cells in pulmonary immunosurveillance. *Front Biosci*. 2013;5:575–587.
196. Barber GN. Host defense, viruses and apoptosis. *Cell Death Differ*. 2001;8(2):113–126.
197. Fairclough L, Urbanowicz RA, Corne J, Lamb JR. Killer cells in chronic obstructive pulmonary disease. *Clin Sci*. 2008;114(8):533–541.
198. Leite-de-Moraes MC, Dy M. Natural killer T cells: a potent cytokine-producing cell population. *Eur Cytokine Netw*. 1997;8(3):229–237.
199. Ballabh P, Simm M, Kumari J, et al. Lymphocyte subpopulations in bronchopulmonary dysplasia. *Am J Perinatol*. 2003;20(8):465–475.
200. Pelkonen AS, Suomalainen H, Hallman M, Turpeinen M. Peripheral blood lymphocyte subpopulations in schoolchildren born very preterm. *Arch Dis Child Fetal Neonatal Ed*. 1999;81(3):F188–F193.
201. Vivier E, Artis D, Colonna M, et al. Innate lymphoid cells: 10 years on. *Cell*. 2018;174(5):1054–1066.
202. Kortekaas Krohn I, Bal SM, Golebski K. The role of innate lymphoid cells in airway inflammation: evolving paradigms. *Curr Opin Pulm Med*. 2018;24(1):11–17.
203. Marashian SM, Mortaz E, Jamaati HR, et al. Role of innate lymphoid cells in lung disease. *Iran J Allergy, Asthma Immunol*. 2015;14(4):346–360.
204. Barlow JL, McKenzie ANJ. Innate lymphoid cells of the lung. *Annu Rev Physiol*. 2019;81:429–452.
205. Kim BS, Wojno ED, Artis D. Innate lymphoid cells and allergic inflammation. *Curr Opin Immunol*. 2013;25(6):738–744.
206. de Kleer IM, Kool M, de Bruijn MJ, et al. Perinatal activation of the interleukin-33 pathway promotes type 2 immunity in the developing lung. *Immunity*. 2016;45(6):1285–1298.
207. Loering S, Cameron GJM, Starkey MR, Hansbro PM. Lung development and emerging roles for type 2 immunity. *J Pathol*. 2019;247(5):686–696.
208. Van Maele L, Carnoy C, Cayet D, et al. Activation of Type 3 innate lymphoid cells and interleukin 22 secretion in the lungs during Streptococcus pneumoniae infection. *J Infect Dis*. 2014;210(3):493–503.
209. Cai T, Qiu J, Ji Y, et al. IL-17-producing ST2(+) group 2 innate lymphoid cells play a pathogenic role in lung inflammation. *J Allergy Clin Immunol*. 2019;143(1), 229-244 e229.

210. O'Dwyer DN, Dickson RP, Moore BB. The lung microbiome, immunity, and the pathogenesis of chronic lung disease. *J Immunol*. 2016;196(12):4839–4847.
211. Man WH, de Steenhuijsen Piters WA, Bogaert D. The microbiota of the respiratory tract: gatekeeper to respiratory health. *Nat Rev Microbiol*. 2017;15(5):259–270.
212. Lal CV, Travers C, Aghai ZH, et al. The airway microbiome at birth. *Sci Rep*. 2016;6:31023.
213. Mathieu E, Escribano-Vazquez U, Descamps D, et al. Paradigms of lung microbiota functions in health and disease, particularly, in asthma. *Front Physiol*. 2018;9:1168.
214. Duranti S, Lugli GA, Milani C, et al. Bifidobacterium bifidum and the infant gut microbiota: an intriguing case of microbe-host co-evolution. *Environ Microbiol*. 2019; 21(10):3683–3695.
215. Moossavi S, Sepehri S, Robertson B, et al. Composition and variation of the human milk microbiota are influenced by maternal and early-life factors. *Cell Host Microbe*. 2019;25(2), 324-335 e324.
216. Wostmann BS. The germfree animal in nutritional studies. *Annu Rev Nutr*. 1981;1:257–279.
217. Yun Y, Srinivas G, Kuenzel S, et al. Environmentally determined differences in the murine lung microbiota and their relation to alveolar architecture. *PLoS One*. 2014;9(12):e113466.
218. Budden KF, Gellatly SL, Wood DL, et al. Emerging pathogenic links between microbiota and the gut-lung axis. *Nat Rev Microbiol*. 2017;15(1):55–63.
219. Anand S, Mande SS. Diet, microbiota and gut-lung connection. *Front Microbiol*. 2018;9:2147.
220. Pammi M, Lal CV, Wagner BD, et al. Airway microbiome and development of bronchopulmonary dysplasia in preterm infants: a systematic review. *J Pediatr*. 2019; 204, 126-133 e122.

CHAPTER 10

The Airway Microbiome and Bronchopulmonary Dysplasia

CHARITHARTH VIVEK LAL, MD • KALSANG DOLMA, MD • NAMASIVAYAM AMBALAVANAN, MBBS, MD

INTRODUCTION

The human microbiome refers to the diverse microbial population that resides within or on various surfaces of the human body.[1] It is estimated that 10–100 trillion microbes are harbored by each human in the gastrointestinal tract alone.[2] The Human Microbiome Project was added to the National Institutes of Health Roadmap for Medical Research in 2007 and since then, several human body sites including the nares, oral cavity, skin, gastrointestinal tract, and urogenital tract have been studied.[2] Recent data have established that host-microbe interactions influence the host immune system and play an important role in modulating the risk of various disease states. Most studies on human microbiome have so far focused on the role of the gut microbiome,[3,4] while the study of the airway microbiome is an area of emerging field of research.[5] The pathogenic role of airway microbial dysbiosis has been demonstrated in lung diseases such as cystic fibrosis (CF), chronic obstructive pulmonary disease, and asthma. Recent studies by us and other investigators[5–7] have established that airway microbiome is present at birth in both term and preterm infants. The role of the airway microbiome in the fetus and newborn infant in lung development, injury, and repair will be discussed in the chapter, although much needs to be discovered.

THE RESPIRATORY MICROBIOME

Historically, the lungs were considered sterile in the normal individual, due to the failure of detection of organisms by standard bacterial culture methods.[8] However, molecular sequencing technologies that assay microbial nucleic acids and antigens have identified large numbers of microbial organisms that reside in healthy human lungs.[9,10] Also, some studies suggest the presence of a lower airway microbiome that is distinct from the microbiome found in the upper airways.[11–14] It is now generally accepted that although at much lower density (than the gut microbiome), a distinct microbiome does exist in the respiratory tract.

CHALLENGES IN THE STUDIES OF THE NEONATAL AIRWAY MICROBIOME

Airway microbiome studies have to overcome multiple challenges, some of which are common to the microbiome field in general and others are unique to the airway microbiome, especially related to technical difficulties in sample collection, contamination of samples with upper airway or reagent, and the low bacterial mass in the lungs. In neonates, airway microbiome studies are even more difficult because of the additional ethical and practical challenges.

The primary challenge in neonatal airway microbiome study is the lack of accessibility of the lower airways for sample collection. Various methods are used to obtain samples of the lower airways. In adults, sputum,[15–18] tracheal aspirates, and endoscopic bronchoalveolar lavage (BAL) samples[19–21] have been used to evaluate the airway microbiome. However, in neonates, owing to the nonavailability of bronchoscopes suitable for tiny preterm infants with smaller airways, tracheal aspirates[22,23] or nonbronchoscopic BAL[24] is widely used to sample more distal airways. There is therefore the risk of sample contamination from upper airways, or from tracheal tube biofilms for ventilated patients. This can be assessed by comparing samples from the lower airways with samples taken simultaneously from the upper airways. Adult studies have found that despite the markedly divergent microbiota of the mouth and nose, the route of bronchoscope insertion (oral vs. nasal) has no detectable influence on BAL microbiota.[19,25] However, it is not clear if this finding can be extrapolated to neonates/children.

Updates on Neonatal Chronic Lung Disease. https://doi.org/10.1016/B978-0-323-68353-1.00010-5

Also, unlike the intestinal or upper airway microbiome, the healthy lung harbors low bacterial mass. This makes it difficult to detect the lower signal of the airway microbiome amidst the background noise. There is also a concern for contamination from the environment, including from laboratory reagents. Thus concurrent sequencing of laboratory reagents as negative controls is of importance to ensure validity of the results.

Overall, despite multiple challenges in the analysis of the airway microbiome, much accumulated evidence indicates the presence of low bacterial mass in healthy human lungs as early as at birth.

WHEN IS THE RESPIRATORY MICROBIOME ESTABLISHED?

The timing of microbial exposure is particularly relevant during early critical developmental windows. Studies in germ-free mice have demonstrated abnormal immune development including underdeveloped Peyer patches and mesenteric lymph nodes, defects in antibody production, and impaired maturation of lymphoid follicles.[26] Historically, fetuses have been considered to be sterile in utero unless infected. However, recent studies showing the presence of microbiota in the placenta,[27,28] fetal membranes,[29] and amniotic fluid[30] of healthy pregnancies have placed the concept of "sterile fetus" in jeopardy. Also, studies have detected low numbers of bacteria in the first-pass meconium samples from healthy term-born infants[31] and in cord blood samples.[32] These studies have refuted the notion that the fetus normally develops in a germ-free environment and have raised the strong possibility of establishment of human microbiome before birth (Fig. 10.1).

There are to date no definitive studies that establish the origin of the respiratory microbiota. Studies have established the presence of microbial signatures in the oral cavity and nose soon after birth,[33,34] suggesting the start of upper airway colonization soon after birth or perhaps even before birth. Similarly, bacterial DNA has also been detected from a larger proportion of

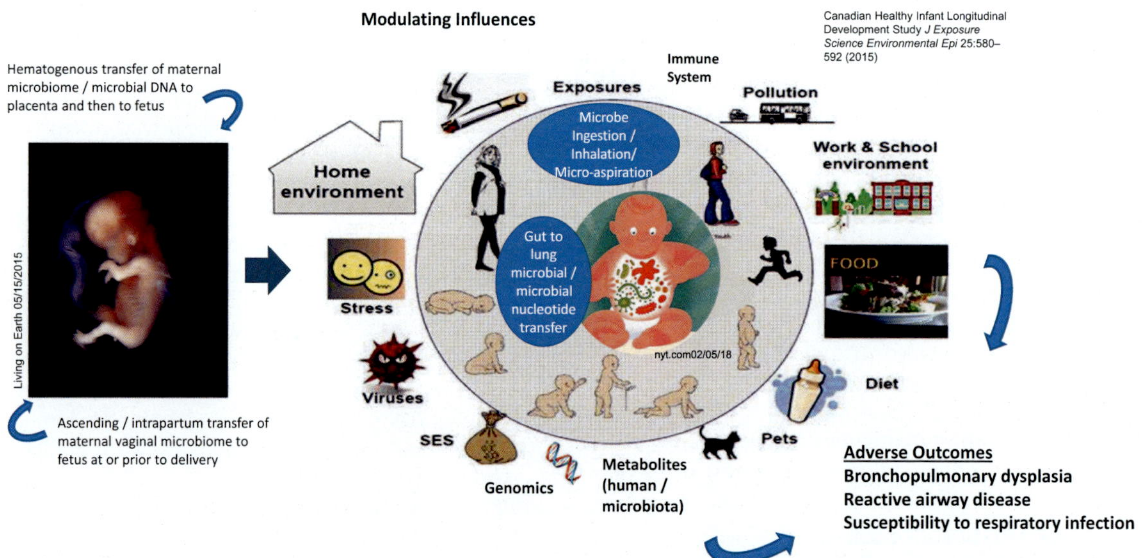

FIG. 10.1 The evolution of the microbiome from acquisition in the fetus to establishment and modulation in the infant and child, in combination with other environmental influences. Acquisition of the microbiome occurs during the fetal period either by hematogenous transfer of maternal microbiome/microbial DNA to placenta and then to the fetus or by ascending/intrapartum transfer of maternal vaginal microbiome to the fetus at or before delivery. In the neonate and infant, ingestion, inhalation, or microaspiration of microbes contributes to the respiratory microbiome, perhaps with contributions from gut to lung microbial or microbial DNA transfer. Environmental influences such as antimicrobial exposure, metabolites, genomic influences, immunity, and diet modulate the microbiome. The microbiome in turn modulates multiple respiratory outcomes depending on host susceptibilities, including bronchopulmonary dysplasia, reactive airway disease, and recurrent respiratory infections. SES, Socio economic status. (Canadian Healthy Infant Longitudinal Development Study. *J Exposure Sci Environ Epi.* 2015;25:580–592.)

preterm infant lungs and/or gastric fluid samples within 24 h of birth if delivered due to prelabor premature rupture of membranes or spontaneous preterm labor.[35] One study has also identified bacterial DNA in all tracheal aspirate samples taken immediately after intubation on day 1 after birth from 25 preterm neonates at ≤32 weeks of gestation.[22] Another study reported early bacterial colonization with varied species only after the first 3 days after birth in the airways of all intubated preterm infants.[36] However, the presence of a diverse array of bacterial DNA in the lower respiratory tract of all intubated preterm babies was demonstrated within the first postnatal week.[23] In our earlier study, we detected the presence of a low biomass airway microbiome in all intubated term and preterm infants at or within 6 hours of birth.[7] Our study also demonstrated that at birth the airway microbiome in both term and preterm infants is similar in microbial diversity and abundance.[7] Recent systemic review analysis by Pammi et al.[37] also concluded that airway microbiome signatures are present *early after birth*. With the recent novel findings of the presence of an airway microbiome signature at birth or very soon after birth,[7,37] it has become imperative to consider the implications of fetal origins of the lung microbiome.

WHAT CONSTITUTES THE NORMAL LUNG MICROBIOME?

Lung microbiome communities are thought to evolve over a period. In healthy adult lungs, the phyla Bacteroidetes (*Prevotella* spp.) and Firmicutes (*Streptococcus* and *Veillonella* spp.) comprise around 80% of the lung microbiome and Proteobacteria (*Pseudomonas, Haemophilus,* and *Neisseria* spp.) represents only about 10%.[11,14,38,39] It remains to be determined if these bacterial communities are established early in childhood or if they change during transition to adulthood. Only limited information is available regarding the airway microbiota in the early days of life. Studies done so far have shown that in term infants, analysis of nasopharyngeal samples at 6 weeks demonstrated predominance of *Staphylococcus, Streptococcus, Moraxella, Corynebacterium,* or *Corynebacterium* and *Dolosigranulum,*[40,41] whereas by 2 years, *Moraxella, Streptococcus,* and *Haemophilus* predominated.[42,43] Grier et al.[44] demonstrated with nasopharyngeal, throat, and rectal swab samples obtained monthly over the first year of postnatal life corrected for gestational age from 38 preterm and 44 full-term infants that the microbial composition in each site was highly dissimilar and unlikely to solely represent inoculation from one site to the other but that at any point in time the composition at one site predicted the composition in the other sites. There also appeared to be a typical order of progression, in each body site, of community state types (CSTs) defined by clustering that reduces microbiota variation and places relative abundance of specific operational taxonomic units into commonly observed archetypal summary representations. Longitudinal CST occurrence was seen in one of the three patterns: (1) chronologic, occurring at consistent postnatal intervals and frequencies independent of the gestational age at birth; (2) idiosyncratic, with maturity at birth occurring at consistent postnatal intervals but with frequency dependent on the gestational age at birth; or (3) convergent, with occurrence dependent on postmenstrual age with convergence upon approaching 1 year of age corrected for prematurity, suggestive of response to innate host developmental maturity.[44] The pre- and full-term infants were colonized with distinct CSTs in the first weeks after birth, with the preterm infants more persistently dominated by staphylococci as compared with the predominance of streptococci in the full-term infants.[44] A study of 25 preterm infants born at <32 weeks of gestation who were intubated within 24 hours of birth demonstrated prevalence of Proteobacteria (*Acinetobacter* spp.) and Firmicutes in their tracheal aspirates.[22] Another study done on tracheal aspirate samples collected from 10 preterm infants with gestational age ≤34 weeks at birth showed seven dominant organisms (>50% of total sequences) in 31 out of 32 samples with positive sequences and demonstrated that *Staphylococcus, Ureaplasma parvum,* and *Ureaplasma urealyticum* were the most frequently identified dominant organisms.[36] Another observational study of 55 premature infants with birth weight <1.3 kg found prevalent coagulase-negative staphylococci in tracheal aspirate samples.[23] A cross-sectional study on tracheal aspirates of 152 preterm infants at 7 days of age also found dominance of *Staphylococcus* and *Ureaplasma.*[45] Our study in tracheal aspirates of both preterm and term newborns identified a predominance of the bacterial phyla Firmicutes and Proteobacteria. In addition, these tracheal aspirate samples showed the presence of Actinobacteria, Bacteroidetes, Tenericutes, *Fusobacterium*, Cyanobacteria, and Verrucomicrobia.[7] A systematic review on the neonatal airway microbiome has also demonstrated that Firmicutes and Proteobacteria are the predominant bacterial phyla and *Staphylococcus* and *Ureaplasma* are the predominant genera of the early airway microbiome. Although the neonatal airway microbiome is distinct at different centers at the species level, it appears to be predominantly constituted by Firmicutes and Proteobacteria at the bacterial phyla level.

WHAT FACTORS AFFECT THE LUNG MICROBIOME?

It has been shown that the establishment of intestinal microbiota and its composition are affected by the delivery mode, feeding choices, and the perinatal use of antibiotics.[46] However, our understanding of the role of different factors on the lung microbiome is minimal. The predominant factor in longitudinal progression of microbial community states is age, both developmental postmenstrual age and chronologic postnatal age.[44] Evidence also suggests that the respiratory microbiome is affected by multiple environmental factors. The primary determining factor of a newborn infant's postnatal microbial colonization was the mode of delivery.[33,47] Regardless of the delivery mode, newborn infants had bacterial communities that were essentially undifferentiated across the skin, oral, nasopharyngeal, and gut habitats, and infants delivered vaginally acquired bacterial communities similar to their mother's vaginal microbiota, with a predominance of *Lactobacillus*, *Prevotella*, and *Sneathia* spp., whereas C-section-born infants have bacterial communities similar to those found on the skin surface, dominated by *Staphylococcus*, *Corynebacterium*, and *Propionibacterium* spp.[33] However, in our neonatal airway microbiome study, we found similar bacterial abundance and diversity between the neonates born via C-section and vaginal delivery.[7] Other postnatal exposures including environmental microorganisms and the infant skin and gut microbiota may also significantly influence microbial colonization of the lung. Studies also demonstrated that the lung bacterial microbiome of healthy individuals shared more communal relationship with the oral microbiome but not with the nose and was found at lower concentrations, with lower membership and a different community composition.[25] This similarity suggests that the upper respiratory tract could be the source of microbial colonization to the lungs, perhaps via microaspiration in later life[48,49] (Fig. 10.1).

Lohmann et al.[22] showed that infants who are mechanically ventilated and exposed to chorioamnionitis have a trend toward decreased diversity in the initial specimens when compared with the unexposed infants (25 vs. 33 species). In our previous study in extremely preterm infants, tracheal aspirate samples showed a decreased abundance of the genus *Lactobacillus* in infants exposed to chorioamnionitis as compared with the infants not exposed to chorioamnionitis,[7] indicating the influence of the in utero environment on the neonatal airway microbiome.

Antimicrobials are commonly used in the neonates, especially in preterm infants admitted in the NICU. Studies have demonstrated that antimicrobial exposure in the early postnatal period influences the development of intestinal microbiota with less diversity and the attenuation of the bacterial colonization of some bacterial groups, especially *Bifidobacterium*.[50] In nasopharyngeal samples from children, antibiotic usage in the 4 weeks before sampling was associated with higher abundances of *Haemophilus*, *Streptococcus*, and *Moraxella* and lower abundances of *Alloiococcus* and *Corynebacterium*.[51] The effect of antibiotic therapy on neonatal lung microbiome has not yet been accurately defined. In our previous study, we did not find a large effect with prenatal antibiotic exposure on the variations in microbiota of the airways of infants at birth.[7] Interestingly, increased Gammaproteobacteria and decreased *Lactobacillus* abundances were associated with the development of severe bronchopulmonary dysplasia (BPD), irrespective of the exposure to the type of antibiotics.[7]

THE GUT-LUNG AXIS

Recent evidence has suggested the role of gut microbiota in modifying many chronic disorders such as asthma, other allergic diseases, and obesity.[52] The gut microbiome has the ability to impact distant mucosal sites via immunologic modulation of mucosal immune response and indirect effects by bacterial byproducts.[53] In addition, interactions between the gut and lung exist due to direct physical transfer of bacteria through reflux and microaspiration.[54]

Clinical evidence has supported the presence of a gut-lung axis. Alteration in gastric acid secretion by using acid reducers may affect lung colonization by affecting the composition of bacteria transferred by microaspiration.[55] Studies have reported the association between use of H2 blockers and the risk of pneumonia in preterm newborn infants.[56] Epidemiologic studies have also linked differences in the intestinal microbiota to allergic and asthmatic manifestations.[57–59] Children at risk of asthma exhibit transient gut microbial dysbiosis with decreased relative abundance of the bacterial genera *Lachnospira*, *Veillonella*, *Faecalibacterium*, and *Rothia* in their first 100 days of life.[6] Also, administration of *Lactobacillus* GG reduced respiratory infections in both healthy children[60] and hospitalized children.[61] However, any effects of oral probiotics on neonatal respiratory health have not yet been determined.

The gut microbiota may also affect respiratory functions through metabolic byproducts, such as short-chain fatty acids (SCFAs). SCFAs act directly on both epithelial cells and immune cells by significantly affecting the immune response.[62] In an in vivo study, mice fed on a high-fiber diet had increased proportions of Bacteroidetes in the gut and higher circulating SCFA levels, whereas animals fed on low-fiber diets had increased proportions of Firmicutes and decreased circulating SCFA levels. Previous reports show that SCFAs may stimulate T-regulatory cells to protect against airway inflammation via activation of GPR43 (G-protein-coupled receptor 43; acetate and propionate) or inhibition of HDAC (histone deacetylase; butyrate).[63,64] Animals with increased circulating SCFA levels were protected from allergic airway inflammation.[62,63]

It is now clear that there is a cross talk between gut and lung compartments. However, the full extent of gut-lung interactions requires further elucidation, especially in infancy. Future research is needed to explore mechanistic pathways and the therapeutic potential of oral probiotics for the prevention or treatment of respiratory diseases.

THE ROLE OF RESPIRATORY MICROBIOME IN DIFFERENT LUNG DISEASES

Associations between alterations in airway microbiota and airway diseases are being reported at an increasing rate.[65] It has been postulated that asthma and allergy represent interplay among consequences of abnormalities in microbial colonization and the composition of bronchial airway microbiota[66] (Fig. 10.1). Numerous studies have demonstrated that the composition of airway microbiota in asthmatic patients are different from those of healthy controls.[9,67] There are more frequent Proteobacteria prevalence and less frequent Bacteroidetes prevalence in patients with asthma. In CF, studies have found a critical relationship between the airway bacterial community structure, disease stage, and clinical state at the time of the sample collection and the decrease in the bacterial diversity over time in patients with typically progressive lung disease.[68]

The Role of Airway Microbiome in Bronchopulmonary Dysplasia

BPD persists as a major cause of morbidity and mortality in extremely preterm infants. The pathogenesis of BPD is multifactorial and results from the complex interplay between an immature lung and lung injury from perinatal insults such as infection, mechanical ventilation-induced lung injury, and oxidative stress due to supplemental oxygen. Studies have shown that inflammation has a central role in the multifactorial and complex pathogenesis of BPD.[69–72] Pulmonary colonization of *Ureaplasma* in preterm infants has been shown to be associated with the development of BPD at both 36 weeks of postmenstrual age and at 28 days of life.[73,74] Infants with BPD demonstrated decreasing bacterial diversity with decreasing proportions of *Acinetobacter* spp. and increasing proportions of *Staphylococcus* spp. in tracheal aspirate samples over the first 3 weeks.[22] Our study demonstrated that BPD-predisposed extremely preterm infants have decreased airway *Lactobacillus* abundance at birth as compared with BPD-resistant infants.[7] Also, infants with established BPD have a distinct bacterial dysbiosis marked by increased proteobacteria and decreased lactobacilli abundance in comparison to age-matched term infants. Consistent temporal dysbiotic changes in the airway microbiome were seen from birth to the development of severe BPD.[7] In a longitudinal study, infants who developed severe BPD exhibited greater bacterial community turnover with age, acquired less *Staphylococcus* in the first days after birth, and had higher initial relative abundance of *Ureaplasma*.[45] Another study done in 169 extremely premature infants demonstrated that *Corynebacterium* species were more frequently detected in the infants with severe BPD than in those with non-severe BPD.[75]

Despite these studies demonstrating an association between the development of BPD and dysbiosis, the direction of causality between airway injury during development and respiratory colonization by specific microorganisms remains unsettled. Our study on exosomal microRNA (miR)-876-3p provides insights into the pathogenesis of BPD.[76] We found that tracheal aspirate samples from infants with BPD have an increased number of exosomes but they are of smaller size. Also, tracheal aspirate samples collected from extremely low-birth-weight infants showed reduced miR-876-3p expression in BPD-predisposed infants compared with BPD-resistant infants, indicating the strong predictive biomarker potential of miR-876-3p in severe BPD.[76] We noted gain of function of miR-876-3p resulted in improvement in alveolar architecture in a murine BPD model.[76] We also observed that miR-876 expression was reduced by both lipopolysaccharide (LPS) exposure and hyperoxia and that addition of LPS led to a larger reduction in exosomal miR-876-3p expression in both hyperoxia and normoxia compared with hyperoxia alone.[76] This suggests that a potential mechanism by which airway microbial dysbiosis can result in BPD is by suppression of miR-876-3p expression. In our subsequent microbial metagenomic analysis,[77] we also found that BPD-predisposed infants had increases in microbial metabolite concentrations involved in fatty acid activation and estrogen and androgen biosynthesis, thus suggesting that the airway microbiome may alter lung development via alterations in metabolites and dysregulation of downstream signaling pathways. Taken together, our data suggest that the early airway microbiome modulates exosomal content of miR[76] and induces changes in multiple metabolites.[77] Progression of lung injury and development of BPD leads to further changes in the microbiome, which may be associated with additional changes in biomarkers.

The association and the possible causal relationship of dysbiosis with BPD suggests a need to determine if probiotics or other attempts to "repair," "replace," or "normalize" the airway microbiota would improve lung development and prevent or reduce severity of BPD. Prebiotics have been shown to improve lung vascular endothelial growth factor signaling in neonatal rat models of BPD.[78] Enteral supplementation of probiotics has not been shown to reduce the occurrence of BPD[79] but airway administration has not yet been attempted. There is increasing interest in probiotics for the airways for chronic airway diseases because of the potential to improve epithelial and immune homeostasis.[80]

Overall, the airway microbiome may have a role in lung development and the airway microbial dysbiosis is associated with BPD. However, the interaction between the airway microbiome and lung development or maturation is not currently well understood.

The Role of Airway Microbiome in Reactive Airway Disease

The composition of the airway microbiome changes during the different stages of life and is influenced by the environment, health status, and age. Several epidemiologic studies have shown an inverse relationship between early life exposure to a diverse microbial environment and the risk of asthma.[81–83] Children who grow up on a farm and are exposed to a wide variety of environmental microorganisms are less likely to have asthma as compared with children who do not grow up on farms.[81] Also, the Copenhagen Prospective Study on Asthma in Childhood (n = 321, children born to mothers with asthma) found that children colonized in the hypopharynx at 1 month post birth with *Streptococcus pneumoniae, Moraxella catarrhalis,* and *Haemophilus influenzae* but not *Staphylococcus aureus* had a higher rate of wheeze and hospitalization for wheeze.[84] In general, exposure to increased bacterial diversity is protective against asthma development but studies have also reported that patients with asthma have increased diversity of opportunistic pathogens, which significantly correlates with bronchial hyperresponsiveness.[66,67] BAL fluid (BALF) samples from asthmatic patients as compared with healthy controls have shown increased Proteobacteria abundance (especially *Haemophilus* spp.).[9] In the upper respiratory tract, alteration in the nasal microbiota composition rather than the oral microbiota was associated with asthma.[85]

Alterations in the airway microbiome have also been studied in relation to the severity of asthma. Studies in human adults have shown that the airway microbiome differs with the severity of asthma. A study found significant differences in the bronchial microbiome among cases of healthy controls, patients with mild-moderate asthma, and patients with severe asthma.[86] Severe asthmatic patients have increased abundance of *Klebsiella* spp. compared with healthy controls and mild-moderate cases of asthma. Another study using sputum samples showed significant increase in Firmicutes abundance in severe asthmatic patients compared with nonsevere asthmatic patients and controls.[87] Past studies have shown strong similarities between adult and pediatric asthmatic patients and controls.[9] Hence, it is likely that results of studies of airway microbiome diversity in relation to asthma severity in adults may be extrapolatable to children with asthma.

Animal studies have demonstrated a direct relation of the establishment of the microbiome in early life with the severity and development of allergic airway inflammation.[88,89] The association between specific predominant microbes and the typical airway inflammatory response provides strong evidence for the role of airway dysbiosis in asthma and requires further mechanistic investigation.

The Role of Airway Microbiome in Cystic Fibrosis

Differences in the lower airway microbiota of healthy children and those with CF are evident from early childhood. BALF examination from children with CF revealed less richness and evenness of microbial community than in controls.[90] Studies of adult patients with CF have demonstrated an association among microbial diversity in the lower airway, clinical stability, and better pulmonary function.[91,92] Sputum samples from children and adults with CF demonstrated the presence of five core microbial genera: *Streptococcus, Prevotella, Rothia, Veillonella,* and *Actinomyces*. They also showed that CF-associated pathogens such as *Pseudomonas, Burkholderia, Stenotrophomonas,* and *Achromobacter* are less prevalent than the core genera but have a strong tendency to dominate the bacterial community when present.[91] A study also suggests that changes in microbial composition within the CF-affected lower airways during the first years of life are associated with the progression of early CF lung disease.[93] Further longitudinal studies are needed to understand how changes in healthy lung microbiome during infancy and early childhood contribute to the pathogenesis of CF lung disease.

The Role of Airway Microbiome in Respiratory Infections

The role of the airway microbiome in respiratory infections has been investigated in a few studies. A cohort study of healthy individuals found that the early upper respiratory microbiota composition at 10 weeks of life correlated strongly with the stability of the microbiota over the first 2 years of life, and these early microbiota profiles were related to the overall respiratory health of the child.[40] Studies also find that the early presence of high abundance of *Moraxella* and *Corynebacterium/Dolosigranulum* in the airway microbiome is protective against respiratory infections in the first 2 years of life.[94] Also, in children with persistent bacterial bronchitis, the airway microbiome was less diverse in terms of richness and evenness. They predominantly have Proteobacteria, and indicator species analysis showed *Haemophilus* and *Neisseria* were significantly associated with the patient group.[95] Similarly, in infants with bronchiolitis, those with *Haemophilus*-dominant nasopharyngeal profile require higher rates of intensive care.[96] In a prospective cohort study in children born to mothers with asthma, neonatal airway colonization with *S. pneumoniae, H. influenzae*, or *M. catarrhalis* was associated with an increased risk of pneumonia and bronchiolitis in early life. This result suggests that airway microbial dysbiosis in infancy may modify susceptibility to respiratory infections.[97]

The Potential Role of Probiotics in Respiratory Disease Prevention and/or Treatment

The role of probiotics in gastrointestinal disorders by modulating intestinal microbiota has been extensively studied.[98] Many studies have demonstrated the role of gut microbiota in respiratory disorders via the gut-lung axis. As mentioned earlier, this has raised speculation that interventions such as oral administration of probiotics to modulate the intestinal microbiota might represent a promising strategy for prevention and/or treatment of various respiratory disorders. So far, there is evidence from mouse models that oral probiotic administration ameliorates allergic airway inflammation by altering the gut microbiota.[99] However, human studies to date have reported conflicting findings, with two studies showing no effect of *Lactobacillus* supplementation on markers of T_H2 inflammation[100] but two other studies demonstrating beneficial improvements in clinical symptoms,[101] lung function,[101] and exacerbation frequency. Further studies to explore the therapeutic role of probiotics/prebiotics given either orally or via inhalation in altering gut or respiratory microbiome is needed.

CONCLUSION

Microbiome research has been a "hot" field for more than a decade. The recent development of culture-independent techniques has confirmed the existence of a low-biomass pulmonary microbiome. However, understanding the composition and diversity of the airway microbiome only touches the top of the iceberg of more important issues. There is a strong need to understand the functional importance of the presence of airway or lung microbiome. Also, more in-depth knowledge of mechanistic pathways involved with the airway microbiome in terms of lung development, maturation, and respiratory health is crucial. Future intervention trials of specific antimicrobials, prebiotics, and probiotics are needed to identify the potential therapeutic benefits of manipulating airway microbiome in various respiratory diseases.

REFERENCES

1. Ursell LK, Metcalf JL, Parfrey LW, Knight R. Defining the human microbiome. *Nutr Rev*. 2012;70(Suppl 1):S38–S44. https://doi.org/10.1111/j.1753-4887.2012.00493.x. PubMed PMID: 22861806; PMCID: 3426293.
2. Turnbaugh PJ, Ley RE, Hamady M, Fraser-Liggett CM, Knight R, Gordon JI. The human microbiome project. *Nature*. 2007;449(7164):804–810. https://doi.org/10.1038/nature06244. PubMed PMID: 17943116; PMCID: 3709439.
3. Morrow AL, Lagomarcino AJ, Schibler KR, et al. Early microbial and metabolomic signatures predict later onset of necrotizing enterocolitis in preterm infants. *Microbiome*. 2013;1(1):13. https://doi.org/10.1186/2049-2618-1-13. PubMed PMID: 24450576; PMCID: 3971624.
4. Mai V, Young CM, Ukhanova M, et al. Fecal microbiota in premature infants prior to necrotizing enterocolitis. *PLoS One*. 2011;6(6):e20647. https://doi.org/10.1371/journal.pone.0020647. PubMed PMID: 21674011; PMCID: 3108958.
5. Mu J, Pang Q, Guo YH, et al. Functional implications of microRNA-215 in TGF-beta1-induced phenotypic transition of mesangial cells by targeting CTNNBIP1. *PLoS One*. 2013;8(3):e58622. https://doi.org/10.1371/

journal.pone.0058622. PubMed PMID: 23554908; PMCID: 3595285.
6. Arrieta MC, Stiemsma LT, Dimitriu PA, et al. Early infancy microbial and metabolic alterations affect risk of childhood asthma. *Sci Transl Med.* 2015;7(307). https://doi.org/10.1126/scitranslmed.aab2271, 307ra152. PubMed PMID: 26424567.
7. Lal CV, Travers C, Aghai ZH, et al. The airway microbiome at birth. *Sci Rep.* 2016;6:31023. https://doi.org/10.1038/srep31023. PubMed PMID: 27488092; PMCID: PMC4973241.
8. Kiley JP, Caler EV. The lung microbiome. A new frontier in pulmonary medicine. *Ann. Am. Thorac. Soc.* 2014; 11(Suppl 1):S66–S70. https://doi.org/10.1513/AnnalsATS.201308-285MG. PubMed PMID: 24437410; PMCID: 5475396.
9. Hilty M, Burke C, Pedro H, et al. Disordered microbial communities in asthmatic airways. *PLoS One.* 2010; 5(1):e8578. https://doi.org/10.1371/journal.pone.0008578. PubMed PMID: 20052417; PMCID: 2798952.
10. Dickson RP, Erb-Downward JR, Martinez FJ, Huffnagle GB. The microbiome and the respiratory tract. *Annu Rev Physiol.* 2016;78:481–504. https://doi.org/10.1146/annurev-physiol-021115-105238. PubMed PMID: 26527186; PMCID: 4751994.
11. Erb-Downward JR, Thompson DL, Han MK, et al. Analysis of the lung microbiome in the "healthy" smoker and in COPD. *PLoS One.* 2011;6(2), e16384. https://doi.org/10.1371/journal.pone.0016384. PubMed PMID: 21364979; PMCID: 3043049.
12. Goddard AF, Staudinger BJ, Dowd SE, et al. Direct sampling of cystic fibrosis lungs indicates that DNA-based analyses of upper-airway specimens can misrepresent lung microbiota. In: *Proceedings of the National Academy of Sciences of the United States of America.* Vol. 109 (34). 2012: 13769–13774. https://doi.org/10.1073/pnas.1107435109. PubMed PMID: 22872870; PMCID: 3427132.
13. Yun Y, Srinivas G, Kuenzel S, et al. Environmentally determined differences in the murine lung microbiota and their relation to alveolar architecture. *PLoS One.* 2014;9(12):e113466. https://doi.org/10.1371/journal.pone.0113466. PubMed PMID: 25470730; PMCID: 4254600.
14. Marsland BJ, Gollwitzer ES. Host-microorganism interactions in lung diseases. *Nat Rev Immunol.* 2014;14(12): 827–835. https://doi.org/10.1038/nri3769. PubMed PMID: 25421702.
15. Cox MJ, Allgaier M, Taylor B, et al. Airway microbiota and pathogen abundance in age-stratified cystic fibrosis patients. *PLoS One.* 2010;5(6):e11044. https://doi.org/10.1371/journal.pone.0011044. PubMed PMID: 20585638; PMCID: 2890402.
16. Rogers GB, van der Gast CJ, Cuthbertson L, et al. Clinical measures of disease in adult non-CF bronchiectasis correlate with airway microbiota composition. *Thorax.* 2013; 68(8):731–737. https://doi.org/10.1136/thoraxjnl-2012-203105. PubMed PMID: 23564400.
17. Zhao J, Murray S, Lipuma JJ. Modeling the impact of antibiotic exposure on human microbiota. *Sci Rep.* 2014;4: 4345. https://doi.org/10.1038/srep04345. PubMed PMID: 24614401; PMCID: 3949250.
18. Stamenkovic I, Seed B. CD19, the earliest differentiation antigen of the B cell lineage, bears three extracellular immunoglobulin-like domains and an Epstein-Barr virus-related cytoplasmic tail. *J Exp Med.* 1988;168(3): 1205–1210. PubMed PMID: 2459292; PMCID: 2189043.
19. Dickson RP, Erb-Downward JR, Freeman CM, et al. Changes in the lung microbiome following lung transplantation include the emergence of two distinct Pseudomonas species with distinct clinical associations. *PLoS One.* 2014;9(5):e97214. https://doi.org/10.1371/journal.pone.0097214. PubMed PMID: 24831685; PMCID: 4022512.
20. Dickson RP, Erb-Downward JR, Freeman CM, et al. Spatial variation in the healthy human lung microbiome and the adapted Island model of lung biogeography. *Ann. Am. Thorac. Soc.* 2015;12(6):821–830. https://doi.org/10.1513/AnnalsATS.201501-029OC. PubMed PMID: 25803243; PMCID: 4590020.
21. Segal LN, Alekseyenko AV, Clemente JC, et al. Enrichment of lung microbiome with supraglottic taxa is associated with increased pulmonary inflammation. *Microbiome.* 2013;1(1):19. https://doi.org/10.1186/2049-2618-1-19. PubMed PMID: 24450871; PMCID: 3971609.
22. Lohmann P, Luna RA, Hollister EB, et al. The airway microbiome of intubated premature infants: characteristics and changes that predict the development of bronchopulmonary dysplasia. *Pediatr Res.* 2014;76(3): 294–301. https://doi.org/10.1038/pr.2014.85. Epub 2014/06/19, PubMed PMID: 24941215.
23. Payne MS, Goss KC, Connett GJ, et al. Molecular microbiological characterization of preterm neonates at risk of bronchopulmonary dysplasia. *Pediatr Res.* 2010; 67(4):412–418. https://doi.org/10.1203/PDR.0b013e3181d026c3. PubMed PMID: 20035248.
24. de Blic J, Midulla F, Barbato A, et al. Bronchoalveolar lavage in children. ERS Task Force on bronchoalveolar lavage in children. European Respiratory Society. *Eur Respir J.* 2000;15(1):217–231. PubMed PMID: 10678650.
25. Bassis CM, Erb-Downward JR, Dickson RP, et al. Analysis of the upper respiratory tract microbiotas as the source of the lung and gastric microbiotas in healthy individuals. *mBio.* 2015;6(2):e00037. https://doi.org/10.1128/mBio.00037-15. PubMed PMID: 25736890; PMCID: 4358017.
26. Round JL, Mazmanian SK. The gut microbiota shapes intestinal immune responses during health and disease. *Nat Rev Immunol.* 2009;9(5):313–323. https://doi.org/10.1038/nri2515. PubMed PMID: 19343057; PMCID: 4095778.

27. Aagaard K, Ma J, Antony KM, Ganu R, Petrosino J, Versalovic J. The placenta harbors a unique microbiome. *Sci Transl Med.* 2014;6(237):237ra65. https://doi.org/10.1126/scitranslmed.3008599. PubMed PMID: 24848255; PMCID: 4929217.
28. Parnell LA, Briggs CM, Cao B, Delannoy-Bruno O, Schrieffer AE, Mysorekar IU. Microbial communities in placentas from term normal pregnancy exhibit spatially variable profiles. *Sci Rep.* 2017;7(1):11200. https://doi.org/10.1038/s41598-017-11514-4. PubMed PMID: 28894161; PMCID: 5593928.
29. Jones HE, Harris KA, Azizia M, et al. Differing prevalence and diversity of bacterial species in fetal membranes from very preterm and term labor. *PLoS One.* 2009;4(12): e8205. https://doi.org/10.1371/journal.pone.0008205. PubMed PMID: 19997613; PMCID: 2785424.
30. DiGiulio DB, Romero R, Amogan HP, et al. Microbial prevalence, diversity and abundance in amniotic fluid during preterm labor: a molecular and culture-based investigation. *PLoS One.* 2008;3(8):e3056. https://doi.org/10.1371/journal.pone.0003056. PubMed PMID: 18725970; PMCID: 2516597.
31. Hansen R, Scott KP, Khan S, et al. First-pass meconium samples from healthy term vaginally-delivered neonates: an analysis of the microbiota. *PLoS One.* 2015;10(7): e0133320. https://doi.org/10.1371/journal.-pone.0133320. PubMed PMID: 26218283; PMCID: 4517813.
32. Jimenez E, Fernandez L, Marin ML, et al. Isolation of commensal bacteria from umbilical cord blood of healthy neonates born by cesarean section. *Curr Microbiol.* 2005;51(4):270–274. https://doi.org/10.1007/s00284-005-0020-3. PubMed PMID: 16187156.
33. Dominguez-Bello MG, Costello EK, Contreras M, et al. Delivery mode shapes the acquisition and structure of the initial microbiota across multiple body habitats in newborns. *Proc Natl Acad Sci USA.* 2010;107(26): 11971–11975. https://doi.org/10.1073/pnas.1002601107. PubMed PMID: 20566857; PMCID: 2900693.
34. Bosch A, Levin E, van Houten MA, et al. Development of upper respiratory tract microbiota in infancy is affected by mode of delivery. *EBioMedicine.* 2016;9:336–345. https://doi.org/10.1016/j.ebiom.2016.05.031. PubMed PMID: 27333043; PMCID: 4972531.
35. Miralles R, Hodge R, McParland PC, et al. Relationship between antenatal inflammation and antenatal infection identified by detection of microbial genes by polymerase chain reaction. *Pediatr Res.* 2005;57(4):570–577. https://doi.org/10.1203/01.PDR.0000155944.48195.97. PubMed PMID: 15695603.
36. Mourani PM, Harris JK, Sontag MK, Robertson CE, Abman SH. Molecular identification of bacteria in tracheal aspirate fluid from mechanically ventilated preterm infants. *PLoS One.* 2011;6(10), e25959. https://doi.org/10.1371/journal.pone.0025959. PubMed PMID: 22016793; PMCID: 3189942.
37. Pammi M, Lal CV, Wagner BD, et al. Airway microbiome and development of bronchopulmonary dysplasia in preterm infants: a systematic review. *J Pediatr.* 2018. https://doi.org/10.1016/j.jpeds.2018.08.042. PubMed PMID: 30297287.
38. Morris A, Beck JM, Schloss PD, et al. Comparison of the respiratory microbiome in healthy nonsmokers and smokers. *Am J Respir Crit Care Med.* 2013;187(10): 1067–1075. https://doi.org/10.1164/rccm.201210-1913OC. PubMed PMID: 23491408; PMCID: 3734620.
39. Charlson ES, Bittinger K, Haas AR, et al. Topographical continuity of bacterial populations in the healthy human respiratory tract. *Am J Respir Crit Care Med.* 2011;184(8): 957–963. https://doi.org/10.1164/rccm.201104-0655OC. PubMed PMID: 21680950; PMCID: 3208663.
40. Biesbroek G, Bosch AA, Wang X, et al. The impact of breastfeeding on nasopharyngeal microbial communities in infants. *Am J Respir Crit Care Med.* 2014;190(3): 298–308. https://doi.org/10.1164/rccm.201401-0073OC. PubMed PMID: 24921688.
41. Tsai MH, Huang SH, Chen CL, et al. Pathogenic bacterial nasopharyngeal colonization and its impact on respiratory diseases in the first year of life: the PATCH Birth Cohort Study. *Pediatr Infect Dis J.* 2015;34(6):652–658. https://doi.org/10.1097/INF.0000000000000688. PubMed PMID: 25973941.
42. Biesbroek G, Tsivtsivadze E, Sanders EA, et al. Early respiratory microbiota composition determines bacterial succession patterns and respiratory health in children. *Am J Respir Crit Care Med.* 2014;190(11):1283–1292. https://doi.org/10.1164/rccm.201407-1240OC. PubMed PMID: 25329446.
43. Yan M, Pamp SJ, Fukuyama J, et al. Nasal microenvironments and interspecific interactions influence nasal microbiota complexity and *S. aureus* carriage. *Cell Host & Microbe.* 2013;14(6):631–640. https://doi.org/10.1016/j.chom.2013.11.005. PubMed PMID: 24331461; PMCID: 3902146.
44. Grier A, McDavid A, Wang B, et al. Neonatal gut and respiratory microbiota: coordinated development through time and space. *Microbiome.* 2018;6(1):193. https://doi.org/10.1186/s40168-018-0566-5. PubMed PMID: 30367675; PMCID: PMC6204011.
45. Wagner BD, Sontag MK, Harris JK, et al. Airway microbial community turnover differs by BPD severity in ventilated preterm infants. *PLoS One.* 2017;12(1):e0170120. https://doi.org/10.1371/journal.pone.0170120. PubMed PMID: 28129336; PMCID: 5271346.
46. Itani T, Ayoub Moubareck C, Melki I, et al. Establishment and development of the intestinal microbiota of preterm infants in a Lebanese tertiary hospital. *Anaerobe.* 2017;43: 4–14. https://doi.org/10.1016/j.anaerobe.2016.11.001. PubMed PMID: 27833033.
47. Gregory KE, LaPlante RD, Shan G, Kumar DV, Gregas M. Mode of birth influences preterm infant intestinal colonization with Bacteroides over the early neonatal period. *Adv Neonatal Care.* 2015;15(6):386–393. https://

doi.org/10.1097/ANC.0000000000000237. PubMed PMID: 26551793; PMCID: 4658307.

48. Gleeson K, Eggli DF, Maxwell SL. Quantitative aspiration during sleep in normal subjects. *Chest*. 1997;111(5): 1266–1272. PubMed PMID: 9149581.
49. Huxley EJ, Viroslav J, Gray WR, Pierce AK. Pharyngeal aspiration in normal adults and patients with depressed consciousness. *Am J Med*. 1978;64(4):564–568. PubMed PMID: 645722.
50. Tanaka S, Kobayashi T, Songjinda P, et al. Influence of antibiotic exposure in the early postnatal period on the development of intestinal microbiota. *FEMS Immunol Med Microbiol*. 2009;56(1):80–87. https://doi.org/10.1111/j.1574-695X.2009.00553.x. PubMed PMID: 19385995.
51. Teo SM, Mok D, Pham K, et al. The infant nasopharyngeal microbiome impacts severity of lower respiratory infection and risk of asthma development. *Cell Host Microbe*. 2015;17(5):704–715. https://doi.org/10.1016/j.chom.2015.03.008. PubMed PMID: 25865368; PMCID: 4433433.
52. West CE, Renz H, Jenmalm MC, et al. The gut microbiota and inflammatory noncommunicable diseases: associations and potentials for gut microbiota therapies. *J Allergy Clin Immunol*. 2015;135(1):3–13. https://doi.org/10.1016/j.jaci.2014.11.012. quiz 4, PubMed PMID: 25567038.
53. Russell SL, Finlay BB. The impact of gut microbes in allergic diseases. *Curr Opin Gastroenterol*. 2012;28(6): 563–569. https://doi.org/10.1097/MOG.0b013e3283573017. PubMed PMID: 23010680.
54. Gill N, Wlodarska M, Finlay BB. The future of mucosal immunology: studying an integrated system-wide organ. *Nat Immunol*. 2010;11(7):558–560. https://doi.org/10.1038/ni0710-558. PubMed PMID: 20562837.
55. Gupta RW, Tran L, Norori J, et al. Histamine-2 receptor blockers alter the fecal microbiota in premature infants. *J Pediatr Gastroenterol Nutr*. 2013;56(4):397–400. https://doi.org/10.1097/MPG.0b013e318282a8c2. PubMed PMID: 23254444.
56. Terrin G, Passariello A, De Curtis M, et al. Ranitidine is associated with infections, necrotizing enterocolitis, and fatal outcome in newborns. *Pediatrics*. 2012;129(1): e40–e45. https://doi.org/10.1542/peds.2011-0796. PubMed PMID: 22157140.
57. Bjorksten B, Naaber P, Sepp E, Mikelsaar M. The intestinal microflora in allergic Estonian and Swedish 2-year-old children. *Clin Exp Allergy*. 1999;29(3):342–346. PubMed PMID: 10202341.
58. Ouwehand AC, Isolauri E, He F, Hashimoto H, Benno Y, Salminen S. Differences in Bifidobacterium flora composition in allergic and healthy infants. *J Allergy Clin Immunol*. 2001;108(1):144–145. PubMed PMID: 11447399.
59. van Nimwegen FA, Penders J, Stobberingh EE, et al. Mode and place of delivery, gastrointestinal microbiota, and their influence on asthma and atopy. *J Allergy Clin Immunol*. 2011;128(5). https://doi.org/10.1016/j.jaci.2011.07.027, 948-955 e1-3. PubMed PMID: 21872915.
60. Hatakka K, Savilahti E, Ponka A, et al. Effect of long term consumption of probiotic milk on infections in children attending day care centres: double blind, randomised trial. *BMJ*. 2001;322(7298):1327. PubMed PMID: 11387176; PMCID: 32161.
61. Hojsak I, Abdovic S, Szajewska H, Milosevic M, Krznaric Z, Kolacek S. Lactobacillus GG in the prevention of nosocomial gastrointestinal and respiratory tract infections. *Pediatrics*. 2010;125(5):e1171–e1177. https://doi.org/10.1542/peds.2009-2568. PubMed PMID: 20403940.
62. Geuking MB, Koller Y, Rupp S, McCoy KD. The interplay between the gut microbiota and the immune system. *Gut Microbes*. 2014;5(3):411–418. https://doi.org/10.4161/gmic.29330. PubMed PMID: 24922519; PMCID: 4153781.
63. Trompette A, Gollwitzer ES, Yadava K, et al. Gut microbiota metabolism of dietary fiber influences allergic airway disease and hematopoiesis. *Nat Med*. 2014; 20(2):159–166. https://doi.org/10.1038/nm.3444. PubMed PMID: 24390308.
64. Thorburn AN, McKenzie CI, Shen S, et al. Evidence that asthma is a developmental origin disease influenced by maternal diet and bacterial metabolites. *Nat Commun*. 2015;6:7320. https://doi.org/10.1038/ncomms8320. PubMed PMID: 26102221.
65. Rogers GB, Shaw D, Marsh RL, Carroll MP, Serisier DJ, Bruce KD. Respiratory microbiota: addressing clinical questions, informing clinical practice. *Thorax*. 2015; 70(1):74–81. https://doi.org/10.1136/thoraxjnl-2014-205826. PubMed PMID: 25035125; PMCID: 4283665.
66. Huang YJ, Nelson CE, Brodie EL, et al. Airway microbiota and bronchial hyperresponsiveness in patients with suboptimally controlled asthma. *J Allergy Clin Immunol*. 2011;127(2). https://doi.org/10.1016/j.jaci.2010.10.048, 372–381 e1-3. PubMed PMID: 21194740; PMCID: 3037020.
67. Marri PR, Stern DA, Wright AL, Billheimer D, Martinez FD. Asthma-associated differences in microbial composition of induced sputum. *J Allergy Clin Immunol*. 2013;131(2). https://doi.org/10.1016/j.jaci.2012.11.013, 346–352 e1-3. PubMed PMID: 23265859; PMCID: 4403876.
68. Zhao J, Schloss PD, Kalikin LM, et al. Decade-long bacterial community dynamics in cystic fibrosis airways. *Proc Natl Acad Sci USA*. 2012;109(15):5809–5814. https://doi.org/10.1073/pnas.1120577109. PubMed PMID: 22451929. PMCID: 3326496.
69. Speer CP. Pulmonary inflammation and bronchopulmonary dysplasia. *J Perinatol*. 2006;26(Suppl 1):S57–S62. https://doi.org/10.1038/sj.jp.7211476. discussion S3-4. PubMed PMID: 16625227.
70. Speer CP. New insights into the pathogenesis of pulmonary inflammation in preterm infants. *Biol Neonate*. 2001;79(3–4):205–209. https://doi.org/10.1159/000047092. PubMed PMID: 11275652.

71. Ryan RM, Ahmed Q, Lakshminrusimha S. Inflammatory mediators in the immunobiology of bronchopulmonary dysplasia. *Clin Rev Allergy Immunol*. 2008;34(2): 174–190. https://doi.org/10.1007/s12016-007-8031-4. PubMed PMID: 18330726.
72. Speer CP. Chorioamnionitis, postnatal factors and proinflammatory response in the pathogenetic sequence of bronchopulmonary dysplasia. *Neonatology*. 2009;95(4): 353–361. https://doi.org/10.1159/000209301. PubMed PMID: 19494557.
73. Da Silva O, Gregson D, Hammerberg O. Role of Ureaplasma urealyticum and *Chlamydia trachomatis* in development of bronchopulmonary dysplasia in very low birth weight infants. *Pediatr Infect Dis J*. 1997;16(4): 364–369. PubMed PMID: 9109137.
74. Lowe J, Watkins WJ, Edwards MO, et al. Association between pulmonary ureaplasma colonization and bronchopulmonary dysplasia in preterm infants: updated systematic review and meta-analysis. *Pediatr Infect Dis J*. 2014;33(7):697–702. https://doi.org/10.1097/INF.0000000000000239. PubMed PMID: 24445836.
75. Imamura T, Sato M, Go H, et al. The microbiome of the lower respiratory tract in premature infants with and without severe bronchopulmonary dysplasia. *Am J Perinatol*. 2017;34(1):80–87. https://doi.org/10.1055/s-0036-1584301. PubMed PMID: 27240094.
76. Lal CV, Olave N, Travers C, et al. Exosomal microRNA predicts and protects against severe bronchopulmonary dysplasia in extremely premature infants. *JCI Insight*. 2018;3(5). https://doi.org/10.1172/jci.insight.93994. PubMed PMID: 29515035.
77. Lal CV, Kandasamy J, Dolma K, et al. Early airway microbial metagenomic and metabolomic signatures are associated with development of severe bronchopulmonary dysplasia. *Am J Physiol Lung Cell Mol Physiol*. 2018. https://doi.org/10.1152/ajplung.00085. Epub 2018/08/17. PubMed PMID: 30113227; PMCID: PMC6295508.
78. Ahmad A, Cai CL, Kumar D, et al. Benefits of pre-, pro- and Syn-biotics for lung angiogenesis in malnutritional rats exposed to intermittent hypoxia. *Am J Tourism Res*. 2014;6(5):459–470. PubMed PMID: 25360212; PMCID: 4212922.
79. Villamor-Martinez E, Pierro M, Cavallaro G, Mosca F, Kramer B, Villamor E. Probiotic supplementation in preterm infants does not affect the risk of bronchopulmonary dysplasia: a meta-analysis of randomized controlled trials. *Nutrients*. 2017;9(11). https://doi.org/10.3390/nu9111197. Epub 2017/11/01. PubMed PMID: 29088103; PMCID: PMC5707669.
80. Martens K, Pugin B, De Boeck I, et al. Probiotics for the airways: potential to improve epithelial and immune homeostasis. *Allergy*. 2018;73(10):1954–1963. https://doi.org/10.1111/all.13495. Epub 2018/06/06. PubMed PMID: 29869783.
81. Ege MJ, Mayer M, Normand AC, et al. Exposure to environmental microorganisms and childhood asthma. *N Engl J Med*. 2011;364(8):701–709. https://doi.org/10.1056/NEJMoa1007302. PubMed PMID: 21345099.
82. Riedler J, Braun-Fahrlander C, Eder W, et al. Exposure to farming in early life and development of asthma and allergy: a cross-sectional survey. *Lancet*. 2001;358(9288): 1129–1133. https://doi.org/10.1016/S0140-6736(01)06252-3. PubMed PMID: 11597666.
83. Omland O, Hjort C, Pedersen OF, Miller MR, Sigsgaard T. New-onset asthma and the effect of environment and occupation among farming and nonfarming rural subjects. *J Allergy Clin Immunol*. 2011;128(4):761–765. https://doi.org/10.1016/j.jaci.2011.06.006. PubMed PMID: 21752438.
84. Bisgaard H, Hermansen MN, Buchvald F, et al. Childhood asthma after bacterial colonization of the airway in neonates. *N Engl J Med*. 2007;357(15):1487–1495. https://doi.org/10.1056/NEJMoa052632. PubMed PMID: 17928596.
85. Depner M, Ege MJ, Cox MJ, et al. Bacterial microbiota of the upper respiratory tract and childhood asthma. *J Allergy Clin Immunol*. 2017;139(3). https://doi.org/10.1016/j.jaci.2016.05.050, 826–834 e13. PubMed PMID: 27576124.
86. Huang YJ, Nariya S, Harris JM, et al. The airway microbiome in patients with severe asthma: associations with disease features and severity. *J Allergy Clin Immunol*. 2015;136(4):874–884. https://doi.org/10.1016/j.jaci.2015.05.044. PubMed PMID: 26220531; PMCID: 4600429.
87. Zhang Q, Cox M, Liang Z, et al. Airway microbiota in severe asthma and relationship to asthma severity and phenotypes. *PLoS One*. 2016;11(4):e0152724. https://doi.org/10.1371/journal.pone.0152724. PubMed PMID: 27078029; PMCID: 4831690.
88. Herbst T, Sichelstiel A, Schar C, et al. Dysregulation of allergic airway inflammation in the absence of microbial colonization. *Am J Respir Crit Care Med*. 2011;184(2): 198–205. https://doi.org/10.1164/rccm.201010-1574OC. PubMed PMID: 21471101.
89. Gollwitzer ES, Saglani S, Trompette A, et al. Lung microbiota promotes tolerance to allergens in neonates via PD-L1. *Nat Med*. 2014;20(6):642–647. https://doi.org/10.1038/nm.3568. PubMed PMID: 24813249.
90. Renwick J, McNally P, John B, et al. The microbial community of the cystic fibrosis airway is disrupted in early life. *PLoS One*. 2014;9(12):e109798. https://doi.org/10.1371/journal.pone.0109798. PubMed PMID: 25526264; PMCID: 4272276.
91. Coburn B, Wang PW, Diaz Caballero J, et al. Lung microbiota across age and disease stage in cystic fibrosis. *Sci Rep*. 2015;5:10241. https://doi.org/10.1038/srep10241. PubMed PMID: 25974282; PMCID: 4431465.
92. Delhaes L, Monchy S, Frealle E, et al. The airway microbiota in cystic fibrosis: a complex fungal and bacterial community–implications for therapeutic management. *PLoS One*. 2012;7(4):e36313. https://doi.org/10.1371/journal.pone.0036313. PubMed PMID: 22558432; PMCID: 3338676.
93. Muhlebach MS, Zorn BT, Esther CR, et al. Initial acquisition and succession of the cystic fibrosis lung

microbiome is associated with disease progression in infants and preschool children. *PLoS Pathogens*. 2018; 14(1):e1006798. https://doi.org/10.1371/journal.-ppat.1006798. PubMed PMID: 29346420; PMCID: 5773228.
94. Hasegawa K, Linnemann RW, Mansbach JM, et al. Nasal airway microbiota profile and severe bronchiolitis in infants: a case-control study. *Pediatr Infect Dis J*. 2017; 36(11):1044–1051. https://doi.org/10.1097/INF.0000000000001500. PubMed PMID: 28005692; PMCID: 5479744.
95. Cuthbertson L, Craven V, Bingle L, Cookson W, Everard ML, Moffatt MF. The impact of persistent bacterial bronchitis on the pulmonary microbiome of children. *PLoS One*. 2017;12(12):e0190075. https://doi.org/10.1371/journal.pone.0190075. PubMed PMID: 29281698; PMCID: 5744971.
96. Hasegawa K, Mansbach JM, Ajami NJ, et al. Association of nasopharyngeal microbiota profiles with bronchiolitis severity in infants hospitalised for bronchiolitis. *Eur Respir J*. 2016;48(5):1329–1339. https://doi.org/10.1183/13993003.00152-2016. PubMed PMID: 27799386; PMCID: 5459592.
97. Vissing NH, Chawes BL, Bisgaard H. Increased risk of pneumonia and bronchiolitis after bacterial colonization of the airways as neonates. *Am J Respir Crit Care Med*. 2013;188(10):1246–1252. https://doi.org/10.1164/rccm.201302-0215OC. Epub 2013/10/05. PubMed PMID: 24090102.
98. Floch MH, Walker WA, Sanders ME, et al. Recommendations for probiotic use—2015 update: proceedings and consensus opinion. *J Clin Gastroenterol*. 2015;49(Suppl 1):S69–S73. https://doi.org/10.1097/MCG.0000000000000420. PubMed PMID: 26447969.
99. Kim H, Kwack K, Kim DY, Ji GE. Oral probiotic bacterial administration suppressed allergic responses in an ovalbumin-induced allergy mouse model. *FEMS Immunol Med Microbiol*. 2005;45(2):259–267. https://doi.org/10.1016/j.femsim.2005.05.005. PubMed PMID: 15963706.
100. Wheeler JG, Shema SJ, Bogle ML, et al. Immune and clinical impact of Lactobacillus acidophilus on asthma. *Ann Allergy Asthma Immunol*. 1997;79(3):229–233. https://doi.org/10.1016/S1081-1206(10)63007-4. PubMed PMID: 9305229.
101. Chen YS, Jan RL, Lin YL, Chen HH, Wang JY. Randomized placebo-controlled trial of lactobacillus on asthmatic children with allergic rhinitis. *Pediatr Pulmonol*. 2010;45(11):1111–1120. https://doi.org/10.1002/ppul.21296. PubMed PMID: 20658483.

CHAPTER 11

Postnatal Infections and Adaptive Immunology of Bronchopulmonary Dysplasia

KRISTIN SCHEIBLE, MD

INTRODUCTION

Bronchopulmonary dysplasia (BPD), although diagnosed at a fixed time in a premature newborn's life, is not a static disease. Through the course of a newborn's early life, multiple exposures converge on the developing lung to promote or prevent normal growth. The outcome of chronic lung disease (CLD) after a diagnosis of BPD is not easily predicted with one variable or exposure alone. Epidemiologic studies consistently show an important interaction between BPD, respiratory infection, and the adaptive immune response and the outcome of respiratory health in infants born prematurely. Understanding the mechanisms underlying lung injury secondary to a failed or poorly regulated adaptive immune response to viral infection in the premature neonate is essential to clinicians and researchers involved in optimizing post–neonatal intensive care unit (NICU) lung recovery. The existing paradigm holds that newborns are more susceptible to severe respiratory viral illnesses (RVIs) due to the absence of immune priming. Essentially every exposure is a new lesson for newborn lymphocytes so that memory induction and early pathogen clearance by the adaptive immune system may be impossible. Preterm infants, by extension of this paradigm, are considered even *more* naïve and therefore more vulnerable to severe RVIs. However, it also appears that this lack of prior experience not only causes delayed or inadequate pathogen clearance but also likely results in a less specific and less well-controlled response with secondary host injury. Deficiencies in either the activation or regulation of inflammation can lead to tissue damage mediated both by uncontrolled viral pathogen (immunocompromise) and by the immune system itself (immunopathology). This chapter will cover developmentally specific adaptive immune system responses governing the balance between protection and pathology in neonates and how both immunocompromise and immunopathology place a preemie at risk for BPD and subsequent CLD (Fig. 11.1).

RESPIRATORY VIRUSES IN PREMATURE INFANTS

Respiratory Viruses in the Neonatal Intensive Care Unit and the Risk for Bronchopulmonary Dysplasia

A premature infant's viral exposures may actually begin in the NICU. Several retrospective studies beginning in the 1990s show that the burden of RVI in the NICU can be substantial, accounting for an estimated 1%–8% of cases of suspected late-onset sepsis.[1–3] Bennett and colleagues[4] found that 26 of 50 NICU patients (52%) tested positive by multiplex PCR for at least one respiratory virus during their NICU stay. The distribution of viruses was varied, including parainfluenza virus 3 (PIV3, n = 13), human metapneumovirus (n = 9), respiratory syncytial virus (RSV, n = 15), PIV2 (n = 7), human enterovirus/rhinovirus (hRV, n = 7), and influenza B (n = 4), and 28% were positive for more than one virus. Infants in whom virus was detected had longer length of stay as well as increased risk of BPD diagnosis. Risk for viral exposure may vary by NICU, however, as another contemporary study detected few viruses in weekly, multiplex reverse transcriptase PCR (TLDA [TaqMan low-density array]) nasal and oropharyngeal swab surveillance of a birth cohort of premature infants, despite frequent detection after discharge.[5] This study also demonstrated that NICU care teams readily identified infants with viral syndromes, and asymptomatic viral infection in the NICU was very rare. Nosocomial respiratory virus infection studies have since been repeated

Updates on Neonatal Chronic Lung Disease. https://doi.org/10.1016/B978-0-323-68353-1.00011-7

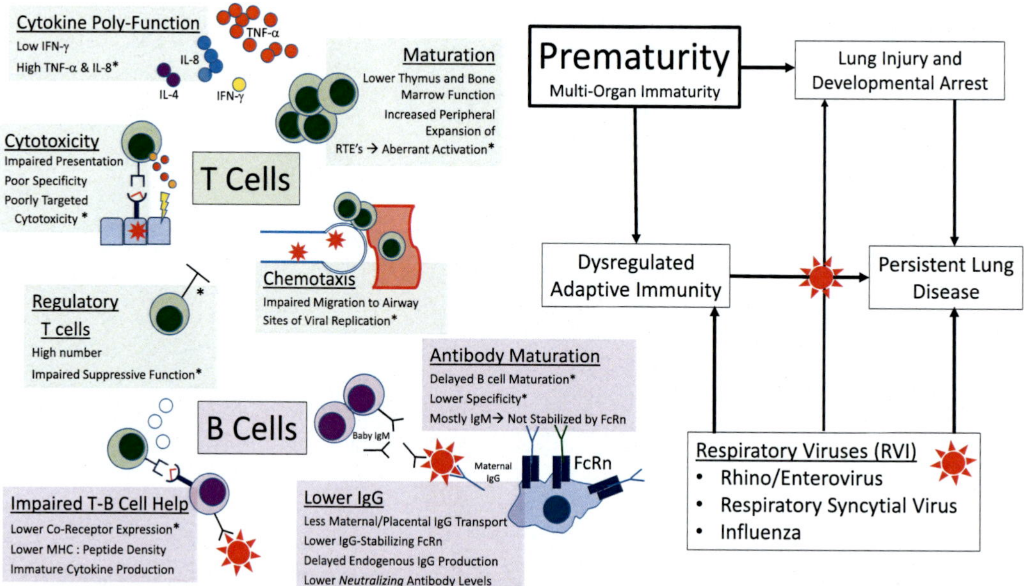

FIG. 11.1 Persistent or chronic lung disease in former preterm infants occurs as a result of immature lung structure susceptible to injury and developmental arrest exacerbated by immature T- and B–lymphocyte-mediated adaptive immune responses to the ex utero environment, including common respiratory viral infections. *Recent data support mediation and complexity due to these factors yet their precise roles remain unclear. *FcRn*, neonatal Fc receptor; *IFN*, interferon; *Ig*, immunoglobulin; *IL*, interleukin; *MHC*, major histocompatibility complex; *RTEs*, recent thymic emigrants; *TNF*, tumor necrosis factor.

by several groups, and given the association with BPD and increased length of hospital stay, there is good reason to test for bacterial and viral infections in cases of acute respiratory decompensation in the NICU and to identify preventive and therapeutic measures to limit RVI-induced injury.[6,7]

Respiratory Viruses Post–Neonatal Intensive Care Unit Discharge

The first year after discharge from NICU represents a period of vulnerability to infections owing to known risk factors, including close contact with siblings and/or daycare. Other factors that contribute to higher rates of infection are younger gestational age at birth, male sex, white race, and singleton birth.[5] Preterm infants are more likely than infants born at term to present with any respiratory virus, but the most common viruses, as in term infants, are hRV and RSV.[8] In a prospective study of 153 infants born at <36 weeks, 32% suffered from lower respiratory tract infection with either hRV or RSV in the first year.[9] The burden of influenza virus is small compared with that of hRV and RSV, but prematurity is a significant risk factor for complicated influenza infection, requiring intensive care.[10,11] Based on the viral epidemiology in preterm infants, hRV, RSV, and influenza are the most commonly studied, both in terms of pathogenesis and outcome. In their retrospective cohort study investigating the impact of clinically assessed RVIs and bacterial illnesses on respiratory symptoms in extremely low-gestational-age newborns diagnosed with BPD, Taylor et al. found that an increasing number of viral infections were associated with increased oxygen, diuretic, and inhaled steroid use and that the effect was enhanced in those with severe BPD. The authors used logistic regression models to predict supplemental oxygen use and found an odds ratio of 15.6 (confidence interval 3.4–71.3) for those who tested positive for viral infection compared with 6.3 (1.1–35.0) for subjects with severe BPD but no documented viral infection.[12] This chapter will return to these three most commonly identified and well-studied pathologic viruses to understand the impact of the adaptive immune response to early infection on later respiratory morbidity.

Respiratory Viruses and Adaptive Immunity

The first line of defense against invading viruses is neutralizing antibody, and placental transfer of maternal antibodies plays an essential role in protecting the less than about 6-month-old naïve infant host from severe diseases. To clear intracellular pathogens that have escaped neutralizing antibodies, however, the immune system needs to recognize the presence of pathogen, localize to the site of infection, coordinate the appropriate balance of cells and mediators to neutralize the virus, and ultimately restore tissue homeostasis. Miscalculation in the quality, quantity, or duration of the immune response results in collateral tissue damage. In fact, there is abundant evidence that severe RVI is only partly due to virulence factors of the pathogen itself but is in large part driven by immunopathology. Several comprehensive reviews outline host- and viral-specific factors that tip the balance either in favor of or by limiting tissue damage.[13–15] An excessive $CD8^+$ (cytotoxic) T-cell response relative to viral load exacerbates lung injury in models of influenza and RSV infection.[16–19] Injury can be mediated through the bystander effect (cytokines promoting inflammation) or the direct antigen-specific cytotoxic effect. Many previous animal and human studies have supported a model in which a lower helper T (Th) 1 (interferon [IFN]-γ) to Th2 (interleukin [IL]-4, IL-5, and IL-13) effector ratio is most harmful.[20–24] Neonatal T cells are naïve, however, and are not yet programmed to be strongly polarized toward either Th1 or Th2. Therefore studies examining the relationship between RVIs and host response need to be placed in this unique context of the developing immune system.

RESPIRATORY VIRUSES AND THE DEVELOPING ADAPTIVE IMMUNE SYSTEM

B Cells, Antibodies, and Passive Immunity in Chronic Lung Disease of Prematurity

Neutralization of pathogens by circulating antibodies is arguably the most critical mechanism of protection provided by the adaptive immune system in young infants and children. The time between infection and the series of molecular events that precede plasma cell differentiation and antibody production is approximately 10–14 days, leaving a naïve host vulnerable to progressive illness in the interim. In the naïve infant, circulating antibody concentrations are entirely dependent on the active transfer of maternal IgG antibody by the placenta, most of which occurs after 28 weeks of gestation.[25] A low antibody state in the preterm, recognized as hypogammaglobulinemia of prematurity, is seen in 81% of infants with BPD[26] and is exaggerated in premature infants born small for gestational age.[27–29] In addition to starting at a lower immunoglobulin (Ig) G level, a more rapid rate of decay for passively acquired antibody and ongoing phlebotomy losses for the preterm in the NICU account for a precipitous decline postnatally.[28] The neonatal Fc receptor (FcRn), an Fc receptor similar in structure to the major histocompatibility complex (MHC) class I molecule, that associates with β_2-microglobulin and that stabilizes circulating Ig and inhibits its degradation is not fully expressed until later in gestation.[30,31] Systemic steroid treatment for BPD further suppresses a premature infant's endogenous antibody response and can increase the duration of antibody deficiency, even beyond the first year of life.[26] The effect of inhaled corticosteroids (ICSs) on antiviral humoral immunity is unknown, but in their investigation, Singanayagam and colleagues[32] showed that mice exposed to ICSs had lower rhinovirus-specific serum IgG levels and neutralizing antibodies. The deficiency of neutralizing antibodies, both physiologic and iatrogenic, places a premature infant at risk for recurrent, prolonged, and severe respiratory infections.

Premature infants with prolonged hypogammaglobulinemia, particularly those with BPD, suffer from more frequent respiratory exacerbations post discharge,[26,33,34] but efforts to provide passive immunity through intravenous immunoglobulin (IVIG) infusion have failed to improve infectious outcomes.[35] At present, there are no published trials supporting IVIG infusion for the prevention of either BPD or CLD. In contrast to the questionable benefit of IVIG, it is quite clear that targeted virus-specific antibodies can prevent severe RVI and subsequent lung injury. The best evidence for this is found in the remarkable success of the anti-RSV monoclonal antibody (palivizumab) in preventing hospitalization of preterm infants post discharge. In fact, the population most likely to benefit from palivizumab is premature infants aged <29 weeks at birth, and premature infants born <32 weeks who develop BPD, emphasizing the central role that prevention plays in decreasing respiratory morbidity in the premature population.[36,37] The benefit of passive immunity in preventing respiratory morbidity in premature infants is likely broader than what is known and has been accomplished specifically for RSV. Prematurity comes with a fourfold higher risk for influenza-related complications among infants with documented influenza infection,[38,39] and any clinical RVI is associated with increased oxygen, steroid, and diuretic use at 12 months in premature infants diagnosed with BPD.[12] Inactivated influenza vaccine, which is strongly recommended for pregnant women, reduces premature delivery, influenza infection, and all-cause mortality in infants whose mothers were vaccinated against influenza during pregnancy.[40] The extent to which boosted humoral immunity using maternal vaccination strategy can prevent or mitigate CLD in premature infants with or without BPD has yet to be studied.

A neonate's ability to generate active antibody production and B-cell memory is dependent on adequate and sustained antigen delivery to initiate a germinal center reaction in the lymph node. There is scant data to inform our understanding of a premature infant's endogenous B-cell responses and their role, either protective or pathologic, in BPD and CLD outcomes. B-cell number, identified by CD19 surface expression, appears to be similar between premature infants with and without BPD.[41] The chemokine receptor CXCR5 promotes germinal center reaction by directing T cells to the follicular compartment of the lymph node, but is not highly expressed on newborn T and B cells.[42] There may be some benefit to a premature infant's low maternal antibody titer, as maternal antibodies can neutralize antigen before initiation of a germinal center reaction. This phenomenon was observed in a cohort recruited for a placebo-controlled trial of RSVIG between 1990 and 1994; 25% of infants with measurable neutralizing maternal antibody titers at enrollment had increased titers after RSV infection, compared with 76% of children who were seronegative at the study entry.[34] In two separate studies performed by D'Angio et al.,[43,44] premature infants generated higher peak antibody titers, as measured by hemagglutinin inhibition assay, in response to their first inactivated influenza vaccine than full terms. However, the antibody levels in preterm infants were lower than those of full terms at a later memory timepoint. Further studies are needed to better characterize how initial B-cell priming events affect a preterm infant's native antibody production and how these early events can be modulated to improve the durability of virus-specific antibodies.

T-Cell Development and Homeostasis in the Premature Infant

T cells are essential in clearing intracellular pathogens that have escaped innate defenses and neutralizing antibodies. A sufficient number of lymphocytes are needed to mount a protective immune response, and preterm infants have marginally lower absolute counts of both T and B cells than full terms at birth.[45] Recent thymic emigrants (RTEs) populate the periphery with new mature, naïve T cells and their numbers directly correlate with gestational age. In a review of 11 state-run newborn screening programs, 13% of positive results for severe combined immunodeficiency (SCID) were from premature infants without evidence of SCID.[46] Transient thymic involution and loss of new T cells also occurs during times of physiologic stress and from exogenous steroid administration, two states that associate with BPD and CLD. The delicate balance between protection and pathology can go awry in chronic lymphopenic and inflammatory states, such as that occurs with BPD or CLD. The diversity and function of T cells expanding after autologous stem cell transplant is similarly compromised, particularly in older individuals without full thymic potential.[47,48] The impact of necessary homeostatic T-cell expansion on a preterm infant's ability to mount a well-regulated and protective response against infection has not been directly studied in preterm humans.

There is some evidence that altered T-cell homeostasis plays a role in preterm humans with BPD and CLD. Early thymic involution was seen in premature infants with respiratory distress syndrome and a small thymus predicted BPD.[49,50] Ballabh et al.[41] found that persistently lower $CD4^+$ T-cell counts over 1 month after birth correlated with the later diagnosis of BPD. In our study from the Prematurity and Respiratory Outcomes Program longitudinal birth cohort, extremely premature infants who were found to have normal $CD4^+$ numbers but *persistently* reduced $CD31^+$ $CD4^+$ T-cell fraction, a population enriched for RTEs, were 3.5-times more likely to experience respiratory exacerbations in their first year post discharge,[51] even after controlling for gestational age, BPD status, and male sex. Animal models can also offer an insight into the pathogenic effect of dysmature T cells on the developing lung. As an example, premature baboons with BPD showed early thymic involution, accelerated peripheral maturation, and lung-autoreactive T cells. Pathologic findings in the lung were attenuated in animals treated with anti-bombesin antibody that preserved normal thymic architecture, suggesting that abnormal development of the adaptive immune system played an important role in this model of BPD.[52] Respiratory viral infections were not included in this model. Further research is indicated to decipher mechanisms by which naïve, RTE, T-cell populations and normal T-cell homeostasis promote healthy respiratory development.

Viral Pathogen Recognition by T Cells in Premature Infants

Failure of T cells to recognize the presence of a respiratory viral infection, or their activation by sterile inflammatory signals in the recovering lung, can place the infant at risk for CLD. In the lung, virus-infected epithelial cells present antigen via class I MHC to $CD8^+$ T cells and the viruses taken up by antigen-presenting cells (APCs) are presented to $CD4^+$ T cells in class II MHC. Patients with MHC I or II deficiencies suffer from recurrent, severe respiratory tract infections and class I deficiencies occur in association with bronchiectasis.[53] Airway epithelial expression of MHC genes is not upregulated until the end of normal human gestation,[54,55] which could contribute to delayed recognition and clearing of respiratory viruses in infants born prematurely. Based on this indirect data, it is likely that impaired antigen presentation plays a role in blunted adaptive immunity, but to date, there are no studies examining the lung epithelial MHC expression postnatally in preterm infants or the potential role of impaired airway antigen presentation in mediating susceptibility to respiratory viruses in patients with BPD.

Although it is unclear whether or not lung MHC expression is developmentally regulated, there is direct evidence of diminished antigen presentation in circulating cells. Early molecular initiators of MHC upregulation, including type I IFN, are suppressed in preterm circulating APC's. In a study comparing cord blood cells collected from infants ≤32 and ≥37 weeks' gestation, isolated dendritic cells (DCs, a specialized APC) were stimulated in vitro with the retinoic acid-inducible gene I protein (RIG-I) agonist 5′ppp-dsRNA (triphosphate double-stranded RNA). 5′ppp-dsRNA is a pathogen-associated molecular pattern expressed on RNA viruses, such as RSV and influenza, and is recognized through RIG-I on APCs. DCs from newborns had lower type I IFN responses than adults, and type I IFN responses in preterm infants were significantly reduced compared with full-term infants.[56] Perez et al.[57] showed monocytes from preterm infants, when compared with monocytes from full-term infants, had fewer MHC-expressing cells and lower per-cell MHC upregulation in response to in vitro lipopolysaccharide (LPS) challenge. Countering the significance of this point, however, in a study using T-cell hybridoma IL-2 production as a functional readout, authors found no correlation between cord blood monocyte MHC II surface expression and T-cell IL-2 production.[58] In a study comparing DCs from newborns and adults, antigen uptake, processing, loading, and presentation with MHC I appeared similar between age cohorts.[59] It seems that the result of reduced MHC expression in circulating preterm infant cells remains unclear.

There are many coreceptors, both stimulatory and inhibitory, that localize to the immunologic synapse upon T-cell receptor (TCR)-MHC engagement and concentrate appropriate TCR-initiated signal transduction. Tumor necrosis factor family receptors, which include CD154 (also named CD40 ligand), BAFF, B7, and CD28, are important in reinforcing T-cell activation in response to respiratory virus. This family of coreceptors, expressed on T and B cells (and other APCs), localizes to the immunologic synapse, and their engagement produces multiple downstream effects, including B-cell Ig class switching and Th1 memory T-cell differentiation.[60] The general consensus among published reports is that CD40L and other tumor necrosis factor receptor family members are lower in newborn T and B cells than in those of adults and are even lower in those of preterm infants than in those of full-term infants.[61–65] When stimulated with CD40 or CD40L, B cell Ig class switching from IgM to IgG and IgA was also diminished in preterm infants compared with full-term infants, and in all newborns compared with adults, suggesting simply deficits in not only coreceptor expression but also coreceptor function.[66] Diminished MHC and coreceptor expression and function in early infancy places a preterm neonate at high risk for severe RVI and sequelae from the delayed mobilization of adaptive immune cells.

Localization of T Cells to Lung in Premature Infants Infected with Respiratory Virus

The ability of rare pathogen-specific naïve neonatal T cells to be directed toward and successfully migrate into the infected tissue is difficult to measure in human infants, but it is modeled in mouse studies. Alferink et al.[67] found T-cell trafficking through lungs in neonatal mice was more permissive than in adults, but the effector response was biased toward immune tolerance. In another study, neonatal T-cell peak in the lung interstitium in response to influenza was delayed but equal in number and percentage when compared to adult mice, yet fewer neonatal T cells were able to reach the air spaces. T cells localized to air spaces early after infection in neonatal mice also did not bear a highly activated antigen-specific phenotype and did not produce adult levels of IFN-γ.[68] In an RSV mouse study, priming of T cells in the mediastinal lymph node was impaired due to age-dependent reduction in stimulatory coreceptors.[19,69] Together, these results suggest specific T-cell migration and functional deficits in neonatal mice, although these deficits are likely to be influenced by both T-cell-intrinsic epithelial mechanisms and APC-related mechanisms.

T-cell migration in response to respiratory infection is studied in humans mostly through autopsy or bronchoalveolar lavage (BAL). Cells localized to airway in neonates with severe RSV infection are predominantly neutrophils, particularly in the upper airway. In an original study published in 1994 examining the cellular contents of BAL from intubated infants with RSV infection, $CD4^+$ T cell numbers were higher than $CD8^+$ T cell numbers, and few, if any, γδ T cells were found. In contrast to neonatal mouse studies, eosinophils were not detected. These results called into question the notion that lymphocyte infiltrates were responsible for the immunopathologic effects associated with RSV.[70] A 2007 study countered this doubt after applying updated techniques to study lung tissue stored from infants who died from atypical pneumonia. Lung pathologic examination revealed airway plugging by sloughed epithelium and macrophage debris. Bronchiolar inflammation was composed of lymphoid aggregates around the bronchial arteries supplying terminal bronchioles. Organized bronchus-associated lymphoid tissue containing organized T-B cell structures was a prominent feature, and the lymphoid nodules extended into the bronchiolar lumens. $CD8^+$ T-cell numbers exceeded $CD4^+$ T-cell numbers in these lymphoid aggregates.[71]

In a 2003 study, cellularity was measured in BAL samples collected from 24 full-term and 23 preterm infants diagnosed with RSV bronchiolitis, none of whom had received passive immunization with RSV monoclonal antibody. Overall cellularity was increased in full-term samples compared with preterm samples and was enriched for neutrophils and macrophages but contained T cells as well. Over the week-long study period, cell numbers remained high in preterm infants in contrast to full-term infants who had rapid reduction in cell numbers following intubation. Interestingly, there was no difference in cell composition between preterm infants with and without CLD, although infants with CLD were intubated for a longer duration.[72] Another study found a similar distribution of cells in BAL collected in RSV-infected infants. In their cohort of 37 intubated infants, from 1 to 10 weeks of age, $CD8^+$ T cells localized to airways displayed markers consistent with an effector phenotype. Airway $CD8^+$ T cells were not enriched for antigen-specific clones until at least several weeks after infection, indicating that a significant proportion of early $CD8^+$ T-cell effectors may accumulate as a result of bystander cytokine-mediated activation.[18] Connors et al. found that children <4 years of age intubated for severe RVIs have accumulation of effector $CD8^+$ T cells in the airway, suggesting that the harm of localized cytotoxic, but nonspecific, $CD8^+$ T cells may outweigh their benefit.[17] Combined, these results are consistent with delayed localization and specificity of lymphocytes to airways in preterm newborns during an acute respiratory infection, which may enhance and prolong a cytopathic effect.

T-Cell Effector Differentiation in Response to Respiratory Virus in Premature Infants

Naïve T cells, once activated by their cognate antigen, differentiate into effector and memory cells. Effector cells, as the name suggests, will localize to infected sites and carry out a variety of tasks, including cytokine secretion ($CD4^+$ and $CD8^+$), cytotoxic functions ($CD8^+$), and immune regulation ($CD4^+$ T-regulatory cells [Tregs]). Differentiated conventional $CD4^+$ Th cells are defined by transcription factors and predominant cytokine profile; in brief, Th1 cells are Tbet-positive and produce IFN-γ; Th2 cells are Gata3-positive and produce IL-4, IL-5, and IL-13; and Th17 cells are RORγt-positive and produce IL-17.[73] There is clear evidence that Th1 cells are indispensable for protection against severe RVIs and for the promotion of durable memory for future infections.[74,75] Several published studies show evidence that a blunted IFN-γ response in the airway associates with more severe symptoms during RSV bronchiolitis, in both preterm and full-term patients.[56,76–79] Th1 and Th2 differentiation pathways are counter-regulated, and the enhanced disease caused by formalin-inactivated RSV vaccine in the 1960s is attributed to an induction of pathologic Th2 mediators, including eosinophils and IL-4-producing $CD4^+$ T cells, and the suppression of Th1 mediators.[80] The mechanism causing poor IFN-γ induction in neonates is related to epigenetic control of cytokines, which favors a more tolerogenic (Th2) immune function.[81] Naïve, cord blood $CD4^+$ and $CD8^+$ T cells are hypermethylated in the IFN-γ promotor site, and IFN-γ responses are therefore dependent on sufficient priming to initiate chromatin remodeling. A similar hypermethylation pattern is not seen in Th2 cytokine regions of neonatal T cells, which supports the notion that newborns are Th2 permissive, although the Th2 response is also relatively blunted in neonates as compared to adults.[24,51,82] It is not known whether or not the methylation pattern changes across gestation or if fetal developmental patterns are modified by premature birth. Th2 induction and Th1 suppression in the context of respiratory viral infection is a well-studied phenomenon that raises the risk for chronic post-RSV and post-hRV wheezing and asthma.[83–85] Compared with full-term infants, however, preterm infants carry a lower risk of developing Th2-mediated allergy and atopy later in life,[86,87] an observation that argues against a straightforward Th1/Th2 model.

Gibbons et al.[88] reported that naïve neonatal CD4+ T cells have a dominant IL-8 (also named CXCL8) cytokine profile and that IL-8-positive T cell levels were elevated in premature infants with infection. IL-8 is a predominantly neutrophil chemoattractant that is produced in high abundance by innate cells, including monocytes and macrophages. In high doses, IL-8 can potentiate excessive, pathologic neutrophil-associated pulmonary inflammation, but at low homeostatic levels, it also mediates angiogenesis.[89–91] Premature infants with higher early tracheal and blood levels of IL-8 had greater ventilator days and increased risk for developing BPD.[92–95] Single nucleotide polymorphisms that enhance IL-8 expression are associated with increased risk for viral bronchiolitis, which is shown in both hRV and RSV infections.[96,97] Full-term infants hospitalized with bronchiolitis have high IL-8 levels in their nasal washes, but interestingly, this relationship does not hold up with preterm infants.[98,99] The absence of a correlation between severe viral bronchiolitis and IL-8 levels in preterm neonates is curious, given the strong association in full-term infants, and warrants some caution in extrapolating what is known about the pathophysiology in the full-term population down to the preterm population. Also, there is no evidence that IL-8-producing naïve T cells, as opposed to innate-cell-derived IL-8, are pathogenic. Our data would suggest that the principle IL-8 producers, naïve CD31+ CD4+ T cells, may be beneficial in preventing CLD, in that preterm infants who recovered this population to levels in full-term infants were at lower risk for the composite respiratory morbidity of persistent respiratory disease.[51] Further research is warranted to elucidate the harmful and protective roles of IL-8-positive T cells in the newborn.

Another, less common, polarized T-cell population, Th17 cells, has received much attention recently as a Th2-alternative mediator of chronic pulmonary inflammation. In a mouse model of LPS lung priming, neonatal lungs showed little to no IL-17 production. Weanling IL-17-positive CD4+ T cells were enriched in lungs conditioned with LPS as neonates, but the Th17 population did not increase following a viral challenge.[100] In human neonates, IL-17-producing T cells are not found in the periphery until later in infancy and they still remain lower in abundance than the other T-cell subsets.[51,101,102] In parallel to IL-8 studies, IL-17 cell numbers are elevated in RSV-positive bronchiolitis compared with non-RSV pneumonia.[103] Similar to IL-8, IL-17 associates with the mucosal inflammatory condition of the intestines in preterm infants, i.e., necrotizing enterocolitis.[104,105] Unlike IL-8, however, IL-17 protein level is increased in peripheral blood samples of preterm infants who survived without BPD.[92] More research is needed to support a role for Th17 cells in the pathogenesis of post-viral respiratory morbidity in preterm infants.

T-Regulatory Cells and Control of Inflammation in Premature Infants with Respiratory Virus Infection

Tregs, as their name suggests, are responsible for downregulating the immune response, and they are critical in transitioning the lung back to homeostatic conditions following a respiratory virus infection. Absence of Treg populations in patients with the immunodysregulation polyendocrinopathy enteropathy X-linked syndrome, caused by FOXP3 mutations, leads to an early, aggressive, and fatal autoimmune disease.[106] It would be logical to hypothesize that human fetal T cells develop in such a way to control the mucosal immune response in preparation of rapid bacterial colonization. In fact, a propensity for fetal lymphoid progenitor cells to differentiate into Tregs in the thymus and in the periphery was shown by Mold et al.[107] Consistent with more robust Treg differentiation during early gestation is the observation that cord blood Tregs decrease linearly with advancing gestational age.[108,109]

Despite their natural abundance in preterm infants, Tregs from neonates were found to be less suppressive of DC activity than from adults, and the balance of inhibitory mechanisms utilized by Tregs from preterm infants is different from full-term infants.[110] Phenotypic variation in naive Treg populations observed in preterm and full-term infants suggest that naive Tregs may be differentially molded in the periphery across gestational ages.[109] Subtle, untested functional differences during early human development may explain the conflicting reports on the role of Tregs in the pathogenesis of severe RVIs. Although an imperfect model, there are observations in mice that inform our general understanding about the function of Tregs in a naïve host. Influenza infection was more efficiently cleared from lungs in mice with intact Tregs when compared to mice depleted of Tregs.[111] In further support of protection by Tregs, RSV vaccine-induced illness enhancement was abrogated by experimentally enhanced lung recruitment of Tregs.[112] In another neonatal mouse RSV model, authors showed that conditional knockout of FOXP3 enhanced illness severity associated with increased and prolonged Th2-biased T cells and eosinophils in the airways.[113] On the other hand, repeated RSV infections (as occurs in human infants) induced a dysregulated Th2 effector Treg population that sensitized animals to the previously tolerated ovalbumin antigen.[114] Induction of IL-10, IL-13, and IL-5 cytokine responses consistent with a Th2/Treg predominance was associated with subsequent wheezing in infants infected with hRV.[115] Together, these findings suggest that the developmental enrichment for Tregs in premature infants may control immunopathology but can, under some experimental conditions, contribute to the pathogenesis of post-viral respiratory morbidity.

Effects of Immature Immune Conditioning by Microbial Exposures on Later Lung Adaptive Immunity in Premature Infants

Epidemiologic studies definitively show that respiratory viruses increase the risk for BPD, and preemies with or without BPD are at increased risk for virus-induced persistent or intermittent pulmonary symptoms. Despite existing strong epidemiologic evidence and dozens of comprehensive reviews on the topic, there are surprisingly few mechanistic studies that can explain the pathophysiology of post-viral respiratory morbidity in preterm infants. In humans, the temporal path from BPD to virus to CLD is difficult to prove, as infants predisposed to wheezing by prematurity will have increased respiratory symptoms and viral loads, which increases the inflammatory response and subsequent respiratory morbidity.[83,84,116,117] Correlative human studies between a premature infant's dysregulated immune response to viral infection, illness severity, and subsequent wheeze are therefore highly confounded by preexisting lung disease and abnormalities of lung development.[118] Some evidence of causation in humans can be inferred from the palivizumab RSV prevention studies, in which palivizumab administration to premature infants resulted in a 61% reduction in wheezing days and a 10% reduction in patients presenting with recurrent wheeze.[36] In a birth cohort of 285 infants, higher cord blood IFN-γ production by peripheral blood mononuclear cells predicted lower rates of viral infections in the first year.[85] These studies support the hypothesis that early, appropriate immune protection against respiratory viruses, whether passively acquired or endogenous, can prevent CLD. The cascade from early respiratory infection to CLD has been reproduced in multiple small animal models using several respiratory viruses.[119] Neonatal mice infected with rhinovirus undergo long-term airway mucous metaplasia, and this early response is followed by the establishment of Th2-resident memory T-cell population. Th2 priming by IL-25 increases sensitivity to allergens in rhinovirus-infected mice. These observations were not seen in mice infected as adults, suggesting that mechanisms relating immune priming by respiratory viruses to subsequent hyperresponsive airway may be unique to newborns.[120,121]

Based on murine models, early priming of an immature lung and immune system by viruses influences later resistance and cytopathogenic response. Mice infected with influenza A within 1 week of birth showed enhanced airway hyperreactivity, chronic pulmonary inflammation, and diffuse emphysematous-type lesions as adults. An adaptive immune insufficiency in the neonate was most apparent in the CD8 T cells. Adoptive transfer of naive CD8 cells, from wild-type but not from IFN-γ-deficient donors, significantly lowered pulmonary viral titers and greatly improved pulmonary function as adults, supporting the importance of IFN-γ from CD8 T cells in controlling the infection and in determining disease outcome.[122] Newborn infection was associated with reduced and delayed IFN-γ responses as compared to infection in older animals. RSV-infected neonatal mice recruited CD8 T cells defective in IFN-γ production in association with mild symptoms. Reinfection as adults however resulted in limited viral replication but enhanced inflammation and T-cell recruitment, including Th2 cells and eosinophils.[23,123] Depletion of CD8 T cells (but not CD4) cells during the primary neonatal infection was protective against the adult challenge. Recall responses from neonate-primed and adult-primed mice were associated with IFN-γ secretion, indicative of a Th1 response. However, IL-4 and IL-5 secretion was enhanced only in neonate-primed mice. Rechallenge of these mice, primed as newborns, was also associated with increased concentrations of the chemokines monocyte chemoattractant protein 1, macrophage inflammatory protein 1α, and RANTES in the lung. It is suggested then that neonatal T cells, in particular IFN-γ-deficient CD8 T cells, play a crucial role in regulation of immune responses after a neonatal infection. It is unclear if these responses are virus specific or if other forms of CD8 T-cell stimulation in the neonatal period also alter immune responses to distant secondary stimuli.

There is mounting evidence that the mucosal microbiome at the time of respiratory infection can also modify both disease severity and risk of subsequent wheezing. The hygiene hypothesis posits that early microbial exposures prime immunity for a Th1-biased response, thereby preventing asthma and atopy. On the other hand, the respiratory microbiome may potentiate inflammation and disease severity during a viral infection. Man et al.,[124] in their study of children aged

4 weeks to 5 years hospitalized for lower respiratory tract infection and age-matched controls, showed improved prediction for lower respiratory tract infection when accounting for virus and microbiome together when compared with individual pathogens. Wouter et al. also showed in their cohort of 132 children that colonization with specific bacteria modified RSV disease severity and inflammatory gene expression. *Streptococcus pneumoniae* and *Haemophilus influenzae* associated with toll-like receptor signaling and enhanced disease, as well as predicted increased disease severity.[125] This was also shown by Ederveen et al., who reported an association between *Haemophilus* colonization and hospitalization with RSV. Mucosal IL-8 levels were increased in these subjects, indicating that the increase in IL-8 (and increased symptoms) levels may be mediated by bacterial colonization rather than virus alone.[126] Studies were not stratified by gestational age, making it difficult to assert that the association between microbiome and illness severity affects all gestational ages equally. However, there is evidence that preterm infants exposed to antibiotics are at increased risk of being colonized with *Haemophilus* species, and colonization is associated with later risk of CLD.[127,128] It is not known whether or not the adaptive immune system is part of this pathway, although T and B cells are certainly able to form memory against both bacteria and viruses and their fates are informed by the inflammatory milieu. More research will be helpful in deciphering the complex interplay between the developing immune system, respiratory viruses, bacterial colonization, and respiratory morbidity.

SUMMARY

Respiratory viruses are a significant risk factor for a preterm infant's development of BPD and persistent respiratory disease. A targeted and regulated adaptive immune response is essential for controlling and clearing viruses from infected lungs, particularly in the absence of passively acquired neutralizing antibodies. The newborn adaptive immune system is naïve, and delayed activation is a direct consequence of this naïve immune physiology, as is the unique requirement to tightly control the inflammatory response during early mucosal colonization events. Molecular mechanisms governing age-related regulation of a newborn's adaptive immune system are very poorly understood, but they globally impact pathogen recognition, cell activation, differentiation, localization, and regulation. Preterm T and B cells may be suited for the relatively pathogen-free fetal environment but may be poorly regulated during postnatal respiratory viral infection. Bacterial exposures and balance of colonization also play a role in modulating lung injury and protection from respiratory viruses, but these mechanisms have not been clarified in preterm infants. Delayed and poorly regulated T- and B-cell responses to viruses during a time of ongoing lung development result in virus- and immune-mediated tissue damage that increase the risk for persistent respiratory disease. Given the substantial morbidity caused by respiratory viruses in preterm infants, more research is indicated to understand the mechanisms underlying the pathogenesis in humans.

REFERENCES

1. Cerone JB, Santos RP, Tristram D, et al. Incidence of respiratory viral infection in infants with respiratory symptoms evaluated for late-onset sepsis. *J Perinatol.* 2017; 37:922–926.
2. Verboon-Maciolek MA, Krediet TG, Gerards LJ, et al. Clinical and epidemiologic characteristics of viral infections in a neonatal intensive care unit during a 12-year period. *Pediatr Infect Dis J.* 2005;24:901–904.
3. Gelber SE, Ratner AJ. Hospital-acquired viral pathogens in the neonatal intensive care unit. *Semin Perinatol.* 2002;26:346–356.
4. Bennett NJ, Tabarani CM, Bartholoma NM, et al. Unrecognized viral respiratory tract infections in premature infants during their birth hospitalization: a prospective surveillance study in two neonatal intensive care units. *J Pediatr.* 2012;161:814–818.
5. Caserta MT, Yang H, Gill SR, et al. Viral respiratory infections in preterm infants during and after hospitalization. *J Pediatr.* 2017;182:53–58 e53.
6. Kidszun A, Klein L, Winter J, et al. Viral infections in neonates with suspected late-onset bacterial sepsis-A prospective cohort study. *Am J Perinatol.* 2017;34:1–7.
7. Zinna S, Lakshmanan A, Tan S, et al. Outcomes of nosocomial viral respiratory infections in high-risk neonates. *Pediatrics.* 2016;138.
8. Yeo KT, de la Puerta R, Tee NWS, et al. Burden, etiology, and risk factors of respiratory virus infections among symptomatic preterm infants in the tropics: a retrospective single-center cohort study. *Clin Infect Dis.* 2018;67: 1603–1609.
9. Drysdale SB, Alcazar-Paris M, Wilson T, et al. Rhinovirus infection and healthcare utilisation in prematurely born infants. *Eur Respir J.* 2013;42:1029–1036.
10. Kaczmarek MC, Ware RS, Coulthard MG, et al. Epidemiology of Australian influenza-related paediatric intensive care unit admissions, 1997–2013. *PLoS One.* 2016;11: e0152305.
11. Resch B, Kurath-Koller S, Eibisberger M, et al. Prematurity and the burden of influenza and respiratory syncytial virus disease. *World J Pediatr.* 2016;12:8–18.

12. Taylor JB, Nyp MF, Norberg M, et al. Impact of intercurrent respiratory infections on lung health in infants born <29 weeks with bronchopulmonary dysplasia. *J Perinatol*. 2014;34:223–228.
13. Braciale TJ, Sun J, Kim TS. Regulating the adaptive immune response to respiratory virus infection. *Nat Rev Immunol*. 2012;12:295–305.
14. Rouse BT, Sehrawat S. Immunity and immunopathology to viruses: what decides the outcome? *Nat Rev Immunol*. 2010;10:514–526.
15. Bruder D, Srikiatkhachorn A, Enelow RI. Cellular immunity and lung injury in respiratory virus infection. *Viral Immunol*. 2006;19:147–155.
16. Anderson KG, Sung H, Skon CN, et al. Cutting edge: intravascular staining redefines lung CD8 T cell responses. *J Immunol*. 2012;189:2702–2706.
17. Connors TJ, Ravindranath TM, Bickham KL, et al. Airway CD8(+) T cells are associated with lung injury during infant viral respiratory tract infection. *Am J Respir Cell Mol Biol*. 2016;54:822–830.
18. Heidema J, Lukens MV, van Maren WW, et al. CD8+ T cell responses in bronchoalveolar lavage fluid and peripheral blood mononuclear cells of infants with severe primary respiratory syncytial virus infections. *J Immunol*. 2007;179:8410–8417.
19. Ruckwardt TJ, Malloy AM, Morabito KM, et al. Quantitative and qualitative deficits in neonatal lung-migratory dendritic cells impact the generation of the CD8+ T cell response. *PLoS Pathog*. 2014;10:e1003934.
20. Carroll MC. The complement system in regulation of adaptive immunity. *Nat Immunol*. 2004;5:981–986.
21. Drysdale SB, Alcazar M, Wilson T, et al. Respiratory outcome of prematurely born infants following human rhinovirus A and C infections. *Eur J Pediatr*. 2014;173:913–919.
22. Gadgil A, Duncan SR. Role of T-lymphocytes and pro-inflammatory mediators in the pathogenesis of chronic obstructive pulmonary disease. *Int J Chronic Obstr Pulm Dis*. 2008;3:531–541.
23. Tregoning JS, Yamaguchi Y, Harker J, et al. The role of T cells in the enhancement of respiratory syncytial virus infection severity during adult reinfection of neonatally sensitized mice. *J Virol*. 2008;82:4115–4124.
24. White GP, Watt PM, Holt BJ, et al. Differential patterns of methylation of the IFN-gamma promoter at CpG and non-CpG sites underlie differences in IFN-gamma gene expression between human neonatal and adult CD45RO- T cells. *J Immunol*. 2002;168:2820–2827.
25. Malek A, Sager R, Kuhn P, et al. Evolution of maternofetal transport of immunoglobulins during human pregnancy. *Am J Reprod Immunol*. 1996;36:248–255.
26. Wheeler W, Kurachek S, McNamara J, et al. Consequences of hypogammaglobulinemia and steroid therapy in severe bronchopulmonary dysplasia. *Pediatr Pulmonol*. 1996;22:96–100.
27. Alkan Ozdemir S, Ozer EA, Kose S, et al. Reference values of serum IgG and IgM levels in preterm and term newborns. *J Matern Fetal Neonatal Med*. 2016;29:972–976.
28. Conway SP, Dear PR, Smith I. Immunoglobulin profile of the preterm baby. *Arch Dis Child*. 1985;60:208–212.
29. Sharma S, Lal H, Saigal RK. Immunoglobulins IgG, IgM and IgA levels in preterm and small for date newborns. *Indian Pediatr*. 1991;28:741–744.
30. Jacobsen B, Hill M, Reynaud L, et al. FcRn expression on placenta and fetal jejunum during early, mid-, and late gestation in minipigs. *Toxicol Pathol*. 2016;44:486–491.
31. Pyzik M, Rath T, Lencer WI, et al. FcRn: the architect behind the immune and nonimmune functions of IgG and albumin. *J Immunol*. 2015;194:4595–4603.
32. Singanayagam A, Glanville N, Girkin JL, et al. Corticosteroid suppression of antiviral immunity increases bacterial loads and mucus production in COPD exacerbations. *Nat Commun*. 2018;9:2229.
33. Lederman HM, Metz SJ, Zuckerberg AL, et al. Antibody deficiency complicating severe bronchopulmonary dysplasia. *Pediatr Pulmonol*. 1989;7:52–54.
34. Wright PF, Gruber WC, Peters M, et al. Illness severity, viral shedding, and antibody responses in infants hospitalized with bronchiolitis caused by respiratory syncytial virus. *J Infect Dis*. 2002;185:1011–1018.
35. Sandberg K, Fasth A, Berger A, et al. Preterm infants with low immunoglobulin G levels have increased risk of neonatal sepsis but do not benefit from prophylactic immunoglobulin G. *J Pediatr*. 2000;137:623–628.
36. Blanken MO, Rovers MM, Molenaar JM, et al. Respiratory syncytial virus and recurrent wheeze in healthy preterm infants. *N Engl J Med*. 2013;368:1791–1799.
37. Simoes EA, Groothuis JR, Carbonell-Estrany X, et al. Palivizumab prophylaxis, respiratory syncytial virus, and subsequent recurrent wheezing. *J Pediatr*. 2007;151, 34-42, 42 e31.
38. Hardelid P, Verfuerden M, McMenamin J, et al. Risk factors for admission to hospital with laboratory-confirmed influenza in young children: birth cohort study. *Eur Respir J*. 2017;50.
39. Gill PJ, Ashdown HF, Wang K, et al. Identification of children at risk of influenza-related complications in primary and ambulatory care: a systematic review and meta-analysis. *Lancet Respir Med*. 2015;3:139–149.
40. Benowitz I, Esposito DB, Gracey KD, et al. Influenza vaccine given to pregnant women reduces hospitalization due to influenza in their infants. *Clin Infect Dis*. 2010;51:1355–1361.
41. Ballabh P, Simm M, Kumari J, et al. Lymphocyte subpopulations in bronchopulmonary dysplasia. *Am J Perinatol*. 2003;20:465–475.
42. Schatorje EJ, Gemen EF, Driessen GJ, et al. Paediatric reference values for the peripheral T cell compartment. *Scand J Immunol*. 2012;75:436–444.
43. D'Angio CT, Heyne RJ, Duara S, et al. Immunogenicity of trivalent influenza vaccine in extremely low-birth-weight, premature versus term infants. *Pediatr Infect Dis J*. 2011;30:570–574.

44. D'Angio CT, Wyman CP, Misra RS, et al. Plasma cell and serum antibody responses to influenza vaccine in preterm and full-term infants. *Vaccine*. 2017;35:5163–5171.
45. Correa-Rocha R, Perez A, Lorente R, et al. Preterm neonates show marked leukopenia and lymphopenia that are associated with increased regulatory T-cell values and diminished IL-7. *Pediatr Res*. 2012;71:590–597.
46. Kwan A, Abraham RS, Currier R, et al. Newborn screening for severe combined immunodeficiency in 11 screening programs in the United States. *JAMA*. 2014;312: 729–738.
47. Arruda LCM, Lima-Junior JR, Clave E, et al. Homeostatic proliferation leads to telomere attrition and increased PD-1 expression after autologous hematopoietic SCT for systemic sclerosis. *Bone Marrow Transplant*. 2018;53: 1319–1327.
48. Farge D, Arruda LC, Brigant F, et al. Long-term immune reconstitution and T cell repertoire analysis after autologous hematopoietic stem cell transplantation in systemic sclerosis patients. *J Hematol Oncol*. 2017;10(21).
49. Chen CM, Yu KY, Lin HC, et al. Thymus size and its relationship to perinatal events. *Acta Paediatr*. 2000;89: 975–978.
50. De Felice C, Vacca P, Presta G, et al. Small thymus at birth and neonatal outcome in very-low-birth-weight infants. *Eur J Pediatr*. 2003;162:204–206.
51. Scheible KM, Emo J, Laniewski N, et al. T cell developmental arrest in former premature infants increases risk of respiratory morbidity later in infancy. *JCI Insight*. 2018;3.
52. Rosen D, Lee JH, Cuttitta F, et al. Accelerated thymic maturation and autoreactive T cells in bronchopulmonary dysplasia. *Am J Respir Crit Care Med*. 2006;174: 75–83.
53. Hanna S, Etzioni A. MHC class I and II deficiencies. *J Allergy Clin Immunol*. 2014;134:269–275.
54. Stoltenberg L, Thrane PS, Rognum TO. Development of immune response markers in the trachea in the fetal period and the first year of life. *Pediatr Allergy Immunol*. 1993;4:13–19.
55. Buhling F, Waldburg N, Kruger S, et al. Expression of cathepsins B, H, K, L, and S during human fetal lung development. *Dev Dynam*. 2002;225:14–21.
56. Marr N, Wang TI, Kam SH, et al. Attenuation of respiratory syncytial virus-induced and RIG-I-dependent type I IFN responses in human neonates and very young children. *J Immunol*. 2014;192:948–957.
57. Perez A, Bellon JM, Gurbindo MD, et al. Impairment of stimulation ability of very-preterm neonatal monocytes in response to lipopolysaccharide. *Hum Immunol*. 2010; 71:151–157.
58. Canaday DH, Chakravarti S, Srivastava T, et al. Class II MHC antigen presentation defect in neonatal monocytes is not correlated with decreased MHC-II expression. *Cell Immunol*. 2006;243:96–106.
59. Gold MC, Robinson TL, Cook MS, et al. Human neonatal dendritic cells are competent in MHC class I antigen processing and presentation. *PLoS One*. 2007;2:e957.
60. Croft M. The role of TNF superfamily members in T-cell function and diseases. *Nat Rev Immunol*. 2009;9: 271–285.
61. Splawski JB, Nishioka J, Nishioka Y, et al. CD40 ligand is expressed and functional on activated neonatal T cells. *J Immunol*. 1996;156:119–127.
62. Suarez A, Mozo L, Gayo A, et al. Induction of functional CD154 (CD40 ligand) in neonatal T cells by cAMP-elevating agents. *Immunology*. 2000;100:432–440.
63. Trivedi HN, HayGlass KT, Gangur V, et al. Analysis of neonatal T cell and antigen presenting cell functions. *Hum Immunol*. 1997;57:69–79.
64. Velilla PA, Rugeles MT, Chougnet CA. Defective antigen-presenting cell function in human neonates. *Clin Immunol*. 2006;121:251–259.
65. Xu J, Treem WR, Roman C, et al. Ileal immune dysregulation in necrotizing enterocolitis: role of CD40/CD40L in the pathogenesis of disease. *J Pediatr Gastroenterol Nutr*. 2011;52:140–146.
66. Kaur K, Chowdhury S, Greenspan NS, et al. Decreased expression of tumor necrosis factor family receptors involved in humoral immune responses in preterm neonates. *Blood*. 2007;110:2948–2954.
67. Alferink J, Tafuri A, Vestweber D, et al. Control of neonatal tolerance to tissue antigens by peripheral T cell trafficking. *Science*. 1998;282:1338–1341.
68. Lines JL, Hoskins S, Hollifield M, et al. The migration of T cells in response to influenza virus is altered in neonatal mice. *J Immunol*. 2010;185:2980–2988.
69. Malloy AM, Ruckwardt TJ, Morabito KM, et al. Pulmonary dendritic cell subsets shape the respiratory syncytial virus-specific CD8+ T cell immunodominance hierarchy in neonates. *J Immunol*. 2017;198:394–403.
70. Everard ML, Swarbrick A, Wrightham M, et al. Analysis of cells obtained by bronchial lavage of infants with respiratory syncytial virus infection. *Arch Dis Child*. 1994;71: 428–432.
71. Johnson JE, Gonzales RA, Olson SJ, et al. The histopathology of fatal untreated human respiratory syncytial virus infection. *Mod Pathol*. 2007;20:108–119.
72. McNamara PS, Ritson P, Selby A, et al. Bronchoalveolar lavage cellularity in infants with severe respiratory syncytial virus bronchiolitis. *Arch Dis Child*. 2003;88:922–926.
73. Nakayamada S, Takahashi H, Kanno Y, et al. Helper T cell diversity and plasticity. *Curr Opin Immunol*. 2012;24: 297–302.
74. Samuel CE. Antiviral actions of interferons. *Clin Microbiol Rev*. 2001;14:778–809.
75. Swain SL, McKinstry KK, Strutt TM. Expanding roles for CD4(+) T cells in immunity to viruses. *Nat Rev Immunol*. 2012;12:136–148.
76. Semple MG, Dankert HM, Ebrahimi B, et al. Severe respiratory syncytial virus bronchiolitis in infants is associated with reduced airway interferon gamma and substance P. *PLoS One*. 2007;2:e1038.
77. Openshaw PJ, Chiu C. Protective and dysregulated T cell immunity in RSV infection. *Curr Opin Virol*. 2013;3: 468–474.

78. Bont L, Heijnen CJ, Kavelaars A, et al. Peripheral blood cytokine responses and disease severity in respiratory syncytial virus bronchiolitis. *Eur Respir J.* 1999;14:144–149.
79. Legg JP, Hussain IR, Warner JA, et al. Type 1 and type 2 cytokine imbalance in acute respiratory syncytial virus bronchiolitis. *Am J Respir Crit Care Med.* 2003;168: 633–639.
80. Acosta PL, Caballero MT, Polack FP. Brief history and characterization of enhanced respiratory syncytial virus disease. *Clin Vaccine Immunol.* 2015;23:189–195.
81. Reinhard G, Noll A, Schlebusch H, et al. Shifts in the TH1/TH2 balance during human pregnancy correlate with apoptotic changes. *Biochem Biophys Res Commun.* 1998;245:933–938.
82. White GP, Hollams EM, Yerkovich ST, et al. CpG methylation patterns in the IFNgamma promoter in naive T cells: variations during Th1 and Th2 differentiation and between atopics and non-atopics. *Pediatr Allergy Immunol.* 2006;17:557–564.
83. Message SD, Laza-Stanca V, Mallia P, et al. Rhinovirus-induced lower respiratory illness is increased in asthma and related to virus load and Th1/2 cytokine and IL-10 production. *Proc Natl Acad Sci USA.* 2008;105: 13562–13567.
84. Busse WW, Lemanske Jr RF, Gern JE. Role of viral respiratory infections in asthma and asthma exacerbations. *Lancet.* 2010;376:826–834.
85. Copenhaver CC, Gern JE, Li Z, et al. Cytokine response patterns, exposure to viruses, and respiratory infections in the first year of life. *Am J Respir Crit Care Med.* 2004; 170:175–180.
86. Siltanen M, Kajosaari M, Pohjavuori M, et al. Prematurity at birth reduces the long-term risk of atopy. *J Allergy Clin Immunol.* 2001;107:229–234.
87. Liem JJ, Kozyrskyj AL, Huq SI, et al. The risk of developing food allergy in premature or low-birth-weight children. *J Allergy Clin Immunol.* 2007;119:1203–1209.
88. Gibbons D, Fleming P, Virasami A, et al. Interleukin-8 (CXCL8) production is a signatory T cell effector function of human newborn infants. *Nat Med.* 2014;20: 1206–1210.
89. Strieter RM, Kunkel SL, Elner VM, et al. Interleukin-8. A corneal factor that induces neovascularization. *Am J Pathol.* 1992;141:1279–1284.
90. Koch AE, Polverini PJ, Kunkel SL, et al. Interleukin-8 as a macrophage-derived mediator of angiogenesis. *Science.* 1992;258:1798–1801.
91. Mukaida N. Pathophysiological roles of interleukin-8/ CXCL8 in pulmonary diseases. *Am J Physiol Lung Cell Mol Physiol.* 2003;284:L566–L577.
92. Ambalavanan N, Carlo WA, D'Angio CT, et al. Cytokines associated with bronchopulmonary dysplasia or death in extremely low birth weight infants. *Pediatrics.* 2009;123: 1132–1141.
93. Bose CL, Dammann CE, Laughon MM. Bronchopulmonary dysplasia and inflammatory biomarkers in the premature neonate. *Arch Dis Child Fetal Neonatal Ed.* 2008; 93:F455–F461.
94. De Dooy J, Ieven M, Stevens W, et al. High levels of CXCL8 in tracheal aspirate samples taken at birth are associated with adverse respiratory outcome only in preterm infants younger than 28 weeks gestation. *Pediatr Pulmonol.* 2007;42:193–203.
95. Paananen R, Husa AK, Vuolteenaho R, et al. Blood cytokines during the perinatal period in very preterm infants: relationship of inflammatory response and bronchopulmonary dysplasia. *J Pediatr.* 2009;154:39–43 e33.
96. Hull J, Ackerman H, Isles K, et al. Unusual haplotypic structure of IL8, a susceptibility locus for a common respiratory virus. *Am J Hum Genet.* 2001;69:413–419.
97. Hull J, Thomson A, Kwiatkowski D. Association of respiratory syncytial virus bronchiolitis with the interleukin 8 gene region in UK families. *Thorax.* 2000;55: 1023–1027.
98. Assefa D, Amin N, Dozor AJ, et al. Attenuated interleukin-8/leukocyte immunoresponse in preterm infants compared with term infants hospitalized with respiratory syncytial virus bronchiolitis: a pilot study. *Hum Immunol.* 2011;72:708–711.
99. Openshaw PJ, Tregoning JS. Immune responses and disease enhancement during respiratory syncytial virus infection. *Clin Microbiol Rev.* 2005;18:541–555.
100. Gleditsch DD, Shornick LP, Van Steenwinckel J, et al. Maternal inflammation modulates infant immune response patterns to viral lung challenge in a murine model. *Pediatr Res.* 2014;76:33–40.
101. Olin A, Henckel E, Chen Y, et al. Stereotypic immune system development in newborn children. *Cell.* 2018;174: 1277–1292 e1214.
102. Lee AH, Shannon CP, Amenyogbe N, et al. Dynamic molecular changes during the first week of human life follow a robust developmental trajectory. *Nat Commun.* 2019; 10:1092.
103. Li B, Wu FL, Feng XB, et al. Changes and the clinical significance of CD4(+) CD25(+) regulatory T cells and Th17 cells in peripheral blood of infants with respiratory syncytial virus bronchiolitis. *Xi Bao Yu Fen Zi Mian Yi Xue Za Zhi.* 2012;28:426–428.
104. Kan B, Razzaghian HR, Lavoie PM. An immunological perspective on neonatal sepsis. *Trends Mol Med.* 2016; 22:290–302.
105. Lawrence SM, Ruoss JL, Wynn JL. IL-17 in neonatal health and disease. *Am J Reprod Immunol.* 2018;79:e12800.
106. Wildin RS, Smyk-Pearson S, Filipovich AH. Clinical and molecular features of the immunodysregulation, polyendocrinopathy, enteropathy, X linked (IPEX) syndrome. *J Med Genet.* 2002;39:537–545.
107. Mold JE, Venkatasubrahmanyam S, Burt TD, et al. Fetal and adult hematopoietic stem cells give rise to distinct T cell lineages in humans. *Science.* 2010;330: 1695–1699.
108. Takahata Y, Nomura A, Takada H, et al. CD25+CD4+ T cells in human cord blood: an immunoregulatory subset with naive phenotype and specific expression of forkhead box p3 (Foxp3) gene. *Exp Hematol.* 2004;32: 622–629.

109. Luciano AA, Arbona-Ramirez IM, Ruiz R, et al. Alterations in regulatory T cell subpopulations seen in preterm infants. *PLoS One*. 2014;9:e95867.
110. Rueda CM, Moreno-Fernandez ME, Jackson CM, et al. Neonatal regulatory T cells have reduced capacity to suppress dendritic cell function. *Eur J Immunol*. 2015;45: 2582–2592.
111. Oliphant S, Lines JL, Hollifield ML, et al. Regulatory T cells are critical for clearing influenza a virus in neonatal mice. *Viral Immunol*. 2015;28:580–589.
112. Loebbermann J, Durant L, Thornton H, et al. Defective immunoregulation in RSV vaccine-augmented viral lung disease restored by selective chemoattraction of regulatory T cells. *Proc Natl Acad Sci USA*. 2013;110: 2987–2992.
113. Durant LR, Makris S, Voorburg CM, et al. Regulatory T cells prevent Th2 immune responses and pulmonary eosinophilia during respiratory syncytial virus infection in mice. *J Virol*. 2013;87:10946–10954.
114. Krishnamoorthy N, Khare A, Oriss TB, et al. Early infection with respiratory syncytial virus impairs regulatory T cell function and increases susceptibility to allergic asthma. *Nat Med*. 2012;18:1525–1530.
115. Jartti T, Paul-Anttila M, Lehtinen P, et al. Systemic T-helper and T-regulatory cell type cytokine responses in rhinovirus vs. respiratory syncytial virus induced early wheezing: an observational study. *Respir Res*. 2009; 10(85).
116. Carroll KN, Hartert TV. The impact of respiratory viral infection on wheezing illnesses and asthma exacerbations. *Immunol Allergy Clin N AM*. 2008;28: 539–561. viii.
117. Montgomery S, Bahmanyar S, Brus O, et al. Respiratory infections in preterm infants and subsequent asthma: a cohort study. *BMJ Open*. 2013;3. e004034.
118. van der Zalm MM, Uiterwaal CS, Wilbrink B, et al. The influence of neonatal lung function on rhinovirus-associated wheeze. *Am J Respir Crit Care Med*. 2011;183: 262–267.
119. Han M, Rajput C, Ishikawa T, et al. Small animal models of respiratory viral infection related to asthma. *Viruses*. 2018;10.
120. Hong JY, Bentley JK, Chung Y, et al. Neonatal rhinovirus induces mucous metaplasia and airways hyperresponsiveness through IL-25 and type 2 innate lymphoid cells. *J Allergy Clin Immunol*. 2014;134:429–439.
121. Schneider D, Hong JY, Popova AP, et al. Neonatal rhinovirus infection induces mucous metaplasia and airways hyperresponsiveness. *J Immunol*. 2012;188:2894–2904.
122. You D, Ripple M, Balakrishna S, et al. Inchoate CD8+ T cell responses in neonatal mice permit influenza-induced persistent pulmonary dysfunction. *J Immunol*. 2008;181:3486–3494.
123. Tasker L, Lindsay RW, Clarke BT, et al. Infection of mice with respiratory syncytial virus during neonatal life primes for enhanced antibody and T cell responses on secondary challenge. *Clin Exp Immunol*. 2008;153: 277–288.
124. Man WH, van Houten MA, Merelle ME, et al. Bacterial and viral respiratory tract microbiota and host characteristics in children with lower respiratory tract infections: a matched case-control study. *Lancet Respir Med*. 2019 May; 7(5):417–426.
125. de Steenhuijsen Piters WA, Heinonen S, Hasrat R, et al. Nasopharyngeal microbiota, host transcriptome, and disease severity in children with respiratory syncytial virus infection. *Am J Respir Crit Care Med*. 2016;194: 1104–1115.
126. Ederveen THA, Ferwerda G, Ahout IM, et al. Haemophilus is overrepresented in the nasopharynx of infants hospitalized with RSV infection and associated with increased viral load and enhanced mucosal CXCL8 responses. *Microbiome*. 2018;6(10).
127. Beeton ML, Maxwell NC, Davies PL, et al. Role of pulmonary infection in the development of chronic lung disease of prematurity. *Eur Respir J*. 2011;37:1424–1430.
128. Gallacher DJ, Kotecha S. Respiratory microbiome of newborn infants. *Front Pediatr*. 2016;4(10).

CHAPTER 12

Optimal Nutritional Management for Prevention and Treatment of Chronic Lung Disease (or Bronchopulmonary Dysplasia) in Preterm Infants

WILLIAM W. HAY, JR., MD

KEY POINTS

- Suboptimal fetal nutrition and intrauterine growth restriction are associated with an increased risk of chronic lung disease (CLD) in preterm infants.
- Extremely preterm, extremely low-birth-weight infants are at greatest risk of CLD, which is often associated with undernutrition and poor growth during the neonatal intensive care unit (NICU) period and after discharge from the NICU.
- Optimal nutrition of the preterm infant is essential, not only for normal growth and development but also particularly for supporting growth of the lung that is injured by oxygen toxicity, barotrauma, and inflammation.
- Gestational age-specific protein requirements are especially important for growing the lung as well as lean body mass in the preterm infant with CLD.
- Increased levels of antioxidants (minerals and vitamins, as well as long-chain polyunsaturated essential fatty acids [LC-PUFAs]) in nutrient products and prevention and modulation of hyperglycemia are important to counter the frequent hyperoxic conditions and oxygen toxicity that preterm infants have as they progress from respiratory distress and pulmonary insufficiency after birth to the development of CLD.

INTRODUCTION: SPECIAL NUTRITIONAL CONSIDERATIONS FOR INFANTS WITH BRONCHOPULMONARY DYSPLASIA

Chronic lung disease (CLD), often still called bronchopulmonary dysplasia (BPD), persists as one of the most common and serious medical disorders of preterm infants, especially those born extremely preterm (EPT) and those with extremely low birth weight (ELBW).[1] The pathogenesis of CLD is directly related to oxygen toxicity, volu- and barotrauma from respirators, and inflammation associated with chronic intubation and oxygen administration.[2] Such pathologic processes, along with high levels of stress and catabolic hormone secretion, often limit optimal nutrition, such that these infants are not only undernourished but also undergrown. Such undergrowth also includes poor growth and development of the lung and the structure of its airways, alveoli, and vasculature. A variety of clinical studies have shown benefits of selective nutrients in reducing the risk of CLD, although there is limited convincing data from randomized controlled trials (RCTs) to define the specific effects of early nutrition, including protein and energy, as well as micronutrients, on the prevention or development of CLD.[3,4] Although severity of illness and early nutritional practices appear to be independently associated with CLD,[5] there is good evidence that improved diets and nutritional status can improve lung growth and promote healing. Infants who receive more nutritional support during the first 3 weeks of life (and who are less critically ill, with <7 days of mechanical ventilation) are less likely to develop CLD.[6] Most studies, in fact, even when focused on the nutrition of infants who already have CLD, show that improved nutrition during the CLD phase can improve lung growth.[7] More specifically, infants who receive more protein in the first 3 weeks after birth and grow with greater velocity have less severe CLD.[8] In contrast, clinical practice has tended to overemphasize energy/

Updates on Neonatal Chronic Lung Disease. https://doi.org/10.1016/B978-0-323-68353-1.00012-9

low-protein diets that have contributed to these infants developing poorly grown lungs in the presence of excess subcutaneous and intra-abdominal fat.[4] Optimizing nutrition of the ELBW/EPT infant has the potential, therefore, to improve lung growth and development and to limit the impact of some of the insults that contribute to the development of CLD. Nutritional factors that are important to consider for infants who require assisted ventilation and/or who have developed CLD are summarized in Table 12.1.[9] Several reviews of nutrition and CLD have been published.[10–14]

CAUSES OF POOR GROWTH IN INFANTS WITH CHRONIC LUNG DISEASE AND THE NEED FOR NUTRITIONAL INTERVENTIONS TO PREVENT CHRONIC LUNG DISEASE

Intrauterine Growth and Pulmonary Outcomes

Fetal growth restriction is independently associated with the development of CLD.[15] Several observational studies have noted higher rates of CLD in small-for-gestational-age (SGA) neonates,[16,17] most of whom are likely to have had intrauterine growth restriction. Decreased lung growth is a major contributor to CLD, if not the only mechanism. It remains uncertain whether underdeveloped lungs from fetal growth restriction can be reversed with postnatal nutritional strategies or whether nutritional approaches will be helpful but remain limited because of the permanently underdeveloped lung structure.

Severity of Illness and Nutritional Requirements

EPT/ELBW infants who have the greatest degree of respiratory distress and requirements for supplemental oxygen, airway distension, and ventilation are also the least well fed and nourished. Ehrenkranz and colleagues,[18] for example, found that infants receiving mechanical ventilation for the first 7 days after birth received significantly less nutritional support (both parenteral and enteral) during each of the first 3 weeks compared with less critically ill infants who did not require ventilation. The rationale for such nutritional restriction is seldom justified, often reflecting untested or historical concerns for protein toxicity and enteral feeding intolerance. Unfortunately, such concerns have led to both less intravenous (IV) and enteral feedings, which is

TABLE 12.1 Nutritional Influences for the Preterm Infant With Respiratory Insufficiency.
Insufficient poor nutrition is associated with abnormal lung development
Fluid and sodium restriction in the first days after birth may reduce the risk of CLD
RDS and CLD increase the metabolic needs for energy and protein in very preterm infants
Steroid therapy has negative effects on protein balance
Early nutritional support and feeding guidelines can reduce the risk of CLD
Hyperglycemia produces reactive oxygen species, contributing to oxygen toxicity
Lipids (ω3-LCPUFAs) are a good alternative source of concentrated energy and act as antioxidants to reduce the risk of oxygen toxicity and CLD
Adequate supply of IV amino acids and enteral protein prevents catabolism of respiratory muscle protein and promotes growth of alveolar structures
Amino acids and protein promote production of IGF-1, which helps promote alveolar development
Vitamin A supplementation during the first month of life is associated with a reduction in CLD
Vitamins C, D, and E are antioxidants and have the potential to reduce the risk of oxygen toxicity and CLD
Vitamin D has additional benefits of promoting surfactant production, inhibiting smooth airway muscle proliferation, increasing NO production, and being proangiogenic in the lung, all of which might reduce the risk of CLD
The trace minerals zinc, copper, manganese, and selenium are antioxidants that might reduce the risk of oxygen toxicity and CLD

CLD, chronic lung disease; *IGF-1*, insulinlike growth factor 1; *IV*, intravenous; *LCPUFAs*, long-chain polyunsaturated essential fatty acids; *NO*, nitric oxide; *RDS*, respiratory distress syndrome.

Adapted from Brown LD, Bell EF, Hay WW Jr., Nutritional Support. In: Goldsmith, J, Karotkin, E, Keszler, M, Suresh, G, (eds.), *Goldsmith: Assisted Ventilation of the Neonate*, 6th edition. Elsevier, Philadelphia, 2016:322–329 [172].

paradoxical because these infants are clearly those who need earlier and higher rates of nutritional support. Furthermore, CLD is not formally diagnosed until after 36 weeks. Thus efforts to prevent postnatal growth failure and nutrient deficits that can be difficult to recoup must start at the earliest period after birth with the worsening respiratory distress and its ongoing treatment. It is important, therefore, to note that there is no categoric contraindication to either parenteral or enteral nutrition in critically ill infants receiving mechanical ventilation.

Nutrition and Lung Development

In infants who are at the highest risk of CLD, optimal nutrition is fundamental for optimizing cellular proliferation and differentiation in the developing lung and for modulating inflammatory responses[19] that are common in infants with early respiratory distress with oxygen and airway distention treatments. Selected amino acids, such as glutamine, have critical roles in promoting cellular differentiation, particularly noted in the developing lung. Glucose, of course, is essential for energy balance and cellular function, but glucose supplied in excess of normal utilization rates leads to lipid production, a highly energy-consuming process that produces excess CO_2 that can compromise respiratory distress already in place.[20] Furthermore, hyperglycemia is inflammatory because of the production of intracellular reactive oxygen species, especially during intermittent hypoxic episodes. Polyunsaturated essential fatty acids (PUFAs) are necessary for membrane formation, and the ω3-PUFAs are important as antiinflammatory substances that balance the hyperoxic and hyperglycemic conditions that promote oxidant injury and inflammation. Nutritional restriction and hyperoxia can each interfere with alveolarization, and nutritional restriction intensifies damage to the pulmonary architecture caused by hyperoxia.[21,22]

Nutrition and Pathology in Preterm Infants

Preterm infants are also at risk of insufficient nutrition due to a variety of pathologic processes. Unfortunately, there has been little research or quality improvement practice to determine how such pathophysiologic processes in unstable or "sick" EPT infants with respiratory distress affect metabolism and growth and thus the nutrient requirements.[23] Such pathophysiologic processes include increased metabolic rate and intermittent and prolonged hypoxic episodes that increase the infants' requirements for nutrients, especially protein. These infants also are commonly treated with corticosteroids, both to prevent CLD and to improve CLD once established, that reduce protein balance. They also receive diuretics that increase loss of nutrients and minerals from the urinary tract and contribute to acidosis. Episodes of late-onset sepsis and tracheal and pulmonary infections increase catabolic risks from endogenous steroid secretion, inflammation, and deficiencies of anabolic hormones. Many of these infants develop limited gastrointestinal function and feeding intolerance. Concerns for all these problems limit administration of IV and enteral nutrition, which impairs not only somatic and lung growth but also recovery from lung injuries, such as oxygen toxicity, inflammation with protein breakdown, and barotrauma from high airway and intrapulmonary pressures. CLD itself, as well as hypoxic episodes and high-pressure ventilation, leads to pulmonary hypertension and right-sided heart failure.[24] Nutritional support of infants who require assisted ventilation, therefore, is necessary to prevent catabolism and exhaustion of endogenous energy resources, achieve growth in lean body mass, and promote healing, growth, and maturation of the lungs, brain, and other vital organs. Insufficient nutrition also contributes to reduced brain growth and abnormal neurodevelopmental outcomes, an established risk of CLD.[25]

General Nutritional Strategies to Optimize Growth, Including Lung Development and Growth

Prevention of postnatal growth restriction requires sufficient protein and energy intakes in the first few weeks after birth, but beginning as soon as reasonable and as safely after birth as possible. Many studies have now shown that providing recommended intakes of 3.5–4.0 g/kg/day of protein and 110–120 kcal/kg/day to EPT infants in the first week of life reduces the incidence of postnatal growth failure. Such studies clearly document the association between optimal nutritional intake in the first week of life and more rapid growth velocity over the first month of life. Adequate protein intake is especially important for promoting lean body mass and organ growth, including that of the lung. A minimum of 2 g/kg/day of IV amino acids should be provided as soon as possible after birth in EPT infants, especially those with respiratory distress. A target of 3.5–4.0 g/kg/day of amino acids is recommended by day 2, with no need to increase amino acid supply slowly over several days. IV lipids, which have a twofold greater degree of concentrated energy source relative to carbohydrates, should also be started early to ensure optimal energy supply. There is no evidence to support a stepwise increase in lipid intake; a minimum of 2 g/kg/day is recommended with a target of 3.0–4.0 g/kg/day shortly thereafter.[26] Given the association among suboptimal nutrition, growth failure, and impaired pulmonary development, standardized feeding guidelines are fundamental, as they have been shown universally to promote early nutrition and ensure that the sickest infants receive optimal nutritional support.

Evidence is accumulating that demonstrates the benefits of human milk as a source of optimal protein quality, optimal lipid quality, and as of yet undetermined factors that promote an optimal microbiome and reduce the risk of inflammatory conditions, including CLD.[27,28] A recent study documented that high-dose human milk feedings decreased oxidative stress in preterm infants compared with cow milk-derived formula feedings.[29] Urinary F_2-isoprostane concentrations, a marker of oxidant stress, were significantly lower in the predominantly milk fed group. Promoting milk feeding, therefore, might reduce oxidative stress that is associated with a variety of morbidities in preterm infants, including necrotizing enterocolitis, late-onset sepsis, and CLD.

SPECIFIC NUTRIENT REQUIREMENTS FOR INFANTS WITH RESPIRATORY DISTRESS AND CHRONIC LUNG DISEASE

The catabolism of major nutrient substrates, including glucose, amino acids, and fatty acids (especially the PUFAs), provides acetyl CoA for the tricarboxylic acid cycle to generate energy. Adequate nutrition generates a variety of metabolites for the biosynthesis of biomolecules, including nucleotides, proteins, and lipids (anabolism).[19] In catabolism, these nutrient substrates are oxidized into CO_2 and H_2O, producing energy. Adequate nutrient supply also regulates cell proliferation and differentiation during normal development and in the healing phases following an injury.[30] Metabolic dysregulation from insufficient nutrition or malnutrition enhances autophagy, apoptosis, senescence, and inflammatory responses contributing to the pathogenesis of CLDs.

Protein Requirements

The absolute requirement for growth of all cells, tissues, and organs is protein. Protein makes up the structure of all living tissues. While energy is necessary to synthesize amino acids into protein and to organize the protein into cell and tissue structures, no amount of energy will produce growth of new tissue. The provision of parenteral or enteral protein as soon after birth as possible is essential, therefore, to promote positive protein accretion and growth of all parts of the infant's body, including the lung. The minimum amount of protein nutrition in preterm infants is similar to that of a healthy growing fetus of the same gestational age. Both animal and human studies have shown that EPT infants, like the fetus of a similar gestational age, have high fractional protein synthetic rates with high turnover rates of amino acid metabolism and incorporation into relatively high growth rates with net protein accretion. As gestation advances, such high rates of protein synthesis and amino acid and protein requirements decline to those of the healthy term breastfed infant (Fig. 12.1). Providing less protein to ELBW preterm infants, therefore, would clearly limit both fractional and net protein synthesis and growth rates. As all tissues are growing during this period of development, no tissue would be spared if less protein were provided and this would contribute to reduced organ growth, including that of the lung.

Many studies have applied such information to show that preterm infants indeed require high amounts of protein to produce net protein balance and growth rates (Figs. 12.2 and 12.3).

Protein accretion must exceed 1.5 g/kg/day to produce positive nitrogen and protein balance. Even higher rates, up to 3.5–4.0 g/kg/day, are needed in ELBW and EPT infants to produce protein balance that supports structural growth of all parts of the body that approaches or equals the growth of a normally growing fetus of the same gestational age. Thus providing optimal amounts of protein, and energy necessary to support the synthesis of amino acids into protein, is critically important to maximize lean tissue and organ growth.[34] Estimates of the protein requirements of preterm infants are higher than those of the healthy fetus because of the enteral nutrient losses in stool, increased protein turnover, and protein losses from stressful conditions (inflammation, endogenous steroid and catecholamine secretion, sepsis), ranging between 3.5 and 4.5 g/kg/day in enterally fed EPT infants.[35,36]

Preterm infants who require assisted ventilation have additional protein requirements that begin immediately after birth and with the onset of respiratory distress.[37,38] Such increased protein requirements are not just theoretic, as studies have demonstrated that early initiation of IV amino acids enhances growth rates in weight, length, and head circumference.[39] Length and head growth are strong indicators of growth of all lean tissue, including the lung. Most preterm infants with CLD have decreased lean body mass and smaller lungs, indicating that the current protein (and energy) nutrition is insufficient, either as a primary and

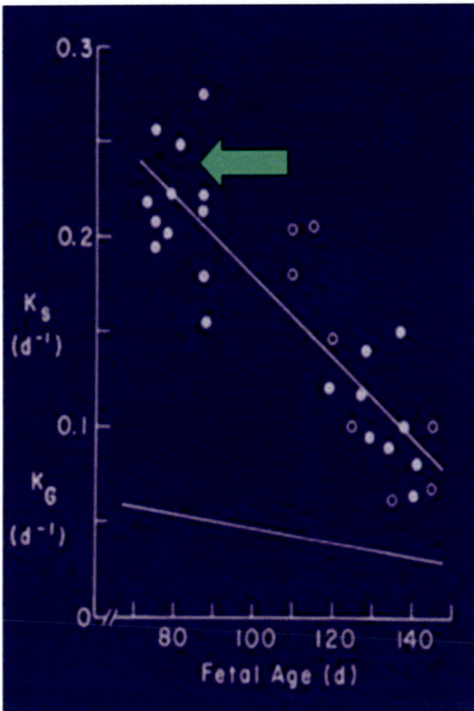

FIGURE 12.1 Fractional protein synthetic rate (K_S) and fractional growth rate (K_G) in fetal sheep over the second half of gestation. The arrow represents the gestational age period in fetal sheep that is equivalent to 20–26 weeks in human gestation. *AA*, amino acid. (Adapted from Hay, WW., Jr, Brown, LD., Regnault, TRH. Fetal requirements and placental transfer of nitrogenous compounds. In: Polin, RA. et al. (eds), *Fetal and Neonatal Physiology*, 5th ed., Elsevier, Philadelphia; 2011:444–458 and Brown, LD., Hendrickson, K., Masor, ML., et al. High-protein formulas: evidence for use in preterm infants. *Clin Perinatol*. 2014;41:383–403.)

independent cause of growth failure or in relation to the increased requirements for protein that are necessary to combat the many stresses that contribute to growth failure independent of nutrition.[40,41] Other studies have shown that enhanced nutrition in the first weeks of life reduces the severity of CLD.[18]

Although total protein intake is fundamental for ensuring a positive anabolic condition and promoting or at least supporting growth, recent evidence suggests that selected amino acids could be important in optimizing lung function. Similar to adults with respiratory distress who demonstrated improved lung function (increased ventilator sensitivity as noted by the decreasing partial pressure of carbon dioxide [P_{CO_2}] and ventilatory response to hypercapnia) with supplemental IV leucine,[42] studies in preterm infants who had higher concentrations of branched-chain amino acids in their parenteral nutrient solutions developed increased dynamic lung compliance, decreased pulmonary resistance, and fewer episodes of apnea.[43] Studies in the neonatal piglet have produced similar results, showing that the addition of 3 g/kg/day rate for 4 hours of an IV amino acid infusion compared with a 10% dextrose infusion increased ventilatory responses to hypoxemia.[44] Thus both lung growth and lung function can be improved in preterm infants with respiratory distress and BPD when they are provided with sufficient amounts of protein, especially protein supplies enriched in essential amino acids.

Selected amino acids

Recent research has shown some promise for selected amino acids to reduce the risk of CLD or improve its treatment. These include glutamine, cysteine, N-acetylcysteine, L-arginine, and L-citrulline.[12]

Glutamine. Glutamine is a conditionally essential amino acid that is important for rapidly dividing cells.[45] In preterm infants, however, glutamine is not a standard component of many IV amino acid solutions

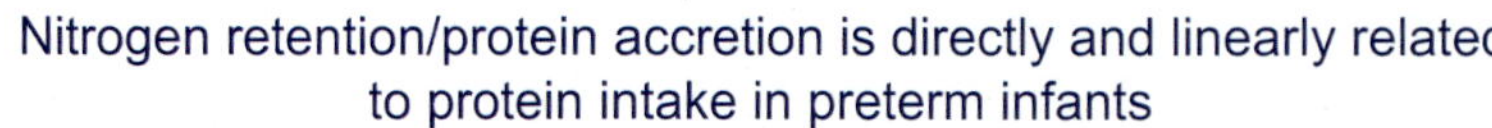

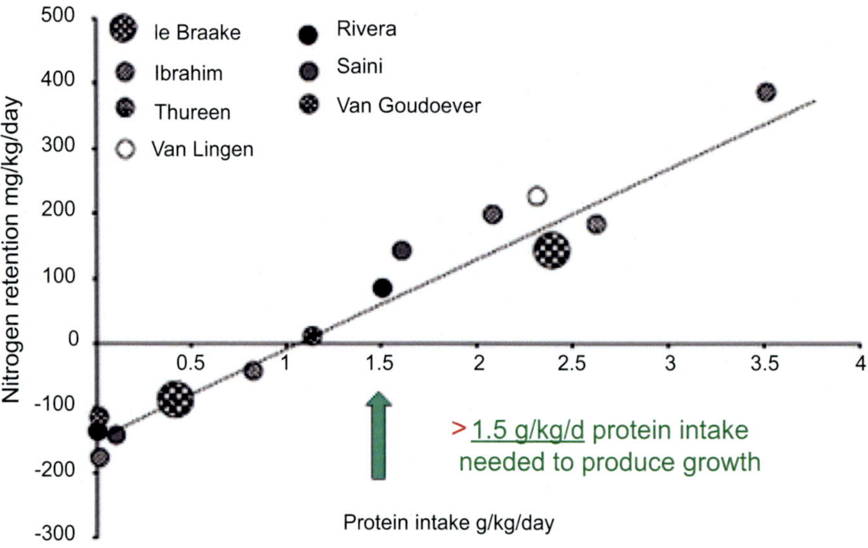

Embleton ND.Ealry Human Development 83: 831-837, 2007.

FIG. 12.2 Nitrogen retention in relationship to protein intake from multiple studies. (Adapted from Embleton ND. Optimal protein and energy intakes in preterm infants. Early Human Development 2007, 83, 831–837 and Te Braake, FW., van den Akker, CH., Wattimena, DJ., et al. Amino acid administration to premature infants directly after birth. *J Pediatr.* 2005;147:457–461.)

owing to its solubility problems in aqueous solution. Requirements for glutamine may be increased during catabolic conditions in very preterm infants with respiratory distress. Glutamine protects mitochondrial structure and function by promoting glutathione that scavenges reactive oxygen species,[46] indicating its potential to ameliorate hyperoxic injury and reduce the risk for BPD.[47] Although there have been several studies of glutamine supplementation in preterm infants, CLD as an outcome has not been sufficiently studied.[48,49] In one study, parenteral nutrition supplemented with glutamine did not decrease mortality, the incidence of late-onset sepsis, or the incidence of CLD in ELBW infants.[50] There is some support from studies in neonatal mice for using the novel dipeptide, arginyl-glutamine, to reduce hyperoxic lung injury, which appears to be better than using either amino acid alone.[51]

Cysteine and N-acetylcysteine. There is rationale, if not experimental evidence, for adding cysteine to generate glutathione and thereby enhance antioxidant defenses, including overexpression of manganese superoxide dismutase messenger RNA (mRNA) and protein.[52] N-acetylcysteine, a precursor of cysteine,[53] is itself a free radical scavenger. Hyperoxia causes increased mortality in animals deficient in cysteine.[54] Cysteine is not added to standard amino acid solutions owing to its poor solubility and instability in aqueous solutions; instead, it is usually added to each daily parenteral nutrition solution. A Cochrane review found a small effect of supplemental cysteine to promote whole-body nitrogen balance, but not enough to affect lung growth.[55] Clinical studies have not convincingly demonstrated that supplemental cysteine can improve lung function (compliance or reduced airway resistance, functional residual capacity, or airway gas mixing capacity) or reduce the development of CLD. In one study, for example, a 6-day course of IV N-acetylcysteine infusion did not prevent death or CLD in ELBW infants.[56]

L-Arginine and L-citrulline. CLD is associated not only with arrested alveolar development but also with abnormal vascular growth. A meta-analysis of inhaled nitric oxide (iNO), a potent vasodilator, did not show benefit in preventing CLD,[57] although an animal study in which iNO was an added therapy showed improved lung alveolar and vascular structure in

Even right after birth, there is a direct correlation between amino acid supply and protein balance, through at least 3 g/kg/day.

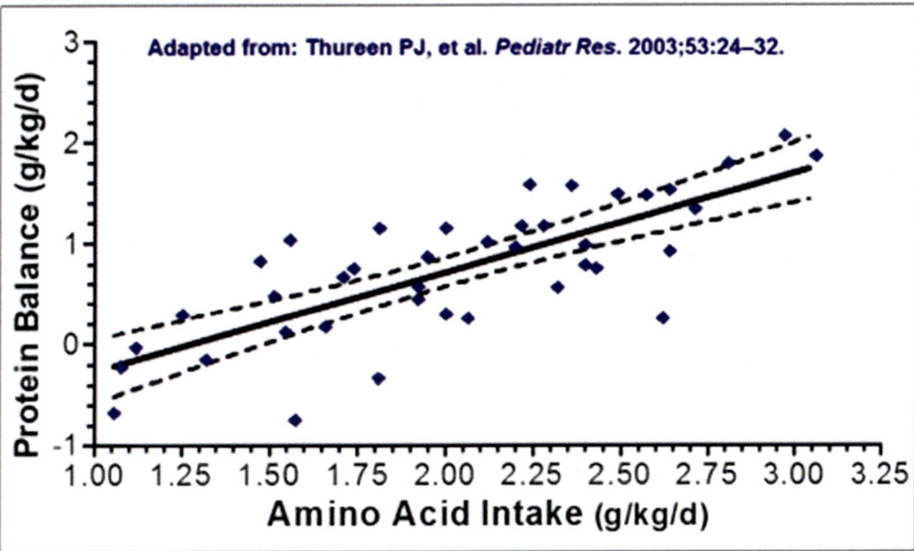

FIG. 12.3 Relationship between protein balance and amino acid intake in very preterm infants in the 1st 48–72 hours after birth. (Adapted from Thureen, PJ., Melara, D., Fennessey, PV. Hay, WW., Jr. Effect of low versus high intravenous amino acid intake on very low birth weight infants in the early neonatal period. *Pediatr Res*, 2003;53:24–32 and Van Goudoever, JB., Colen, T., Wattimena, JL., et al. Immediate commencement of amino acid supplementation in preterm infants: effect on serum amino acid concentrations and protein kinetics on the first day of life. *J Pediatr*. 1995;127:458–465.)

neonatal rats exposed to prolonged hyperoxia.[58] Endogenous NO originates from the metabolism of two amino acids, L-arginine and L-citrulline.[59] Theoretically, L-arginine and L-citrulline supplementation could reduce the severity of CLD. Low plasma arginine concentrations have been reported in acute neonatal diseases, including respiratory distress syndrome (RDS), and in an animal model of CLD.[60] However, plasma arginine levels are not abnormally low in preterm infants with RDS or CLD,[61] indicating that arginine might not be deficient in preterm infants with CLD.

In several animal models of CLD, L-citrulline appears effective in attenuating hyperoxia-induced pulmonary injuries, indicating the pivotal role played by the L-citrulline-L-arginine-NO pathway in the developing lung.[62] For example, in a newborn rat model of CLD, plasma L-arginine and L-citrulline levels were decreased and L-citrulline supplementation attenuated the arrested alveolar growth and pulmonary hypertension.[63] In another newborn rat model of oxygen-induced lung injury, L-citrulline supplementation increased serum L-arginine levels and improved alveolar and vascular growth by enhancing the lung vascular endothelial growth factor (VEGF) and nitric oxide synthase expression and by reversing the damaged relaxation of airways.[64] Although there are no clinical trials yet, these results indicate that L-citrulline supplementation deserves consideration as a potential approach to treat preterm infants at risk of developing pulmonary hypertension or to treat the established chronic, progressive forms of the condition in infants with CLD.

Energy Requirements

Healthy preterm infants need about 110–130 kcal/kg/day to support normal energy metabolism and protein accretion and lean body mass growth when protein intake is sufficient for growth.[65] Basal energy metabolism accounts for about 40%–50% (about 50 kcal/

kg/day) of total energy requirements in preterm infants. Additional energy requirements are highly variable. For example, energy production for thermoregulation depends on the heat and humidity in the incubator. Energy for physical activity is lower than often assumed, only about 1%–3% of total energy production, as very preterm infants are generally tightly wrapped in blankets and do not move much.[66] Additional energy is needed for postprandial or synthetic energy expenditure that is necessary for net protein production and growth.[67] The energy cost of growth is highly variable, depending on protein intake, net protein accretion in lean body mass, and fat production in adipose tissue. Higher amounts of energy may be needed for very preterm infants who are enterally fed to account for stool losses.[68] Most estimates of energy requirements, however, exceed the requirements for normal metabolism and growth, which has led to preterm infants receiving excess energy and thus production of excess body fat by term gestation.[69]

Infants with RDS and those receiving continuous positive airway pressure for such diseases require more energy to support the increased work of breathing.[70] Preterm infants who are treated with caffeine, including those with CLD, also have increased respiratory rates and work of breathing that require more energy.[71] The increased resting metabolic expenditure in patients with CLD, particularly those with growth failure,[70] indicates impaired substrate oxidative metabolism. Sets of genes characteristic of oxidative phosphorylation are reduced in infants with CLD compared with control infants.[72] Human umbilical venous endothelial cells from patients with CLD have lower mitochondrial respiration than the cells from infants who survive without CLD. Such observations indicate that maximal oxygen consumption is a significant predictor of CLD.[73] Indeed, hyperoxic exposure in a rodent model of CLD reduced mitochondrial respiration and complex I activity in neonatal mice.[74] Furthermore, administration of the complex I inhibitor, pyridaben, caused significantly delayed alveolarization compared with control mice, indicating that dysfunction of mitochondrial respiration contributes to hyperoxic lung injury.[19]

In the past, it was assumed that because infants with CLD might have higher energy expenditure than those without CLD owing to the increased work of breathing, such infants might benefit from greater energy intake to achieve sustained growth. One nonrandomized interventional cohort study showed enteral energy intake was positively associated with weight gain velocity during enteral nutrition in infants with CLD, and inversely associated with the severity of CLD,[7] but the increased enteral energy intake was accompanied by increased protein intake, confounding the specific effect of energy. Furthermore, despite some evidence for possibly increased energy requirements to meet increased respiratory rates and effort,[68] there is little evidence that exceeding the normal energy intakes promotes improved lung growth, lung function, or resolution of CLD. Excess energy in these infants produces excess body fat, just as it does in infants without respiratory disorders. Furthermore, increased oxygen consumption in infants with CLD is not entirely due to the increased work of breathing, as approaches to improve pulmonary function (e.g., use of diuretics to reduce lung water) do not necessarily decrease oxygen consumption.[75] As with preterm infants without CLD, overfeeding has produced higher body fat content, particularly in intra-abdominal regions, which has been associated with obesity in later life. Higher protein/energy ratio diets are likely to be more effective in improving lung growth and function than higher energy diets alone.

Lipid Requirements

Lipids are important energy sources for metabolism and growth, particularly after birth because the newborn's diet becomes increasingly enriched in lipids relative to the fetus whose energy supply is mostly glucose and lactate and amino acids. In addition to fatty acids providing energy, essential fatty acids are fundamental for producing normal membrane phospholipid structure in all cells, particularly in lipid components (myelin sheath) of neurons.[76] Only two fatty acids are known to be essential (cannot be synthesized in the body) for humans: α-linolenic acid, an ω3 fatty acid, and linoleic acid, an ω6 fatty acid. Milk and most formulas contain adequate amounts of linoleic acid and α-linolenic acid, from which the long-chain polyunsaturated essential fatty acids (LCPUFAs) arachidonic acid (AA) and docosahexaenoic acid (DHA) are derived, respectively. LCPUFAs may be particularly important as immune modulators of inflammatory conditions in the lung, particularly oxygen toxicity. An increase in the dietary levels of ω6 fatty acids tends to promote, whereas an increase in ω3 LCPUFA levels tends to inhibit, inflammatory responses.[77] Supplementation with ω3 LCPUFAs increases tolerance to acute lung injury induced by intestinal ischemia-reperfusion in rats.[78] In mice with acute lung injury, high concentrations of ω3 PUFAs from supplemental DHA reduced inflammatory responses such as leukocyte infiltration and tissue damage in lungs. These observations suggest that

LCPUFAs might prevent diseases associated with oxidative stress in preterm infants, such as those with respiratory distress from surfactant deficiency and CLD.[51,79] Similarly, maternal DHA supplementation reduces pulmonary leukocyte infiltration in offspring mice exposed to hyperoxia, suggesting a potential route for DHA supplementation to reduce pulmonary inflammation in preterm infants exposed to hyperoxia.[80]

Accretion of LCPUFAs increases markedly during the last trimester of gestation; thus early preterm birth indicates that ELBW/EPT infants have greater LCPUFA requirements.[81] Postnatal concentrations of DHA and AA are low in the blood of preterm infants and are associated with a variety of neonatal morbidities.[80] A meta-analysis of studies in preterm infants, however, did not show a significant association between ω3 LCPUFAs and reduced risk of CLD in infants born at ≤32 weeks' gestation.[82] Nevertheless, a multicenter RCT in Australia showed that DHA supplementation reduced the incidence of CLD in male infants born at <33 weeks' gestation and in all infants with birth weights <1250 g.[83]

IV lipid emulsions are important for infants who require assisted ventilation, providing important energy when enteral feeding is still limited. LCPUFAs are integral components, but they vary according to the lipid source (soy, olive, or fish oils) in IV lipid emulsions.[84] Early introduction of soybean-oil-based emulsions in preterm infants produces detrimental effects on pulmonary gas exchange and hemodynamics,[85] but only in very high dosages, greater than 5 g/kg/day, that are not used clinically. Other studies have not shown either beneficial or adverse effects on growth, death, or the development, severity, or progress of CLD with early introduction of IV lipids. IV lipid preparations based solely on soybean oil such as Intralipid do not contain LCPUFAs, leading to a deficit of DHA in very low-birth-weight (VLBW) infants who are not being fed enterally with milk or formulas. Decreased DHA levels and increased linoleic acid/DHA ratios are associated with an increased risk of CLD in preterm infants.[81] The more recently developed IV lipid emulsions containing fish oil, which are primarily used for treating severe cholestatic disease and hepatic failure, have shown additional benefit in attenuating inflammatory cytokine activity in lungs of very preterm infants with respiratory distress progressing to CLD.[86] Decreased DHA and AA levels in preterm infants are associated with an increased risk of CLD, perhaps through the anti-inflammatory role of DHA and the structural lipid role of AA.[87] DHA or AA supplements via IV lipid emulsion nutrition or as supplements to milk feedings have not shown a consistent benefit to improve CLD development.[88]

Carbohydrate Requirements

Glucose

Glucose is the primary circulating carbohydrate that is fundamental for normal energy metabolism in all cells. Nevertheless, preterm and stressed infants are at risk for developing hyperglycemia, especially those with respiratory distress, mechanical ventilation, and restricted cardiac output and circulation. Complications of hyperglycemia that frequently develop in neonates when the maximal glucose oxidative capacity (>8−10 mg/kg/min) is exceeded include increased energy expenditure (glucose-to-fat synthesis is energy expensive), increased oxygen consumption (and hypoxia), increased CO_2 production,[89] increased fat deposition in excess of lean mass, and increased fatty infiltration of heart and liver.[90,91] Infants with marked hyperglycemia are often intermittently hypoxic, which adds to increased glucagon, adrenalin, and glucocorticoid secretion. These stress-reactive hormones not only reduce insulin secretion and insulin action but also promote glucose production through both glycogenolysis (acutely) and gluconeogenesis (over a sustained period). They also contribute to protein breakdown. Hyperglycemia leads to excess carbon that cannot be fully oxidized, producing increased amounts of reactive oxygen species that cause cellular breakdown.[92] It is worth considering, therefore, that excess hyperglycemia that produces inflammation could contribute to oxygen toxicity and other mechanisms producing lung injury that results in CLD.

Inositol

Inositol is a naturally occurring sugar alcohol that promotes endothelial cell growth, enhances glucocorticoid-mediated lung epithelial cell differentiation, and may serve as an antioxidant. Inositol is particularly important for lung development. It is fundamental for surfactant phospholipid production. A meta-analysis of studies in preterm infants supplemented with inositol demonstrated a statistically significant reduction in the incidence of death or CLD.[93] Possible mechanisms include antioxidant properties and reduced barotrauma, as infants treated with inositol had lower airway pressures and oxygen requirements. Breast milk contains high concentrations of inositol, but most parenteral nutrition solutions contain little or no inositol. Term and late-preterm infants can produce inositol from glucose at rates sufficient to meet nutritional requirements.[94] However, an ELBW infant who is critically ill and requires prolonged parenteral nutrition may not be able to produce enough endogenous inositol to meet requirements. Lower inositol concentrations are associated with more severe RDS. Previous clinical studies showed that providing inositol to preterm infants might decrease the incidence of CLD, but not necessarily its severity.[95]

Water Requirement

Normally, urinary flow rates decline after birth in infants with respiratory distress, with subsequent improvement in renal function as lung function improves. [96] This is also triggered by increased atrial natriuretic peptide levels[97] in response to increased body water balance from aggressive IV fluid administration (both dextrose only and total parenteral nutrition solutions). Excessive water intake in infants with limited renal function, particularly when accompanied by sodium supplements, leads to fluid accumulation in the lung, which worsens lung function and increases the need for potentially injurious oxygen and ventilator support. Pulmonary edema due to fluid overload can contribute to decreased pulmonary compliance and increased airway resistance. A study from the National Institute of Child Health and Human Development (NICHD) Neonatal Research Network documented that higher fluid intake and less weight loss during the first 10 days of life were associated with an increased risk of CLD[98] and a Cochrane review concluded that restricted water intake tended to reduce the risk of CLD.[99] Another study from the NICHD Neonatal Research Network showed that early postnatal weight loss was associated with a lower risk of death or CLD in both ELBW appropriate-for-gestational-age and SGA infants. This observation indicates that the association between early postnatal weight loss and risk of CLD is independent of gestation/birth weight status.[100] Excessive pulmonary fluid from high water intake, along with high sodium intake, also increases the risk and severity of patent ductus arteriosus (PDA), which increase lung blood flow and contribute to pulmonary edema and the risk of CLD.[101]

A recent meta-analysis indicated that the incidence of CLD was reduced with increased use of furosemide.[102] Such treatment, however, has been associated with renal calcinosis and systemic acidosis. Chronic diuretic treatment[103] also reduces lung fluid and oxygen requirements, but at the expense of urinary mineral loss. Although the efficacy of diuretic therapy may be controversial, there is no disputing the increased risk of hyponatremia and hypokalemia in infants who receive diuretics. In animal models, sodium restriction, even with relatively normal serum sodium levels, is associated with poor weight gain and linear growth and can also negatively impact lung growth.[104] If diuretics are given, sodium supplementation may be necessary for optimal growth.

Mineral Requirements

Sodium and potassium

Normally, sodium and potassium requirements for preterm infants are relatively high in the first week of life, but not right after birth in preterm infants with respiratory distress, who have delayed renal water and mineral excretion. During this period, administration of these electrolyte minerals should be restricted to help avoid lung water volume overload that increases the risk of CLD.

Calcium, phosphorus, and vitamin D

Osteopenia of prematurity, a condition due to the nutritional deficiency of calcium and phosphorus rather than problems with vitamin D metabolism, is much more common in infants with CLD. Calcium and phosphorus accretion occurs primarily in the third trimester, increasing the risk of rickets in preterm infants. The limited solubility of calcium and phosphorus in parenteral nutrition limits their intake, compounding low enteral intakes and fluid restriction. Other factors leading to calcium deficiency include the use of loop diuretics and increased urinary losses secondary to inadequate phosphorus intake. Because diuretic use is common, especially in infants with severe CLD, these infants are more prone to develop osteopenia if not supplemented adequately with calcium and phosphorus. Enterally fed infants also receive inadequate calcium and phosphorus with unfortified breast milk, cholestasis, and malabsorption. These infants should receive additional calcium, phosphorus, and vitamin D supplementation with fortification of breast milk or use of preterm formulas. Hypophosphatemia is common in the first few days of life and is associated with a greater risk of CLD, compounded by more days on mechanical ventilation and a higher incidence of PDA.[105]

Trace Mineral Requirements

Zinc, copper, and manganese

Lipid peroxidation can play an important role in the development of CLD. Trace elements such as copper, zinc, and manganese increase pulmonary antioxidant defenses.[106] These trace elements may play a role through synthesis of antioxidant enzymes such as copper-zinc superoxide dismutase and manganese superoxide dismutase. A multicenter study of intratracheal administration of human recombinant copper-zinc superoxide dismutase did not change the incidence of CLD. It was, however, associated with improved pulmonary status in the form of reduced hospital admissions, emergency room visits, and use of asthma medications measured at 1 year of corrected age.[107] More studies are needed for assessing the role of these trace elements on CLD.

Selenium

Selenium is an integral part of the antioxidant, glutathione peroxidase.[108] Selenium and vitamin E act synergistically to prevent peroxide formation. Selenium deficiency leads to rapid metabolism of the antioxidant, vitamin E, producing vitamin E deficiency and increased oxidant injury and inflammation.[109] Experimental animals are more prone to have oxidative and inflammatory lung injury with low selenium levels. Preterm human infants have quite low blood levels of selenium,[110] perhaps increasing their risk of CLD. Selenium supplementation can protect the developing lung of neonatal rats from oxygen-induced injury. Early studies of selenium supplementation in preterm infants showed that large amounts of selenium would be needed to normalize selenium concentrations and reduce the risk of CLD.[111] One study of preterm infants aged less than 30 weeks showed that increased selenium intake during the first week after birth was associated with a decreased need for supplemental oxygen on day 28 and that erythrocyte glutathione peroxidase activity increased, even though plasma and erythrocyte selenium levels decreased.[112] However, another RCT of selenium supplementation in VLBW infants from 1 week of life to 36 weeks' postmenstrual age did not show any difference in oxygen requirement between treated and control infants at either 28 days or 36 weeks' postmenstrual age.[113] A Cochrane review of oral selenium supplementation did not show reduction in oxygen dependency at 28 days or reduction in total days of oxygen dependency.[114] Thus, at present, benefits of selenium supplementation to prevent CLD are unclear.

Vitamin Requirements

Preterm infants have significantly lower cord blood levels of the principal antioxidant vitamins A, E, D, and C, compared with term infants.[115] Infants with fat malabsorption due to cholestatic liver disease or short bowel syndrome are at risk for developing fat-soluble vitamin deficiency. Thus additional fat-soluble vitamin supplementation may be necessary in these patients. This practice is common but has not been tested for its potential to reduce oxidative injury, inflammation, or the development of CLD.

Vitamin A is essential for the growth and differentiation of epithelial tissues, including those in the lung. Preterm infants are at risk for vitamin A deficiency, starting out with low stores at birth. Preterm infants with lung disease have even lower plasma vitamin A levels than those without lung disease,[116] but this observation was made after the infants developed respiratory distress. Because of its antioxidant function, vitamin A deficiency may cause or contribute to the development of CLD. A preterm lamb model showed that daily vitamin A supplementation increased alveolar secondary septation, decreased thickness of the mesenchymal tissue cores between the distal air space walls, and increased alveolar capillary growth in chronically ventilated preterm lambs by regulating expression of tropoelastin, deposition of elastin, and expression of vascular growth factors.[117] Clinical studies of vitamin A supplementation have shown that it can decrease the incidence of CLD,[118,119] but there has been wide variation in practice regarding the use of vitamin A for prevention of CLD.[120] A large randomized clinical trial showed a reduction in the risk of death or CLD (defined as a requirement for supplemental oxygen at 36 weeks' postmenstrual age) with vitamin A supplementation, 5000 IU given intramuscularly 3 times a week for 4 weeks.[121] A systematic review of eight clinical trials of vitamin A supplementation to preterm infants confirmed the beneficial effect of vitamin A in reducing the risk of death or oxygen requirement at 1 month of age, but only by 7%, and neurodevelopmental assessment of the surviving infants at 18–22 months corrected age showed no differences between groups.[122] The principal problem with administering vitamin A is that it must be given by repeated intramuscular injections—it is not absorbed sufficiently from the gastrointestinal tract, which has kept it from common use and gaining an established role in preventing the worsening of respiratory distress or CLD.[123] One study did attempt supplementing the mother with vitamin A, but doing this would require knowing ahead of time that the infant would be born preterm with respiratory distress.[124] A more promising therapeutic strategy combined iNO with vitamin A intramuscular injections in ELBW/EPT infants and showed a reduced incidence of CLD and CLD plus death, as well as improved neurocognitive outcomes at 1 year.[125]

Vitamin E is an antioxidant that protects lipid-containing cell membranes from oxidative injury. Severe vitamin E deficiency has been shown to exacerbate acute hyperoxic lung injury in the presence of oxidative stress and inflammation.[126] The amount of vitamin E required to prevent lipid peroxidation in vulnerable tissues depends on the PUFA content of the tissues and diet. Thus it is advisable to keep the dietary ratio of vitamin E to PUFA at or above the level of 0.6 mg of D-α-tocopherol (0.9 IU) per gram of PUFA.[127] Recommended IV dosages of vitamin E are 2.8 IU/kg/day as α-tocopheryl acetate.[128] Early studies on infants with respiratory distress showed that vitamin E had protective effect on preterm lungs.[129] Later studies did not confirm these findings both in animals exposed to prolonged hyperoxia[130] and in preterm infants.[131] In the later studies, however, the infants in the control group were not vitamin E deficient and the incidence of CLD in controls was low. Further studies are needed before vitamin E supplementation is recommended in preterm infants to prevent oxygen toxicity and CLD.[132]

Vitamin D increases surfactant synthesis and secretion in alveolar type II cells and inhibits airway smooth muscle proliferation.[133] It also improves endothelial cell dysfunction through increased nitric oxide (NO) bioavailability. Increased maternal antenatal vitamin D improves oxygenation and survival in newborn rat pups. Key vitamin D regulatory enzymes that govern its activity are strongly expressed in the late fetal lung and undergo striking developmental regulation immediately before birth.[134] In addition to the maturational effects of vitamin D on the airway, vitamin D has striking proangiogenic effects in the developing lung. Such effects may be partly due to direct effects on endothelial cell growth and increased VEGF and VEGF receptor 2 (KDR) mRNA expression, as well as angiocrine signaling that stimulates and coordinates alveolar growth.[135]

Vitamin C is an established antioxidant, and preterm infants have low plasma concentrations of vitamin C after birth.[136] Supplemental vitamin C has been suggested, but in an animal model of oxygen toxicity, treatment of newborn baboons with high-dose vitamin C did not prevent the development of pulmonary oxygen toxicity in those infant baboons exposed to hyperoxia.[130] There is also the potential for excess vitamin C to cause further oxidant injury, as vitamin C at high doses can act as a pro-oxidant, producing specific adverse effects in the lungs, especially in combination with excess free iron.[2] A randomized clinical trial demonstrated that vitamin C supplementation of cigarette-smoking mothers during pregnancy can improve pulmonary function of mostly term infants.[137] Because dietary iron is necessary to support erythropoiesis, maintain an adequate red cell volume, and prevent iron deficiency anemia as blood volume expands with growth, extra vitamin C is not indicated for preterm infants.[138]

Carotenoids are also important antioxidant vitamins present in human milk. Lutein/zeaxanthin supplementation has been tried in a multicenter double-blinded RCT, but no significant effect was found in the reduction of CLD.[139]

CORTICOSTEROIDS (E.G., DEXAMETHASONE, HYDROCORTISONE, AND PREDNISONE) AND GROWTH

Short- and long-term steroid administration was a common feature of management of infants with CLD during the 1990s, but use of steroids has decreased because of an association between steroid treatment for CLD and cerebral palsy. There has been little recent addition to the literature to guide the use of corticosteroids for the prevention or treatment of CLD. The risks remain significant. Dexamethasone has both transient and long-term negative effects on growth, including slower weight gain and head growth,[140] although some studies evaluating changes in growth rate in infants receiving dexamethasone were conducted before early parenteral nutrition.[141] The reduced growth rate does not seem to be related to increased energy expenditure. Increased rates of protein breakdown are a direct effect of steroids, which would augment suboptimal protein intakes that are common in these infants. Dexamethasone also increases fat accretion.[142] Animal studies have shown that corticosteroids suppress the growth of lung parenchyma.[143] Also, dexamethasone treatment is associated with increased risk of gastrointestinal adverse effects, including ulceration, bleeding, and perforation.[144] Catabolic effects of dexamethasone cause hyperglycemia, potentially contributing to oxidative injury.

REFERENCES

1. Stoll BJ, Hansen NI, Bell EF, et al. Trends in care practices, morbidity, and mortality of extremely preterm neonates, (1993–2012). *JAMA*. 2015;314:1039–1051.
2. Saugstad OD. Bronchopulmonary dysplasia-oxidative stress and antioxidants. *Semin Neonatol*. 2003;8:39–49.
3. Natarajan G, Johnson YR, Brozanski B, et al. Postnatal weight gain in preterm infants with severe bronchopulmonary dysplasia. *Am J Perinatol*. 2014;31:223–230.
4. Lai NM, Rajadurai SV, Tan K. Increased energy intake for preterm infants with (or developing) bronchopulmonary dysplasia/chronic lung disease. *Cochrane Database Syst Rev*. 2006:Cd005093.
5. Ehrenkranz RA. Ongoing issues in the intensive care for the periviable infant–nutritional management and

prevention of bronchopulmonary dysplasia and nosocomial infections. *Semin Perinatol.* 2014;38:25–30.
6. Klevebro S, Westin V, Stoltz Sjöström E, et al. Early energy and protein intakes and associations with growth, BPD, and ROP in extremely preterm infants. *Clin Nutr.* 2019; 38:1289–1295.
7. Gianni ML, Roggero P, Colnaghi MR, et al. The role of nutrition in promoting growth in pre-term infants with bronchopulmonary dysplasia: a prospective non-randomised interventional cohort study. *BMC Pediatr.* 2014;14:235.
8. Theile AR, Radmacher PG, Anschutz TW, et al. Nutritional strategies and growth in extremely low birth weight infants with bronchopulmonary dysplasia over the past 10 years. *J Perinatol.* 2012;32:117–122.
9. Brown LD, Bell EF, Hay Jr WW. Nutritional support. In: Goldsmith J, Karotkin E, Keszler M, Suresh G, eds. *Goldsmith: Assisted Ventilation of the Neonate.* 6th ed. Philadelphia: Elsevier; 2016:322–329.
10. Poindexter BB, Martin CR. Impact of nutrition on bronchopulmonary dysplasia. *Clin Perinatol.* 2015;42:797–806.
11. Biniwale MA, Ehrenkranz RA. The role of nutrition in the prevention and management of bronchopulmonary dysplasia. *Semin Perinatol.* 2006;30:200–208.
12. Ma L, Zhou P, Neu J, Lin H-C. Potential nutrients for preventing or treating bronchopulmonary dysplasia. *Paediatr Respir Rev.* 2017;22:83–88.
13. Atkinson SA. Special nutritional needs of infants for prevention of and recovery from bronchopulmonary dysplasia. *J Nutr.* 2001;131, 942S–6S.
14. Dani C, Poggi C. Nutrition and bronchopulmonary dysplasia. *J Matern Fetal Neonatal Med.* 2012;25(suppl. 3):37–40.
15. Bose C, Van Marter LJ, Laughon M, et al. Fetal growth restriction and chronic lung disease among infants born before the 28th week of gestation. *Pediatrics.* 2009;124. e450–8.
16. Reiss I, Landmann E, Heckmann M, et al. Increased risk of bronchopulmonary dysplasia and increased mortality in very preterm infants being small for gestational age. *Arch Gynecol Obstet.* 2003;269:40–44.
17. Eriksson L, Haglund B, Odlind V, et al. Perinatal conditions related to growth restriction and inflammation are associated with an increased risk of bronchopulmonary dysplasia. *Acta Paediatr.* 2015;10:259–263.
18. Ehrenkranz RA, Das A, Wrage LA, et al. Early nutrition mediates the influence of severity of illness on extremely LBW infants. *Pediatr Res.* 2011;69:522–529.
19. Zhao H, Dennery PA, Yao H. Metabolic reprogramming in the pathogenesis of chronic lung diseases, including CLD, COPD, and pulmonary fibrosis. *Am J Physiol Lung Cell Mol Physiol.* 2018;314:L544–L554.
20. Forsyth JS, Crighton A. Low birthweight infants and total parenteral nutrition immediately after birth. I. Energy expenditure and respiratory quotient of ventilated and non-ventilated infants. *Arch Dis Child Fetal Neonatal Ed.* 1995;73. F4–7.
21. Uberos J, Lardon-Fernandez M, Machado-Casas I, Molina-Oya M, Narbona-Lopez E. Nutrition in very low birth weight infants: impact on bronchopulmonary dysplasia. *Minerva Pediatr.* 2014;68:419–426.
22. Mataloun MM, Rebello CM, Mascaretti RS, et al. Pulmonary responses to nutritional restriction and hyperoxia in premature rabbits. *J Pediatr.* 2006;82:179–185.
23. Ramel SE, Brown LD, K Georgieff M. The impact of neonatal illness on nutritional requirements-one size does not fit all. *Curr Pediatr Rep.* 2014;2:248–254.
24. Moya F. Preterm nutrition and the lung. *World Rev Nutr Diet.* 2014;110:239–252.
25. Isaacs EB, Gadian DG, Sabatini S, et al. The effect of early human diet on caudate volumes and IQ. *Pediatr Res.* 2008;63:308–314.
26. van Goudoever JB, Sulkers EJ, Lafeber HN, et al. Short-term growth and substrate use in very-low-birth-weight infants fed formulas with different energy contents. *Am J Clin Nutr.* 2000;71:816–821.
27. Spiegler J, Preuß M, Gebauer C, et al. German neonatal Network GNN. Does breastmilk influence the development of bronchopulmonary dysplasia? *J Pediatr.* 2016; 169:76–80.
28. Dicky O, Ehlinger V, Montjaux N, et al. Policy of feeding very preterm infants with their mother's own fresh expressed milk was associated with a reduced risk of bronchopulmonary dysplasia. *Acta Paediatr.* 2017;106: 755–762.
29. Chen Y, Fantuzi G, Schoeny M, et al. High-dose human milk feedings decrease oxidative stress in premature infant. *J Parenter Enteral Nutr.* 2019;43:126–132.
30. Agathocleous M, Harris WA. Metabolism in physiological cell proliferation and differentiation. *Trends Cell Biol.* 2013;23:484–492.
31. Hay Jr WW, Brown LD, Regnault TRH. Fetal requirements and placental transfer of nitrogenous compounds. In: Polin R, Abman S, Benetz W, Rowitch D, eds. *Fetal and Neonatal Physiology.* 5th ed. Philadelphia: Elsevier; 2016: 444–458.
32. Embleton ND. Optimal protein and energy intakes in preterm infants. *Early Hum Dev.* 2007;83:831–837.
33. Thureen PJ, Melara D, Fennessey PV, et al. Effect of low versus high intravenous amino acid intake on very low birth weight infants in the early neonatal period. *Pediatr Res.* 2003;53:24–32.
34. Kashyap S, Forsyth M, Zucker C, et al. Effects of varying protein and energy intakes on growth and metabolic response in low birth weight infants. *J Pediatr.* 1986; 108:955–963.
35. Agostoni C, Buonocore G, Carnielli VP, et al. Enteral nutrient supply for preterm infants: commentary from the European society of paediatric gastroenterology, hepatology and nutrition committee on nutrition. *J Pediatr Gastroenterol Nutr.* 2010;50:85–91.
36. Brown LD, Hendrickson K, Masor ML, et al. High-protein formulas: evidence for use in preterm infants. *Clin Perinatol.* 2014;41:383–403.

37. te Braake FW, van den Akker CH, Wattimena DJ, et al. Amino acid administration to premature infants directly after birth. *J Pediatr*. 2005;147:457–461.
38. Van Goudoever JB, Colen T, Wattimena JL, et al. Immediate commencement of amino acid supplementation in preterm infants: effect on serum amino acid concentrations and protein kinetics on the first day of life. *J Pediatr*. 1995;127:458–465.
39. Poindexter BB, Langer JC, Dusick AM, et al. Early provision of parenteral amino acids in extremely low birth weight infants: relation to growth and neurodevelopmental outcome. *J Pediatr*. 2006;148:300–305.
40. Brunton JA, Saigal S, Atkinson SA. Growth and body composition in infants with bronchopulmonary dysplasia up to 3 months corrected age: a randomized trial of a high-energy nutrient-enriched formula fed after hospital discharge. *J Pediatr*. 1988;133:340–345.
41. deRegnier RA, Guilbert TW, Mills MM, et al. Growth failure and altered body composition are established by one month of age in infants with bronchopulmonary dysplasia. *J Nutr*. 1996;126:168–175.
42. Manner T, Wiese S, Katz DP, et al. Branched-chain amino acids and respiration. *Nutrition*. 1992;8:311–315.
43. Blazer S, Reinersman GT, Askanazi J, et al. Branched-chain amino acids and respiratory pattern and function in the neonate. *J Perinatol*. 1994;14:290–295.
44. Soliz A, Suguihara C, Huang J, et al. Effect of amino acid infusion on the ventilatory response to hypoxia in protein-deprived neonatal piglets. *Pediatr Res*. 1994;35: 316–320.
45. Wernerman J. Glutamine supplementation. *Ann Intensive Care*. 2011;1:25.
46. Ahmad S, White CW, Chang LY, et al. Glutamine protects mitochondrial structure and function in oxygen toxicity. *Am J Physiol Lung Cell Mol Physiol*. 2001;280:L779–L791.
47. Perng WC, Huang KL, Li MH, et al. Glutamine attenuates hyperoxia-induced acute lung injury in mice. *Clin Exp Pharmacol Physiol*. 2010;37:56–61.
48. Poindexter BB, Ehrenkranz RA, Stoll BJ, et al. Effect of parenteral glutamine supplementation on plasma amino acid concentrations in extremely low-birth-weight infants. *Am J Clin Nutr*. 2003;77:737–743.
49. Moe-Byrne T, Wagner JV, McGuire W. Glutamine supplementation to prevent morbidity and mortality in preterm infants Cochrane. *Database Syst Rev*. 2016;1:CD001457.
50. Poindexter BB, Ehrenkranz RA, Stoll BJ, et al. Parenteral glutamine supplementation does not reduce the risk of mortality or late-onset sepsis in extremely low birth weight infants. *Pediatrics*. 2004;113:1209–1215.
51. Ma L, Li N, Liu X, et al. Arginyl-glutamine dipeptide or docosahexaenoic acid attenuate hyperoxia-induced lung injury in neonatal mice. *Nutrition*. 2012;28:1186–1191.
52. Nagata K, Iwasaki Y, Yamada T, et al. Overexpression of manganese superoxide dismutase by N-acetylcysteine in hyperoxic lung injury. *Respir Med*. 2007;101:800–807.
53. Moe-Byrne T, Wagner JV, McGuire W. Glutamine supplementation for prevention of morbidity in preterm infants. *Cochrane Database Syst Rev*. 2012;3:CD001457.
54. Faintuch J, Aguilar PB, Nadalin W. Relevance of N-acetylcysteine in clinical practice: fact, myth or consequence? *Nutrition*. 1999;15:177–179.
55. Soghier LM, Brion LP. Cysteine, cystine or N-acetylcysteine supplementation in parenterally fed neonates. *Cochrane Database Syst Rev*. 2006;4:CD004869.
56. Ahola T, Lapatto R, Raivio KO, et al. N-acetylcysteine does not prevent bronchopulmonary dysplasia in immature infants: a randomized controlled trial. *J Pediatr*. 2003;143:713–719.
57. Donohue PK, Gilmore MM, Cristofalo E, et al. Inhaled nitric oxide in preterm infants: a systematic review. *Pediatrics*. 2011;127:e414–e422.
58. Lu A, Sun B, Qian L. Combined iNO and endothelial progenitor cells improve lung alveolar and vascular structure in neonatal rats exposed to prolonged hyperoxia. *Pediatr Res*. 2015;77:784–792.
59. El Sayed M, Sherif L, Said RN, et al. Endothelin-1 and L-Arginine in preterm infants with respiratory distress. *Am J Perinatol*. 2011;28:129–136.
60. Vadivel A, Aschner JL, Rey-Parra GJ. Jet al. L-Citrulline attenuates arrested alveolar growth and pulmonary hypertension in oxygen-induced lung injury in newborn rats. *Pediatr Res*. 2010;68, 519–5.
61. Heckmann M, Kreuder J, Riechers K, et al. Plasma arginine and urinary nitrate and nitrite excretion in bronchopulmonary dysplasia. *Biol Neonate*. 2004;85:173–178.
62. Fike CD, Summar M, Aschner JL. L-citrulline provides a novel strategy for treating chronic pulmonary hypertension in newborn infants. *Acta Paediatr*. 2014;103: 1019–1026.
63. Grisafi D, Tassone E, Dedja A, et al. L-citrulline prevents alveolar and vascular derangement in a rat model of moderate hyperoxia-induced lung injury. *Lung*. 2012; 190:419–430.
64. Sopi RB, Zaidi SI, Mladenov M, et al. L-citrulline supplementation reverses the impaired airway relaxation in neonatal rats exposed to hyperoxia. *Respir Res*. 2012;13: 68.
65. Hay Jr WW, Brown LD, Denne SC. Energy requirements, protein-energy metabolism and balance, and carbohydrates in preterm infants. *World Rev Nutr Diet*. 2014; 110:64–81.
66. Thureen PJ, Phillips RE, Baron KA, et al. Direct measurement of the energy expenditure of physical activity in preterm infants. *J Appl Physiol*. 1985;85:223–230.
67. Roberts SB, Young VR. Energy costs of fat and protein deposition in the human infant. *Am J Clin Nutr*. 1988; 48:951–955.
68. de Meer K, Westerterp KR, Houwen RH, et al. Total energy expenditure in infants with bronchopulmonary dysplasia is associated with respiratory status. *Eur J Pediatr*. 1997; 156:299–304.
69. Denne SC. Energy expenditure in infants with pulmonary insufficiency: is there evidence for increased energy needs? *J Nutr*. 2001;131, 935s-7s.
70. Kurzner SI, Garg M, Bautista DB, et al. Growth failure in infants with bronchopulmonary dysplasia: nutrition and

elevated resting metabolic expenditure. *Pediatrics.* 1988; 81:379–384.
71. Bauer J, Maier K, Linderkamp O, et al. Effect of caffeine on oxygen consumption and metabolic rate in very low birth weight infants with idiopathic apnea. *Pediatrics.* 2001;107:660–663.
72. Cohen J, Van Marter LJ, Sun Y, et al. Perturbation of gene expression of the chromatin remodeling pathway in premature newborns at risk for bronchopulmonary dysplasia. *Genome Biol.* 2007;8:R210.
73. Kandasamy J, Olave N, Ballinger SW, et al. Vascular endothelial mitochondrial function predicts death or pulmonary outcomes in preterm infants. *Am J Respir Crit Care Med.* 2017;196:1040–1049.
74. Ratner V, Starkov A, Matsiukevich D, et al. Mitochondrial dysfunction contributes to alveolar developmental arrest in hyperoxia-exposed mice. *Am J Respir Cell Mol Biol.* 2009;40:511–518.
75. Kao LC, Durand DJ, Nickerson BG. Improving pulmonary function does not decrease oxygen consumption in infants with bronchopulmonary dysplasia. *J Pediatr.* 1988;112:616–621.
76. Lapillonne A, Groh-Wargo S, Gonzalez CH, et al. Lipid needs of preterm infants: updated recommendations. *J Pediatr.* 2013;162:S37–S47.
77. Kelley DS. Modulation of human immune and inflammatory responses by dietary fatty acids. *Nutrition.* 2001; 17:669–673.
78. Jing H, Yao J, Liu X, et al. Fish-oil emulsion (omega-3 polyunsaturated fatty acids) attenuates acute lung injury induced by intestinal ischemia-reperfusion through Adenosine 5′-monophosphate-activated protein kinase-sirtuin1 pathway. *J Surg Res.* 2014;187:252–261.
79. Kinniry P, Amrani Y, Vachani A, et al. Dietary flaxseed supplementation ameliorates inflammation and oxidative tissue damage in experimental models of acute lung injury in mice. *J Nutr.* 2006;136:1545–1551.
80. Rogers LK, Valentine CJ, Pennell M, et al. Maternal docosahexaenoic acid supplementation decreases lung inflammation in hyperoxia-exposed newborn mice. *J Nutr.* 2011;141:214–222.
81. Martin CR, Dasilva DA, Cluette-Brown JE, et al. Decreased postnatal docosahexaenoic and arachidonic acid blood levels in premature infants are associated with neonatal morbidities. *J Pediatr.* 2011;159:743–749.
82. Zhang P, Lavoie PM, Lacaze-Masmonteil T, et al. Omega-3 long-chain polyunsaturated fatty acids for extremely preterm infants: a systematic review. *Pediatrics.* 2014; 134:120–134.
83. Manley BJ, Makrides M, Collins CT, et al. High-dose docosahexaenoic acid supplementation of preterm infants: respiratory and allergy outcomes. *Pediatrics.* 2011;128. e71–7.
84. Skouroliakou M, Konstantinou D, Agakidis C, et al. Cholestasis, bronchopulmonary dysplasia, and lipid profile in preterm infants receiving MCT/omega-3- PUFA-containing or soybean-based lipid emulsions. *Nutr Clin Pract.* 2012;27:817–824.
85. Prasertsom W, Phillipos EZ, Van Aerde JE, et al. Pulmonary vascular resistance during lipid infusion in neonates. *Arch Dis Child Fetal Neonatal Ed.* 1996;74: F95–F98.
86. Hsiao CC, Lin HC, Chang YJ, et al. Intravenous fish oil containing lipid emulsion attenuates inflammatory cytokines and the development of bronchopulmonary dysplasia in very premature infants: a double-blind, randomized controlled trial. *Clin Nutr.* 2019;38: 1045–1052.
87. Fleith M, Clandinin MT. Dietary PUFA for preterm and term infants: review of clinical studies. *Crit Rev Food Sci Nutr.* 2005;45:205–229.
88. Houeijeh A, Aubry E, Coridon H, et al. Effects of n-3 polyunsaturated fatty acids in the fetal pulmonary circulation. *Crit Care Med.* 2011;39:1431–1438.
89. Yunis KA, Oh W. Effects of intravenous glucose loading on oxygen consumption, carbon dioxide production, and resting energy expenditure in infants with bronchopulmonary dysplasia. *J Pediatr.* 1989;115:127–132.
90. Stoll B, Horst DA, Cui L, et al. Chronic parenteral nutrition induces hepatic inflammation, steatosis, and insulin resistance in neonatal pigs. *J Nutr.* 2010;140:2193–2200.
91. Wang H, Khaoustov VI, Krishnan B, et al. Total parenteral nutrition induces liver steatosis and apoptosis in neonatal piglets. *J Nutr.* 2006;136:2547–2552.
92. Picard M, Juster RP, McEwen BS. Mitochondrial allostatic load puts the 'gluc' back in glucocorticoids. *Nat Rev Endocrinol.* 2014;10:303–310.
93. Howlett A, Ohlsson A. Inositol for respiratory distress syndrome in preterm infants. *Cochrane Database Syst Rev.* 2003;4:CD000366.
94. Brown LD, Cheung A, Harwood JE, et al. Inositol and mannose utilization rates in term and late-preterm infants exceed nutritional intakes. *J Nutr.* 2009;139: 1648–1652.
95. Hallman M, Bry K, Hoppu K, et al. Inositol supplementation in premature infants with respiratory distress syndrome. *N Engl J Med.* 1992;326:1233–1239.
96. Quigley R. Developmental changes in renal function. *Curr Opin Pediatr.* 2012;24:184–190.
97. Modi N, Betremieux P, Midgley J, et al. Postnatal weight loss and contraction of the extracellular compartment is triggered by atrial natriuretic peptide. *Early Hum Dev.* 2000;59:201–208.
98. Oh W, Poindexter BB, Perritt R, et al. Association between fluid intake and weight loss during the first ten days of life and risk of bronchopulmonary dysplasia in extremely low birth weight infants. *J Pediatr.* 2005;147:786–790.
99. Bell EF, Acarregui MJ. Restricted versus liberal water intake for preventing morbidity and mortality in preterm infants. *Cochrane Database Syst Rev.* 2014;12:CD000503.
100. Wadhawan R, Oh W, Perritt R, et al. Association between early postnatal weight loss and death or CLD in small and appropriate for gestational age extremely low-birth-weight infants. *J Perinatol.* 2007;27:359–364.
101. Stephens BE, Gargus RA, Walden RV, et al. Fluid regimens in the first week of life may increase risk of patent ductus

arteriosus in extremely low birth weight infants. *J Perinatol.* 2008;28:123–128.

102. Greenberg RG, Gayam S, Savage D, et al. Furosemide exposure and prevention of bronchopulmonary dysplasia in premature infants. *J Pediatr.* 2018;(18): 31690–31691. pii: S0022-3476.
103. Stewart A, Brion LP, Soll R. Diuretics for respiratory distress syndrome in preterm infants. *Cochrane Database Syst Rev.* 2011;12:CD001454.
104. Wassner SJ. Altered growth and protein turnover in rats fed sodium-deficient diets. *Pediatr Res.* 1989;26: 608–613.
105. Ross JR, Finch C, Ebeling M, et al. Refeeding syndrome in very-low-birth-weight intrauterine growth-restricted neonates. *J Perinatol.* 2013;33:717–720.
106. Shaikhkhalil AK, Curtiss J, Puthoff TD, et al. Enteral zinc supplementation and growth in extremely-low-birth-weight infants with chronic lung disease. *J Pediatr Gastroenterol Nutr.* 2014;58:183–187.
107. Davis JM, Parad RB, Michele T, et al. Pulmonary outcome at 1 year corrected age in premature infants treated at birth with recombinant human CuZn superoxide dismutase. *Pediatrics.* 2003;111:469–476.
108. Tindell R, Tipple T. Selenium: implications for outcomes in extremely preterm infants. *J Perinatol.* 2018;38: 197–202.
109. Lee JW, Davis JM. Future applications of antioxidants in premature infants. *Curr Opin Pediatr.* 2011;23:161–166.
110. Mostafa-Gharehbaghi M, Mostafa-Gharabaghi P, Ghanbari F, et al. Determination of selenium in serum samples of preterm newborn infants with bronchopulmonary dysplasia using a validated hydride generation system. *Biol Trace Elem Res.* 2012;147:1–7.
111. Daniels L, Gibson R, Simmer K. Randomised clinical trial of parenteral selenium supplementation in preterm infants. *Arch Dis Child Fetal Neonatal Ed.* 1996;74: F158–F164.
112. Mentro AM, Smith AM, Moyer-Mileur L. Plasma and erythrocyte selenium and glutathione peroxidase activity in preterm infants at risk for bronchopulmonary dysplasia. *Biol Trace Elem Res.* 2005;106:97–106.
113. Darlow BA, Winterbourn CC, Inder TE, et al. The effect of selenium supplementation on outcome in very low birth weight infants: a randomized controlled trial. The New Zealand Neonatal Study Group. *J Pediatr.* 2000;136: 473–480.
114. Darlow BA, Austin NC. Selenium supplementation to prevent short-term morbidity in preterm neonates. *Cochrane Database Syst Rev.* 2003;4:CD003312.
115. Baydas G, Karatas F, Gursu MF, et al. Antioxidant vitamin levels in term and preterm infants and their relation to maternal vitamin status. *Arch Med Res.* 2002;33: 276–280.
116. Shenai JP, Chytil F, Stahlman MT. Vitamin A status of neonates with bronchopulmonary dysplasia. *Pediatr Res.* 1985;19:185–188.
117. Albertine KH, Dahl MJ, Gonzales LW, et al. Chronic lung disease in preterm lambs: effect of daily vitamin A treatment on alveolarization. *Am J Physiol Lung Cell Mol Physiol.* 2010;299:L59–L72.
118. Pearson E, Bose C, Snidow T, et al. Trial of vitamin A supplementation in very low birth weight infants at risk for bronchopulmonary dysplasia. *J Pediatr.* 1992;121: 420–427.
119. Darlow BA, Graham PJ. Vitamin A supplementation to prevent mortality and short- and long-term morbidity in very low birth weight infants. *Cochrane Database Syst Rev.* 2011;10:CD000501.
120. Kaplan HC, Tabangin ME, McClendon D, et al. Understanding variation in vitamin A supplementation among NICUs. *Pediatrics.* 2010;126:e367–e373.
121. Kennedy KA, Stoll BJ, Ehrenkranz RA, et al. Vitamin A to prevent bronchopulmonary dysplasia in very- low-birth-weight infants: has the dose been too low? The NICHD Neonatal Research Network. *Early Hum Dev.* 1997;49: 19–31.
122. Tyson JE, Wright LL, Oh W, et al. Vitamin A supplementation for extremely-low birth-weight infants. National institute of child health and human development neonatal research Network. *N Engl J Med.* 1999;340, 1962–8.
123. Ambalavanan N, Tyson JE, Kennedy KA, et al. Vitamin A supplementation for extremely low birth weight infants: outcome at 18 to 22 months. *Pediatrics.* 2005;115: e249–e254.
124. Babu TA, Sharmila V. Vitamin A supplementation in late pregnancy can decrease the incidence of bronchopulmonary dysplasia in newborns. *J Matern Fetal Neonatal Med.* 2010;23:1468–1469.
125. Gadhia MM, Cutter GR, Abman SH, et al. Effects of early inhaled nitric oxide therapy and vitamin A supplementation on the risk for bronchopulmonary dysplasia in premature newborns with respiratory failure. *J Pediatr.* 2014; 164:744–748.
126. Yamaoka S, Kim HS, Ogihara T, et al. Severe Vitamin E deficiency exacerbates acute hyperoxic lung injury associated with increased oxidative stress and inflammation. *Free Radic Res.* 2008;42:602–612.
127. Bell EF, Filer Jr LJ. The role of vitamin E in the nutrition of premature infants. *Am J Clin Nutr.* 1981;34:414–422.
128. Brion LP, Bell EF, Raghuveer TS, et al. What is the appropriate intravenous dose of vitamin E for very-low-birth-weight infants? *J Perinatol.* 2004;24:205–207.
129. Ehrenkranz RA, Bonta BW, Ablow RC, et al. Amelioration of bronchopulmonary dysplasia after vitamin E administration. A preliminary report. *N Engl J Med.* 1978;299: 564–569.
130. Berger TM, Frei B, Rifai N, et al. Early high dose antioxidant vitamins do not prevent bronchopulmonary dysplasia in premature baboons exposed to prolonged hyperoxia: a pilot study. *Pediatr Res.* 1998;43: 719–726.
131. Watts JL, Milner R, Zipursky A, et al. Failure of supplementation with vitamin E to prevent bronchopulmonary dysplasia in infants less than 1,500 g birth weight. *Eur Respir J.* 1991;4:188–190.

132. Brion LP, Bell EF, Raghuveer TS. Vitamin E supplementation for prevention of morbidity and mortality in preterm infants. *Cochrane Database Syst Rev*. 2003;3: CD003665.
133. Cookson MW, Ryan SL, Seedorf GJ, et al. Antenatal vitamin D preserves placental vascular and fetal growth in experimental chorioamnionitis due to intra-amniotic endotoxin exposure. *Am J Perinatol*. 2018;35:1260–1270.
134. Lykkedegn S, Sorensen GL, Beck-Nielsen SS, et al. The impact of vitamin D on fetal and neonatal lung maturation. A systematic review. *Am J Physiol Lung Cell Mol Physiol*. 2015;308:L587–L602.
135. Mandell E, Seedorf G, Gien J, et al. Vitamin D treatment improves survival and infant lung structure after intra-amniotic endotoxin exposure in rats: potential role for the prevention of bronchopulmonary dysplasia. *Am J Physiol Lung Cell Mol Physiol*. 2014;306. L420–8.
136. Berger TM, Rifai N, Avery ME, et al. Vitamin C in premature and full-term human neonates. *Redox Rep*. 1996;2:257–262.
137. McEvoy CT, Schilling D, Clay N, et al. Vitamin C supplementation for pregnant smoking women and pulmonary function in their newborn infants: a randomized clinical trial. *JAMA*. 2014;311:2074–2082.
138. Ehrenkranz RA. Iron requirements of preterm infants. *Nutrition*. 1994;10:77–78.
139. Manzoni P, Guardione R, Bonetti P, et al. Lutein and zeaxanthin supplementation in preterm very low-birth-weight neonates in neonatal intensive care units: a multicenter randomized controlled trial. *Am J Perinatol*. 2013; 30:25–32.
140. Papile LA, Tyson JE, Stoll BJ, et al. A multicenter trial of two dexamethasone regimens in ventilator-dependent premature infants. *N Engl J Med*. 1998;338:1112–1118.
141. Gibson AT, Pearse RG, Wales JK. Growth retardation after dexamethasone administration: assessment by knemometry. *Arch Dis Child*. 1993;69:505–509.
142. Leitch CA, Ahlrichs J, Karn C, et al. Energy expenditure and energy intake during dexamethasone therapy for chronic lung disease. *Pediatr Res*. 1999;46:109–113.
143. Tschanz SA, Haenni B, Burri PH. Glucocorticoid induced impairment of lung structure assessed by digital image analysis. *Eur J Pediatr*. 2002;161:26–30.
144. Ng PC, Brownlee KG, Dear PR. Gastroduodenal perforation in preterm babies treated with dexamethasone for bronchopulmonary dysplasia. *Arch Dis Child*. 1991;66: 1164–1166.

CHAPTER 13

Control of Breathing

ANDREW M. DYLAG, MD • RICHARD J. MARTIN, MD

INTRODUCTION

The clinical approach to, and investigation of, bronchopulmonary dysplasia (BPD) has appropriately focused on long-term pulmonary morbidity. Meanwhile, the high incidence of BPD remains almost unchanged despite several decades focused on optimizing respiratory care. It is increasingly recognized that inadequate lung maturation is associated with immaturity of respiratory control. This combination likely has an adverse effect on respiratory outcomes.[1] In this chapter, we seek to address this maturational challenge and focus on the cause of immature respiratory control, resultant intermittent hypoxia (IH, largely measured as hypoxemia), and their contributions to the unique short- and long-term vulnerability of infants with BPD.

CONTROL OF BREATHING AND PHYSIOLOGIC CONTRIBUTIONS TO IMMATURE RESPIRATORY CONTROL

Respiratory control and its maturation is under tight regulation, with interplay from the central and peripheral nervous systems and feedback from the lung parenchyma and airway musculature. Our still limited knowledge of the normal and pathophysiologic developmental pathways governing the control of breathing comes from both human and animal studies. Understanding the normal developmental trajectory and maturation of each component coupled with its modification by postnatal environmental factors can inform clinicians about the magnitude of disordered breathing control in preterm and former preterm infants, providing guidelines for monitoring and targets for treatment.

Central Respiratory Control

The human fetus and neonate have progressive maturation of breathing control mainly in the pons and medulla of the brain stem (Fig. 13.1). Respiratory rhythm generation is primarily located in the pre-Bötzinger complex near the CO_2-sensitive areas of the brain stem. Respiratory pattern formation occurs more caudally in the ventral respiratory column and is capable of generating rhythmic activity without sensory feedback, triggering "automatic" breathing efforts that occur throughout life. These patterns, however, can be modified in response to changing metabolic conditions via inhibitory sensory inputs from the peripheral nervous system (i.e., from the upper airway), resulting in apnea. These inhibitory signals are integrated through the nucleus of the solitary tract (NTS) and medullary raphe nuclei. Sensory afferents such as slowly adapting stretch receptors (SARs), rapidly adapting stretch receptors (RARs), and bronchopulmonary C-fibers all terminate in the NTS, which then projects outputs to other respiratory nuclei and spinal phrenic motor neurons to change the motor output pattern (discussed further in the section Peripheral Respiratory Control).[2] In addition, there are separate and complex interactions governing the neurochemical excitation and inhibition of respiratory control, discussed in other texts on this subject.[3]

Fetal breathing can be detected in as early as the 11th gestational week by ultrasonography and is an important stimulus of lung growth and development. There are three phases to breathing movements under control by coordinated firing of different respiratory neurons: inspiration, stage 1 of expiration, and stage 2 of expiration.[4] Placental and environmental exposures can have inhibitory and stimulatory effects on fetal breathing movements. For example, fetal breathing occurs phasically only during rapid eye movement (REM) sleep and ceases during non-REM sleep possibly secondary to inhibitory pontine input to the medullary rhythm-generating center. Additionally, chronic hypoxia (i.e., uteroplacental insufficiency) increases adenosine production thereby inhibiting fetal breathing movements. Conversely, hypercapnic exposure increases the rate and depth of fetal breathing movements, an early indication that a ventilatory response to CO_2 is important for a successful fetal to neonatal transition.[5] There are several CO_2/H^+ chemosensitive neuronal populations

Updates on Neonatal Chronic Lung Disease. https://doi.org/10.1016/B978-0-323-68353-1.00013-0

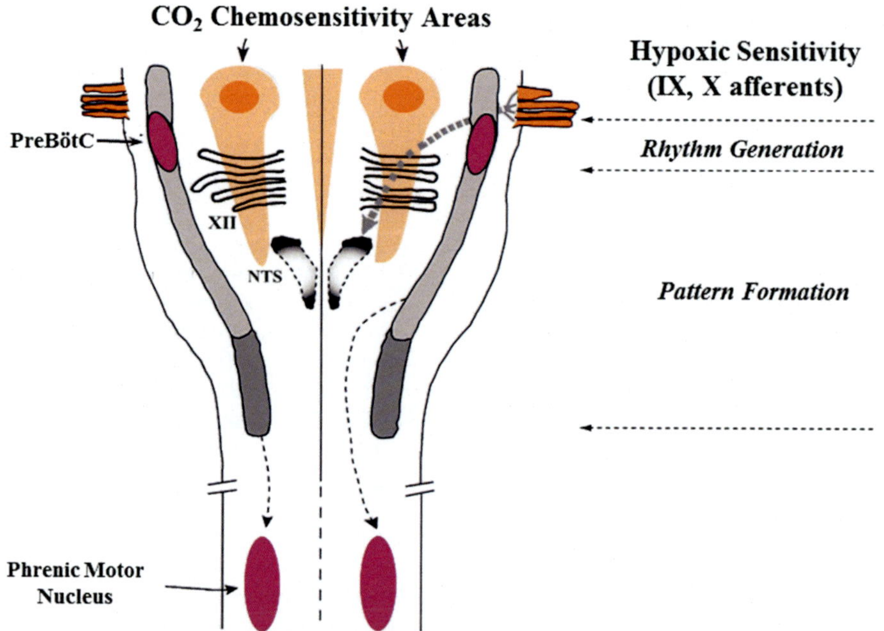

FIG. 13.1 The ventral medullary surface of the pons and medulla highlighting major chemosensory areas and their role in rhythm generation and pattern formation of respiratory neural output. Roman numerals refer to cranial nerves. *NTS*, nucleus of the solitary tract; *Pre-BötC*, pre-Bötzinger complex.

in varied brain stem regions that control ventilatory responses, with the greatest density in the medullary raphe.[5]

Ventilatory responses to CO_2 are present at birth in most mammalian species, including humans. Premature infants have diminished CO_2 sensitivity in the early postnatal period, evidenced by increased tidal volume with a prolonged expiratory period that can be associated with expiratory braking and grunting.[6–8] This is in contrast to older infants and adults who exhibit increased respiratory rate and a shorter expiratory phase in response to a CO_2 stimulus. Furthermore, the premature infant has a different level of partial pressure of arterial carbon dioxide ($PaCO_2$) below which breathing ceases, termed the "apneic threshold." A premature infant's apneic threshold is closer to eupneic levels than that of adults, thereby decreasing their tolerance for swings in $Paco_2$ levels.[9] Furthermore, the $PaCO_2$ in preterm infants fluctuates widely due to lower functional residual capacity (FRC) and longer sleep state periods than older infants and adults. These factors of respiratory instability, chemosensory immaturity, and different CO_2 set points all contribute to apnea of prematurity and result in increased hypoxemic episodes in the preterm population.

Peripheral Respiratory Control

The central nervous system signals are synthesized by end organs that provide feedback via pulmonary and lower airway vagal afferents. The sensory receptors in the lung are either fast-conducting myelinated fibers (SARs and RARs) or slow-conducting unmyelinated fibers (bronchopulmonary C-fibers) that terminate in the NTS. Projections from the NTS then innervate the phrenic motor neurons in the medulla, pons, and spinal cord. The selective activation and inhibition of the SARs, RARs, and C-fibers each separately affect cardiopulmonary reflexes, discussed separately in this section. Premature infants have uniquely distinct developmental features that make their peripheral respiratory control a clinical management challenge.

SARs are activated by lung volume and parenchymal stretch to enhance inspiratory effort, dilate large airways, and increase heart rate.[10] They project to ipsilateral subnuclei within the NTS, which then have second-order neurons that synapse on pump cells (P-cells) and inspiratory-β cells. When stimulated, P-cells induce changes that mimic the Breuer-Hering (B-H) reflex in which pulmonary stretch receptors in the bronchial and bronchiolar walls respond to excessive stretch during large inspirations, preventing overinflation, in turn controlling the duration of inspiration and expiration in relation to lung inflation. Although the B-H reflex does not regulate fetal breathing movements,[11] it contributes significantly to tidal breathing movements in newborns, with decreasing impact through the first year of life.[12] The observation of immediately prolonged expiratory phase with continuous positive airway pressure (CPAP) and the resultant maintenance of FRC is a presumed manifestation of the B-H reflex. The result is an immediate slowing of respiratory rate when infants go on CPAP.

RARs are activated in response to lung deflation, mechanical stimulation, and irritant inhalation, which stimulates coughing, laryngo-/bronchoconstriction, and mucus secretion.[10] RARs also act mainly through ipsilateral, and some contralateral, NTS subnuclei, sending second-order projections to inspiratory neurons in the NTS and bulbospinal neurons, which stimulate lung inflation.[10] RARs are activated by the low lung volumes common in premature and term newborns to activate sigh breaths in an effort to restore lung inflation. Preterm infants respond differently to sigh breaths than adults, as the rapid increase in partial pressure of arterial oxygen (Pao_2) and decrease in partial pressure of carbon dioxide (Pco_2) decreases excitatory input from peripheral arterial chemoreceptors; this can decrease respiratory drive and, somewhat paradoxically, lead to apnea.

Bronchopulmonary C-fibers are unmyelinated vagal afferents activated by physical and environmental stimuli such as capsaicin, carbon dioxide, edema, and hyperthermia, thereby inducing rapid shallow breathing, cough, laryngo-/bronchoconstriction, and bradycardia.[10] They terminate mainly in the ipsilateral NTS and, when stimulated, release neuropeptides, such as substance P, which mediate the aforementioned effects. Additionally, C-fibers can be sensitized by inflammatory mediators from bacterial or viral infections such as respiratory syncytial virus infection, which may explain the apnea observed in infected infants.[13]

The carotid body is responsible for ventilatory control in response to acute, low peripheral oxygen tension, and acid hypercapnia via clusters of Type I (glomus) cells and the surrounding, modulating Type II (glial-like) cells.[14] Peripheral arterial chemoreceptor afferents also synapse in the NTS at the commissural nucleus, sending second-order neurons to the retrotrapezoid nucleus and dorsal/ventral respiratory groups. These chemoreceptors are not thought to influence fetal breathing but are important in establishing and stabilizing postnatal breathing patterns. Notably, denervation results in apnea and death.[15] Near-term fetal chemoreceptor activity in the carotid body is generally reduced with a poor response to hypoxia that improves with age and maturation. Conversely, acute exposure to hyperoxia, common in preterm infants receiving supplemental oxygen, reduces respiratory drive and ventilation.

There is a critical developmental window in the first two postnatal weeks when exposure to chronic hypoxia, chronic hyperoxia, and intermittent hypoxia can lead to persistent alterations in chemoreceptor function and response in animals.[16] The current speculation is that the sensitivity of peripheral chemoreceptors to hypoxia "resets" at birth with only a limited time before neuroplasticity decreases and the changes become permanent. This same 2- to 3-week period is observed in term newborns, coinciding with the period of increased peripheral chemosensitivity and periodic breathing. Preterm infants have the unfortunate circumstance of being born into a relatively hyperoxic extrauterine environment at an immature neuronal developmental stage. More studies are needed to determine the temporal relationship of each of these extrauterine influences to determine whether they have longer-lasting critical consequences in preterm infants, as well as term infants treated for respiratory failure.

In summary, the central mechanisms contributing to immature respiratory control are increased inhibitory neurotransmission limiting inspiration, decreased CO_2 chemosensitivity, and depressed hypoxic ventilatory drive. Peripheral reflexes demonstrate immaturity with altered carotid body activity, increased laryngeal chemoreflexes, and excessive bradycardic responses to hypoxia. When superimposed on inflammatory conditions (sepsis/cytokines), the premature infant demonstrates apnea of prematurity with associated intermittent hypoxia episodes. These periods of hypoxia, as well as the current treatments, can have long-term deleterious effects on the control of breathing and further pulmonary and neurologic development.

APNEA OF PREMATURITY AND RESULTANT INTERMITTENT HYPOXIA

The advancement of neonatal care and survival of more immature babies has brought about challenges in dealing with immature respiratory control. For the reasons outlined earlier, the premature transition from fetal to neonatal life has a large impact on the incidence and severity of hypoventilation, apnea, and intermittent hypoxemia (IH). Apnea of prematurity, typically defined as a cessation of breathing for more than 15–20 s, or shorter if associated with bradycardia and oxygen desaturation, is likely a physiologic rather than pathologic disorder of respiratory control. Apnea can be classified into three categories: central, obstructive, and mixed (Fig. 13.2). Central apnea is a total cessation of respiratory effort with no evidence of airway obstruction. Conversely, obstructive apnea is accompanied by breathing efforts and chest wall movement that do not result in effective airflow due to an obstructed upper airway. Mixed apnea is characterized by obstructed respiratory effort, which typically follows, but might precede, a central pause and is likely the most common type of apnea.

The incidence and magnitude of apneic episodes is difficult to quantify because standard impedance monitoring of chest wall movement does not detect the obstructed inspiratory efforts that commonly occur with central respiratory depression. Therefore clinical trials generally operate under the assumption that IH/desaturation episodes are caused by central apnea events, but event detection is highly dependent on averaging time, monitoring equipment, and NICU-specific alarm protocols.[17] Several studies have quantified desaturation events by pulse oximetry to show relatively few episodes in the first few days of life, an

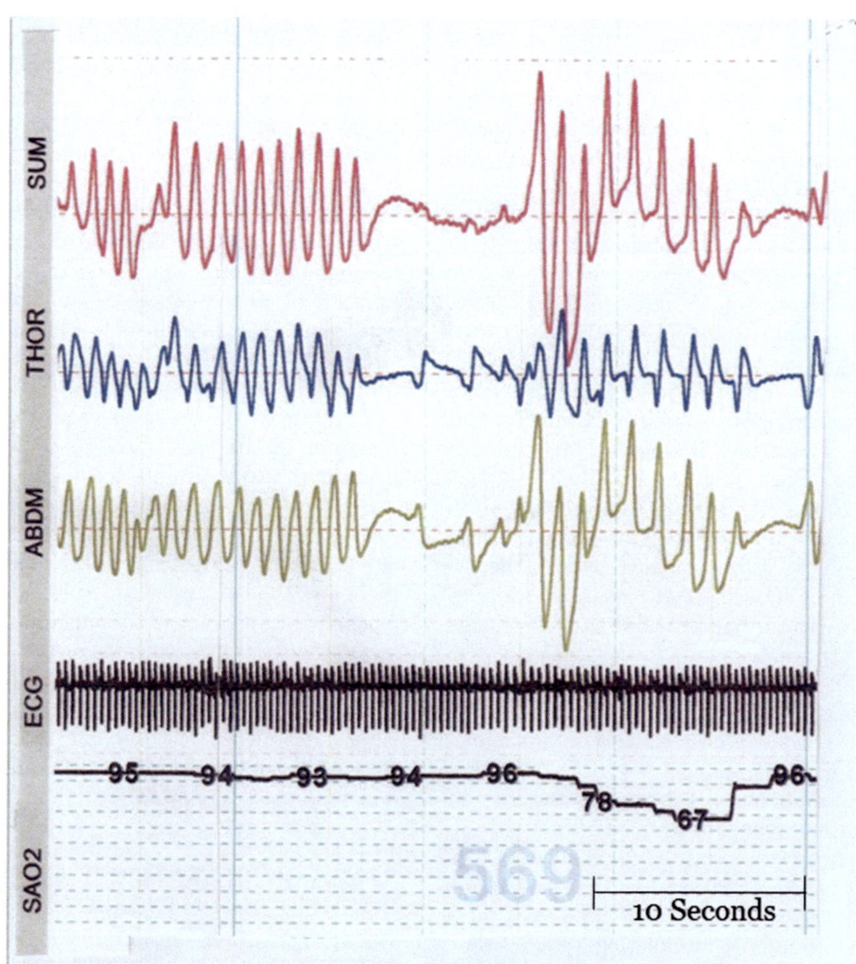

FIG. 13.2 The technique of respiratory inductance plethysmography demonstrates a 10-s absence of airflow (SUM) with obstructed inspiratory efforts (ABDM and THOR) and the resultant desaturation. In this tracing, bradycardia is not apparent. *ABDM*, abdominal motion; *SUM*, noninvasive estimate of tidal volume; *THOR*, thoracic motion.

increase in weeks 2–4 (~50–100 per day), followed by a decrease in weeks 6–8.[18] This phenomenon occurs independent of mechanical ventilation and may mirror the developmental window encompassing a decline in central chemosensitivity observed in animal models during the first few days of postnatal life.[19]

IH can have effects on long-term pulmonary development independent of other factors. Until recently, the temporal relationship of IH with mechanical ventilation and cumulative oxygen exposure was unclear. One analysis of intermittent hypoxia showed that BPD was associated with more frequent, longer, but less severe, IH events that occur toward the end of the first week of life through approximately the first month[20] (Fig. 13.3). The emergence of this IH pattern is consistent with other studies that describe pulmonary deterioration during the second postnatal week, which is worse in the infants receiving already high levels of supplemental oxygen.[21] The infants experiencing more frequent and longer IH are likely treated with more supplemental oxygen, which increases their likelihood of BPD.[22] The pattern and timing of IH events may also be an oxidative stress, given the wide swings in oxygen saturations that occur in relatively close temporal proximity. Animal models of induced IH describe a superoxide burst during hyperoxic recovery lasting up to 20 minutes.[23] In humans, IH events occurring between 1 and 20 minutes apart or lasting >1 minute have been linked to retinopathy of prematurity (ROP) requiring laser surgery and late death or disability.[24,25] Similarly, the treatment response is to increase the supplemental oxygen, which worsens oxidative injury, or to administer mechanical ventilation, with probable deleterious effects on lung function. Finally, there may be longer term impacts of IH on pulmonary outcomes, as increased cumulative oxygen exposure, increased daily IH, and lower mean SpO_2 are associated with increased asthma medication use at the 2-year follow-up.[26]

Intermittent hypoxia is likely a proinflammatory stimulus that when superimposed on other causes of pre- or postnatal inflammation can increase pulmonary and neurodevelopmental morbidity. The underlying mechanisms, including the role of diminished tissue oxygenation, are in need of clarification. The data describing inflammation induced by intermittent hypoxia has been extrapolated from adults with obstructive sleep apnea. Tumor necrosis factor α levels are increased in adults with obstructive sleep apnea and intermittent hypoxia and resolve after CPAP therapy.[27] Additionally, healthy adults experiencing IH have increased levels of reactive oxygen species without a compensatory increase in antioxidant activity.[28] Animal models show similar characteristics with the addition of infection/inflammation further impairing the hypoxic ventilatory response.[29] Taken together, the proinflammatory IH stimulus, superimposed on other causes of pre-and postnatal inflammation, can synergistically inhibit the hypoxic ventilatory response creating a vicious cycle of inflammation and respiratory depression, promoting progressive respiratory failure.

Further analysis of IH events demonstrates long-term extrapulmonary consequences associated with their frequency and severity. Several studies have shown that excessive or persistent apnea of prematurity is associated with long-term neurodevelopmental problems[30]; however, their causal relationship remains unclear. Both the number of days of ventilation for apnea[31]

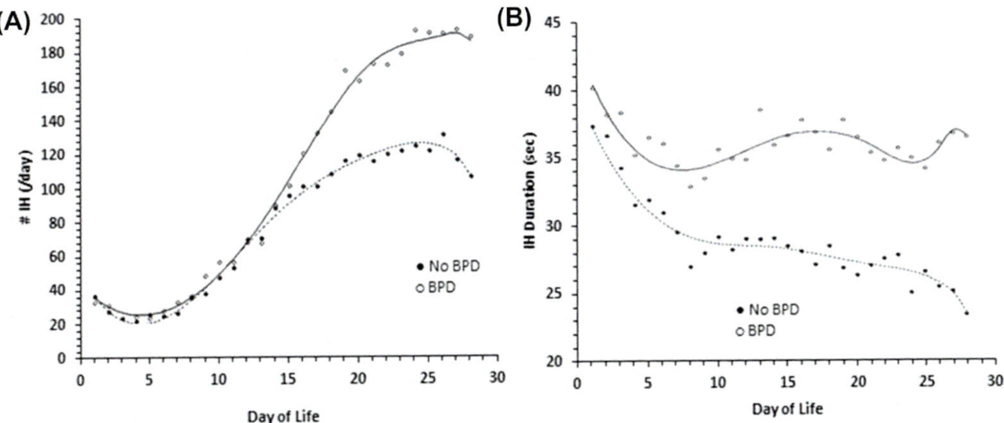

FIG. 13.3 Infants with a subsequent diagnosis of bronchopulmonary dysplasia (BPD) demonstrate a higher incidence of intermittent hypoxia (IH) from approximately 2 weeks of postnatal age **(A)** that are of longer duration **(B)**.[20] Open circles, BPD; closed circles, no BPD.

and the persistence of apnea beyond 36 weeks' corrected age are associated with unfavorable neurodevelopmental outcomes.[30] Such an association may not be causal, as other factors, e.g., intrauterine, may contribute to both postnatal apnea and poor outcome. ROP is also linked to IH through the elevation of hypoxia-induced vascular endothelial growth factor (VEGF) concentration.[32] Indeed, infants who have more IH events are more likely to need ROP laser surgery[18] than those who did not. Compounding this issue, IH events may impact metabolism and growth rates in animal models which are independent risk factors for ROP, triggering recent suggestions for ROP screening proposals based on postnatal weight gain.[33] Finally, IH may contribute to persistent abnormal sleep disordered breathing in former preterm infants, further discussed in the sleep disordered breathing section, that further increases risk of long-term neurodevelopmental outcomes.[34,35]

VULNERABILITY OF INFANTS WITH BRONCHOPULMONARY DYSPLASIA

There are multiple reasons why infants with BPD have high vulnerability to intermittent hypoxic episodes, although all preterm infants are at risk. Risk factors include immature respiratory control, adverse pulmonary function, and predisposition to reactive hypoxemia-induced pulmonary hypertension (Fig. 13.4). Data on maturation of respiratory control in infants with chronic lung disease are limited. Neonatal rodent data provide some insight, especially the consequences of chronic intermittent hypoxia in early postnatal life.[36,37] Intermittent hypoxia superimposed on hyperoxia-induced lung injury appears to enhance the risk of neurologic injury.[38] We have documented that a period of sustained hypoxia, followed by exposure to chronic intermittent hypoxia, resulted in attenuation of ventilation in response to a subsequent hypoxic exposure. These data could provide insight into the consequences of not maintaining adequate levels of oxygen saturation during the neonatal period, especially in vulnerable preterm infants susceptible to the frequent bouts of hypoxemic events that are commonly associated with apnea of prematurity.[39]

Two groups of investigators have studied peripheral chemosensitivity in preterm infants of advanced postnatal age who have developed BPD or chronic neonatal lung disease.[40,41] Such infants with BPD may be exposed to a combination of acute or more chronic hypoxia, although these may coexist. In both studies, BPD was associated with decreased peripheral chemosensitivity. From these studies, it would seem that decreased peripheral chemosensitivity may delay recovery from apnea-induced hypoxia episodes in infants with BPD, thus aggravating the problem.

Adverse pulmonary function is a long-lasting problem in many preterm survivors, especially those with BPD. This is largely addressed in other chapters of this book and manifests clinically as increased airway reactivity and obstructive lung disease. Abnormal lung and airway function may compromise ventilatory responses to hypoxia, and hypoxia may, in turn, induce bronchospasm. Earlier data in infants with BPD demonstrated the potential for hypoxia-induced airway constriction.[42,43] Interestingly, we have shown in rat pups that chronic exposure to intermittent hypoxia

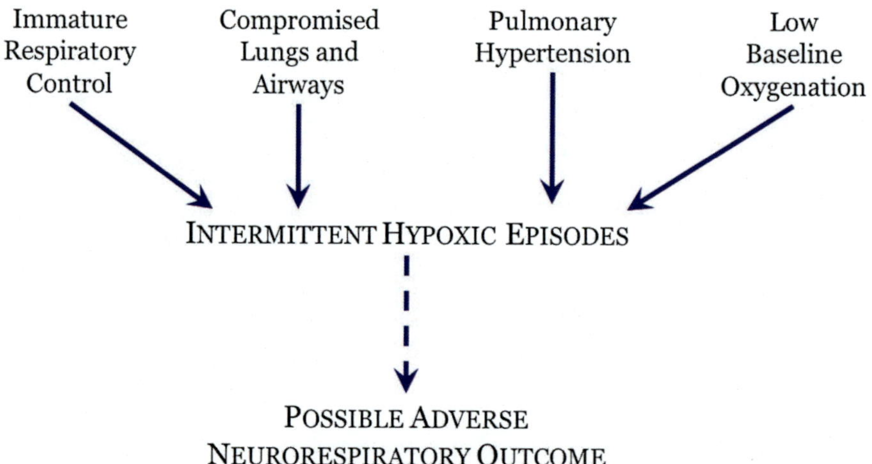

FIG. 13.4 Contributors to intermittent hypoxic episodes and potential longer term adverse outcomes that may be most prominent in infants with bronchopulmonary dysplasia.

only elicits increased airway reactivity if intermittent hypoxic episodes are followed by hyperoxic recovery.[44]

Many factors may contribute to the increased airway reactivity that is seen after neonatal hyperoxic exposure, especially in the face of BPD. Studies have focused on neonatal rodent models exposed to only moderate (e.g., 40%) hyperoxic exposure because this more closely simulates the clinical condition. Our data demonstrate that 40% oxygen exposure elicited a greater increase in airway reactivity than 70% oxygen exposure, associated with greater airway smooth muscle thickness.[45] This might be attributed to a dominant proliferative effect of 40% oxygen on airway smooth muscles versus a predominantly apoptotic effect at high oxygen levels.[46] Epithelial injury with loss of airway relaxant factors may also contribute to the hyperoxia-induced increase in airway contractile responses. It would thus appear that hypoxic episodes, hyperoxic exposure, and adverse pulmonary and airway function are all interrelated.

The contribution of pulmonary vasoconstriction to hypoxic spells in BPD has been recognized from the earliest descriptions of the disease. Vascular remodeling with intimal hyperplasia leads to abnormal vasoreactivity, as evidenced by the vasoconstrictor response seen in even modest episodes of hypoxia. In addition, very preterm infants with BPD may have decreased angiogenesis and this may be a contributing factor to the development of pulmonary hypertension. Reduced vascular growth limits the vascular surface area and further increases pulmonary vascular resistance, especially when cardiac output is increased, such as with exercise or stress. In animal models, Abman's group[47] has demonstrated in a series of elegant experiments that impaired angiogenesis can lead to impaired alveolarization. Thus a primary contributor to the development of BPD is abnormal vascular development. In summary, hypoxic episodes are significant challenges in the shorter and longer term management of former preterm infants. Because the cause may be multifactorial, including immature respiratory control and airway-related and vascular causes, an integrated approach to understand the pathobiology of these events is essential in this high-risk population.

THERAPEUTIC CHALLENGES

Both pharmacologic and nonpharmacologic therapies are key to minimize apnea of prematurity and the resultant intermittent hypoxia. Typically, therapies are initiated depending on clinical practice, nursing documentation of events, overall clinical status, often suboptimal monitoring tools including capillary blood gases, and perceived infant respiratory requirements. Some therapies are shown to be beneficial in larger trials; however, other treatments are based on clinical judgment.[47]

Caffeine is the mainstay therapy used to treat apnea and IH. Caffeine and other methylxanthines have been prescribed in preterm infants for the past 40 years and have been shown to reduce apnea and the need for ventilation. Rhein et al. demonstrated that caffeine, administered to infants of 25–32 weeks' gestation, decreased the number of intermittent hypoxemic events and time with hypoxemia even at 35 and 36 weeks' postmenstrual age. This raises the question of how long caffeine therapy should be continued.[48]

The largest trial of caffeine, the (Caffeine for Apnea of Prematurity [CAP] trial) randomly assigned 2006 infants with birth weights between 500 and 1250 g to caffeine or placebo in the first 10 days of life.[48] Initiation and discontinuation was largely at physician discretion. Although apnea of prematurity was not measured in this clinical trial, caffeine administration was associated with a reduction in the duration of positive-pressure support, oxygen supplementation, and the incidence of BPD. Early caffeine use also significantly improved survival without neurodevelopmental disability at 18–21 months. It additionally improved motor outcomes well into school age.

There are various pharmacologic effects of caffeine on apnea of prematurity. Most importantly, it stimulates the respiratory center in the brain stem and increases sensitivity to CO_2. Mechanisms of action include blockade of adenosine A_1 and A_{2A} receptor subtypes resulting in excitation of respiration neural output.[49] An intravenous loading dose of caffeine evidenced a rapid (within 5 min) and prolonged (2 h) increase in diaphragmatic activity that was associated with an increase in tidal volume.[50] It is also suggested, in a primate model, that inhibition of phosphodiesterase 4 plays a role in caffeine, and other xanthine, respiratory stimulant effects.[51] Lastly, caffeine may have antiinflammatory properties in the lung. For example, rat pups exposed prenatally to lipopolysaccharide had improved lung resistance and cytokine profiles after caffeine treatment.[52] There is evolving evidence for mechanisms of antiinflammatory effects of caffeine, and other methylxanthines, to involve phosphodiesterase 4 and adenosine antagonism, enhanced intracellular cyclic AMP, and inhibitory effects on certain prostaglandins.[53]

TABLE 13.1
Neonatal Caffeine Therapy: Unresolved Issues

	Pros	Cons
Early onset	• Improves various morbidities	• Available data are largely based on associations rather than randomized trials • How early is too early?
Prolongation of therapy	• Decreases duration of intermittent hypoxic episodes • May shorten hospitalization (if discharged on caffeine)	• May provide exposure to unnecessary medication • May prolong hospitalization (if discharged off caffeine)
Higher doses	• More strongly enhance respiratory neural output	• Adenosine receptor subtype inhibition of inflammation is variable and dose dependent, raising safety concerns • Preliminary report of cerebellar injury • Likely need for postnatal dose adjustments

Optimal strategies of caffeine therapy have yet to be determined (Table 13.1). For example, common practice entails a caffeine citrate loading dose of 20 mg/kg followed by 5−10 mg/kg per day, typically begun in the first 24 hours in preterm infants at highest risk for apnea and in need of ventilatory support. Slightly higher maintenance doses are often employed, but a higher loading dose has been associated with an increased incidence of cerebellar hemorrhage and should most likely be avoided.[52]

There have been no randomized control trials to address the optimal time to start or stop treatment with caffeine. The ideal time to start caffeine treatment has been examined by a few retrospective cohort studies. Early caffeine administration during the first 2−3 days of life was associated with reduction of BPD, patent ductus arteriosus requiring treatment, and duration of positive-pressure ventilation.[54,55] The American Academy of Pediatrics guidelines suggest discontinuing caffeine therapy when cardiorespiratory events are insignificant for 5−7 days or at 33−34 weeks' postmenstrual age, whichever comes first.[56] However, it is important to realize that preterm infants born at very young gestational ages may continue to have apnea and IH events even beyond 33−34 weeks' postmenstrual age. Persistent unstable ventilatory control and increased periodic breathing were identified in over 30% of preterm infants tested at approximately 36 weeks' corrected gestational age by a systematic reduction in supplemental oxygen and flow, if still on oxygen support, or by a brief "fitness-to-fly," 15% oxygen exposure test if on room air at time of testing.[57] Over 60% of infants distinguished by the diagnosis of BPD based on at least 28 days of oxygen use before 36 weeks of gestation failed the hypoxia challenge test shortly before NICU discharge; failure was again noted in a few infants retested at up to 17 months' corrected gestational age.[58] The National Institutes of Health Neonatal Research Network has recently (February 2019) begun a randomized study of continuing caffeine dosing after perceived resolution of apnea of prematurity in the NICU, when open-label caffeine use would otherwise be stopped, and after discharge for 28 days to assess the effect on the length of hospital stay, as well as on a number of secondary outcomes including rehospitalization and illness visits (the MoCHA study, ClinicalTrials.gov Identifier: NCT03340727).

As discussed earlier, centrally mediated hypoxic depression is prominent in early postnatal life. It follows that avoidance of hypoxemia should benefit apnea; additionally, hypoxia increases the pauses associated with periodic breathing. Earlier studies found that increases in the fraction of inspired oxygen (FiO_2) decreased apnea of prematurity and periodic breathing.[59] Recent data demonstrated that a lower baseline oxygen saturation (85%−89%) compared with a higher oxygen saturation (91%−95%) was associated with an increased rate of intermittent hypoxemic events in preterm infants.[60] Because major complications of oxygen toxicity include ROP and lung damage with resultant BPD, it is important to balance the level of supplemental oxygen with potential risks associated with hyperoxia.

Nasal CPAP is safe and effective and has a prominent role in treatment for apnea of prematurity. CPAP is a noninvasive form of applying constant distending pressure level during inhalation and exhalation. It supports infants who are spontaneously breathing but who have airway instability, pulmonary edema, and atelectasis. CPAP enhances and stabilizes FRC, reduces work of breathing, and decreases mixed and obstructive apnea.[61]

There is considerable controversy regarding the best mode of CPAP delivery. This is further complicated by the various low- and high-flow cannulas that are widely used for CPAP delivery despite limited comparative studies. Refinement of techniques to both deliver CPAP and provide effective synchronized noninvasive ventilation may be the answer.

DISCHARGE AND POSTDISCHARGE CHALLENGES

There is no evidence basis for practice regarding discharge decisions for infants who have persistence of desaturation events or apnea of prematurity. It is known that infants born at a younger gestational age have delayed resolution of apnea and bradycardia events. In a retrospective cohort study that included 1400 infants at 34 weeks' gestation or earlier, a 5- to 7-day apnea/bradycardia-free interval had a success rate between 94% and 96% of predicting no events after discharge. Success rates were dependent on the gestational age and postmenstrual age of the infant.[62] In most NICU settings, an apnea-event-free period before discharge of 5–7 days is used. Often this is based on nursing observation and monitor alarm thresholds for recording of apnea and bradycardia events. Preterm infants have clinically undetected apnea events that may not be apparent to caregivers unless continuous electronic recording is performed. However, there is no evidence that they predict subsequent infant death. Although it has been recognized since 1982 that infants with BPD are predisposed to sudden infant death syndrome, there are clearly a multitude of contributing factors.[63] Routine home monitoring for resolved apnea of prematurity is not recommended, although this is an option for selected infants who are sent home while using oxygen.[64] In infants who have residual lung disease and are on full oral feeds, discharge on low supplemental oxygen is increasingly employed, although clear guidelines for initiation and maintenance of such therapy do not exist. Infants with BPD are clearly vulnerable to a hypoxic challenge as demonstrated by the "fitness to fly" challenge.[58] This may be due to a combination of hypoxic respiratory depression and impaired lung function. In the PROP study, several infants were observed to have a predictable response to hypoxia with early brief periods of hyperpnea followed by periodic breathing and ultimately hypopnea and hypoxia at the end of the test (Fig. 13.5). As discussed earlier, low baseline oxygen saturation and intermittent hypoxia may aggravate the increased airway reactivity to which former infants, especially those with BPD, are predisposed.[65]

Finally, former preterm infants have a higher prevalence of sleep disordered breathing at 8–10 years of age,

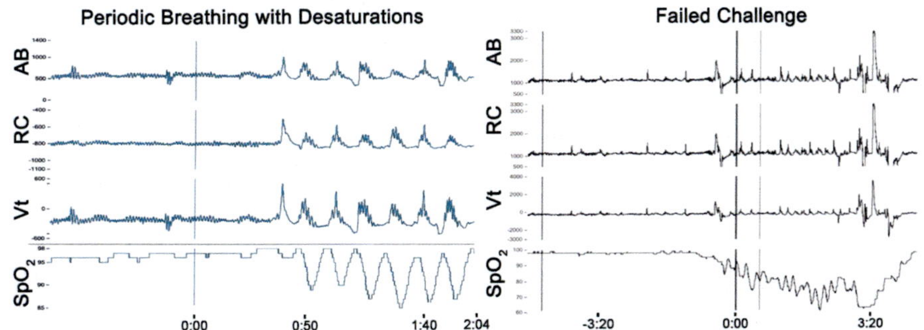

FIG. 13.5 Respiratory inductance plethysmography during a fitness-to-fly, 15% oxygen challenge test of two room-air-stable preterm infants. (AB = abdominal, RC = rib cage, Vt = tidal volume, $SpO_2 > 95\%$ before test begun.) The recording on the left showed periodic breathing with intermittent desaturations and recovery. A failed challenge (right panel) shows periodic breathing, hypopnea, and desaturations below $SpO_2 = 80\%$ resulting in test discontinuation (approximately 3:20). (Courtesy of James Kemp, MD at the Washington University, St Louis, MO, and the Prematurity and Respiratory Outcomes Program NHLBI U01 HL101465, U01 HL101813.)

which may be a manifestation of respiratory control remodeling during early maturation.[34] Recent data have demonstrated an approximate 10% incidence of obstructive sleep apnea in ex-preterm infants, which is considerably higher than that expected in a term population.[66] These data demonstrate a diverse longer term respiratory morbidity in former preterm infants, especially those with BPD, and delayed respiratory control maturation figures prominently in this morbidity. Current and future studies need to address this issue as the preterm population matures beyond childhood and adolescence to adulthood.

ACKNOWLEDGMENT

Supported by the NIH grant HL56470.

REFERENCES

1. Martin RJ. The unfortunate tale of immature respiratory control superimposed on an immature lung. *Pediatr Res.* 2018;84:153–154.
2. Alheid GF, McCrimmon DR. The chemical neuroanatomy of breathing. *Respir Physiol Neurobiol.* 2008;164:3–11.
3. Stryker C, Dylag A, Martin R. Apnea and control of breathing. In: Jobe A, Whitsett J, Abman S, eds. *Fetal and Neonatal Lung Development.* New York, NY: Cambridge: Cambridge University Press; 2016.
4. Smith JC, Abdala AP, Rybak IA, Paton JF. Structural and functional architecture of respiratory networks in the mammalian brainstem. *Philos Trans R Soc Lond B Biol Sci.* 2009;364:2577–2587.
5. Ritchie JW, Lakhani K. Fetal breathing movements in response to maternal inhalation of 5% carbon dioxide. *Am J Obstet Gynecol.* 1980;136:386–388.
6. Eichenwald EC, Ungarelli RA, Stark AR. Hypercapnia increases expiratory braking in preterm infants. *J Appl Physiol (1985).* 1993;75:2665–2670.
7. Frantz 3rd ID, Adler SM, Thach BT, Taeusch Jr HW. Maturational effects on respiratory responses to carbon dioxide in premature infants. *J Appl Physiol.* 1976;41:41–45.
8. Rigatto H, Brady JP, de la Torre Verduzco R. Chemoreceptor reflexes in preterm infants: II. The effect of gestational and postnatal age on the ventilatory response to inhaled carbon dioxide. *Pediatrics.* 1975;55:614–620.
9. Khan A, Qurashi M, Kwiatkowski K, Cates D, Rigatto H. Measurement of the CO_2 apneic threshold in newborn infants: possible relevance for periodic breathing and apnea. *J Appl Physiol (1985).* 2005;98:1171–1176.
10. Kubin L, Alheid GF, Zuperku EJ, McCrimmon DR. Central pathways of pulmonary and lower airway vagal afferents. *J Appl Physiol (1985).* 2006;101:618–627.
11. Hasan SU, Rigaux A. Effect of bilateral vagotomy on oxygenation, arousal, and breathing movements in fetal sheep. *J Appl Physiol (1985).* 1992;73:1402–1412.
12. Rabbette PS, Fletcher ME, Dezateux CA, Soriano-Brucher H, Stocks J. Hering-Breuer reflex and respiratory system compliance in the first year of life: a longitudinal study. *J Appl Physiol (1985).* 1994;76:650–656.
13. Lee LY, Pisarri TE. Afferent properties and reflex functions of bronchopulmonary C-fibers. *Respir Physiol.* 2001;125:47–65.
14. Nurse CA, Leonard EM, Salman S. Role of glial-like type II cells as paracrine modulators of carotid body chemoreception. *Physiol Genom.* 2018;50:255–262.
15. Gauda EB, Lawson EE. Developmental influences on carotid body responses to hypoxia. *Respir Physiol.* 2000;121:199–208.
16. Carroll JL. Developmental plasticity in respiratory control. *J Appl Physiol (1985).* 2003;94:375–389.
17. Martin RJ, Wang K, Koroglu O, Di Fiore J, Kc P. Intermittent hypoxic episodes in preterm infants: do they matter? *Neonatology.* 2011;100:303–310.
18. Di Fiore JM, Bloom JN, Orge F, et al. A higher incidence of intermittent hypoxemic episodes is associated with severe retinopathy of prematurity. *J Pediatr.* 2010;157:69–73.
19. Darnall RA. The role of CO(2) and central chemoreception in the control of breathing in the fetus and the neonate. *Respir Physiol Neurobiol.* 2010;173:201–212.
20. Raffay TM, Dylag AM, Sattar A, et al. Neonatal intermittent hypoxemia events are associated with diagnosis of bronchopulmonary dysplasia at 36 weeks postmenstrual age. *Pediatr Res.* 2019;85:318–323.
21. Laughon M, Allred EN, Bose C, et al. Patterns of respiratory disease during the first 2 postnatal weeks in extremely premature infants. *Pediatrics.* 2009;123:1124–1131.
22. Wai KC, Kohn MA, Ballard RA, et al. Early cumulative supplemental oxygen predicts bronchopulmonary dysplasia in high risk extremely low gestational age newborns. *J Pediatr.* 2016;177, 97-102 e102.
23. Fabian RH, Perez-Polo JR, Kent TA. Extracellular superoxide concentration increases following cerebral hypoxia but does not affect cerebral blood flow. *Int J Dev Neurosci.* 2004;22:225–230.
24. Poets CF, Roberts RS, Schmidt B, et al. Association between intermittent hypoxemia or bradycardia and late death or disability in extremely preterm infants. *J Am Med Assoc.* 2015;314:595–603.
25. Di Fiore JM, Kaffashi F, Loparo K, et al. The relationship between patterns of intermittent hypoxia and retinopathy of prematurity in preterm infants. *Pediatr Res.* 2012;72:606–612.
26. Di Fiore JM, Dylag AM, Honomichl RD, et al. Early inspired oxygen and intermittent hypoxemic events in extremely premature infants are associated with asthma medication use at 2 years of age. *J Perinatol.* 2019;39:203–211.
27. Ryan S, Taylor CT, McNicholas WT. Selective activation of inflammatory pathways by intermittent hypoxia in obstructive sleep apnea syndrome. *Circulation.* 2005;112:2660–2667.
28. Pialoux V, Hanly PJ, Foster GE, et al. Effects of exposure to intermittent hypoxia on oxidative stress and acute hypoxic

ventilatory response in humans. *Am J Respir Crit Care Med.* 2009;180:1002–1009.
29. Balan KV, Kc P, Hoxha Z, Mayer CA, Wilson CG, Martin RJ. Vagal afferents modulate cytokine-mediated respiratory control at the neonatal medulla oblongata. *Respir Physiol Neurobiol.* 2011;178:458–464.
30. Pillekamp F, Hermann C, Keller T, von Gontard A, Kribs A, Roth B. Factors influencing apnea and bradycardia of prematurity - implications for neurodevelopment. *Neonatology.* 2007;91:155–161.
31. Janvier A, Khairy M, Kokkotis A, Cormier C, Messmer D, Barrington KJ. Apnea is associated with neurodevelopmental impairment in very low birth weight infants. *J Perinatol.* 2004;24:763–768.
32. Chen J, Smith LE. Retinopathy of prematurity. *Angiogenesis.* 2007;10:133–140.
33. Binenbaum G, Bell EF, Donohue P, et al. Development of modified screening criteria for retinopathy of prematurity: primary results from the postnatal growth and retinopathy of prematurity study. *JAMA Ophthalmol.* 2018;136: 1034–1040.
34. Rosen CL, Larkin EK, Kirchner HL, et al. Prevalence and risk factors for sleep-disordered breathing in 8- to 11-year-old children: association with race and prematurity. *J Pediatr.* 2003;142:383–389.
35. Urschitz MS, Eitner S, Guenther A, et al. Habitual snoring, intermittent hypoxia, and impaired behavior in primary school children. *Pediatrics.* 2004;114:1041–1048.
36. Pawar A, Peng YJ, Jacono FJ, Prabhakar NR. Comparative analysis of neonatal and adult rat carotid body responses to chronic intermittent hypoxia. *J Appl Physiol (1985).* 2008;104:1287–1294.
37. Julien C, Bairam A, Joseph V. Chronic intermittent hypoxia reduces ventilatory long-term facilitation and enhances apnea frequency in newborn rats. *Am J Physiol Regul Integr Comp Physiol.* 2008;294:R1356–R1366.
38. Ratner V, Kishkurno SV, Slinko SK, et al. The contribution of intermittent hypoxemia to late neurological handicap in mice with hyperoxia-induced lung injury. *Neonatology.* 2007;92:50–58.
39. Mayer CA, Ao J, Di Fiore JM, Martin RJ, MacFarlane PM. Impaired hypoxic ventilatory response following neonatal sustained and subsequent chronic intermittent hypoxia in rats. *Respir Physiol Neurobiol.* 2013;187:167–175.
40. Calder NA, Williams BA, Smyth J, Boon AW, Kumar P, Hanson MA. Absence of ventilatory responses to alternating breaths of mild hypoxia and air in infants who have had bronchopulmonary dysplasia: implications for the risk of sudden infant death. *Pediatr Res.* 1994;35: 677–681.
41. Katz-Salamon M, Jonsson B, Lagercrantz H. Blunted peripheral chemoreceptor response to hyperoxia in a group of infants with bronchopulmonary dysplasia. *Pediatr Pulmonol.* 1995;20:101–106.
42. Teague WG, Pian MS, Heldt GP, Tooley WH. An acute reduction in the fraction of inspired oxygen increases airway constriction in infants with chronic lung disease. *Am Rev Respir Dis.* 1988;137:861–865.
43. Tay-Uyboco JS, Kwiatkowski K, Cates DB, Kavanagh L, Rigatto H. Hypoxic airway constriction in infants of very low birth weight recovering from moderate to severe bronchopulmonary dysplasia. *J Pediatr.* 1989;115: 456–459.
44. Dylag AM, Mayer CA, Raffay TM, Martin RJ, Jafri A, MacFarlane PM. Long-term effects of recurrent intermittent hypoxia and hyperoxia on respiratory system mechanics in neonatal mice. *Pediatr Res.* 2017;81:565–571.
45. Wang H, Jafri A, Martin RJ, et al. Severity of neonatal hyperoxia determines structural and functional changes in developing mouse airway. *Am J Physiol Lung Cell Mol Physiol.* 2014;307:L295–L301.
46. Hartman WR, Smelter DF, Sathish V, et al. Oxygen dose responsiveness of human fetal airway smooth muscle cells. *Am J Physiol Lung Cell Mol Physiol.* 2012;303: L711–L719.
47. Abman SH. Bronchopulmonary dysplasia: "a vascular hypothesis". *Am J Respir Crit Care Med.* 2001;164: 1755–1756.
48. Rhein LM, Dobson NR, Darnall RA, et al. Effects of caffeine on intermittent hypoxia in infants born prematurely: a randomized clinical trial. *JAMA Pediatr.* 2014;168: 250–257.
49. Wilson CG, Martin RJ, Jaber M, et al. Adenosine A2A receptors interact with GABAergic pathways to modulate respiration in neonatal piglets. *Respir Physiol Neurobiol.* 2004; 141:201–211.
50. Kraaijenga JV, Hutten GJ, de Jongh FH, van Kaam AH. The effect of caffeine on diaphragmatic activity and tidal volume in preterm infants. *J Pediatr.* 2015;167:70–75.
51. Howell LL. Comparative effects of caffeine and selective phosphodiesterase inhibitors on respiration and behavior in rhesus monkeys. *J Pharmacol Exp Ther.* 1993;266: 894–903.
52. Koroglu OA, MacFarlane PM, Balan KV, et al. Anti-inflammatory effect of caffeine is associated with improved lung function after lipopolysaccharide-induced amnionitis. *Neonatology.* 2014;106:235–240.
53. Al Reef T, Ghanem E. Caffeine: well-known as psychotropic substance, but little as immunomodulator. *Immunobiology.* 2018;223:818–825.
54. Dobson NR, Patel RM, Smith PB, et al. Trends in caffeine use and association between clinical outcomes and timing of therapy in very low birth weight infants. *J Pediatr.* 2014; 164:992–998 e993.
55. Lodha A, Seshia M, McMillan DD, et al. Association of early caffeine administration and neonatal outcomes in very preterm neonates. *JAMA Pediatr.* 2015;169:33–38.
56. Eichenwald EC, Committee on Fetus and Newborn. Apnea of prematurity. *Pediatrics.* 2016;137.
57. Coste F, Ferkol T, Hamvas A, et al. Ventilatory control and supplemental oxygen in premature infants with apparent chronic lung disease. *Arch Dis Child Fetal Neonatal.* 2015; 100:F233–F237.
58. Vetter-Laracy S, Osona B, Pena-Zarza JA, Gil JA, Figuerola J. Hypoxia challenge testing in neonates for fitness to fly. *Pediatrics.* 2016;137. e20152915.

59. Weintraub Z, Alvaro R, Kwiatkowski K, Cates D, Rigatto H. Effects of inhaled oxygen (up to 40%) on periodic breathing and apnea in preterm infants. *J Appl Physiol (1985)*. 1992;72:116–120.
60. Di Fiore JM, Walsh M, Wrage L, et al. Low oxygen saturation target range is associated with increased incidence of intermittent hypoxemia. *J Pediatr*. 2012;161:1047–1052.
61. Shah V, Di Fiore J, Martin R. Respiratory control and apnea in premature infants. In: Bancalari E, Keszler M, Davis PG, eds. *The Newborn Lung*. Philadelphia: Elsevier; 2018:239–249.
62. Lorch SA, Srinivasan L, Escobar GJ. Epidemiology of apnea and bradycardia resolution in premature infants. *Pediatrics*. 2011;128:e366–373.
63. Werthammer J, Brown ER, Neff RK, Taeusch Jr HW. Sudden infant death syndrome in infants with bronchopulmonary dysplasia. *Pediatrics*. 1982;69:301–304.
64. Moon RY, Task S. Force on sudden infant death, SIDS and other sleep-related infant deaths: evidence base for 2016 updated recommendations for a safe infant sleeping environment. *Pediatrics*. 2016;138.
65. Martin RJ, Di Fiore JM, Walsh MC. Hypoxic episodes in bronchopulmonary dysplasia. *Clin Perinatol*. 2015;42: 825–838.
66. Marcus CL, et al. Long-term effects of caffeine therapy for apnea of prematurity on sleep at school age. *Am J Respir Crit Care Med*. 2014;190:791–799.

CHAPTER 14

Oxyhemoglobin Saturation Targets in Newborns and the Role of Automated Oxygen Delivery Systems

PAYAM VALI, MD • SATYAN LAKSHMINRUSIMHA, MBBS, MD, FAAP

INTRODUCTION

Lack of oxygen delivery can lead to inadequate cellular metabolism and ultimately cell death, in as quickly as a few minutes. It comes without surprise that oxygen therapy, therefore, remains the most abundantly administered drug in the neonatal intensive care unit (NICU). Premature infants have underdeveloped lungs that fail to achieve adequate gas exchange. Several congenital deformities in term newborns may result in lung malformations or cardiac defects, which require supplemental oxygen therapy to prevent hypoxia. Furthermore, oxygen, a potent pulmonary vasodilator, remains the mainstay therapeutic intervention for neonates who have persistent pulmonary hypertension of the newborn (PPHN) owing to an incomplete transition from the fetal circulation as a result of an insufficient drop in pulmonary vascular resistance (PVR) following birth.

At the advent of neonatology, administering 100% oxygen was common practice to treat neonates with respiratory distress. Not long thereafter, research has shown that exposure to high concentrations of oxygen can lead to blindness. The full extent of the deleterious effects of oxygen (even a brief administration during resuscitation) has only recently become apparent. Newborns lack robust antioxidant defense systems and premature infants, in particular, are highly susceptible to free radical damage.

Determining the correct amount of oxygen in premature and sick newborns that avoids anaerobic metabolism at one extreme (hypoxia) and free radical damage at the other extreme (hyperoxia) is an area of active research. The modernization of NICUs has allowed continuous noninvasive measurements of oxygenation by sophisticated pulse oximeters in all neonates. There is currently a tremendous interest to find the optimal oxyhemoglobin saturation target range that would promote health in sick newborns; automated oxygen delivery systems have shown promising results by better maintaining oxyhemoglobin saturations in a desired target range. Does the oxyhemoglobin saturation target range, however, paint the full picture? Blood flow, location of the oximeter probe, and carbon dioxide (CO_2) and hemoglobin concentrations are important variables that, also, influence oxygen delivery and need to be taken into consideration when attempting to optimize tissue perfusion and oxygen delivery.

OXYGENATION IN NEWBORNS

Oxygen is necessary for cellular respiration and aerobic metabolism. Oxygen acts as an electron acceptor in the respiratory chain, which reduces to water. In the absence of oxygen, anaerobic metabolism occurs, which leads to decreased energy production (ATP [adenosine triphosphate]) and metabolic acidosis. Excessive oxygen generates increased reactive oxygen species (ROS), including superoxide radical (O_2^-), hydrogen peroxide (H_2O_2), and hydroxyl radical (OH).[1] Superoxide and hydroxyl radicals are free radicals that are highly toxic and can destroy cell membranes by lipid peroxidation and damage structural and enzymatic proteins, and DNA, by oxidation.[2] As the field of neonatology evolved, providing supplemental oxygen to premature infants was associated with significant improvement in neonatal survival and reduced disability.[3] Oxygen remains the most common therapy used in the care of premature and sick newborns today.

The impact of hyperoxia on cellular metabolism, and the resulting adverse effects on tissue health, however, continues to be recognized. The clinical implications of exposing newborns to high concentrations of

Updates on Neonatal Chronic Lung Disease. https://doi.org/10.1016/B978-0-323-68353-1.00014-2

oxygen became evident over 70 years ago when this practice caused blindness in premature infants, which is known today as retinopathy of prematurity (ROP).[4,5] Following the discovery of this devastating condition, the goal of oxygen therapy shifted to prevent excessive exposure to oxygen that could lead to irreversible tissue damage. The subsequent restriction in oxygen use in NICUs, however, was associated with increased mortality.[6] In the 1960s, the use of oxygen was drastically limited, usually to a fraction of inspired oxygen (FIO_2) < 0.4, even for premature infants with respiratory distress, risking them to become severely hypoxemic and leading to a substantial increase in the incidence of cerebral palsy.[7] By the 1970s, it is estimated that over 150,000 premature babies died of hypoxic respiratory failure.[6,8] Recent evidence suggests that insufficient oxygen therapy also leads to severe morbidity from necrotizing enterocolitis (NEC), while superfluous oxygen use increases the risk of bronchopulmonary dysplasia (BPD); determining the optimal oxygenation is a balance of competing adverse outcomes[9] (Fig. 14.1).

Advancements in medical technology have provided improved and noninvasive means to monitor oxygenation. In the 1940 and 1950s, oxygen status was assessed by the concentration of inspired oxygen. The concentration of oxygen delivered to the alveoli does not necessarily predict the amount that is absorbed into the blood depending on the extent of pulmonary disease and is therefore a poor method of determining the oxygen content in the blood. In the following couple of decades, blood gas analysis allowed measurement of the partial pressure of arterial oxygen (Pao_2); this method is limited by its invasive and mostly intermittent nature (continuous measurement of Pao_2 was possible at the risk of indwelling invasive instrumentation). In the late 1970s, noninvasive measurement by transcutaneous oxygen monitoring became available, but owing to limitations in reliability and risk of injury to the skin, use of these devices fell out of favor with the introduction of pulse oximeters.[10,11] In the 1980s, pulse oximetry measurement of oxyhemoglobin saturation provided a reliable and easier means to continuously monitor oxygenation, compared with transcutaneous oxygen tension measurements, and has become the standard of care across NICUs.[12,13]

Oxyhemoglobin Saturation: Pulse Oximeter Reliability and Clinical Implications

Monitoring oxygenation status by pulse oximeters has become ubiquitous in neonatal care. Premature and sick newborns are continuously monitored by pulse oximetry during their stay in the intensive care unit. Furthermore, all healthy term newborns in the nursery are screened for critical congenital heart diseases with pulse oximeters.[14] Although the pulse oximeter has proven to be an indispensable technology in the care of premature and sick newborns, clinicians need to be cognizant of its limitations.

The differential light absorption of oxyhemoglobin (red spectrum of visible light) and deoxyhemoglobin (infrared spectrum of light) and the distinction between pulsatile and nonpulsatile flow constitute the principles of pulse oximetry. The sensor of the pulse oximeter contains two light-emitting diodes (LEDs), infrared and red light, that transmit light through the applied tissue (hand or foot in neonates) and are received by a phototransistor on the opposing side of the LEDs (Fig. 14.2). Pulsatile blood flow results in fluctuations in blood volume, thus changing the distance the light travels. The pulsatile component of the red to infrared light modulation ratio is calculated, and a microprocessor with built-in algorithms converts this ratio to a saturation of pulsed oxyhemoglobin (SpO_2) value based on a calibration curve.[15,16] Pulse oximeters are calibrated by data collected from healthy adults and correlated to arterial blood samples tested by co-oximetry (absorbance spectroscopy) that measures the actual arterial oxyhemoglobin saturation (SaO_2). Therefore pulse oximeters do not measure oxyhemoglobin saturations directly but generate an SpO_2 value using an algorithm generated from SaO_2 samples. One of the most widely used pulse oximeters, Masimo Radical-7, established the accuracy of its algorithm in neonates using 79 samples collected from 16 neonates over an SpO_2 range of 70%–100%.[17] The accuracy of current pulse oximeters has been shown to be approximately 3%, which represents 1 standard deviation (SD).[18,19] As such, a displayed SpO_2 of 93% may represent a true SaO_2 anywhere from 90% to 96% in 68 percent of cases (1 SD), but may fall outside the range of 87%–99% in 5% of patients (2 SD). In a study of preterm infants comparing postductal SpO_2 to umbilical artery SaO_2, an SpO_2 between 85% and 89% was associated with an SaO_2 <85% in 39% of samples.[20] Furthermore, the translation of SpO_2 to Pao_2 can be difficult to establish. The relationship between SpO_2 and Pao_2 depends on various physiologic variables such as affinity of hemoglobin for oxygen, which is significantly greater in fetal hemoglobin.[21] Thus the higher the fetal hemoglobin concentration, the higher the SpO_2 would be for any given Pao_2 value. Furthermore, because of the nonlinear relationship between SpO_2 and Pao_2 on the oxygen-hemoglobin equilibrium curve, a greater rise

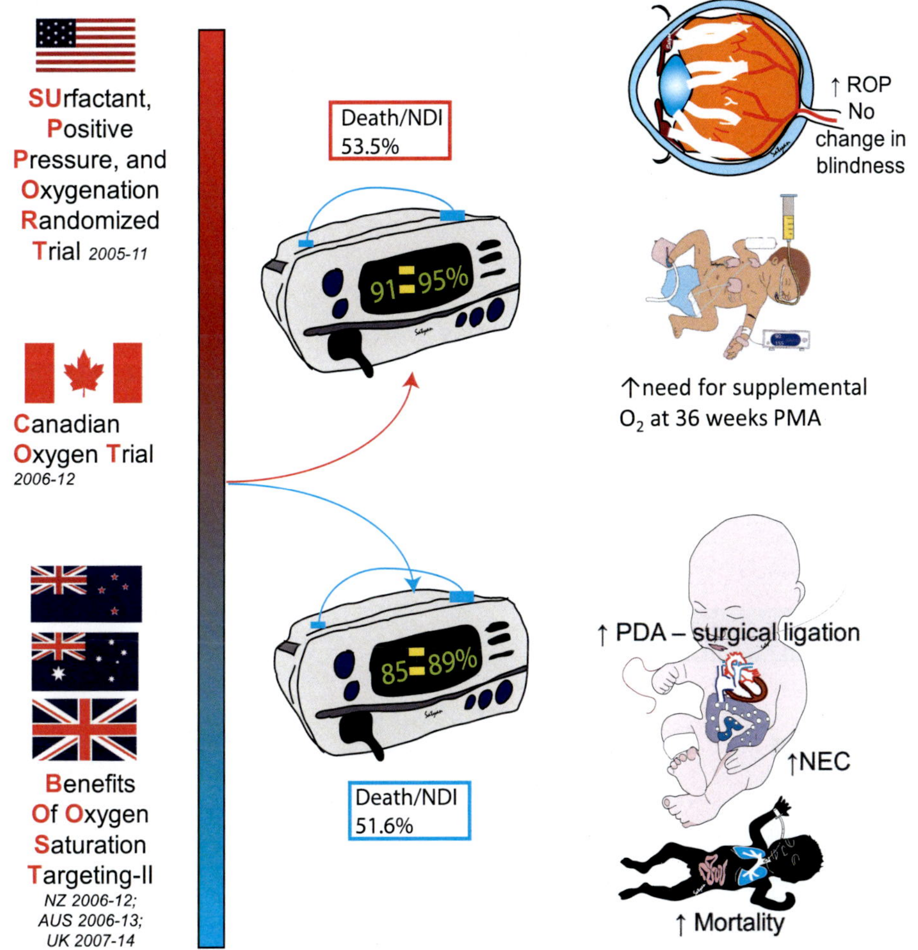

FIG. 14.1 **Results of the Neonatal Oxygen Prospective Meta-Analysis (NeOProM) collaboration.** Analysis includes data of almost 5000 premature infants from five large randomized clinical trials. Premature infants born at <28 weeks' gestation who were randomized to a higher saturation of pulsed oxyhemoglobin (SpO_2) target range (91%–95%) had increased risk of retinopathy of prematurity (ROP) and need for supplemental oxygen at 36 weeks of postmenstrual age (PMA). Infants randomized to the lower SpO_2 target range had increased incidence of patent ductus arteriosus (PDA) surgical ligation, necrotizing enterocolitis (NEC), and mortality. The combined outcome of death and neurodevelopmental impairment was not different between the groups. *NDI*, neurodevelopmental impairment. (Modified from Saugstad OD, Oei JL, Lakshminrusimha S, Vento M. Oxygen therapy of the newborn from molecular understanding to clinical practice. *Pediatr Res*. 2018. Copyright Satyan Lakshminrusimha.)

in Pao_2 occurs at higher SpO_2 values.[22] Despite these shortcomings, the quick, reliable, and continuous SpO_2 measurement obtained by pulse oximetry provides the advantage to rapidly adjust FIO_2 in an attempt to prevent hypoxemia and hyperoxemia.

SUPPLEMENTAL OXYGEN USE IN THE DELIVERY ROOM

Establishing and maintaining adequate breathing and gas exchange at birth is essential to sustain oxygenation and life. During this transition from fetal to neonatal

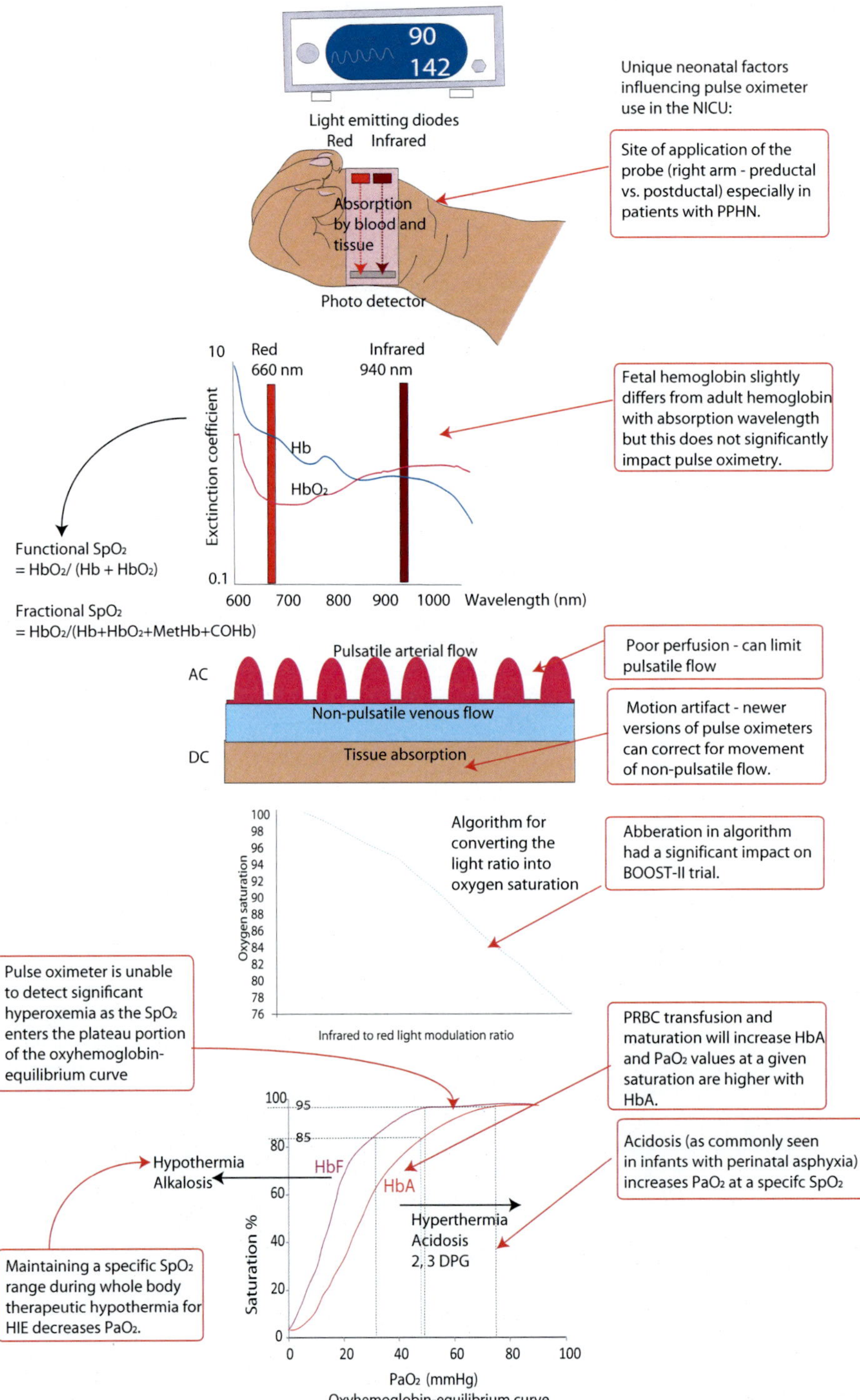

FIG. 14.2 Infographic detailing of the basic principles of pulse oximetry and its limitations in neonates. The pulse oximeter probe has diodes that emit light in the red and infrared spectra. After absorption of this light by pulsatile arterial blood, venous blood, and tissue, it is detected by photodetectors in the pulse oximeter

life, gas replaces fluid in the lungs, which results in a drop in PVR leading to an increase in pulmonary blood flow. The lungs take on the role of the placenta as the organ of gas exchange: hemoglobin inside red blood cells flowing to the alveolar capillaries absorbs oxygen from the air inside the alveoli. The oxygen bound to hemoglobin circulates through the body and is released at the level of the tissues. The use of supplemental oxygen in the resuscitation of newborns has been practiced since the early 19th century[23] and has remained in favor for over 200 years until recently, when the harmful effects associated with hyperoxia have become better understood. The need for supplemental oxygen during resuscitation of newborns remains uncertain, particularly in premature infants, and the recommendation on the optimal FIO_2 to administer has undergone several revisions over the past decade. Current guidelines recommend resuscitation in 21% O_2 for newborns born at >35 weeks' gestation,[24] and the use of 21%–30% O_2 in newborns born at <35 weeks' gestation remains a weak recommendation based on a very low certainty of evidence.[1,24–26]

The goal of oxygen therapy in the delivery room is to maintain sufficient oxygenation to ensure a constant and adequate supply of oxygen at the cellular level. When exposed to insufficient oxygen, cells undergo anaerobic metabolism that results in production of lactic acidosis. The production of ATP is reduced, and over time, purine derivatives accumulate in the cytoplasm and extracellular spaces.[27] Prolonged energy failure results in membrane depolarization, followed by cellular injury or death. Conversely, exposure to excessive oxygen generates ROS that overwhelm the antioxidant defense system of newborns and increase the risk of oxidative stress, which can leave long-lasting negative effects on a person's health.[28–30]

In utero, the fetus thrives in a relative hypoxemic environment. The oxyhemoglobin saturation in the ascending aorta of the fetus is approximately 65%.[31,32] Nevertheless, the fetus maintains tissue normoxia owing to the higher oxygen affinity of hemoglobin F, the elevated hemoglobin concentration, and the high cardiac output.[33,34] Normoxia in newborns undergoing transition is poorly understood. Therefore the threshold at which insufficient or excessive oxygen leads to hypoxia or hyperoxia has not been determined. Interquartile ranges derived from preductal SpO_2 measurements collected during the first 10 minutes from healthy term newborns delivered vaginally can serve as a guide[35,36] and have been adopted by the neonatal resuscitation program (NRP) guidelines.[37]

Supplemental Oxygen in the Resuscitation of Term and Early-Term (>35 Weeks' Gestation) Newborns

In 1998 the World Health Organization recommended that air could be used instead of pure oxygen for basic newborn resuscitation. In 2010, the International Liaison Committee on Resuscitation (ILCOR) revised their guidelines to recommend resuscitation of term and early-term infants in 21% O_2. Several clinical studies have shown that initiation of resuscitation in room air results in a shorter time to first breath, higher Apgar scores, decreased oxidative stress, and lower mortality at 1 week and 1 month of age.[38–41] Furthermore, even a brief exposure to 100% oxygen in the delivery room has been reported to increase the risk of childhood leukemia.[30,42] Current evidence supports that resuscitation in room air is better than using 100% O_2; however, there are no studies that have explored the effect of initiating resuscitation with an intermediate oxygen concentration.

In newborns in respiratory distress in need for oxygen supplementation, the evidence on how to titrate FIO_2 to meet the NRP SpO_2 target goals is lacking. In addition, the proposed SpO_2 target goals represent measurements from vaginally delivered infants from a period when early umbilical cord clamping was common practice. A recent study suggests that delayed cord clamping results in slightly higher SpO_2 values in the first 10 minutes of age,[43] and SpO_2 curves from newborns with delayed cord clamping are currently nonexistent. One needs to be mindful that the current SpO_2 target goals are derived from healthy newborns and that it is unclear whether titrating supplemental oxygen in newborns suffering from anoxic injury to meet these SpO_2 goals is appropriate. Asphyxiated lambs

probe. The extinction coefficients for hemoglobin (Hb) and HbO_2 are different at red and infrared spectra. The infrared-to-red light modulation ratio is converted to a saturation of pulsed oxyhemoglobin (SpO_2) number using an algorithm. The SpO_2 is usually within ±3% of arterial oxyhemoglobin saturation (SaO_2). The relationship between partial pressure of arterial oxygen (Pao_2) and SaO_2 describes the oxyhemoglobin-equilibrium curve. Limitations of pulse oximetry are shown in red boxes. *2,3-DPG*, 2,3-diphosphoglycerate; *BOOST*, Benefits of Oxygen Saturation Targeting; *HIE*, hypoxic-ischemic encephalopathy; *NICU*, neonatal intensive care unit; *PRBC*, packed red blood cell; *PPHN*, persistent pulmonary hypertension of the newborn. (Modified from Essentials of Neonatal Ventilation–Editors–Rajiv PK, Vidyasagar D and Lakshminrusimha S, Elsevier 2018. Copyright Satyan Lakshinrusimha.)

with meconium aspiration achieve low Pa_{O_2} levels and a smaller degree of pulmonary vasodilation when resuscitated with 21% oxygen. Titration of inspired oxygen to achieve the target SpO_2 recommended by NRP maintains physiologic Pa_{O_2} levels and higher pulmonary blood flow than resuscitation with 21% oxygen.[44] Resuscitation with 100% oxygen results in higher pulmonary blood flow but supraphysiologic Pa_{O_2} levels. However, 100% oxygen resuscitation for 30 minutes in lambs asphyxiated by umbilical cord occlusion increases superoxide anion levels in pulmonary arteries and increases their contractility.[45] Excess oxygen exposure after hypoxemia may exacerbate free radical damage and reperfusion injury.[46] The speed at which "normoxia" needs to be established in sick term newborns has not been studied. Hyperoxia in the first hour after birth has been associated with worse neurologic outcomes in infants with moderate to severe hypoxic-ischemic encephalopathy.[47,48]

Supplemental Oxygen in the Resuscitation of Preterm Infants

The current NRP guidelines recommend resuscitation of preterm infants to begin at 21%–30% O_2 and that FIO_2 should be titrated to maintain SpO_2 within the same target range as defined for full-term newborns.[24] Studies comparing initiation of supplemental oxygen at different FIO_2 in the resuscitation of preterm infants have demonstrated that 21% O_2 is not sufficient to achieve the target SpO_2 ranges and that most infants need approximately 30% O_2 by the time of stabilization.[49–53] Possible mechanisms that may explain the need for higher FIO_2 in premature infants in the delivery room include (1) an underdeveloped airspace-capillary interface, (2) immature fluid-filled lungs in the canalicular stage of development, (3) pulmonary vascular smooth muscle cells that are less responsive to oxygen, and (4) surfactant deficiency[1] (Fig. 14.3).

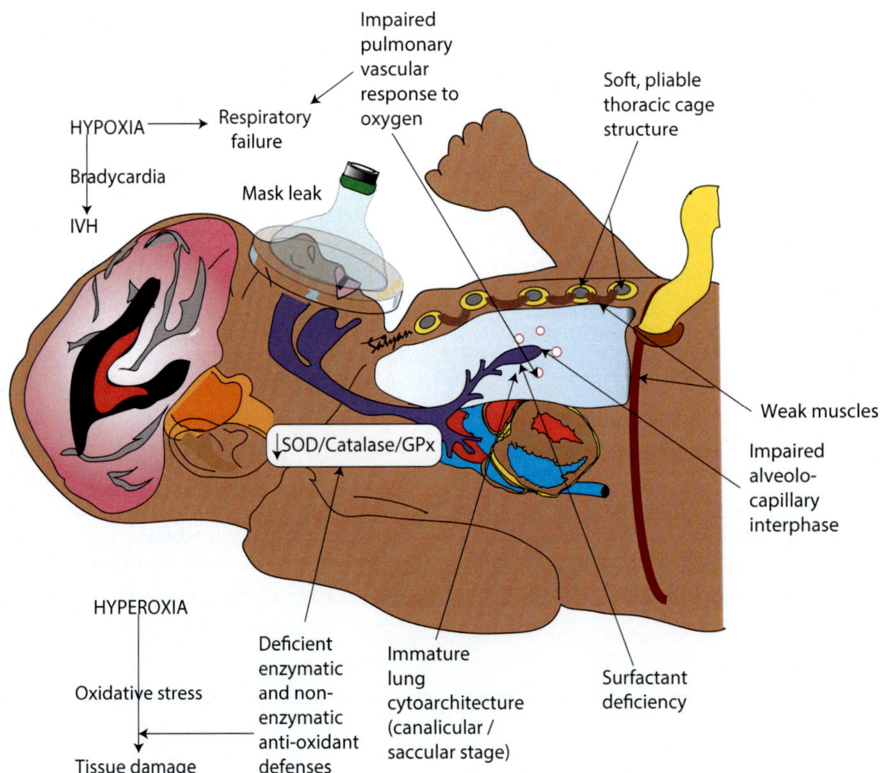

FIG. 14.3 **Infographic describing characteristics of premature infants that explain the need for supplemental oxygen in the delivery room.** Inadequate ventilation or mask leak can cause hypoxia and worsen bradycardia. Conversely, too much oxygen can lead to hyperoxia and oxidative stress. *GPx*, glutathione peroxidase; *IVH*, intraventricular hemorrhage; *SOD*, superoxide dismutase. (Copyright Satyan Lakshminrusimha.)

A meta-analysis including approximately 500 premature infants from eight studies comparing high versus low oxygen use in the delivery room showed no difference in death or major morbidities (intraventricular hemorrhage [IVH], BPD, ROP, and patent ductus arteriosus).[54] A Cochrane review including 914 infants from 10 trials, also, concluded no evidence of an effect from the use of a lower rather than a higher initial oxygen concentration targeted to SpO_2 on mortality or other newborn health outcomes.[55] One study showed an increased mortality rate in infants born at <28 weeks' gestation resuscitated with lower (0.21) rather than higher (1.0) initial FIO_2. However, the study only enrolled 292 out of the 1976 intended subjects owing to loss of equipoise in using 100% O_2,[56] and, therefore, the findings of increased mortality based on a non-prespecified post hoc analysis need to be interpreted with caution. Analysis of data from 768 preterm infants (<32 weeks' gestation) showed that regardless of the initial FIO_2, infants who did not reach an SpO_2 of 80% by 5 min of age were at significantly increased risk of bradycardia, IVH, and death.[57] Whether these findings can be explained by the failure to reach an SpO_2 >80% owing to inadequate oxygen use or the inherent clinical instability of the infants is uncertain and needs to be examined in randomized trials.

A review of 45 international clinical practice guidelines on current recommendations for oxygen management of preterm infants in the delivery room identified 17 guidelines that recommend initiating resuscitation at an FIO_2 of 0.21–0.3, 8 that recommend an FIO_2 of 0.21, 9 that recommend an FIO_2 of 0.3, 6 that recommend an FIO_2 of 0.3–0.4, and 1 country each that recommend 0.21–1.0, 0.21–0.4, and 0.3–0.5.[58] Recommendations for five-minute SpO_2 targets ranged from 70% to 90%. Until stronger evidence from ongoing and future randomized trials are reported, it is reasonable to initiate resuscitation of preterm infants with low FIO_2 (<0.4) and adjust oxygen concentration to maintain the NRP-recommended SpO_2 target goals.

OXYHEMOGLOBIN SATURATION TARGETS IN THE NEONATAL INTENSIVE CARE UNIT

Optimal SpO_2 Target in Premature Infants

Despite the exceedingly common use of supplemental oxygen in premature infants, there is little consensus on the optimal oxygen concentration that maximizes growth and development and minimizes harm. Previous clinical guidelines in the recent era were mainly based on observational studies and data that suggested that lower oxyhemoglobin saturation protects immature infants against ROP without increasing mortality.[59,60] Two randomized clinical trials addressed whether higher SpO_2 targets could prevent progression of ROP.[61,62] The STOP-ROP (Supplemental Therapeutic Oxygen for Prethreshold Retinopathy of Prematurity) trial randomized preterm infants with prethreshold ROP at 35 weeks corrected gestational age to an SpO_2 target range of 89%–94% or 96%–99%. No difference in ROP was found, but patients randomized to the higher target range required increased need for oxygen supplementation and prolonged hospitalization.[61] The BOOST (Benefits of Oxygen Saturation Targeting) trial randomized premature infants on supplemental oxygen at 32 weeks corrected gestational age to a lower (91%–94%) or higher (95%–98%) SpO_2 target range. There were no significant differences between the groups regarding ROP, growth, or neurodevelopmental outcomes, but patients randomized to the higher SpO_2 target range had a greater likelihood to be discharged from the hospital on supplemental oxygen.[62] The aforementioned studies used relatively higher SpO_2 target ranges in both the lower and higher groups, and although the results proved helpful in defining an upper SpO_2 limit, the ideal lower limit remained elusive. Hence, the findings of these studies exposed the urgent need to better understand the impact oxygenation has on the health of premature infants, and the importance to conduct large randomized clinical trials to determine the optimal SpO_2 target. Accordingly, five clinical studies were initiated with similar protocols in order to undertake a prospective individual patient meta-analysis: the NeOProM (Neonatal Oxygen Prospective Meta-Analysis) study randomized babies born at <28 weeks' gestation to a low (85%–89%) or a high (91%–95%) SpO_2 target.[63]

In total, almost 5000 infants were enrolled in these studies (Fig. 14.1). The final analysis of the NeOProM collaboration revealed no significant difference between the lower and higher SpO_2 target ranges on the primary composite outcome of death or major disability (neurodevelopmental impairment as defined by blindness, deafness, cognitive impairment, or cerebral palsy) at a corrected age of 18–24 months.[64] However, infants randomized to the lower SpO_2 target range had a significantly higher risk of death (relative risk [RR], 1.17) and NEC (requiring surgery or causing death; RR, 1.33), but a lower incidence of BPD (as defined by oxygen use at 36 weeks corrected gestation; RR 0.81) and ROP requiring treatment (RR 0.77). In other terms, the number needed to harm leading to one extra death with lower SpO_2 targeting is 31, and for NEC the number needed to harm is 37.[65] On the other hand, for infants with lower SpO_2 targeting, the number needed to prevent one case of severe ROP is 34 and the number needed to prevent one case of BPD is 20.[65] A post hoc analysis of data from the Surfactant Positive Airway Pressure and Pulse Oximetry Trial (SUPPORT) on small for gestational age (SGA) infants (defined as <tenth centile of weight) has shown that SGA infants had a significantly higher risk of mortality (38.5%), which was more than a twofold increase in the lower (56.1%) compared with the higher (25.5%) SpO_2 target group.[66,67] A Cochrane analysis, however, did not confirm a higher risk of mortality in SGA infants.[65] These data are impressive and compelling. The results of these studies suggest that a SpO_2 target range of 91%–95% may be safer than a range of 85%–89% in some extremely preterm infants. Despite these findings, the optimal SpO_2 target range for premature infants remains uncertain. Furthermore, whether SGA infants need higher SpO_2 targets and whether the target ranges need to be changed as the infants mature require future trials.

Readers should also know that changes in the algorithms of the pulse oximeters occurred during the study period in centers of three trials (BOOST-II Australia, BOOST-II United Kingdom, and Canadian Oxygen Trial), which make interpretation and analysis of the data more complicated. Interim analysis of the BOOST-II data suggested that patients randomized to the lower SpO_2 group were observed to have significantly higher saturations than expected. Inquiry into the pulse oximeters revealed that the algorithm initially merged two curves (one derived from the higher saturation range and the other from the lower saturation range) that inadvertently generated higher SpO_2 values by 2% in the range of 87%–90% where the two curves merged.[18] The algorithm has since been revised to include a single curve. This change in algorithm had an impact on results obtained from the BOOST-II trial in the United Kingdom and Australia.[68]

Optimal SpO_2 Target in Persistent Pulmonary Hypertension of the Newborn

During gestation, the fetus has evolved to divert a large proportion of the circulation away from the lungs toward the placenta, which serves as the organ of gas exchange, by maintaining an elevated PVR and a low placental vascular resistance. The onset of breathing at birth results in a dramatic drop in PVR and establishes the necessary blood flow from the right ventricle to the postnatal gas-filled lungs. Adverse in utero events or abnormalities in the pulmonary vascular bed that prevent a fall in PVR at birth result in PPHN, which limits sufficient pulmonary blood flow to participate in adequate gas exchange. PPHN represents an important proportion of newborns admitted to the NICU and is associated with an increased risk of morbidity and mortality. Oxygen remains the mainstay therapeutic intervention in the management of PPHN. Knowledge gaps on what constitutes the optimal oxygenation target, however, leads to a wide variation in practices and often leads to excessive oxygen use.

The pulmonary vessels of the fetus nearing term develop oxygen sensitivity and contract or relax in response to hypoxemia or hyperoxemia, respectively.[69] PVR is predominantly regulated by pulmonary artery smooth muscle cells in precapillary resistance arterioles, but alveolar oxygen tension exerts a greater effect on these vessels than Pao_2,[70] which explains the important vasodilatory role of oxygen on the pulmonary vascular bed to mitigate increased PVR. High concentrations of oxygen, however, may be detrimental. In a lamb PPHN ductal ligation model, PVR steadily increases when Pao_2 falls below ≈60 mm Hg with a very steep increase in PVR at Pao_2 values below ≈14 mm Hg.[71] In normal term lambs and asphyxiated lambs with meconium aspiration and PPHN, PVR increases with Pao_2 levels below 45 mm Hg. Furthermore, an increase from 50% to 100% inspired oxygen does not produce any further decrease in pulmonary arterial pressure or PVR in this model. Although lambs with PPHN that are resuscitated with 100% oxygen compared to 21% oxygen marginally enhance the decrease in PVR at birth, the effect is not sustained, and 100% oxygen induces oxidative stress, decreases subsequent response to inhaled nitric oxide, and increases pulmonary artery reactivity.[45,72]

The goal of oxygen therapy in PPHN is to (1) relax the pulmonary vasculature by decreasing PVR and to prevent hypoxemia, which would further exacerbate hypoxic pulmonary vasoconstriction; (2) provide adequate oxygen delivery to vital tissues such as the brain and heart while maintaining tissue oxygen demand; (3) avoid anaerobic metabolism and lactic acidosis; and (4) minimize oxidative stress (Fig. 14.4). The evidence strongly suggests that hypoxemia and hyperoxemia can exacerbate hypoxic respiratory failure in PPHN, but the optimal SpO_2 (or Pao_2) range whereby a balance is achieved where either extreme can be avoided has not yet been established. A recent survey of neonatologists working in level 3 or 4 NICUs across the United States evaluating oxygen management in neonates with PPHN has shown wide practice variations regarding the optimal SpO_2 or Pao_2 targets.[73] About 70% of respondents chose SpO_2 targets >95%,

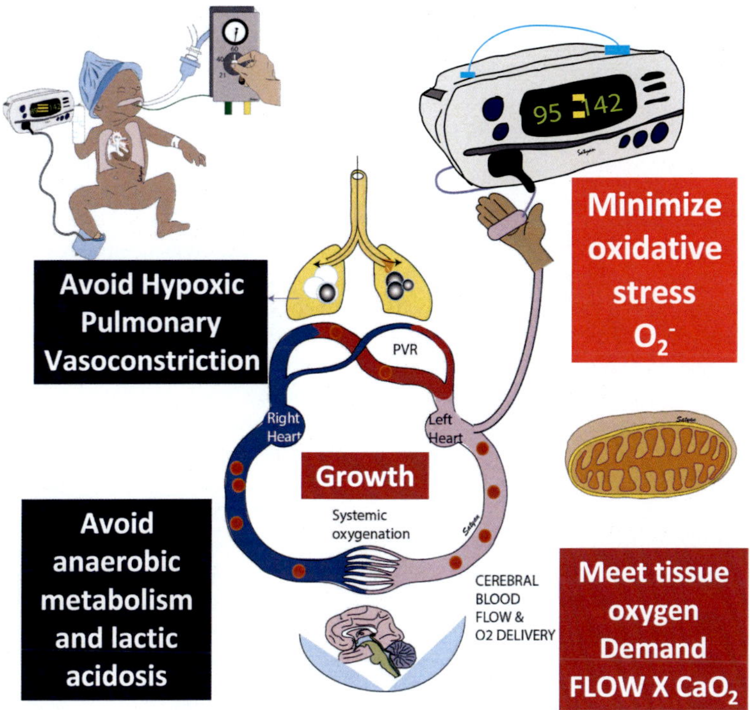

FIG. 14.4 **Infographic summarizing goals of oxygen therapy.** Optimizing oxygenation is a balance between avoiding hypoxia and hyperoxia to promote growth free of side effects. *CaO_2*, arterial oxygen content; *PVR*, pulmonary vascular resistance. (Copyright Satyan Lakshminrusimha.)

and 11% aimed to achieve Pao_2 > 120 mm Hg, while as many as 6% of respondents preferred to treat with 100% oxygen until they were confident that the pulmonary vascular reactivity had stabilized and did not wean FIO_2 despite an SpO_2 of 100%. Only 28% reported using specific oxygen titration guidelines. Furthermore, in an international survey of neonatologists, 22% of respondents indicated that they target Pao_2 > 81 mm Hg, 38% target SpO_2 > 96%, and 56% aim between 91% and 95%.[74] The wide practice variation and the tendency to hyperoxygenate newborns with PPHN highlight the importance of studying the optimal oxygen target range for this patient population in the clinical setting.

Optimal SpO_2 Target in Bronchopulmonary Dysplasia with Pulmonary Hypertension

With increased survival of extremely preterm infants, the incidence of BPD, the form of chronic lung disease associated with prematurity, is increasing. The Pediatric Pulmonary Hypertension Network published clinical guidelines to assist management of infants with BPD associated with pulmonary hypertension.[75] Optimal ventilator care and oxygenation are crucial in managing infants with severe BPD with associated pulmonary hypertension. Chronic or intermittent hypoxia is a common cause of pulmonary hypertension and avoiding hypoxemia is important to prevent progression of disease. Brief "spot checks" are not sufficient for making decisions regarding the level of supplemental oxygen. Long-term monitoring or the use of home pulse oximeter sleep studies may be helpful to determine the presence of intermittent hypoxemia. Targeting oxygen saturations to 92%–95% should be sufficient to prevent adverse effects of hypoxia without increasing the risk of oxygen toxicity to the lung and enhance growth[75] (Fig. 14.4).

PULSE OXIMETER ALARM SETTINGS AND AUTOMATED CLOSED LOOPED CONTROL OF FIO_2

Challenges in determining the optimal SpO_2 target range are not only complicated by the limitations of current pulse oximeters but, also, the potential pitfalls of frequent alarm notifications that can lead to desensitization, as well as the implausible task for medical care providers to constantly adjust FIO_2 in patients with labile oxyhemoglobin saturations. Systems for automated closed loop control of FIO_2 (A-FIO_2) have been developed for use in neonates with promising clinical applications, which may help the seemingly daunting task toward defining and maintaining the optimal SpO_2 target range.

Alarms and Alarm Fatigue

Clinical alarms are meant to alert clinicians when one of the parameters being monitored has moved outside the range that was set as normal for the patient. The ECRI (Emergency Care Research Institute) defines alarm fatigue as a condition of sensory overload for staff members who are exposed to an excessive number of alarms.[76] In the NICU, the majority of alarms occur due to low or high SpO_2 values. Exposure to frequent alarm noise can desensitize staff members who may silence alarms without checking the patient, and alarm fatigue may lead to failure to respond to important and critical alarms (Fig. 14.5).[77,78] Improving alarm management has been identified as a priority for patient safety for over a decade.[79]

Pulse oximeters average the measured data (SpO_2) over several heartbeats. The number displayed on the screen is an average of the SpO_2 value over a previous set number of seconds. Pulse oximeters from different manufacturers have varying default settings for averaging times and alarm delays. For example, the Masimo Radical pulse oximeter has user-adjustable averaging times that range from 2 to 16 seconds and alarm delays of 0, 5, 10, and 15 seconds.[17] Regardless of the averaging time set, a new number is displayed every 2 seconds. When setting a 2-second or 16-second averaging time, the number displayed on the monitor represents the average of the previous 2 or 16 seconds, respectively. Shorter averaging time increases the saturation fidelity, where quick changes in saturation will be captured more frequently. Conversely, the longer the averaging time, the slower the oximeter's reaction to rapidly changing SpO_2 values, and therefore a decrease in alarm frequency. Longer averaging times, however, may result in an underestimation of desaturations (Fig. 14.6). Setting an alarm delay enables a wait period before the alarm triggers. The set alarm delay allows a period during which the measured SpO_2 is outside the SpO_2 alarm parameters without being set off. For example, a pulse oximeter that has an alarm delay set at 10 seconds with a low SpO_2 alarm set at 90% will only set off the alarm if the average SpO_2 remains below 90% for >10 seconds.

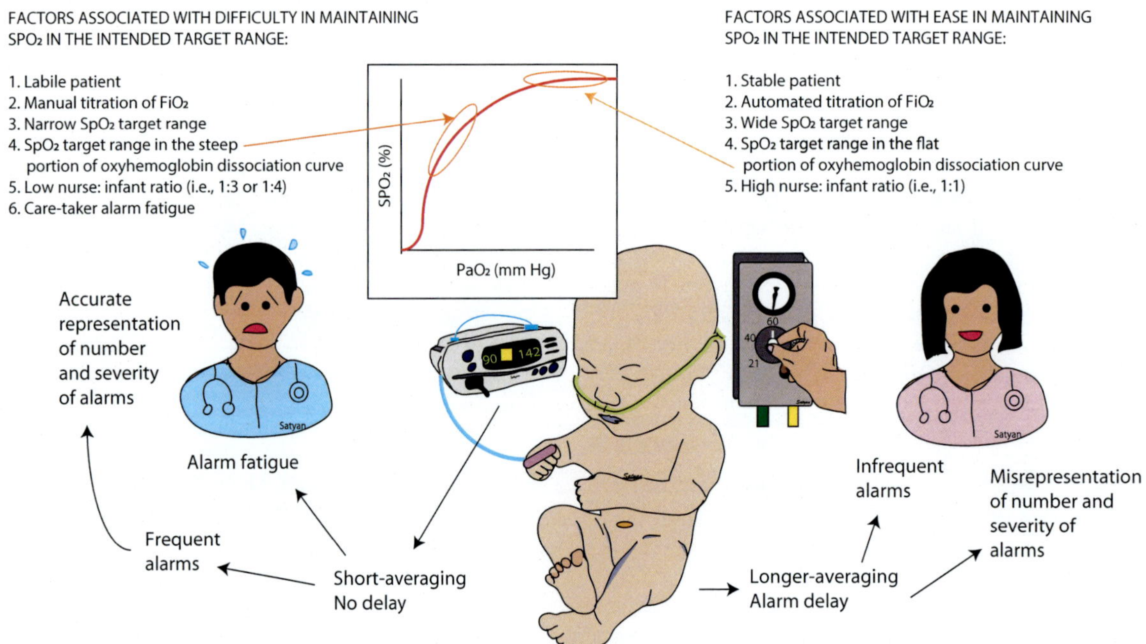

FIG. 14.5 Challenges in maintaining saturation of pulsed oxyhemoglobin (SpO_2) in the target range and alarm fatigue. A summary of the factors that are associated with difficulty in maintaining SpO_2 and steps that can be taken to facilitate maintaining SpO_2 in the desired range. (Copyright Satyan Lakshminrusimha.)

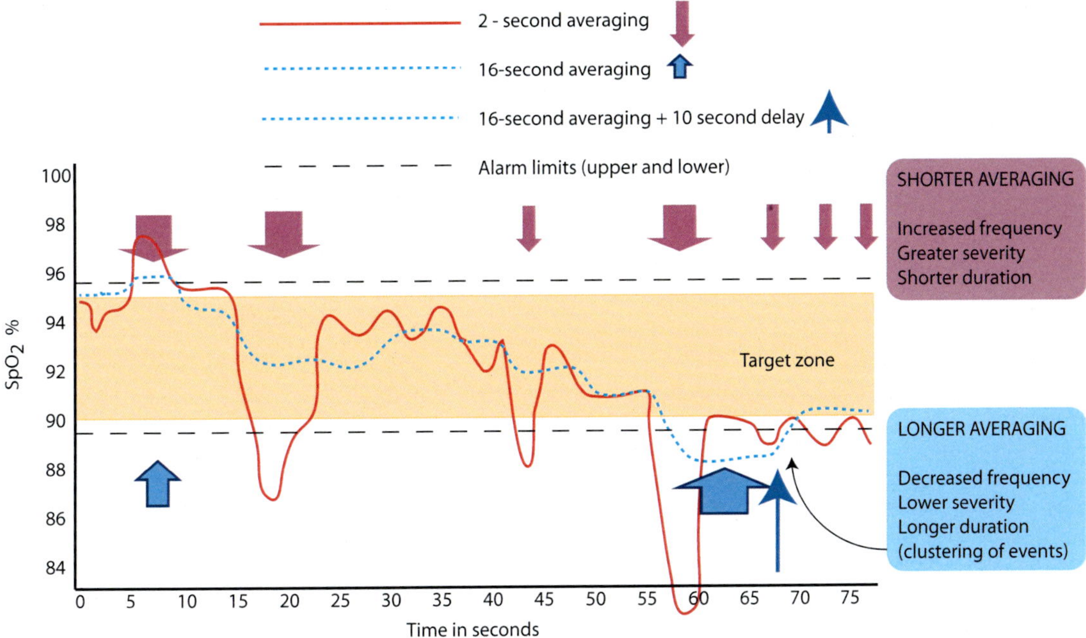

FIG. 14.6 **Effect of averaging time and alarm delay on saturation of pulsed oxyhemoglobin (SpO_2) display and alarm trigger.** Shorter averaging times capture quick changes in SpO_2 thereby increasing fidelity. Longer averaging times will underestimate the frequency of fluctuations. Arrows represent alarm trigger; the width represents alarm duration. The effects of shorter and longer averaging times on alarm trigger are shown in the purple and blue boxes, respectively. *FIO_2*, fraction of inspired oxygen; *Pao_2*, partial pressure of arterial oxygen. (Copyright Satyan Lakshminrusimha.)

Clinical studies have supported that longer averaging times not only lead to fewer SpO_2 alarms but also misrepresent the number and severity of low SpO_2 events.[80,81] In one study, 22 premature infants (<32 weeks' gestation) had simultaneous SpO_2 measurements taken from the lower extremities over a 24 hours-period using averaging times of either 2 or 16 seconds.[80] The shorter averaging time showed more frequent and severe desaturations, whereas the longer averaging time overestimated the duration of hypoxia by interpreting a cluster of desaturations as a single prolonged event. In another study of 15 extremely premature infants (gestation at birth, 24–27 weeks; gestation during study period, 32–33 weeks), 168 hours of SpO_2 data was analyzed using seven different averaging times to determine the number of desaturations below four hypoxemia thresholds.[81] The total number of desaturations to <80% was 1958 with an averaging time of 3 seconds and 339 with an averaging time of 16 seconds. However, the duration of hypoxemia was longer when setting greater averaging times: 96% of desaturations were <20 seconds and 4% were ≥20 seconds when using an averaging time of 3 seconds, whereas approximately 70% of desaturations were <20 seconds and ≈30% were ≥20 seconds when using an averaging time of 16 seconds. In both studies, the total time spent within a targeted SpO_2 range was not significantly affected by different averaging times. In addition, in a study to estimate the impact of extended SpO_2 averaging times and alarm delays, investigators found that incorporating an alarm delay with shorter SpO_2 averaging times can reduce alarm number and duration.[82] These observations were corroborated by another study in which nonactionable alarms were significantly reduced in the NICU following a quality improvement initiative that explored different alarm settings.[83]

Automated Closed Looped Control of FIO_2 Systems (A-FIO_2)

Newborns in respiratory distress have frequent fluctuations in SpO_2 that require constant titration of FIO_2 and make SpO_2 targeting a clinical challenge. Studies in premature infants have shown that patients spend considerable periods with SpO_2 outside the intended target range.[84–86] A multinational prospective study revealed that premature infants (<28 weeks' gestation) on respiratory support and supplemental oxygen maintain SpO_2 within the intended target range only 48% of the time, whereas 36% and 16% of the time is spent above and below the intended range, respectively.[85] Maintaining accurate SpO_2 is affected by limitations in staff availability to respond to frequent SpO_2 fluctuations, as well as a tolerance of higher SpO_2 values.[87–89] The proportion of time with SpO_2 within the target range declined from 38% to 15% with a 1:3 compared to a 1:1 nurse-to-infant ratio.[87] To overcome the challenges faced by clinicians to adjust FIO_2 and to provide respite to neonatal nursing staff, A-FIO_2 systems have been developed and are increasingly incorporated into standard neonatal ventilators. These systems have the potential to improve the precision of SpO_2 targeting and may provide a solution to the conundrum posed by the increasing acceptance of the importance of targeting a desired SpO_2 range and the recognition that such targeting cannot be achieved by bedside caregivers. The first reported case of using an FIO_2 control system in premature infants dates back to the 1970s, when Pao_2 measured by indwelling umbilical electrodes served as the feedback signal to the ventilator to adjust FIO_2.[90] More recently, the noninvasive and calibration-free characteristics of SpO_2, as well as the advance of motion-resistant pulse oximeters, make SpO_2 measurement the preferred feedback signal for A-FIO_2 systems.

A-FIO_2 systems generally consist of an oxygenation monitoring device (pulse oximeter), gas (air/oxygen mixing) delivery device, and a software algorithm that determines the timing, frequency, and magnitude of the FIO_2 adjustments.[91] Most A-FIO_2 systems currently available are rule-based and respond to any deviation from the target SpO_2 according to a set of predefined rules.[92] In most simple terms, the measured SpO_2 is compared to the set target and the FIO_2 adjustments made by the algorithm are inversely related to their difference[91] (Fig. 14.7). For example, the algorithm can be designed to increase or decrease FIO_2 by a set amount (e.g., ±0.05 or ±0.02) depending on the magnitude of deviation of the measured SpO_2 from the target SpO_2 (e.g., ±6% or ±3%).[93] A determined "wait-and-see" (lockout) period may be observed by the software to assess the response to the FIO_2 adjustment before any further changes are made.[94] Rule-based algorithms, however, have limitations where, for instance, a system designed to respond only to slow-changing fluctuations in SpO_2 is unlikely to provide a timely response during acute and rapid changes in SpO_2.[95] The ideal algorithm,

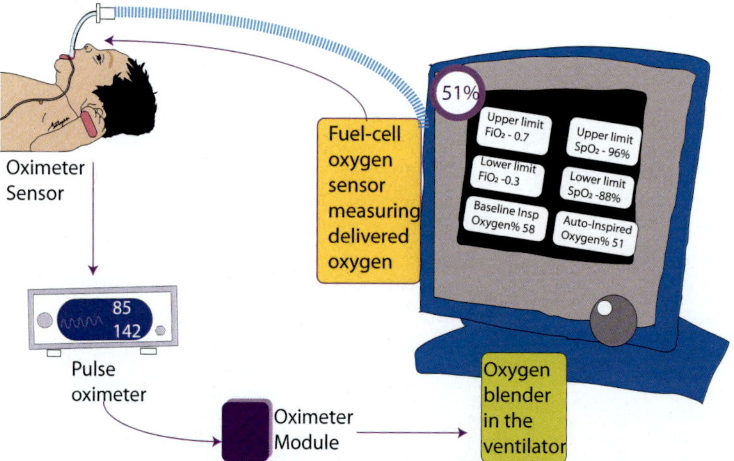

FIG. 14.7 Ventilator closed loop inspired oxygen control. The system is equipped with a fuel-cell oxygen sensor that measures delivered fraction of inspired oxygen (FIO_2). Feedback on patient oxygenation is obtained by saturation of pulsed oxyhemoglobin (SpO_2) measurement by pulse oximetry that connects to an oximeter interface module, which interacts with the integrated oxygen blender in the ventilator. Parameters for upper and lower SpO_2 targets, upper and lower alarm SpO_2 limits, and the maximum and minimum FIO_2 to be delivered can be set. The system's algorithm can be adjusted to increase or decrease FIO_2 by a set amount depending on the magnitude of deviation of the measured SpO_2 from the desired target SpO_2. The auto-inspired oxygen is the instantaneous command to the blender, while the monitored FIO_2 is measured by the patient's airway by the fuel cell; a slight difference between the auto-FIO_2 command and the monitored value for a few seconds after any change in FIO_2 can be expected. (Copyright Satyan Lakshminrusimha.)

therefore, would be rapidly responsive and, also, deal with the nonlinearity of the SpO_2-PaO_2 relationship (PaO_2 changes by only 1–2 mm Hg for each 1% step change in SpO_2 on the linear portion of the oxyhemoglobin dissociation curve, but by >20 mm Hg toward the asymptote[22]). Different software algorithms are being designed to optimize A-FIO_2 systems that would need to be tested in clinical trials.[92,95,96]

Clinical Trials Studying the Efficacy of A-FIO_2 Systems

To date, most trials have used the automated A-FIO_2 system built into the Avea (CareFusion, Yorba Linda, CA) infant ventilator.[97–102] Other systems include the software linked to the Radical-7 (Masimo Inc), the Auto-Mixer algorithm (Centro Medico Imbanaco, Cali, Colombia), and the VDL 1.0 algorithm.[93,103,104] Several studies have shown that A-FIO_2 systems are consistently more effective than manual control in maintaining SpO_2 in the target range.[105] The percentage of time spent in the target range, however, varied widely between 32% and 82% for manual control and from 40% to 91% for automated control.[92] A systematic review of clinical trials comparing automated versus manual FIO_2 control to target SpO_2 identified 10 studies and concluded that automated FIO_2 adjustment provides significant improvement of time in target saturations and reduces periods of hyperoxemia and severe hypoxemia (defined as $SpO_2 < 80\%$).[106] The quality of evidence of the studies, however, was deemed "very low" to "moderate" based on the GRADE (Grading of Recommendations, Assessment, Development and Evaluation) assessment. A recent study comparing an A-FIO_2 system to manual adjustments of FIO_2 in preterm infants on high-flow nasal cannula found similar observations: the automated system maintained SpO_2 in the desired target range 80% of the time compared with 49% of the time under manual control.[107] In addition, fewer episodes of severe hypoxemia ($SpO_2 < 80\%$) occurred under automated control. A study of preterm infants on noninvasive ventilation has shown that narrowing the target range (SpO_2, 89%–91%) compared with a wider range (86% –94%) during A-FIO_2 reduces the time spent in hypoxemia, but it does not result in an increased time spent within the clinically set wider range.[108] Owing to a rule-based algorithm design, when using a narrower target range during automated control, the FIO_2 increase starts earlier and the magnitude of the FIO_2 increase will be greater as the SpO_2 starts to drop.

The results from several clinical trials that A-FIO_2 systems are efficient in improving precision of SpO_2 targets have shown great promise. The impact of these observations on clinical outcomes of premature infants, however, remains unknown. The association between intermittent hypoxemia and long-term outcomes seems to be stronger for episodes occurring at 6–10 weeks of age than in the first few postnatal weeks, suggesting that the brain may become more sensitive to the deleterious effects of intermittent hypoxemia as it becomes more mature.[109] This raises concern that the effects of A-FIO_2 on clinical outcomes may be smaller than expected because most infants may already be in room air or on little respiratory support by 6–10 weeks. Well-conducted, large trials are necessary to assess the impact A-FIO_2 systems have on neonatal outcomes such as death, severe ROP, BPD, and NEC. The results of an ongoing large multicenter parallel group trial (funded by the German Ministry of Research and Education) that tests if automated FIO_2 control can provide better patient outcomes[92] than standard manual adjustments will be enthusiastically awaited.

CONCLUSION

Once thought to be innocuous, oxygen is now known to be highly toxic when administered in excess. Over the past several decades, basic science, translational, and clinical trial research on oxygen has led to some extraordinary discoveries, while at the same time exposing many gaps in knowledge that spurred new interests to determine the optimal oxygen target for newborns in need of supplemental oxygen. Current evidence suggests that hypoxemia increases the risk of mortality and NEC and that hyperoxemia increases the risk of ROP and BPD; either extreme may impair neurodevelopmental outcomes. The task to define the optimal SpO_2 target is further complicated by two major challenges: (1) feasibility of maintaining SpO_2 within an intended target range owing to the frequent fluctuations in SpO_2 and (2) variability across different NICUs in pulse oximeter averaging times and alarm delay settings, which influences the displayed SpO_2 values and impacts FIO_2 titration. The former problem may be addressed with the advent of automated oxygen delivery systems, which have shown to better maintain SpO_2 in the desired target range. In respect to the latter issue, investigators of future clinical trials must ensure that similar pulse oximeter settings are used in order to accurately interpret the results and improve generalizability of their findings.

REFERENCES

1. Saugstad OD, Oei JL, Lakshminrusimha S, Vento M. Oxygen therapy of the newborn from molecular understanding to clinical practice. *Pediatr Res*. 2019 Jan;85(1):20–29.
2. Halliwell B, Gutteridge JM. Oxygen toxicity, oxygen radicals, transition metals and disease. *Biochem J*. 1984; 219(1):1–14.
3. Avery ME. Recent increase in mortality from hyaline membrane disease. *J Pediatr*. 1960;57:553–559.
4. Campbell K. Intensive oxygen therapy as a possible cause of retrolental fibroplasia; a clinical approach. *Med J Aust*. 1951;2(2):48–50.
5. Silverman WA. A cautionary tale about supplemental oxygen: the albatross of neonatal medicine. *Pediatrics*. 2004; 113(2):394–396.
6. Bolton DP, Cross KW. Further observations on cost of preventing retrolental fibroplasia. *Lancet*. 1974;1(7855): 445–448.
7. Usher RH. Clinical investigation of the respiratory distress syndrome of prematurity. Interim report. *N Y State J Med*. 1961;61:1677–1696.
8. Cross KW. Cost of preventing retrolental fibroplasia? *Lancet*. 1973;2(7835):954–956.
9. Cummings JJ, Polin RA, Committee on Fetus and Newborn. Oxygen targeting in extremely low birth weight infants. *Pediatrics*. 2016;138(2).
10. Cassady G. Transcutaneous monitoring in the newborn infant. *J Pediatr*. 1983;103(6):837–848.
11. Saugstad OD. Oxygenation of the immature infant: a commentary and recommendations for oxygen saturation targets and alarm limits. *Neonatology*. 2018;114(1):69–75.
12. Durand M, Ramanathan R. Pulse oximetry for continuous oxygen monitoring in sick newborn infants. *J Pediatr*. 1986;109(6):1052–1056.
13. Van Meter A, Williams U, Zavala A, et al. Beat to beat: a measured look at the history of pulse oximetry. *J Anesth Hist*. 2017;3(1):24–26.
14. Ewer AK, Granelli AD, Manzoni P, Sánchez Luna M, Martin GR. Pulse oximetry screening for congenital heart defects. *Lancet*. 2013;382(9895):856–857.
15. Chan ED, Chan MM. Pulse oximetry: understanding its basic principles facilitates appreciation of its limitations. *Respir Med*. 2013;107(6):789–799.
16. Tin W, Lal M. Principles of pulse oximetry and its clinical application in neonatal medicine. *Semin Fetal Neonatal Med*. 2015;20(3):192–197.
17. Masimo Radical 7 Signal Extraction Pulse CO-OXimeter with Rainbow Technology —Operator's Manual 2010.
18. Johnston ED, Boyle B, Juszczak E, King A, Brocklehurst P, Stenson BJ. Oxygen targeting in preterm infants using the Masimo SET Radical pulse oximeter. *Arch Dis Child Fetal Neonatal Ed*. 2011;96(6):F429–F433.
19. Milner QJ, Mathews GR. An assessment of the accuracy of pulse oximeters. *Anaesthesia*. 2012;67(4):396–401.
20. Rosychuk RJ, Hudson-Mason A, Eklund D, Lacaze-Masmonteil T. Discrepancies between arterial oxygen saturation and functional oxygen saturation measured with pulse oximetry in very preterm infants. *Neonatology*. 2012;101(1):14–19.
21. Vali P, Underwood M, Lakshminrusimha S. Hemoglobin oxygen saturation targets in the neonatal intensive care unit: is there a light at the end of the tunnel? *Can J Physiol Pharmacol*. 2018:1–9.
22. Severinghaus JW. Simple, accurate equations for human blood O2 dissociation computations. *J Appl Physiol Respir Environ Exerc Physiol*. 1979;46(3):599–602.
23. Obladen M. History of neonatal resuscitation. Part 2: oxygen and other drugs. *Neonatology*. 2009;95(1):91–96.
24. Wyckoff MH, Aziz K, Escobedo MB, et al. Part 13: neonatal resuscitation: 2015 American heart association guidelines update for cardiopulmonary resuscitation and emergency cardiovascular care. *Circulation*. 2015; 132(18 suppl 2):S543–S560.
25. Kapadia V, Rabi Y, Oei JL. The Goldilocks principle. Oxygen in the delivery room: when is it too little, too much, and just right? *Semin Fetal Neonatal Med*. 2018 Oct;23(5): 347–354.
26. Oei JL, Saugstad OD, Vento M. Oxygen and preterm infant resuscitation: what else do we need to know? *Curr Opin Pediatr*. 2018;30(2):192–198.
27. Saugstad OD. Hypoxanthine as an indicator of hypoxia: its role in health and disease through free radical production. *Pediatr Res*. 1988;23(2):143–150.
28. Vento M, Escobar J, Cernada M, Escrig R, Aguar M. The use and misuse of oxygen during the neonatal period. *Clin Perinatol*. 2012;39(1):165–176.
29. Eden A, Gaudet F, Waghmare A, Jaenisch R. Chromosomal instability and tumors promoted by DNA hypomethylation. *Science*. 2003;300(5618):455.
30. Naumburg E, Bellocco R, Cnattingius S, Jonzon A, Ekbom A. Supplementary oxygen and risk of childhood lymphatic leukaemia. *Acta Paediatr*. 2002;91(12): 1328–1333.
31. Rudolph A. The fetal circulation. In: *Congenital Diseases of the Heart: Clinical-Physiological Considerations*. 3rd ed. Hoboken, NJ, USA: Wiley-Blackwell; 2009:1–24.
32. Prsa M, Sun L, van Amerom J, et al. Reference ranges of blood flow in the major vessels of the normal human fetal circulation at term by phase-contrast magnetic resonance imaging. *Circ Cardiovasc Imaging*. 2014;7(4):663–670.
33. Maurer HS, Behrman RE, Honig GR. Dependence of the oxygen affinity of blood on the presence of foetal or adult haemoglobin. *Nature*. 1970;227(5256):388–390.
34. Mielke G, Benda N. Cardiac output and central distribution of blood flow in the human fetus. *Circulation*. 2001; 103(12):1662–1668.
35. Mariani G, Dik PB, Ezquer A, et al. Pre-ductal and post-ductal O_2 saturation in healthy term neonates after birth. *J Pediatr*. 2007;150(4):418–421.
36. Dawson JA, Kamlin CO, Vento M, et al. Defining the reference range for oxygen saturation for infants after birth. *Pediatrics*. 2010;125(6):e1340–e1347.
37. Weiner GM, Zaichkin J, eds. *Textbook of Neonatal Resuscitation (NRP)*. 7th ed. 2016, 326 pp.

38. Vento M, Asensi M, Sastre J, Lloret A, García-Sala F, Viña J. Oxidative stress in asphyxiated term infants resuscitated with 100% oxygen. *J Pediatr.* 2003;142(3):240–246.
39. Vento M, Saugstad OD. Oxygen as a therapeutic agent in neonatology: a comprehensive approach. *Semin Fetal Neonatal Med.* 2010;15(4):185.
40. Saugstad OD. Resuscitation of newborn infants: from oxygen to room air. *Lancet.* 2010;376(9757):1970–1971.
41. Rabi Y, Rabi D, Yee W. Room air resuscitation of the depressed newborn: a systematic review and meta-analysis. *Resuscitation.* 2007;72(3):353–363.
42. Spector LG, Klebanoff MA, Feusner JH, Georgieff MK, Ross JA. Childhood cancer following neonatal oxygen supplementation. *J Pediatr.* 2005;147(1):27–31.
43. Smit M, Dawson JA, Ganzeboom A, Hooper SB, van Roosmalen J, te Pas AB. Pulse oximetry in newborns with delayed cord clamping and immediate skin-to-skin contact. *Arch Dis Child Fetal Neonatal Ed.* 2014;99(4): F309–F314.
44. Rawat M, Chandrasekharan PK, Swartz DD, et al. Neonatal resuscitation adhering to oxygen saturation guidelines in asphyxiated lambs with meconium aspiration. *Pediatr Res.* 2016 Apr;79(4):583–588.
45. Lakshminrusimha S, Steinhorn RH, Wedgwood S, et al. Pulmonary hemodynamics and vascular reactivity in asphyxiated term lambs resuscitated with 21 and 100% oxygen. *J Appl Physiol (1985).* 2011;111(5):1441–1447.
46. Saugstad OD. The oxygen paradox in the newborn: keep oxygen at normal levels. *J Pediatr.* 2013;163(4):934–935.
47. Klinger G, Beyene J, Shah P, Perlman M. Do hyperoxaemia and hypocapnia add to the risk of brain injury after intrapartum asphyxia? *Arch Dis Child Fetal Neonatal Ed.* 2005;90(1):F49–F52.
48. Kapadia VS, Chalak LF, DuPont TL, Rollins NK, Brion LP, Wyckoff MH. Perinatal asphyxia with hyperoxemia within the first hour of life is associated with moderate to severe hypoxic-ischemic encephalopathy. *J Pediatr.* 2013;163(4):949–954.
49. Kapadia VS, Chalak LF, Sparks JE, Allen JR, Savani RC, Wyckoff MH. Resuscitation of preterm neonates with limited versus high oxygen strategy. *Pediatrics.* 2013; 132(6):e1488–e1496.
50. Wang CL, Anderson C, Leone TA, Rich W, Govindaswami B, Finer NN. Resuscitation of preterm neonates by using room air or 100% oxygen. *Pediatrics.* 2008;121(6):1083–1089.
51. Escrig R, Arruza L, Izquierdo I, et al. Achievement of targeted saturation values in extremely low gestational age neonates resuscitated with low or high oxygen concentrations: a prospective, randomized trial. *Pediatrics.* 2008; 121(5):875–881.
52. Rabi Y, Singhal N, Nettel-Aguirre A. Room-air versus oxygen administration for resuscitation of preterm infants: the ROAR study. *Pediatrics.* 2011;128(2):e374–e381.
53. Rook D, Schierbeek H, Vento M, et al. Resuscitation of preterm infants with different inspired oxygen fractions. *J Pediatr.* 2014;164(6), 1322–1326.e3.
54. Oei JL, Vento M, Rabi Y, et al. Higher or lower oxygen for delivery room resuscitation of preterm infants below 28 completed weeks gestation: a meta-analysis. *Arch Dis Child Fetal Neonatal Ed.* 2017;102(1):F24–F30.
55. Lui K, Jones LJ, Foster JP, et al. Lower versus higher oxygen concentrations titrated to target oxygen saturations during resuscitation of preterm infants at birth. *Cochrane Database Syst Rev.* 2018;5. CD010239.
56. Oei JL, Saugstad OD, Lui K, et al. Targeted oxygen in the resuscitation of preterm infants, a randomized clinical trial. *Pediatrics.* 2017;139(1).
57. Oei JL, Finer NN, Saugstad OD, et al. Outcomes of oxygen saturation targeting during delivery room stabilisation of preterm infants. *Arch Dis Child Fetal Neonatal Ed.* 2018;103(5):F446–F454.
58. Wilson A, Vento M, Shah PS, et al. A review of international clinical practice guidelines for the use of oxygen in the delivery room resuscitation of preterm infants. *Acta Paediatr.* 2018;107(1):20–27.
59. Tin W, Milligan DW, Pennefather P, Hey E. Pulse oximetry, severe retinopathy, and outcome at one year in babies of less than 28 weeks gestation. *Arch Dis Child Fetal Neonatal Ed.* 2001;84(2):F106–F110.
60. Chow LC, Wright KW, Sola A, CSMC Oxygen Administration Study Group. Can changes in clinical practice decrease the incidence of severe retinopathy of prematurity in very low birth weight infants? *Pediatrics.* 2003; 111(2):339–345.
61. Supplemental therapeutic oxygen for prethreshold retinopathy of prematurity (STOP-ROP), a randomized, controlled trial. I: primary outcomes. *Pediatrics.* 2000; 105(2):295–310.
62. Askie LM, Henderson-Smart DJ, Irwig L, Simpson JM. Oxygen-saturation targets and outcomes in extremely preterm infants. *N Engl J Med.* 2003;349(10):959–967.
63. Askie LM, Brocklehurst P, Darlow BA, et al. NeOProM: neonatal oxygenation prospective meta-analysis collaboration study protocol. *BMC Pediatr.* 2011;11:6.
64. Askie LM, Darlow BA, Finer N, et al. Association between oxygen saturation targeting and death or disability in extremely preterm infants in the neonatal oxygenation prospective meta-analysis collaboration. *JAMA.* 2018; 319(21):2190–2201.
65. Askie LM, Darlow BA, Davis PG, et al. Effects of targeting lower versus higher arterial oxygen saturations on death or disability in preterm infants. *Cochrane Database Syst Rev.* 2017;4. CD011190.
66. Walsh MC, Di Fiore JM, Martin RJ, Gantz M, Carlo WA, Finer N. Association of oxygen target and growth status with increased mortality in small for gestational age infants: further analysis of the surfactant, positive pressure and pulse oximetry randomized trial. *JAMA Pediatr.* 2016;170(3):292–294.
67. Di Fiore JM, Martin RJ, Li H, et al. Patterns of oxygenation, mortality, and growth status in the surfactant positive pressure and oxygen trial cohort. *J Pediatr.* 2017;186, 49-56.e1.

68. Tarnow-Mordi W, Stenson B, Kirby A, et al. Outcomes of two trials of oxygen-saturation targets in preterm infants. *N Engl J Med*. 2016;374(8):749–760.
69. Fineman JR, Soifer SJ, Heymann MA. Regulation of pulmonary vascular tone in the perinatal period. *Annu Rev Physiol*. 1995;57:115–134.
70. Moudgil R, Michelakis ED, Archer SL. Hypoxic pulmonary vasoconstriction. *J Appl Physiol (1985)*. 2005;98(1):390–403.
71. Lakshminrusimha S, Swartz DD, Gugino SF, et al. Oxygen concentration and pulmonary hemodynamics in newborn lambs with pulmonary hypertension. *Pediatr Res*. 2009;66(5):539–544.
72. Lakshminrusimha S, Russell JA, Steinhorn RH, et al. Pulmonary arterial contractility in neonatal lambs increases with 100% oxygen resuscitation. *Pediatr Res*. 2006;59(1):137–141.
73. Alapati D, Jassar R, Shaffer TH. Management of supplemental oxygen for infants with persistent pulmonary hypertension of newborn: a survey. *Am J Perinatol*. 2017;34(3):276–282.
74. Nakwan N, Chaiwiriyawong P. An international survey on persistent pulmonary hypertension of the newborn: a need for an evidence-based management. *J Neonatal Perinat Med*. 2016;9(3):243–250.
75. Krishnan U, Feinstein JA, Adatia I, et al. Evaluation and management of pulmonary hypertension in children with bronchopulmonary dysplasia. *J Pediatr*. 2017;188, 24-34.e1.
76. ECRI Institute. Alarm related terms. In: *The Advancing Safety in Medical Science Clinical Alarms 2011 Summit*. October 4–5, 2011. Herndon, VA, USA.
77. Bonafide CP, Lin R, Zander M, et al. Association between exposure to nonactionable physiologic monitor alarms and response time in a children's hospital. *J Hosp Med*. 2015;10(6):345–351.
78. Brockmann PE, Wiechers C, Pantalitschka T, Diebold J, Vagedes J, Poets CF. Under-recognition of alarms in a neonatal intensive care unit. *Arch Dis Child Fetal Neonatal Ed*. 2013;98(6):F524–F527.
79. Critical alarms and patient safety. ECRI's guide to developing effective alarm strategies and responding to JCAHO's alarm-safety goal. *Health Devices*. 2002;31(11):397–417.
80. Ahmed SJ, Rich W, Finer NN. The effect of averaging time on oximetry values in the premature infant. *Pediatrics*. 2010;125(1):e115–e121.
81. Vagedes J, Poets CF, Dietz K. Averaging time, desaturation level, duration and extent. *Arch Dis Child Fetal Neonatal Ed*. 2013;98(3):F265–F266.
82. McClure C, Jang SY, Fairchild K. Alarms, oxygen saturations, and SpO_2 averaging time in the NICU. *J Neonatal Perinat Med*. 2016;9(4):357–362.
83. Johnson KR, Hagadorn JI, Sink DW. Reducing alarm fatigue in two neonatal intensive care units through a quality improvement collaboration. *Am J Perinatol*. 2018;35(13):1311–1318.
84. Hagadorn JI, Sink DW, Buus-Frank ME, et al. Alarm safety and oxygen saturation targets in the Vermont Oxford Network iNICQ 2015 collaborative. *J Perinatol*. 2017;37(3):270–276.
85. Hagadorn JI, Furey AM, Nghiem TH, et al. Achieved versus intended pulse oximeter saturation in infants born less than 28 weeks' gestation: the AVIOx study. *Pediatrics*. 2006;118(4):1574–1582.
86. Lim K, Wheeler KI, Gale TJ, et al. Oxygen saturation targeting in preterm infants receiving continuous positive airway pressure. *J Pediatr*. 2014;164(4), 730-736.e1.
87. Sink DW, Hope SA, Hagadorn JI. Nurse:patient ratio and achievement of oxygen saturation goals in premature infants. *Arch Dis Child Fetal Neonatal Ed*. 2011;96(2):F93–F98.
88. Clucas L, Doyle LW, Dawson J, Donath S, Davis PG. Compliance with alarm limits for pulse oximetry in very preterm infants. *Pediatrics*. 2007;119(6):1056–1060.
89. Sola A, Golombek SG, Montes Bueno MT, et al. Safe oxygen saturation targeting and monitoring in preterm infants: can we avoid hypoxia and hyperoxia? *Acta Paediatr*. 2014;103(10):1009–1018.
90. Beddis IR, Collins P, Levy NM, Godfrey S, Silverman M. New technique for servo-control of arterial oxygen tension in preterm infants. *Arch Dis Child*. 1979;54(4):278–280.
91. Claure N, Bancalari E. Automated closed loop control of inspired oxygen concentration. *Respir Care*. 2013;58(1):151–161.
92. Poets CF, Franz AR. Automated FiO_2 control: nice to have, or an essential addition to neonatal intensive care? *Arch Dis Child Fetal Neonatal Ed*. 2017;102(1):F5–F6.
93. Hallenberger A, Poets CF, Horn W, Seyfang A, Urschitz MS, Group CS. Closed-loop automatic oxygen control (CLAC) in preterm infants: a randomized controlled trial. *Pediatrics*. 2014;133(2):e379–e385.
94. Urschitz MS, Horn W, Seyfang A, et al. Automatic control of the inspired oxygen fraction in preterm infants: a randomized crossover trial. *Am J Respir Crit Care Med*. 2004;170(10):1095–1100.
95. Dargaville PA, Sadeghi Fathabadi O, Plottier GK, et al. Development and preclinical testing of an adaptive algorithm for automated control of inspired oxygen in the preterm infant. *Arch Dis Child Fetal Neonatal Ed*. 2017;102(1):F31–F36.
96. Fathabadi OS, Gale T, Wheeler K, et al. Hypoxic events and concomitant factors in preterm infants on non-invasive ventilation. *J Clin Monit Comput*. 2017;31(2):427–433.
97. Claure N, D'Ugard C, Bancalari E. Automated adjustment of inspired oxygen in preterm infants with frequent fluctuations in oxygenation: a pilot clinical trial. *J Pediatr*. 2009;155(5), 640-645.e1-2.
98. Claure N, Gerhardt T, Everett R, Musante G, Herrera C, Bancalari E. Closed-loop controlled inspired oxygen concentration for mechanically ventilated very low birth

weight infants with frequent episodes of hypoxemia. *Pediatrics.* 2001;107(5):1120–1124.

99. Lal M, Tin W, Sinha S. Automated control of inspired oxygen in ventilated preterm infants: crossover physiological study. *Acta Paediatr.* 2015;104(11):1084–1089.
100. Claure N, Bancalari E, D'Ugard C, et al. Multicenter crossover study of automated control of inspired oxygen in ventilated preterm infants. *Pediatrics.* 2011;127(1):e76–83.
101. van Kaam AH, Hummler HD, Wilinska M, et al. Automated versus manual oxygen control with different saturation targets and modes of respiratory support in preterm infants. *J Pediatr.* 2015;167(3), 545-550.e1-2.
102. Waitz M, Schmid MB, Fuchs H, Mendler MR, Dreyhaupt J, Hummler HD. Effects of automated adjustment of the inspired oxygen on fluctuations of arterial and regional cerebral tissue oxygenation in preterm infants with frequent desaturations. *J Pediatr.* 2015; 166(2), 240-244.e1.
103. Zapata J, Gómez JJ, Araque Campo R, Matiz Rubio A, Sola A. A randomised controlled trial of an automated oxygen delivery algorithm for preterm neonates receiving supplemental oxygen without mechanical ventilation. *Acta Paediatr.* 2014;103(9):928–933.
104. Plottier GK, Wheeler KI, Ali SK, et al. Clinical evaluation of a novel adaptive algorithm for automated control of oxygen therapy in preterm infants on non-invasive respiratory support. *Arch Dis Child Fetal Neonatal Ed.* 2017; 102(1):F37–F43.
105. Claure N, Bancalari E. Closed-loop control of inspired oxygen in premature infants. *Semin Fetal Neonatal Med.* 2015;20(3):198–204.
106. Mitra S, Singh B, El-Naggar W, McMillan DD. Automated versus manual control of inspired oxygen to target oxygen saturation in preterm infants: a systematic review and meta-analysis. *J Perinatol.* 2018;38(4):351–360.
107. Reynolds PR, Miller TL, Volakis LI, et al. Randomised cross-over study of automated oxygen control for preterm infants receiving nasal high flow. *Arch Dis Child Fetal Neonatal Ed.* 2019 Jul;104(4):F366–F371.
108. van den Heuvel MEN, van Zanten HA, Bachman TE, Te Pas AB, van Kaam AH, Onland W. Optimal target range of closed-loop inspired oxygen support in preterm infants: a randomized cross-over study. *J Pediatr.* 2018; 197:36–41.
109. Poets CF, Roberts RS, Schmidt B, et al. Association between intermittent hypoxemia or bradycardia and late death or disability in extremely preterm infants. *JAMA.* 2015;314(6):595–603.

CHAPTER 15

Noninvasive Ventilation: Does it Reduce BPD? What Is the Evidence?

OSAYAME A. EKHAGUERE, MBBS, MPH • K. LIM KUA, MD • PETER G. DAVIS, MD • HARESH KIRPALANI, BM, MSC

INTRODUCTION

The modern era of neonatal intensive care may be considered to date from the detailed descriptions of the pathophysiology of respiratory distress syndrome (RDS) and the infant's own strategies to prevent lung collapse.[1,2] As the physiologic lessons of laryngeal braking (manifested clinically by "grunting") were understood, they were quickly translated into therapeutic strategies. This was particularly so for noninvasive approaches for RDS, including continuous positive airway pressure (CPAP) and negative pressure ventilation.[3,4] Yet there were also parallel developments in the early 1950s, as servo controlled respirators were first used for preterm infants with RDS.[5,6] The ensuing decades witnessed rising rates of mechanical ventilation (MV). Most equipment were conscripted from adult or pediatric intensive care units and often used as a last resort.[7] In this era, survival rates of mechanically ventilated preterm neonates were low. Furthermore, deleterious long-term effects on premature lungs were first observed.[8] Radiographic, pathologic, and clinical evidence implicated prolonged MV of preterm infants as the cause of respiratory failure from pulmonary fibrosis.[2,8] This condition was later termed bronchopulmonary dysplasia (BPD).[2] It soon became obvious that the promise of invasive mechanical support was accompanied by major pulmonary complications.

Early randomized clinical trials of noninvasive respiratory support (NRS) showed reduced need for MV.[9] However, inadequate devices and interfaces which led to serious complications limited their widespread adoption.[9–11] Furthermore, the development of ventilators specifically designed for neonates,[12] the introduction of surfactant[13,14] and antenatal corticosteroids[15] significantly improved outcomes for the most premature viable neonates.[16] Invasive ventilation remained the standard of care and a necessary prerequisite to surfactant therapy. Survival rates rose but were accompanied by an increase in the incidence of BPD, which was associated with poor short- and long-term outcomes.[16] Interest in NRS was rekindled when it was observed in 1987 that a center which used CPAP frequently had a reduced incidence of BPD compared with similar North American units.[17] But only much later, in 2008 was the first substantive trial evaluating NRS in the delivery room performed to answer the question—"does NRS reduce the incidence of BPD?[18]"

In this chapter, we discuss the strategy of avoiding intubation to prevent BPD; we review the physiologic principles of NRS, including peculiarities of the different modalities; and finally, we review the evidence available on the relationship between modes of respiratory support and rates of BPD. We focus primarily on evidence from randomized controlled trials (RCTs).

BRONCHOPULMONARY DYSPLASIA

Definition

The clinical definition of BPD has changed over time—necessitated by changes in survival rates and infant demographics.[19,20] Definitions have aimed to predict long-term respiratory outcomes,[21] and severity of illness[20]; and to grapple with considerable variation in rates reported by different centers arising from differing BPD definitions.[22] The current definition is stratified by severity—as mild (if breathing room air), moderate (if on <30% supplemental oxygen), or severe (if on ≥30% supplemental oxygen) at 36 weeks' postmenstrual age.[20] Attempts to precisely quantify degree of functional effects, include the "physiologic definition" which uses the oxygen reduction test. This assesses infants managed on supplemental oxygen in the range of 21%–30% and determines whether oxygen saturations of <90% can be maintained asymptomatically for

Updates on Neonatal Chronic Lung Disease. https://doi.org/10.1016/B978-0-323-68353-1.00015-4

60 minutes after reducing the fraction of inspired oxygen to 21%.[23] However, it is difficult to apply and is not universally used. Moreover, contemporary changes in management of infants, such as provision of continuous distending pressure (CDP) in 21% oxygen, limit the application of existing definitions and increases the risk misclassification.[24] In response to this, a recent Eunice Kennedy Shriver National Institute of Child Health and Human Development (NICHD) workshop proposed a new classification to account for the amount of respiratory support.[25] Moreover, other new definitions are based upon their accuracy in predicting specified 2-year clinical outcomes.[26]

Epidemiology of BPD

With an annual incidence between 10,000 and 15,000 in the United States, BPD is the most common adverse outcome of premature infants.[27] The incidence is inversely related to the degree of prematurity and approximately 40% of infants with birth weight <1000 g will develop BPD.[16] Despite improved rates of neonatal survival, large registry data in the United States suggest that the incidence of BPD has remained unchanged over the last 20 years.[16,28] However, for infants born at 26–27 weeks gestation the incidence rose between 2009 and 2012.[16] Because BPD is closely tied to poor later neurodevelopment[29], rehospitalization[30], mortality[31], and increased healthcare cost[32], it is a major health burden.

Pathophysiology of BPD

Increasing survival of more immature infants prompted a paradigm shift in our concept of the pathogenesis of BPD since its first description in 1967.[2,20] We now consider that BPD is best characterized as an arrest of pulmonary development. This concept now supplements the prior emphasis on chronic airway injury and inflammation with resultant parenchymal fibrosis.[20,33,34] In infants <30 weeks gestation, emphysematous changes, with fewer terminal air sacs alveoli, and a superimposed fibrosis in severe BPD are now the typical morphological characteristics. One reason for these observed changes in histological appearance of BPD may have been the shift from invasive to noninvasive respiratory therapies. However, there are reports of similar morphology in extreme premature infants never exposed to positive pressure or supplemental oxygen.[35]

This confirms that the pathogenesis of BPD is multifactorial and involves genetic, intrauterine, and postnatal factors. Nonetheless, prolonged exposure to MV and oxygen toxicity remains important modifiable postnatal risk factors.[2,36] MV causes lung injury through volutrauma and barotrauma (together comprising Ventilator Induced Lung Injury), atelectotrauma, rheotrauma (inappropriate airway flow), and biotrauma.[37,38] In lamb studies, markers of lung injury such as alveolar neutrophil influx, hydrogen peroxide production, and protein accumulation—hallmarks of lung injury that predispose to BPD—are elevated in MV compared to noninvasive forms of respiratory support.[39,40] The correlation between the duration of MV and severity of BPD further underscores this relationship.[41–44] On this account, a consensus exists that the use of NRS to avoid or limit exposure to MV in preterm infants is likely to decrease BPD.[45]

NONINVASIVE RESPIRATORY SUPPORT

NRS is the provision of assisted ventilation without the use of an endotracheal tube. Although CPAP was first delivered via an ETT[3], alternate interfaces are now used. A fundamental mechanism of action is the provision of CDP to overcome atelectasis in spontaneously breathing neonates. The same principle is applied in invasive ventilation through the use of Positive End Expiratory Pressure (PEEP). Today, NRS is available as CPAP, nasal intermittent positive pressure ventilation (NIPPV), HHFNC, and noninvasive high frequency ventilation (nHFV).

Physiologic Principles of Noninvasive Respiratory Support

The generation of CDP helps maintain a functional residual capacity.[46–48] Being at or just above this optimal lung volume reduces elastic, flow resistive, and inertial resistance properties of the respiratory system.[47,49] It prevents collapse of the very compliant premature chest wall and diminishes thoracoabdominal synchrony.[50,51] The physiologic consequences are improvements in ventilation perfusion mismatch, oxygenation, and work of breathing.[47,51,52] Moreover at these lung volumes, pulmonary vascular resistance is lowest.[53] At the same time, CDP reduces supraglottic resistance to airflow and prevents oropharyngeal collapse, reducing obstructive apnea.[54] CPAP and HHFNC utilize these principles, however, with different techniques and modalities.

Noninvasive Respiratory Support Modalities

CPAP

CPAP can generate CDP either through a variable or continuous flow system.[55] In the variable flow CPAP system, entrained airflow generates pressure using Bernoulli's principle, with the presence of an adaptive "flip" valve at the nasal interface.[55] The Infant Flow LP CPAP system (Care Fusion, Yorba Linda, CA, USA) is an example of a variable flow CPAP. Alternatively, the continuous flow devices generate flow by preventing gas egress by an expiratory limb resistance or titratable PEEP valve.[55] Ventilator derived and bubble CPAP (bCPAP) are both continuous flow CPAP devices. In animal studies, the bCPAP delivered via an ETT generates low-amplitude, high-frequency oscillations to the lungs and improves ventilation.[56] However, in a randomized crossover trial that involved 26 preterm infants, ventilation and oxygenation did not differ between vigorous, high amplitude, or slow bubbling.[57] Moreover, trials comparing bubble CPAP with machine delivered CPAP do not show clinically important differences.[58] The common interfaces used to deliver CPAP are nasal masks, binasal prongs, and nasopharyngeal tubes.

HHFNC

HHFNC generates CDP by delivering heated, humidified high gas flow at rates > 1L/min. Other physiologic attributes of HHFNC include improved airway conductance, washout of nasopharyngeal dead space, and reduction of inspiratory resistance.[59] Any nasal cannula can deliver HHFNC. However, soft, malleable silicone-based nasal cannula are most commonly used in practice.

NIPPV

NIPPV superimposes peak inspiratory pressure (PIP) on a background of PEEP (similar to that generated by conventional CPAP).[55] The cycled PIPs may be low (between 9 and 11 cmH_20) during bilevel NIPPV or high (>11 cmH_20) when NIPPV is provided by a ventilator.[60] They also may be synchronized with the infant's spontaneous breathing (S—NIPPV) or nonsynchronized (NS—NIPPV).[61,62] Synchronization requires special sensors which are presently only available in some countries.[60] Common devices used to synchronize, include pneumatic capsules that detect abdominal wall movement and airflow sensors. More recently, neurally adjusted ventilator assist (NAVA) which utilizes diaphragmatic electromyogram signals has been used.[60] The proposed physiologic advantages of NIPPV over conventional CPAP is that the generated PIP increases tidal volume, improves gas exchange, and reduces work of breathing. However, evidence to support the benefits of NIPPV is inconsistent.[60] NIPPV may also induce Head's paradoxical reflex which is of potential benefit in apnea of prematurity.[55] Delivery interfaces are similar to those used to deliver CPAP.

nHFV

nHFV superimposes high-frequency oscillatory pressure over a set PEEP.[63] The mechanism of gas exchange is assumed similar to HFV via an ETT, i.e., Taylor dispersion and molecular diffusion (augmented dispersion).[64] Another touted advantage is its ability to provide support without requiring synchronization with the patient.[65] Any ventilator capable of providing HFV can deliver nHFV. Nasopharyngeal endotracheal tubes, short binasal prongs, and heated humidified nasal prongs are used to administer nHFV.

METHODS

Search Strategy

We conducted this umbrella review using the methods of the Cochrane handbook for systematic reviews of interventions, Version 5.1.0.[66] We searched PubMed, Embase, the Cumulative Index to Nursing and Allied Health Literature (CINAHL), the Cochrane library for relevant studies (see appendix 1 for search strategy).

We chose the primary outcomes of (1) BPD, (2) the composite outcome death or BPD, and (3) treatment failure and/or need for intubation when NRS treatment was used as initial treatment for preterm infants with RDS or postextubation respiratory support. We included studies that reported BPD as the requirement for supplemental oxygen at either 28 days of life or at 36-week PMA. Definitions of treatment failure varied across the included studies. Moreover, we have not attempted to explore potential differences by type of interface used. We included any RCTs that recruited neonates <37 weeks gestation at birth and reported any of the prespecified primary outcomes. We excluded trials not published in English and those testing surfactant. In a sensitivity analysis we also included studies where surfactant usage was coupled to MV and extubation. Very few studies used the most recent classification of BPD, hence subgroup analyses by severity were not possible for all. We also excluded study protocols, cohort studies, retrospective studies, review articles, abstracts, editorials, and animal studies. Where a Cochrane review exists which had obtained data from the author of a referenced article, we included those data in our analysis.

We wished to provide comparison both between major modalities of NRS, and within different subtypes within a modality. In order to be comprehensive and yet informative we have used the following definitions:

1) Initial respiratory support: The use of NRS for respiratory support soon after birth

2) Postextubation support: The use of NRS following extubation from MV. Note that this pools together studies where varying durations of time free of reintubation are used. In fact there is considerable variation between these times, which range from 48 hours to 7 days.

The literature search was conducted independently by (OAE and HC), titles and abstracts of all retrieved articles were screened by (OAE), and data abstraction was independently performed (OAE and KLK). Discrepancies were resolved by discussion and consensus. Included studies were stratified by treatment intention (initial or postextubation support), and grouped by intervention tested. We reference findings from the relevant Cochrane reviews if study inclusion criteria matched those of this review. When no Cochrane review existed for an intervention, or the review did not include all identified studies, we conducted or updated a pooled analysis. Reports are in accordance with the PRISMA (Preferred Reporting Items for Systematic Reviews and Meta-Analyses) guidelines.[67]

Risk of Bias Assessment

Using the Cochrane Collaboration tool, we assessed bias in the following domains, randomization, allocation concealment, blinding and adherence to intention.

Statistical Analysis

The principal outcome measures are reported as relative risk (RR), risk difference (RD), and number needed to treat (NNT)—when statistically significant differences exist—with their corresponding 95% confidence intervals (CIs). Fixed or random effect models were used when heterogeneity between studies was less or greater than 50%, respectively. All analyses were performed using RevMan version 5.3.[68]

RESULTS

We identified 3810 articles in the search conducted on February 26, 2019. We included an additional 66 studies identified from reference list. After excluding duplicates and studies not meeting inclusion criteria, a full text review was conducted on 200 studies and 78 were included in the final analysis.

The composite outcome death or BPD was not frequently reported in the majority of the studies reviewed. It is a relatively new outcome measure in clinical practice. In studies where both death and BPD were reported, it was impossible to distinguish those who survived with BPD from those who did not. To avoid the risk of double inclusion, we only report those trials that specified the composite outcome, death, or BPD.

CPAP

Any CPAP device compared to supplemental oxygen for initial respiratory support

We identified eight eligible studies which included 789 infants.[69–76] Five studies reported BPD, defined as supplemental oxygen requirement at 28 days of life, as an outcome. However, data for one study were obtained from a Cochrane review.[76] Only one study reported the composite outcome death or BPD.[75] CPAP or continuous negative pressure constituted the study intervention which we accepted as a form of CDP. Supplemental oxygen was provided by headbox oxygen or regular nasal cannula. The INSURE (INtubation-SURfactant-Extubation) technique was included in one study.[75] Intubating for resuscitation was allowed in three studies.[71,73,75]

Two Cochrane reviews have examined this question.[77,78] One evaluated the prophylactic use of CDP,[77] and the other as treatment for established respiratory distress syndrome.[78] We made no separation based on treatment intent. Furthermore, we excluded five studies included in the Cochrane reviews, for the following reasons. One compared CPAP to intubation[18]; one included intubation or CPAP as part of its standard care[79]; while three compared CPAP with or without surfactant.[80–82]

In pooled analysis of the five studies that reported BPD (N = 695) the risk of BPD was not different between groups (RR, 1.01; 95% CI, 0.73–1.40; RD, 0.00; 95% CI, −0.05 to 0.05) (Fig. 15.1). There was no difference in the incidence of death or BPD in the one study that reported this outcome (RR, 0.72; 95% CI, 0.41–1.25; RD, −0.05; 95% CI, −0.15 to 0.04). The incidence of respiratory failure was, significantly reduced by CDP when compared to supportive care (RR, 0.75; 95% CI, 0.56–1.00; RD, −0.14; 95% CI, −0.27 to −0.1; NNT, 7), however, with borderline significance (Fig. 15.1).

Any CPAP device compared to supplemental oxygen for postextubation support

We identified nine studies recruiting 726 infants which met our inclusion criteria in this category.[83–91] Supplemental oxygen was provided by headbox and extubation failure was determined on or before postextubation day 7 in all included studies. Six studies reported BPD defined as the need for supplemental oxygen at 28 days,[84,86–89,91] of these, two also reported

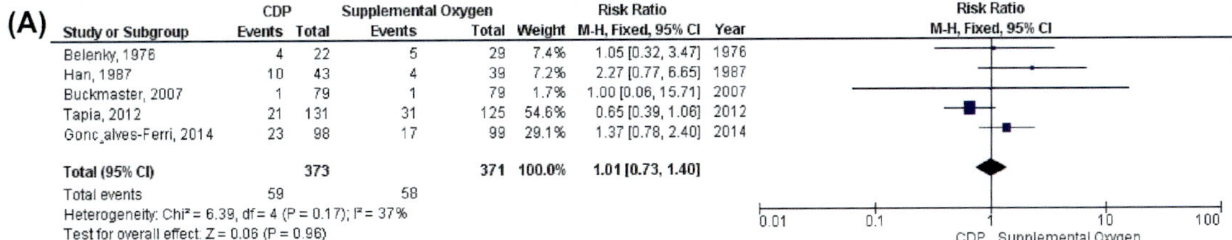

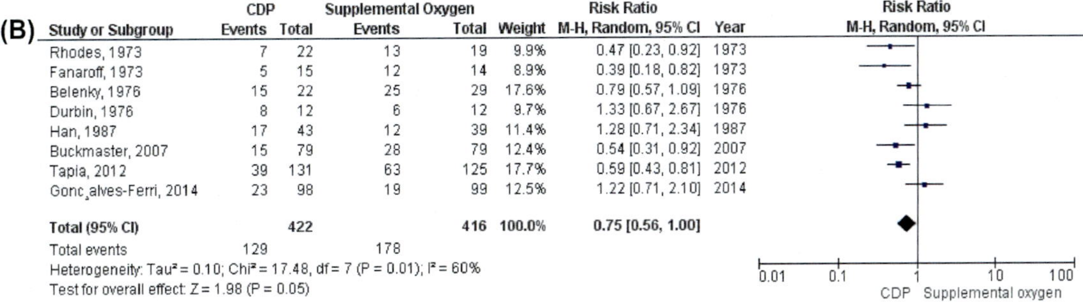

A, BPD at 28 days of life. B, Respiratory failure within 7 days.

FIG. 15.1 Forrest plot of CPAP or CDP versus supplemental oxygen as initial respiratory support. **A**, BPD at 28 days of life. **B**, Respiratory failure within 7 days. *BPD*, bronchopulmonary dysplasia; *CDP*, continuous distending pressure; *CPAP*, continuous positive airway pressure.

BPD rates at 36 weeks' PMA.[89,92] Only one study reported the composite outcome death or BPD.[88] All studies were included in a Cochrane review.[88]

There was no difference between CPAP and headbox for the outcome BPD (RR, 0.94; 95% CI, 0.64–1.37; RD, −0.03; 95% CI, −0.16 to 0.11), and for the composite outcome death or BPD (RR, 1.29; 95% CI, 0.91–1.83; RD, 0.15; 95% CI, −0.05 to 0.35). Extubation failure was, however, significantly reduced by CPAP compared to headbox (RR, 0.63; 95% CI, 0.51–0.77; RD, −0.16; 95% CI, −0.23 to −0.10; NNT 6). When we assessed the two studies that reported supplemental oxygen use at 36 weeks PMA, no difference was observed (RR, 1.17; 95% CI, 0.69–1.98; RD, 0.03; 95% CI, −0.07 to 0.12) (Fig. 15.2).

Any CPAP device compared to mechanical ventilation for initial respiratory support

Surfactant therapy by the INSURE technique has become an integral part of current neonatal practice. Hence we had two categories of comparison. The first category included studies where CPAP alone was compared with either MV or INSURE. We identified four studies in this category that included 2782 infants.[18,80–82] The incidence of BPD was similar in both the CPAP and MV or INSURE group (RR, 0.91; 95% CI, 0.82–1.01; RD, −0.03; 95% CI, −0.11 to 0.00). The composite outcome death or BPD was not different between both groups (RR, 0.92; 95% CI, 0.84–1.00; RD, −0.04; 95% CI, −0.07 to 0.00) (Fig. 15.3).

The second category included studies where CPAP (with or without INSURE) was compared with MV. We identified four studies in this category that included 1289 infants.[18,81,93,94] CPAP (with or without INSURE) significantly reduced the incidence of BPD compared to MV (RR, 0.81; 95% CI, 0.68–0.96; RD, −0.06; 95% CI, −0.11 to −0.01; NNT, 17). Of the two studies that reported the composite outcome death or BPD,[18,81] no difference in the outcome death or BPD was observed (RR, 0.86; 95% CI, 0.74–1.01; RD, −0.05; 95% CI, −0.11 to 0.00) (Fig. 15.4).

Comparison of CPAP devices

Continuous compared to variable flow CPAP devices for initial respiratory support. We identified four eligible studies which included 450 infants.[95–98] Two studies reported rates of BPD.[97,98] None of the studies reported the composite outcome death or BPD. Continuous CPAP was provided by bubble CPAP in three studies and ventilator CPAP in one.[98] Variable flow was provided by the IFD CPAP device in three studies,[95,96,98] and the fourth utilized a JET CPAP (Phoenix Medical Systems Private, Chennai, India).[97] There was potential sources of bias in the study

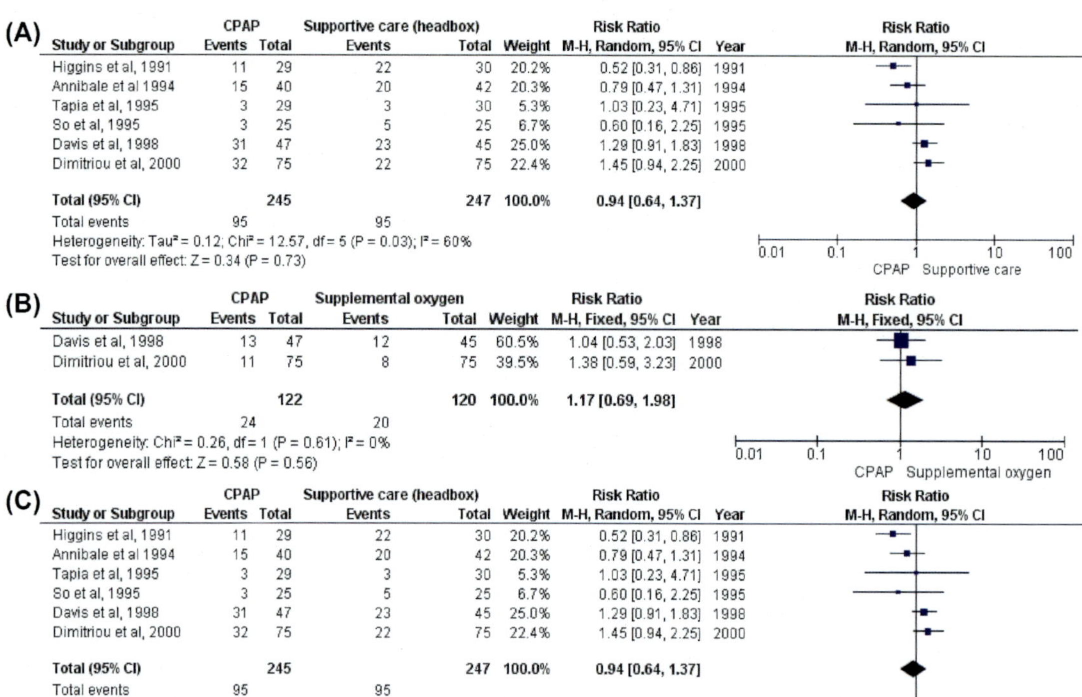

A, BPD at 28 days of life. B, BPD at 28 days of life. C, Respiratory failure within 7 days.

FIG. 15.2 Forrest plot of CPAP or CDP versus supplemental oxygen as postextubation respiratory support. **A**, BPD at 28 days of life. **B**, BPD at 28 days of life. **C**, Respiratory failure within 7 days. *BPD*, bronchopulmonary dysplasia; *CDP*, continuous distending pressure; *CPAP*, continuous positive airway pressure.

that utilized the JET CPAP as some subjects were excluded from the study because study equipment were not available after randomization.

The incidence of BPD did not differ between groups (RR, 1.13; 95% CI, 0.67–1.92; RD, 0.02; 95% CI, −0.06 to 0.10). Likewise, the incidence of respiratory failure (RR, 1.02; 95% CI, 0.70–1.48; RD, 0.00; 95% CI, −0.07 to 0.07).

Continuous compared to variable flow CPAP devices for postextubation respiratory support. We identified three studies in this category that included 459 infants.[58,98,99] Bubble CPAP was used in one study.[58] There were two additional studies available only as abstracts which are not included.[100,101] Moderate heterogeneity existed between the included studies ($I^2 = 62\%$). At least in part this may arise from variable end points that defined extubation failure, ranging from 72 hours in two studies, up to 7 days in the third study. Only two studies reported on the composite outcome death or BPD.[58,99] In pooled analysis, the incidence of BPD did not differ between groups (RR, 0.81; 95% CI, 0.59–1.11; RD, −0.10; 95% CI, −0.22 to 0.02) and (RR, 0.97; 95% CI, 0.77–1.22; RD, −0.02; 95% CI, −0.12 to 0.09), respectively. Extubation failure rates were also similar between the groups (RR, 1.07; 95% CI, 0.65–1.78; RD, 0.02; 95% CI, −70.13 to 0.17). It is worth noting that one study had a significant proportion of infants with mild BPD.[98] We restricted the analysis to include only moderate to severe BPD or death and no difference was observed.

NIPPV

Any NIPPV Device Compared to Supplemental Oxygen for Initial Respiratory Support

Only one trial has compared NIPPV to headbox.[9] The study randomized 44 infants with mean gestational age and birth weight of 33 weeks and 1892 g, respectively. Treatment failure, defined as having a partial pressure of oxygen <45 mm Hg in 100% oxygen,

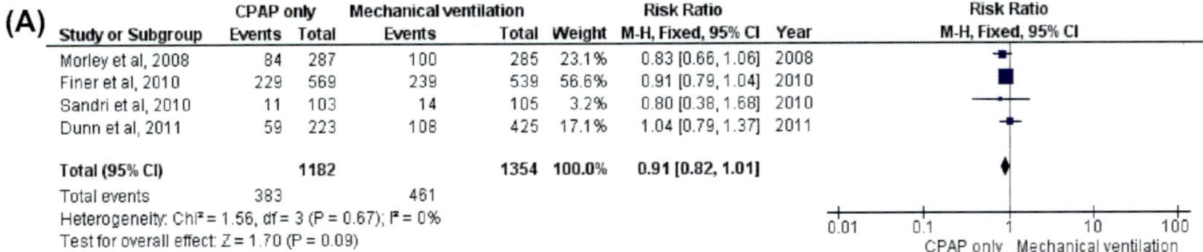

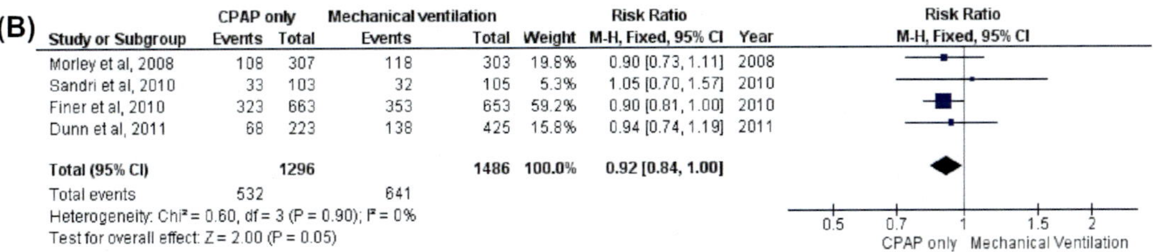

A, BPD. B, Death or BPD

FIG. 15.3 Forrest plot of CPAP versus mechanical ventilation or CPAP after INSURE as initial respiratory support. **A**, BPD. **B**, Death or BPD. *BPD*, bronchopulmonary dysplasia; *CPAP*, continuous positive airway pressure; *INSURE*, Intubate surfactant and extubate.

(A)

Study or Subgroup	CPAP or INSURE Events	Total	Mechanical Ventilation Events	Total	Weight	Risk Ratio M-H, Fixed, 95% CI	Year
Tooley et al, 2003	1	21	4	21	2.1%	0.25 [0.03, 2.05]	2003
Dani et al, 2004	0	13	3	14	1.8%	0.15 [0.01, 2.71]	2004
Morley et al, 2008	84	287	100	285	52.7%	0.83 [0.66, 1.06]	2008
Dunn et al, 2011	106	439	61	209	43.4%	0.83 [0.63, 1.08]	2011
Total (95% CI)		**760**		**529**	**100.0%**	**0.81 [0.68, 0.96]**	
Total events	191		168				

Heterogeneity: Chi² = 2.58, df = 3 (P = 0.46); I² = 0%
Test for overall effect: Z = 2.37 (P = 0.02)

Risk Ratio M-H, Fixed, 95% CI: 0.01 0.1 1 10 100 — CPAP or INSURE / Mechanical ventilation

(B)

Study or Subgroup	CPAP or INSURE Events	Total	Mechanical Ventilation Events	Total	Weight	Risk Ratio M-H, Fixed, 95% CI	Year
Morley et al, 2008	108	307	118	303	53.6%	0.90 [0.73, 1.11]	2008
Dunn et al, 2011	130	439	76	209	46.4%	0.81 [0.65, 1.03]	2011
Total (95% CI)		**746**		**512**	**100.0%**	**0.86 [0.74, 1.01]**	
Total events	238		194				

Heterogeneity: Chi² = 0.43, df = 1 (P = 0.51); I² = 0%
Test for overall effect: Z = 1.89 (P = 0.06)

Risk Ratio M-H, Fixed, 95% CI: 0.01 0.1 1 10 100 — CPAP or INSURE / Mechanical ventilation

A, BPD. B, Death or BPD

FIG. 15.4 Forrest plot of CPAP alone or CPAP after INSURE versus mechanical ventilation as initial respiratory support. **A**, BPD. **B**, Death or BPD. *CPAP*, continuous positive airway pressure; *INSURE*, Intubate surfactant and extubate; *BPD*, bronchopulmonary dysplasia.

occurred in 13 of 22 infants (59%) and 20 of 22 infants (91%) in the NIPPV and headbox group, respectively (RR, 0.65; 95% CI, 0.45–0.94; RD, −0.32; 95% CI, −0.56 to −0.08). BPD was not assessed and mortality did not differ between groups.[9]

Any NIPPV Device Compared to Supplemental Oxygen for Postextubation Support

A single trial compared NS-NIPPV to headbox.[102] The authors did not report rates of death or BPD. It randomized 95 infants with birth weight less than 2 kg. Infants received MV for at least 24 hours and were under 28 days of age. The outcome measure was reintubation within 72 hours. NIPPV significantly reduced extubation failure compared to headbox (RR, 0.25; 95% CI, 0.12−0.51; RD, −0.47; 95%CI, −0.64 to −0.29; NNT 2).

Comparison of NIPPV Devices for Initial Respiratory Support

We identified one studies in this category that randomized 124 infants.[103] NS-NIPPV was compared with bilevel CPAP. The study allowed sustained inflation (application of PIP of 20−30 cm H_2O during resuscitation for 10−20 seconds)[104] and INSURE during resuscitation. The composite outcome death or BPD was not reported in this study. The incidence of BPD was similar between interventions (RR, 1.00; 95% CI, 0.37−2.68; RD, 0.00; 95%CI, −0.11 to 0.11). The incidence of respiratory failure was not also significantly different (RR, 1.25; 95% CI, 0.53−2.96; RD, 0.03; 95%CI, −0.09 to 0.16).

As primary respiratory support for preterm infants with or without respiratory distress syndrome, there are no RCTs directly comparing N- to S-NIPPV.

Comparison of NIPPV devices for postextubation support

There are no studies comparing NS- with S-NIPPV or trials of NS- or S-NIPPV versus bilevel CPAP for the prevention of extubation failure.

NIPPV Devices Compared to Other Mode of NRS

Any form of NIPPV (NS- S-NIPPV and Bilevel CPAP) compared to CPAP for initial respiratory support

This is the most pragmatic approach, but suffers from lack of a specific ventilatory modality. We identified 16 studies which include 2,014 infants.[105−120] This added six new studies and 762 more subjects to the 2016 Cochrane review which included 10 studies (N = 1096).[121] We excluded one of the studies from the 2016 Cochrane review as it is only available as an abstract.[122] However, we also included one trial excluded in the Cochrane review, which utilized DuoPAP (Hamilton Medical, Bonaduz, Switzerland), which is a form of bilevel CPAP.[119] Three studies did not report BPD.[106,118,120] Only two studies reported the composite outcome death or BPD.[112,113] Most of the trials allowed for INSURE. One trial allowed the use of minimally invasive surfactant therapy (MIST).[113]

When pooled, there was no difference between NIPPV and CPAP for the outcome BPD (RR, 0.77; 95% CI, 0.58−1.01; RD, −0.03; 95% CI, −0.06 to 0.00) or the composite outcome death or BPD (RR, 0.79; 95% CI, 0.59−1.08; RD, −0.06; 95% CI, −0.15 to 0.02). The incidence of respiratory failure was reduced significantly by NIPPV (RR, 0.55; 95% CI, 0.46−0.65; RD, −0.12; 95% CI, −0.16 to −0.09; NNT, 8) (Fig. 15.5). These findings are similar to those reported in the 2016 Cochrane review.

NS-NIPPV compared to CPAP for initial respiratory support. Seven studies, which when pooled include 1077 infants, tested NS-NIPPV against CPAP.[106,107,112,113,116,118,120] Three did not report BPD.[106,118,120] One pragmatic study was classified as ineligible because it allowed various modes of NIPPV.[109] When pooled, the incidence of BPD was similar in both the NS-NIPPV and CPAP groups (RR, 0.75; 95% CI, 0.49−1.15; RD, −0.04; 95% CI, −0.20 to 0.10). There was, however, a significant reduction in the incidence of respiratory failure with the use of NS-NIPPV (RR, 0.57; 95% CI, 0.44−0.73; RD, −0.12; 95% CI, −0.17 to −0.07; NNT 8).

S−NIPPV compared to CPAP for initial respiratory support. There were four studies testing S-NIPPV, which when pooled include 338 infants.[108,110,114,117] S-NIPPV was superior to CPAP in the prevention of BPD (RR, 0.49; 95% CI, 0.30−0.81; RD, −0.11; 95% CI, −0.19 to −0.04; NNT, 9) and respiratory failure (RR, 0.40; 95% CI, 0.26−0.62; RD, −0.20; 95% CI, −0.29 to −0.12; NNT, 5).

Bilevel CPAP compared to CPAP for initial respiratory support. We identified four eligible studies that included 415 infants.[105,111,115,119] Only two reported rates of BPD.[105,111] Bilevel CPAP was associated with a significant reduction in respiratory failure (RR, 0.59; 95% CI, 0.38−0.94; RD, −0.08; 95% CI, −0.15 to −0.01, NNT 12) but had effect on BPD compared to CPAP (RR, 1.22; 95% CI, 0.49−3.01; RD, 0.01; 95% CI, −0.03 to 0.05).

Any form of NIPPV (NS-, S-NIPPV, and Bilevel CPAP) compared to CPAP for postrespiratory extubation support

We identified 12 eligible studies that included 2072 infants.[109,123−133] This added 2 studies and 641 more infants than the 2017 Cochrane review.[134] Only one study reported the composite outcome death or BPD.[130] Three studies did not report the outcome

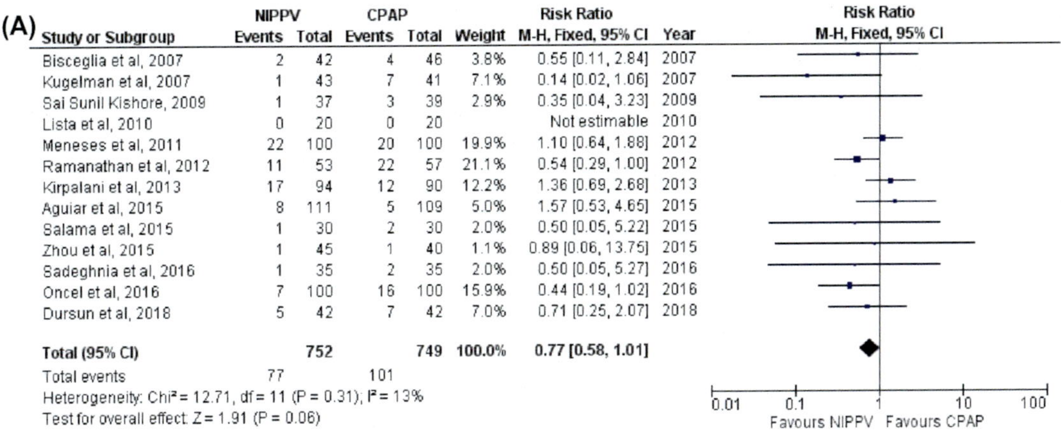

(B)

Study or Subgroup	NIPPV Events	NIPPV Total	CPAP Events	CPAP Total	Weight	Risk Ratio M-H, Fixed, 95% CI	Year
Kugelman et al, 2007	11	43	20	41		Not estimable	2007
Bisceglia et al, 2007	1	42	1	46		Not estimable	2007
Sai Sunil Kishore, 2009	7	37	16	39	7.0%	0.46 [0.21, 0.99]	2009
Lista et al, 2010	2	20	3	20	1.3%	0.67 [0.12, 3.57]	2010
Meneses et al, 2011	25	100	34	100	15.2%	0.74 [0.48, 1.14]	2012
Ramanathan et al, 2012	4	53	14	57	6.0%	0.31 [0.11, 0.87]	2012
Kirpalani et al, 2013	20	94	26	90	11.9%	0.74 [0.44, 1.22]	2013
Armanina et al, 2014	2	44	1	54	0.4%	2.45 [0.23, 26.18]	2014
Shi et al, 2014	7	71	14	73	6.2%	0.51 [0.22, 1.20]	2014
Zhou et al, 2015	2	45	9	40	4.3%	0.20 [0.05, 0.86]	2015
Aguiar et al, 2015	16	111	20	109	9.0%	0.79 [0.43, 1.43]	2015
Salama et al, 2015	3	30	6	30	2.7%	0.50 [0.14, 1.82]	2015
Silvera et al, 2015	12	40	25	40	11.2%	0.48 [0.28, 0.82]	2015
Oncel et al, 2016	13	100	29	100	13.0%	0.45 [0.25, 0.81]	2016
Sadeghnia et al, 2016	5	35	9	35	4.0%	0.56 [0.21, 1.49]	2016
Dursun et al, 2018	5	42	17	42	7.6%	0.29 [0.12, 0.72]	2018
Total (95% CI)		**822**		**829**	**100.0%**	**0.55 [0.45, 0.67]**	
Total events	123		223				

Heterogeneity: Chi² = 11.77, df = 13 (P = 0.55); I² = 0%
Test for overall effect: Z = 6.01 (P < 0.00001)

Risk Ratio M-H, Fixed, 95% CI: 0.01 0.1 1 10 100 — Favours NIPPV Favours CPAP

A, BPD. B, Respiratory failure

FIG. 15.5 Forrest plot of NIPPV (all types) versus CPAP as initial respiratory support. **A**, BPD. **B**, Respiratory failure. *NIPPV*, nasal intermittent positive pressure ventilation; *CPAP*, continuous positive airway pressure; *BPD*, bronchopulmonary dysplasia.

BPD. In the pooled analysis, the incidence of BPD was similar in both the NIPPV and CPAP groups (RR, 0.92; 95% CI, 0.82–1.03; RD, −0.03; 95% CI, −0.08 to 0.01) (Fig. 15.6). There was no difference in the composite outcome death or BPD (RR, 1.39; 95% CI, 0.90–2.16; RD, 0.18; 95% CI, −0.06 to 0.42). However, NIPPV significantly reduced the rate of postextubation failure (RR, 0.60; 95% CI, 0.45–0.81; RD, −0.15; 95% CI, −0.23 to −0.08; NNT 7) (Fig. 15.6). These findings are similar to that in the 2017 Cochrane review.

NS-NIPPV compared to CPAP for postextubation respiratory support. Only four studies that utilized NS-NIPPV exclusively were found, which when pooled included 279 infants.[127,130,131,133] The incidence of BPD was significantly reduced in the NS-NIPPV compared to CPAP group (RR, 0.60; 95% CI, 0.36–0.99; RD, −0.12; 95% CI, −0.22 to −0.01; NNT 8). Extubation failure was also significantly reduced in the NS-NIPPV compared to the CPAP group (RR, 0.53; 95% CI, 0.32–0.88; RD, −0.12; 95% CI, −0.22 to −0.03; NNT, 8).

S-NIPPV compared to CPAP for postextubation respiratory support. We identified five studies in this category, which included 272 infants.[123–126,128] Three assessed BPD[124–126] and showed a significant benefit of S-NIPPV compared to CPAP (RR, 0.64; 95%

(A)

Study or Subgroup	NIPPV Events	NIPPV Total	CPAP Events	CPAP Total	Weight	Risk Ratio M-H, Fixed, 95% CI	Year
Khalaf et al, 2001	12	34	16	30	4.6%	0.66 [0.38, 1.16]	2001
Barrington et al, 2001	12	27	15	27	4.1%	0.80 [0.47, 1.37]	2001
Moretti et al, 2008	2	32	7	31	1.9%	0.28 [0.06, 1.23]	2008
O'Brien et al, 2012	21	64	22	64	6.0%	0.95 [0.59, 1.55]	2012
Kahramaner et al, 2013	8	28	16	36	3.8%	0.64 [0.32, 1.28]	2013
Kirpalani et al, 2013	144	394	130	380	36.0%	1.07 [0.88, 1.29]	2013
Victor et al, 2016	132	270	143	270	38.9%	0.92 [0.78, 1.09]	2016
Jasani et al, 2016	2	31	9	32	2.4%	0.23 [0.05, 0.98]	2016
Ribeiro et al, 2017	6	36	12	65	2.3%	0.90 [0.37, 2.20]	2017
Total (95% CI)		**916**		**935**	**100.0%**	**0.92 [0.82, 1.03]**	
Total events	339		370				

Heterogeneity: Chi² = 11.00, df = 8 (P = 0.20); I² = 27%
Test for overall effect: Z = 1.44 (P = 0.15)

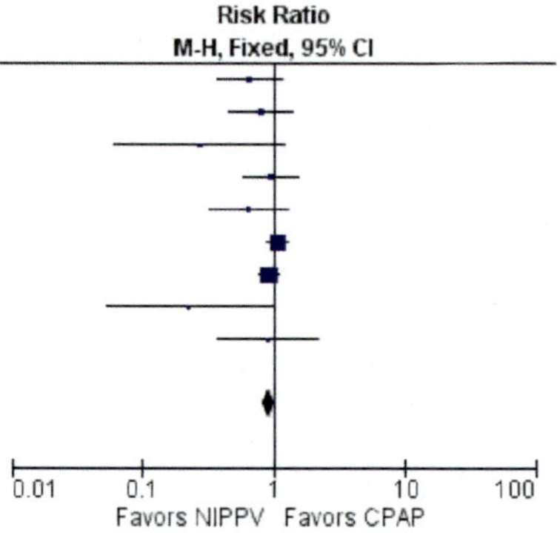

Risk Ratio M-H, Fixed, 95% CI: 0.01 0.1 1 10 100 — Favors NIPPV Favors CPAP

(B)

Study or Subgroup	NIPPV Events	NIPPV Total	CPAP Events	CPAP Total	Weight	Risk Ratio M-H, Fixed, 95% CI	Year
Friedlich et al, 1999	1	22	7	19	1.9%	0.12 [0.02, 0.91]	1999
Barrington et al, 2001	4	27	12	27	3.1%	0.33 [0.12, 0.90]	2001
Khalaf et al, 2001	2	34	12	30	3.3%	0.15 [0.04, 0.60]	2001
Moretti et al, 2008	2	32	12	31	3.1%	0.16 [0.04, 0.66]	2008
Khorana et al, 2009	2	24	4	24	1.0%	0.50 [0.10, 2.48]	2009
Gao et al, 2010	6	25	12	25	3.1%	0.50 [0.22, 1.12]	2010
O'Brien et al, 2012	22	67	29	69	7.4%	0.78 [0.50, 1.21]	2012
Kahramaner et al, 2013	5	39	10	28	3.0%	0.36 [0.14, 0.94]	2013
Kirpalani et al, 2013	156	423	182	422	47.0%	0.86 [0.72, 1.01]	2013
Victor et al, 2016	92	270	85	270	21.9%	1.08 [0.85, 1.38]	2016
Jasani et al, 2016	6	31	9	32	2.3%	0.69 [0.28, 1.70]	2016
Ribeiro et al, 2017	5	36	15	65	2.8%	0.60 [0.24, 1.52]	2017
Total (95% CI)		**1030**		**1042**	**100.0%**	**0.78 [0.69, 0.89]**	
Total events	303		389				

Heterogeneity: Chi² = 28.61, df = 11 (P = 0.003); I² = 62%
Test for overall effect: Z = 3.92 (P < 0.0001)

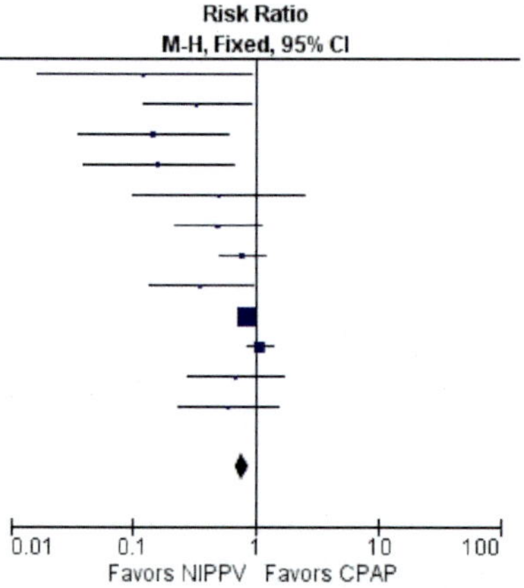

Risk Ratio M-H, Fixed, 95% CI: 0.01 0.1 1 10 100 — Favors NIPPV Favors CPAP

A, BPD. B, Respiratory failure

FIG. 15.6 Forrest plot of NIPPV (all types) versus CPAP as postextubation respiratory support. **A**, BPD. **B**, Respiratory failure. *NIPPV*, nasal intermittent positive pressure ventilation; *CPAP*, continuous positive airway pressure; *BPD*, bronchopulmonary dysplasia.

CI, 0.44–0.95; RD, −0.15; 95% CI, −0.28 to −0.02; NNT, 7) in reducing the incidence of BPD. In the five studies, extubation failure incidence was significantly reduced with S-NIPPV compared to CPAP (RR, 0.26; 95% CI, 0.16–0.44; RD, −0.31; 95% CI, −0.40 to −0.21; NNT, 3).

Bilevel CPAP compared to CPAP for postextubation respiratory support. In the two trials that utilized bilevel CPAP, when pooled included 679 infants.[129,132] The incidence of BPD did not differ between group (RR, 0.93; 95% CI, 0.79–1.09; RD, −0.04; 95% CI, −0.11 to 0.04. The incidence of postextubation respiratory failure also did not differ between groups (RR, 1.01; 95% CI, 0.81–1.24; RD, 0.00; 95% CI, −0.07 to 0.07).

HHFNC

HHFNC Compared to CPAP for Initial Respiratory Support

We identified six studies in this category which when pooled included 1539 infants.[135–140] Our analysis differs from that of a 2016 Cochrane review, in our selection of articles for inclusion.[141] We excluded two studies that are only available as abstracts.[142,143] We included one study not published in English.[139] The authors had provided data for the 2016 Cochrane review. Three studies reported the outcome BPD. In the analysis of the pooled data, BPD rates were similar in the HHFNC and CPAP groups (RR, 1.02; 95% CI, 0.60–1.74; RD, −0.00; 95% CI, −0.03 to 0.03). Only one study reported the composite outcome death or BPD,[135] which was not significant between the groups (RR, 1.03; 95% CI, 0.55–1.94; RD,

0.00; 95% CI, −0.04 to 0.04). However, CPAP significantly reduced the incidence of primary respiratory failure compared to HHFNC (RR, 1.86; 95% CI, 1.46−2.37; RD, 0.10; 95% CI, 0.06 to 0.13; NNT, 17) (Fig. 15.7).

HHFNC Compared to CPAP for PostExtubation Respiratory Support

We included seven trials in this category that included 943 infants.[136,144−148] Of these, two trial utilized the INSURE technique.[146,148] We excluded one study that was included in the 2016 Cochrane review. The study was not published in English and data from the published abstract differed from that of the Cochrane review which included six studies with 934 infants.[149] Four trials reported rates of BPD.[136,145,146,150] When pooled, there was no difference in the incidence of BPD (RR, 0.99; 95% CI, 0.77−1.26; RD, −0.00; 95% CI, −0.06 to 0.06), or respiratory failure (RR, 1.35; 95% CI, 0.86−2.11; RD, 0.07; 95% CI, −0.00 to 0.17) (Fig. 15.8).

HHFNC Compared to NIPPV for Initial Respiratory Support

In the one trial that compared HHFNC to NIPPV for primary respiratory support, there was no difference in intubation rates (RR, 0.96; 95% CI, 0.49−1.88; RD, −0.01; 95% CI, −0.01 to 0.08). No infant died in the study, and BPD rates did not differ (RR, 0.57; 95% CI, 0.05−5.99; RD, −0.02; 95% CI, −0.10 to 0.06) between groups.[151]

NHFV EVALUATIONS

Trials comparing nHFV to other forms of NRS in preterm infants are sparse. We identified three trials in the category that involved 239 infants. Two compared nHFV to CPAP[152,153] and one to bilevel CPAP.[154] In the study of nHFV versus bilevel CPAP, both modalities were applied as rescue for CPAP failure. Two assessed BPD.[152,154] When pooled, there were no significant differences in the incidence of BPD (RR, 0.92; 95% CI, 0.61−1.38; RD, −0.03; 95% CI, −0.16 to 0.10) (Fig. 15.9). nHFV significantly reduced the incidence of respiratory failure compared to CPAP (including bilevel CPAP) (RR, 0.47; 95% CI, 0.30−0.73; RD, −0.19; 95% CI, −0.29 to −0.09; NNT 5) (Fig. 15.9) and CPAP (excluding bilevel CPAP) (RR, 0.43; 95% CI, 0.25−0.75; RD, −0.17; 95% CI, −0.28 to −0.10; NNT 6).

CONCLUSION

BPD is associated with an increased incidence of morbidity and mortality. NRS to prevent lung injury

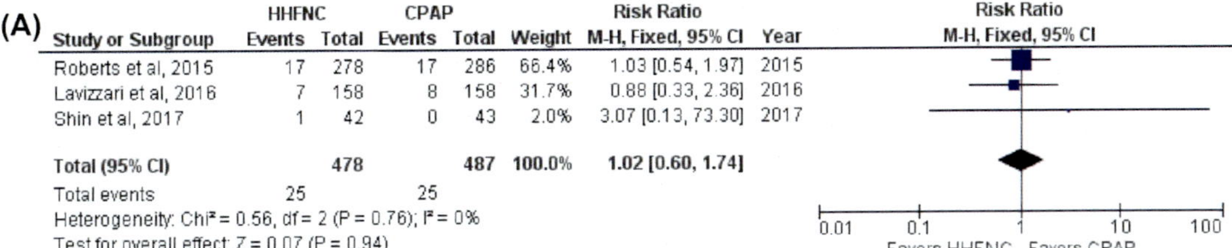

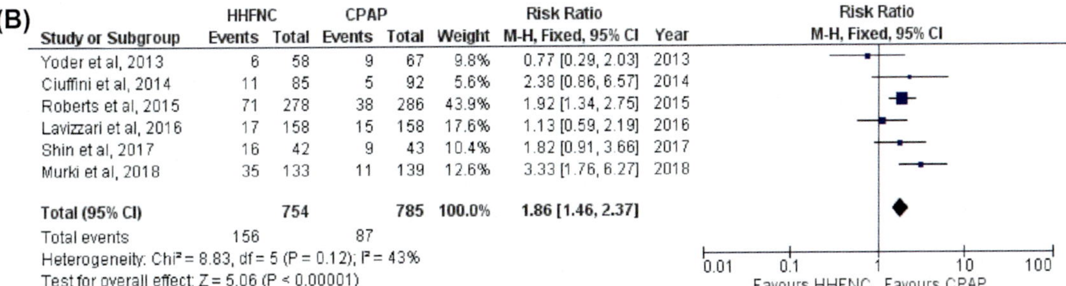

A, BPD. B, Respiratory failure

FIG. 15.7 Forrest plot of HHFNC versus CPAP as Initial respiratory support. **A**, BPD. **B**, Respiratory failure. *HHFNC*, heated humidified high flow nasal cannula; *CPAP*, continuous positive airway pressure; *BPD*, bronchopulmonary dysplasia.

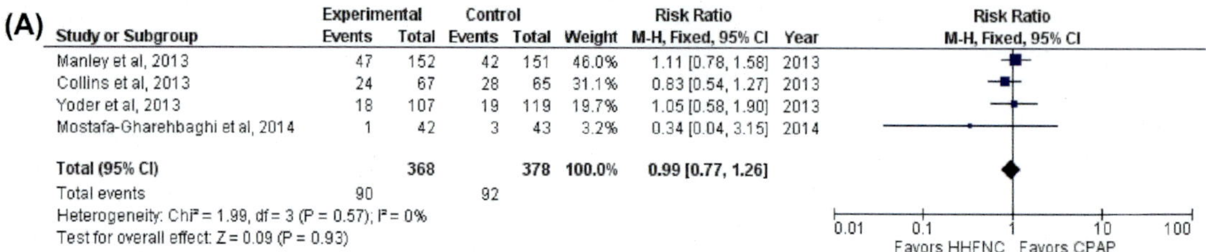

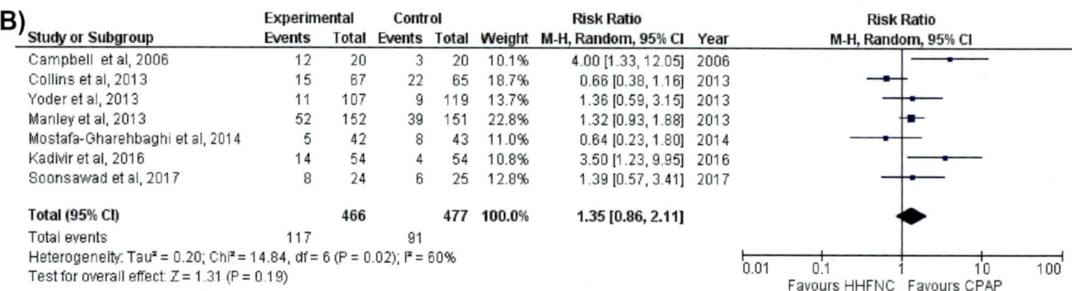

A, BPD. B, Respiratory failure

FIG. 15.8 Forrest plot of HHFNC versus CPAP as postextubation respiratory support. **A**, BPD. **B**, Respiratory failure. *HHFNC*, heated humidified high flow nasal cannula; *CPAP*, continuous positive airway pressure; *BPD*, bronchopulmonary dysplasia.

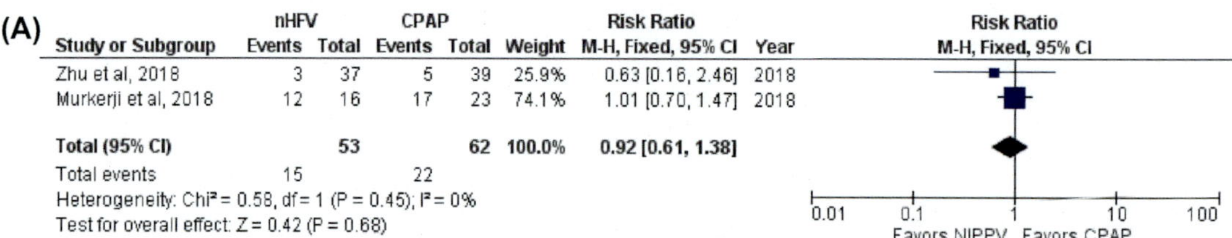

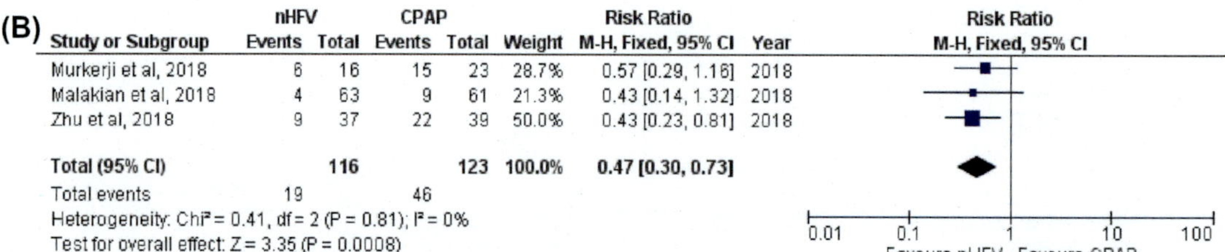

A, BPD. B, Respiratory failure

FIG. 15.9 Forrest plot of nHFV versus CPAP as initial respiratory support. **A**, BPD. **B**, Respiratory failure. *nHFV*, noninvasive high-frequency ventilation; *CPAP*, continuous positive airway pressure; *BPD*, bronchopulmonary dysplasia.

mediated by exposure to MV has become standard practice in modern neonatal medicine. NRS is available as CPAP, HHFNC, NIPPV, and nHFV. Available evidence from RCTs (Table 15.1) suggest that the incidence of BPD is significantly reduced when S-NIPPV is used for initial and postextubation support. NS-NIPPV is only superior to CPAP when used for postextubation support. Respiratory failure is significantly reduced when NIPPV is used for initial and postextubation respiratory support in preterm infants compared to CPAP, when all are grouped together, but segregated, only NS-NIPPV and S-NIPPV resulted in significant reduction. HHFNC

TABLE 15.1
Summary of Comparison on Noninvasive Support for the Prevention of BPD and Respiratory Failure.

Comparison	# Of Included Studies	# Of Subjects	Effect Size and Number Needed to Treat for the Outcome BPD	Effect Size and Number Needed to Treat for the Outcome Failure of Non-invasive Support
CPAP versus supplemental oxygen for initial respiratory support	8[69–76]	789	RR, 0.72; 95% CI, 0.41–1.25	RR, 0.75; 95% CI, 0.56–1.00; NNT 7
CPAP versus supplemental oxygen for postextubation respiratory support	9[83–91]	726	RR, 0.94; 95% CI, 0.64–1.37	RR, 0.63; 95% CI, 0.51–0.77; NNT 6
CPAP alone versus MV or INSURE for initial respiratory support	4[18,80–82]	2782	RR, 0.91; 95% CI, 0.82–1.01	NA
CPAP (with or without INSURE) versus MV for initial respiratory support	4[18,81,93,94]	1289	RR, 0.81; 95% CI, 0.68–0.96; NNT, 17	NA
Continuous versus variable flow CPAP devices for initial respiratory support	4[95–98]	450	RR, 1.13; 95% CI, 0.67–1.92	RR, 1.02; 95% CI, 0.70–1.48
Continuous versus variable flow CPAP devices for postextubation respiratory support	3[58,98,99]	459	RR, 0.97; 95% CI, 0.77–1.22	RR, 1.07; 95% CI, 0.65–1.78
NIPPV versus supplemental oxygen for initial respiratory support	1[9]	44	NA	RR, 0.65; 95% CI, 0.45–0.94
NIPPV versus supplemental oxygen for postextubation respiratory support	1[102]	95	NA	RR, 0.25; 95% CI, 0.12–0.51; NNT 2
NS-NIPPV versus bilevel CPAP for initial respiratory support	1[103]	124	RR, 1.00; 95% CI, 0.37–2.68	RR, 1.25; 95% CI, 0.53–2.96
Any form of NIPPV (NS-S-NIPPV and Bi-level CPAP) versus CPAP for initial respiratory support	16[105–120]	2014	RR, 0.77; 95% CI, 0.58–1.01	RR, 0.55; 95% CI, 0.46–0.65; NNT 8
NS-NIPPV versus CPAP for initial respiratory support	7[106,107,112,113,116,118,120]	1077	RR, 0.75; 95% CI, 0.49–1.15	RR, 0.57; 95% CI, 0.44–0.73; NNT 8
S–NIPPV versus CPAP for initial respiratory support	4[108,110,114,117]	338	RR, 0.49; 95% CI, 0.30–0.81; NNT 9	RR, 0.40; 95% CI, 0.26–0.62; NNT 5
Bilevel CPAP versus CPAP for initial respiratory support	4	415	RR, 1.22; 95% CI, 0.49–3.01	RR, 0.59; 95% CI, 0.38–0.94; NNT, 12

Continued

TABLE 15.1
Summary of Comparison on Noninvasive Support for the Prevention of BPD and Respiratory Failure.—cont'd

Comparison	# Of Included Studies	# Of Subjects	Effect Size and Number Needed to Treat for the Outcome BPD	Effect Size and Number Needed to Treat for the Outcome Failure of Non-invasive Support
Any form of NIPPV (NS-S-NIPPV and Bilevel CPAP) versus CPAP for postextubation respiratory support	12[109,123–133]	2072	RR, 0.92; 95% CI, 0.82–1.03	RR, 0.60; 95% CI, 0.45–0.81; NNT 7
NS-NIPPV versus CPAP for postextubation respiratory support	4[127,130,131,133]	279	RR, 0.60; 95% CI, 0.36–0.99; NNT 8	RR, 0.53; 95% CI, 0.32–0.88; NNT 8
S-NIPPV versus CPAP for postextubation respiratory support	5[123–126,128]	272	RR, 0.64; 95% CI, 0.44–0.95; NNT 7	RR, 0.26; 95% CI, 0.16–0.44, NNT 3
Bilevel CPAP versus CPAP for postextubation respiratory support	2[129,132]	679	RR, 0.93; 95% CI, 0.79–1.09	RR, 1.01; 95% CI, 0.81–1.24
HHFNC versus CPAP for initial respiratory support	6[135–140]	1539	RR, 1.02; 95% CI, 0.60–1.74	RR, 1.86; 95% CI, 1.46–2.37; NNT 15
HHFNC versus CPAP for postextubation respiratory support	7[136,144–148]	943	RR, 0.83; 95% CI, 0.67–1.03	RR, 1.35; 95% CI, 0.86–2.11
HHFNC versus NIPPV for initial respiratory support	1[151]	76	RR, 0.57; 95% CI, 0.05–5.99	RR, 0.96; 95% CI, 0.49–1.88
nHFV versus CPAP for initial respiratory support	3[152–154]	239	RR, 0.92; 95% CI, 0.61–1.38	RR, 0.47; 95% CI, 0.30–0.73; NNT

CI, confidence interval; *CPAP*, continuous positive airway pressure; *HHFNC*, heated humidified high flow nasal cannula; *INSURE*, Intubate surfactant and extubate; *MV*, mechanical ventilation; *nHFV*, noninvasive high-frequency ventilation; *NIPPV*, nasal intermittent positive pressure ventilation; *NNT*, number needed to treat; *RR*, relative risk.

and CPAP appear to have similar efficacy when used for postextubation support. CPAP only showed superiority over HHFNC in preventing respiratory failure when used as primary respiratory support. The few trials on nHFV suggest potential benefit over CPAP in the prevention of primary respiratory failure. Rigorous evaluation of efficacy and safety before widespread adoption into practice is required.

The superiority of one mode of NIPPV over another is undetermined due to scarcity of trials comparing different NIPPV modalities. Furthermore, restricted availability of some synchronized modes of NIPPV limits its application in clinical practices.

DISCLOSURE STATEMENT

None of the authors have any conflict of interest to declare.

REFERENCES

1. Harrison V, Heese HV, Klein M. The significance of grunting in hyaline membrane disease. *Pediatrics*. 1968;41(3): 549–559.
2. Northway Jr WH, Rosan RC, Porter DY. Pulmonary disease following respirator therapy of hyaline-membrane disease: bronchopulmonary dysplasia. *N Engl J Med*. 1967;276(7):357–368.
3. Gregory GA, Kitterman JA, Phibbs RH, Tooley WH, Hamilton WK. Treatment of the idiopathic respiratory-

distress syndrome with continuous positive airway pressure. *N Engl J Med.* 1971;284(24):1333–1340.
4. Stern L, Ramos AD, Outerbridge EW, Beaudry PH. Negative pressure artificial respiration: use in treatment of respiratory failure of the newborn. *Can Med Assoc J.* 1970; 102(6):595.
5. Donald I, Lord J. Augmented respiration studies in atelectasis neonatorum. *Lancet.* 1953;261(6749):e1.
6. Donald I. Augmented respiration: an emergency positive-pressure patient-cycled respirator. *Lancet.* 1954; 263(6818):895–899.
7. Delivoria-Papadopoulos M, Swyer PR. Assisted ventilation in terminal hyaline membrane disease. *Arch Dis Child.* 1964;39(207):481.
8. Shepard F, Gray J, Stahlman M. The occurrence of pulmonaryfibrosis in children who had idiopathic respiratory distress syndrome. *J Pediatr.* 1964;65(6): 1078–1079.
9. Llewellyn M, Tilak K, Swyer P. A controlled trial of assisted ventilation using an oro-nasal mask. *Arch Dis Child.* 1970;45(242):453–459.
10. Pape KE, Armstrong DL, Fitzhardinge PM. CNS pathology associated with mask ventilation. *Pediatrics.* 1977; 60(5):787–788.
11. Garland JS, Nelson DB, Rice T, Neu J. Increased risk of gastrointestinal perforations in neonates mechanically ventilated with either face mask or nasal prongs. *Pediatrics.* 1985;76(3):406–410.
12. Kirby R, Robison E, Schulz J. Continuous-flow ventilation as an alternative to assisted or controlled ventilation in infants. *Anesth Analg.* 1972;51(6):871–875.
13. Fujiwara T, Chida S, Watabe Y, Maeta H, Morita T, Abe T. Artificial surfactant therapy in hyaline-membrane disease. *Lancet.* 1980;315(8159):55–59.
14. Jobe A, Ikegami M. Surfactant for the treatment of respiratory distress syndrome. *Am J Respir Crit Care Med.* 1987; 136(5):1256–1275.
15. Liggins GC, Howie RN. A controlled trial of antepartum glucocorticoid treatment for prevention of the respiratory distress syndrome in premature infants. *Pediatrics.* 1972; 50(4):515–525.
16. Stoll BJ, Hansen NI, Bell EF, et al. Trends in care practices, morbidity, and mortality of extremely preterm neonates, 1993-2012. *JAMA.* 2015;314(10):1039–1051.
17. Avery ME, Tooley WH, Keller JB, et al. Is chronic lung disease in low birth weight infants preventable? A survey of eight centers. *Pediatrics.* 1987;79(1):26–30.
18. Morley CJ, Davis PG, Doyle LW, Brion LP, Hascoet JM, Carlin JB. Nasal CPAP or intubation at birth for very preterm infants. *N Engl J Med.* 2008;358(7):700–708.
19. Tooley WH. Epidemiology of bronchopulmonary dysplasia. *J Pediatr.* 1979;95(5 Pt 2):851–858.
20. Jobe AH, Bancalari E. Bronchopulmonary dysplasia. *Am J Respir Crit Care Med.* 2001;163(7):1723–1729.
21. Shennan AT, Dunn MS, Ohlsson A, Lennox K, Hoskins EM. Abnormal pulmonary outcomes in premature infants: prediction from oxygen requirement in the neonatal period. *Pediatrics.* 1988;82(4):527–532.
22. Walsh MC, Wilson-Costello D, Zadell A, Newman N, Fanaroff A. Safety, reliability, and validity of a physiologic definition of bronchopulmonary dysplasia. *J Perinatol.* 2003;23(6):451–456.
23. Walsh M, Laptook A, Kazzi SN, et al. A cluster-randomized trial of benchmarking and multimodal quality improvement to improve rates of survival free of bronchopulmonary dysplasia for infants with birth weights of less than 1250 grams. *Pediatrics.* 2007; 119(5):876–890.
24. Poindexter BB, Feng R, Schmidt B, et al. Comparisons and limitations of current definitions of bronchopulmonary dysplasia for the prematurity and respiratory outcomes program. *Ann Am Thor Soc.* 2015;12(12): 1822–1830.
25. Higgins RD, Jobe AH, Koso-Thomas M, et al. Bronchopulmonary dysplasia: executive summary of a workshop. *J Pediatr.* 2018;197:300–308.
26. Jensen EA, Wright CJ. *Bronchopulmonary Dysplasia: The Ongoing Search for One Definition to Rule Them All.* Elsevier; 2018.
27. Jensen EA, Schmidt B. Epidemiology of bronchopulmonary dysplasia. *Birth Defects Res A Clin Mol Teratol.* 2014;100(3):145–157.
28. Horbar JD, Edwards EM, Greenberg LT, et al. Variation in performance of neonatal intensive care units in the United States. *JAMA Pediatr.* 2017;171(3):e164396.
29. Schmidt B, Asztalos EV, Roberts RS, et al. Impact of bronchopulmonary dysplasia, brain injury, and severe retinopathy on the outcome of extremely low-birth-weight infants at 18 months: results from the trial of indomethacin prophylaxis in preterms. *JAMA.* 2003;289(9): 1124–1129.
30. Smith VC, Zupancic JA, McCormick MC, et al. Rehospitalization in the first year of life among infants with bronchopulmonary dysplasia. *J Pediatr.* 2004;144(6): 799–803.
31. Stoll BJ, Hansen NI, Bell EF, et al. Neonatal outcomes of extremely preterm infants from the NICHD Neonatal Research Network. *Pediatrics.* 2010;126(3):443–456.
32. Stroustrup A, Trasande L. Epidemiological characteristics and resource use in neonates with bronchopulmonary dysplasia: 1993–2006. *Pediatrics.* 2010;126(2):291–297.
33. Baraldi E, Filippone M. Chronic lung disease after premature birth. *N Engl J Med.* 2007;357(19):1946–1955.
34. Husain AN, Siddiqui NH, Stocker JT. Pathology of arrested acinar development in postsurfactant bronchopulmonary dysplasia. *Hum Pathol.* 1998;29(7):710–717.
35. O'reilly M, Sozo F, Harding R. Impact of preterm birth and bronchopulmonary dysplasia on the developing lung: long-term consequences for respiratory health. *Clin Exp Pharmacol Physiol.* 2013;40(11):765–773.
36. Philip AG. Oxygen plus pressure plus time: the etiology of bronchopulmonary dysplasia. *Pediatrics.* 1975;55(1): 44–50.
37. Dreyfuss D, Saumon G. Ventilator-induced lung injury: lessons from experimental studies. *Am J Respir Crit Care Med.* 1998;157(1):294–323.

38. Donn S, Sinha S. Minimising ventilator induced lung injury in preterm infants. *Arch Dis Child Fetal Neonatal Ed*. 2006;91(3):F226–F230.
39. Groneck P, Speer CP. Inflammatory mediators and bronchopulmonary dysplasia. *Arch Dis Child Fetal Neonatal Ed*. 1995;73(1):F1.
40. Jobe AJ. The new BPD: an arrest of lung development. *Pediatr Res*. 1999;46(6):641.
41. Laughon M, Bose C, Allred EN, et al. Antecedents of chronic lung disease following three patterns of early respiratory disease in preterm infants. *Arch Dis Child Fetal Neonatal Ed*. 2011;96(2):F114–F120.
42. Jensen EA, DeMauro SB, Kornhauser M, Aghai ZH, Greenspan JS, Dysart KC. Effects of multiple ventilation courses and duration of mechanical ventilation on respiratory outcomes in extremely low-birth-weight infants. *JAMA Pediatr*. 2015;169(11):1011–1017.
43. Van Marter LJ, Allred EN, Pagano M, et al. Do clinical markers of barotrauma and oxygen toxicity explain interhospital variation in rates of chronic lung disease? The Neonatology Committee for the Developmental Network. *Pediatrics*. 2000;105(6):1194–1201.
44. Oh W, Poindexter BB, Perritt R, et al. Association between fluid intake and weight loss during the first ten days of life and risk of bronchopulmonary dysplasia in extremely low birth weight infants. *J Pediatr*. 2005;147(6):786–790.
45. Papile L-A, Baley JE, Benitz W, et al. Respiratory support in preterm infants at birth. *Pediatrics*. 2014;133(1): 171–174.
46. Morley C. Continuous distending pressure. *Arch Dis Child Fetal Neonatal Ed*. 1999;81(2):F152–F156.
47. da Silva WJ, Abbasi S, Pereira G, Bhutani VK. Role of positive end-expiratory pressure changes on functional residual capacity in surfactant treated preterm infants. *Pediatr Pulmonol*. 1994;18(2):89–92.
48. Saunders RA, Milner AD, Hopkin IE. The effects of continuous positive airway pressure on lung mechanics and lung volumes in the neonate. *Biol Neonate*. 1976; 29(3–4):178–186.
49. Miller M, DiFiore J, Strohl K, Martin R. Effects of nasal CPAP on supraglottic and total pulmonary resistance in preterm infants. *J Appl Physiol*. 1990;68(1):141–146.
50. Agostoni E. Statics of the respiratory system. In: handbook of physiology. *Am Physiol Soc*. 1964;1:387–409.
51. Chernick V. Hyaline-membrane disease: therapy with constant lung-distending pressure. *N Engl J Med*. 1973; 289(6):302–304.
52. Polin RA, Sahni R. Newer experience with CPAP. *Semin Neonatol*. 2002;7(5):379–389.
53. Gal TJ. Nunn's applied respiratory physiology. *Anesth Analg*. 2000;90(4):1010.
54. Miller MJ, Carlo WA, Martin RJ. Continuous positive airway pressure selectively reduces obstructive apnea in preterm infants. *J Pediatr*. 1985;106(1):91–94.
55. Courtney SE, Barrington KJ. Continuous positive airway pressure and noninvasive ventilation. *Clin Perinatol*. 2007;34(1):73–92.
56. Pillow JJ, Hillman N, Moss TJ, et al. Bubble continuous positive airway pressure enhances lung volume and gas exchange in preterm lambs. *Am J Respir Crit Care Med*. 2007;176(1):63–69.
57. Morley CJ, Lau R, De Paoli A, Davis PG. Nasal continuous positive airway pressure: does bubbling improve gas exchange? *Arch Dis Child Fetal Neonatal Ed*. 2005;90(4): F343–F344.
58. Gupta S, Sinha SK, Tin W, Donn SM. A randomized controlled trial of post-extubation bubble continuous positive airway pressure versus Infant Flow Driver continuous positive airway pressure in preterm infants with respiratory distress syndrome. *J Pediatr*. 2009;154(5), 645-650. e2.
59. Mikalsen IB, Davis P, Øymar K. High flow nasal cannula in children: a literature review. *Scand J Trauma Resusc Emerg Med*. 2016;24(1):93.
60. Nasal intermittent positive pressure ventilation in preterm infants: equipment, evidence, and synchronization. In: Owen LS, Manley BJ, eds. *Seminars in Fetal and Neonatal Medicine*. Elsevier; 2016.
61. Owen LS, Morley CJ, Davis PG. Neonatal nasal intermittent positive pressure ventilation: what do we know in 2007? *Arch Dis Child Fetal Neonatal Ed*. 2007;92(5): F414–F418.
62. Dumpa V, Katz K, Northrup V, Bhandari V. SNIPPV vs NIPPV: does synchronization matter? *J Perinatol*. 2012; 32(6):438.
63. High-frequency ventilation for non-invasive respiratory support of neonates. In: Yoder BA, Albertine K, Null Jr D, eds. *Seminars in Fetal and Neonatal Medicine*. Elsevier; 2016.
64. Pillow JJ. High-frequency oscillatory ventilation: mechanisms of gas exchange and lung mechanics. *Crit Care Med*. 2005;33(3):S135–S141.
65. Mukerji A, Dunn M. High-frequency ventilation as a mode of noninvasive respiratory support. *Clin Perinatol*. 2016;43(4):725–740.
66. Higgins JP. *Cochrane Handbook for Systematic Reviews of Interventions*. version 5.0. 1. The Cochrane Collaboration; 2008. http://www_cochrane-handbook_org.
67. Moher D, Liberati A, Tetzlaff J, Altman DG, Group P. Preferred reporting items for systematic reviews and meta-analyses: the PRISMA statement. *PLoS Medicine*. 2009;6(7):e1000097.
68. Collaboration C. *Review Manager (RevMan) 5.3 [program]. 5.3. 5 (Build Date: 30/10/14 11: 54) Version*. Copenhagen: The Nordic Cochrane Centre, The Cochrane Collaboration; 2014.
69. Fanaroff AA, Cha CC, Sosa R, Crumrine RS, Klaus MH. Controlled trial of continuous negative external pressure in the treatment of severe respiratory distress syndrome. *J Pediatr*. 1973;82(6):921–928.
70. Rhodes PG, Hall RT. Continuous positive airway pressure delivered by face mask in infants with the idiopathic respiratory distress syndrome: a controlled study. *Pediatrics*. 1973;52(1):1–5.

71. Durbin G, Hunter N, McIntosh N, Reynolds E, Wimberley P. Controlled trial of continuous inflating pressure for hyaline membrane disease. *Arch Dis Child.* 1976;51(3):163–169.
72. Belenky DA, Orr RJ, Woodrum DE, Hodson WA. Is continuous transpulmonary pressure better than conventional respiratory management of hyaline membrane disease? A controlled study. *Pediatrics.* 1976;58(6): 800–808.
73. Han VK, Beverley DW, Clarson C, et al. Randomized controlled trial of very early continuous distending pressure in the management of preterm infants. *Early Human Dev.* 1987;15(1):21–32.
74. Buckmaster AG, Arnolda G, Wright IM, Foster JP, Henderson-Smart DJ. Continuous Positive Airway Pressure Therapy for infants with respiratory distress in non–tertiary care centers: a randomized, controlled trial. *Pediatrics.* 2007;120(3):509–518.
75. Tapia JL, Urzua S, Bancalari A, et al. Randomized trial of early bubble continuous positive airway pressure for very low birth weight infants. *J Pediatr.* 2012;161(1): 75–80.e1.
76. Gonçalves-Ferri W, Martinez FE, Caldas J, et al. Application of continuous positive airway pressure in the delivery room: a multicenter randomized clinical trial. *Braz J Med Biol Res.* 2014;47(3):259–264.
77. Subramaniam P, Ho JJ, Davis PG. Prophylactic nasal continuous positive airway pressure for preventing morbidity and mortality in very preterm infants. *Cochrane Database Syst Rev.* 2016;(6).
78. Ho JJ, Subramaniam P, Davis PG. Continuous distending pressure for respiratory distress in preterm infants. *Cochrane Database Syst Rev.* 2015;(7). Cd002271.
79. Samuels MP, Raine J, Wright T, et al. Continuous negative extrathoracic pressure in neonatal respiratory failure. *Pediatrics.* 1996;98(6 Pt 1):1154–1160.
80. Finer NN, Carlo WA, Walsh MC, et al. Early CPAP versus surfactant in extremely preterm infants. *N Engl J Med.* 2010;362(21):1970–1979.
81. Dunn MS, Kaempf J, de Klerk A, et al. Randomized trial comparing 3 approaches to the initial respiratory management of preterm neonates. *Pediatrics.* 2011;128(5): e1069–e1076.
82. Sandri F, Plavka R, Ancora G, et al. Prophylactic or early selective surfactant combined with nCPAP in very preterm infants. *Pediatrics.* 2010;125(6):e1402–e1409.
83. Engelke SC, Roloff DW, Kuhns LR. Postextubation nasal continuous positive airway pressure: a prospective controlled study. *Am J Dis Child.* 1982;136(4):359–361.
84. Higgins RD, Richter SE, Davis JM. Nasal continuous positive airway pressure facilitates extubation of very low birth weight neonates. *Pediatrics.* 1991;88(5):999–1003.
85. Chan V, Greenough A. Randomised trial of methods of extubation in acute and chronic respiratory distress. *Arch Dis Child.* 1993;68(5 Spec No):570–572.
86. Annibale DJ, Hulsey TC, Engstrom PC, Wallin LA, Ohning BL. Randomized, controlled trial of nasopharyngeal continuous positive airway pressure in the extubation of very low birth weight infants. *J Pediatr.* 1994;124(3):455–460.
87. So B-H, Tamura M, Mishina J, Watanabe T, Kamoshita S. Application of nasal continuous positive airway pressure to early extubation in very low birthweight infants. *Arch Dis Child Fetal Neonatal Ed.* 1995;72(3):F191–F193.
88. Davis PG, Henderson-Smart DJ. Nasal continuous positive airways pressure immediately after extubation for preventing morbidity in preterm infants. *Cochrane Database Syst Rev.* 2003;(2). Cd000143.
89. Dimitriou G, Greenough A, Kavvadia V, et al. Elective use of nasal continuous positive airways pressure following extubation of preterm infants. *Eur J Pediatr.* 2000; 159(6):434–439.
90. Peake M, Dillon P, Shaw N. Randomized trial of continuous positive airways pressure to prevent reventilation in preterm infants. *Pediatr Pulmonol.* 2005;39(3):247–250.
91. Tapia JL, Bancalari A, González A, Mercado ME. Does continuous positive airway pressure (CPAP) during weaning from intermittent mandatory ventilation in very low birth weight infants have risks or benefits? A controlled trial. *Pediatr Pulmonol.* 1995;19(5):269–274.
92. Davis P, Jankov R, Doyle L, Henschke P. Randomised, controlled trial of nasal continuous positive airway pressure in the extubation of infants weighing 600 to 1250 g. *Arch Dis Child Fetal Neonatal Ed.* 1998;79(1):F54–F57.
93. Tooley J, Dyke M. Randomized study of nasal continuous positive airway pressure in the preterm infant with respiratory distress syndrome. *Acta Paediatr.* 2003;92(10): 1170–1174.
94. Dani C, Bertini G, Pezzati M, Cecchi A, Caviglioli C, Rubaltelli FF. Early extubation and nasal continuous positive airway pressure after surfactant treatment for respiratory distress syndrome among preterm infants <30 weeks' gestation. *Pediatrics.* 2004;113(6): e560–e563.
95. Mazzella M, Bellini C, Calevo M, et al. A randomised control study comparing the Infant Flow Driver with nasal continuous positive airway pressure in preterm infants. *Arch Dis Child Fetal Neonatal Ed.* 2001;85(2):F86–F90.
96. Mazmanyan P, Mellor K, Doré C, Modi N. A randomised controlled trial of flow driver and bubble continuous positive airway pressure in preterm infants in a resource-limited setting. *Arch Dis Child Fetal Neonatal Ed.* 2016;101(1):16–20.
97. Bhatti A, Khan J, Murki S, Sundaram V, Saini SS, Kumar P. Nasal Jet-CPAP (variable flow) versus Bubble-CPAP in preterm infants with respiratory distress: an open label, randomized controlled trial. *J Perinatol.* 2015;35(11): 935–940.
98. Bober K, Swietlinski J, Zejda J, et al. A multicenter randomized controlled trial comparing effectiveness of two nasal continuous positive airway pressure devices in very-low-birth-weight infants. *Pediatr Crit Care Med.* 2012;13(2):191–196.
99. Stefanescu BM, Murphy WP, Hansell BJ, Fuloria M, Morgan TM, Aschner JL. A randomized, controlled trial comparing two different continuous positive airway

pressure systems for the successful extubation of extremely low birth weight infants. *Pediatrics*. 2003; 112(5):1031–1038.

100. Sun SC, Tien HC. Randomized controlled trial of two methods of nasal CPAP(NCPAP): flow driver vs conventional NCPAP. *Pediatr Res*. 1999;45:322A.
101. Roukema H, O'Brien K, Nesbitt K, Zaw W. A randomized controlled trial of infant flow continuous positive airway pressure (CPAP) versus nasopharyngeal CPAP in the extubation of babies ≤ 1250 grams. *Pediatr Res*. 1999; 45:318A.
102. Kumar M, Avasthi S, Ahuja S, Malik G, Singh S. Unsynchronized nasal intermittent positive pressure ventilation to prevent extubation failure in neonates: a randomized controlled trial. *Indian J Pediatr*. 2011; 78(7):801–806.
103. Salvo V, Lista G, Lupo E, et al. Noninvasive ventilation strategies for early treatment of RDS in preterm infants: an RCT. *Pediatrics*. 2015;135(3):444–451.
104. Foglia EE, Te Pas AB. Sustained lung inflation: physiology and practice. *Clin Perinatol*. 2016;43(4):633–646.
105. Aguiar T, Macedo I, Voutsen O, Silva P, Nona J, Araujo C. Nasal bilevel versus continuous positive airway pressure in preterm infants: a randomized controlled trial. *J Clin Trials*. 2015;5(3):221.
106. Armanian A-m, Badiee Z, Heidari G, Feizi A, Salehimehr N. Initial treatment of respiratory distress syndrome with nasal intermittent mandatory ventilation versus nasal continuous positive airway pressure: a randomized controlled trial. *Int J Prev Med*. 2014;5(12): 1543.
107. Bisceglia M, Belcastro A, Poerio V, et al. A comparison of nasal intermittent versus continuous positive pressure delivery for the treatment of moderate respiratory syndrome in preterm infants. *Minerva Pediatrica*. 2007; 59(2):91–95.
108. Dursun M, Uslu S, Bulbul A, Celik M, Zubarioglu U, Bas EK. Comparison of early nasal intermittent positive pressure ventilation and nasal continuous positive airway pressure in preterm infants with respiratory distress syndrome. *J Trop Pediatr*. 2018.
109. Kirpalani H, Millar D, Lemyre B, Yoder BA, Chiu A, Roberts RS. A trial comparing noninvasive ventilation strategies in preterm infants. *N Engl J Med*. 2013; 369(7):611–620.
110. Kugelman A, Feferkorn I, Riskin A, Chistyakov I, Kaufman B, Bader D. Nasal intermittent mandatory ventilation versus nasal continuous positive airway pressure for respiratory distress syndrome: a randomized, controlled, prospective study. *J Pediatr*. 2007;150(5), 521-526, 6.e1.
111. Lista G, Castoldi F, Fontana P, et al. Nasal continuous positive airway pressure (CPAP) versus bi-level nasal CPAP in preterm babies with respiratory distress syndrome: a randomised control trial. *Arch Dis Child Fetal Neonatal Ed*. 2010;95(2):F85–F89.
112. Meneses J, Bhandari V, Alves JG, Herrmann D. Noninvasive ventilation for respiratory distress syndrome: a randomized controlled trial. *Pediatrics*. 2011;127(2): 300–307.
113. Oncel MY, Arayici S, Uras N, et al. Nasal continuous positive airway pressure versus nasal intermittent positive-pressure ventilation within the minimally invasive surfactant therapy approach in preterm infants: a randomised controlled trial. *Arch Dis Child Fetal Neonatal Ed*. 2016;101(4):F323–F328.
114. Ramanathan R, Sekar K, Rasmussen M, Bhatia J, Soll R. Nasal intermittent positive pressure ventilation after surfactant treatment for respiratory distress syndrome in preterm infants< 30 weeks' gestation: a randomized, controlled trial. *J Perinatol*. 2012;32(5):336.
115. Sadeghnia A, Barekateyn B, Badiei Z, Hosseini SM. Analysis and comparison of the effects of N-BiPAP and Bubble-CPAP in treatment of preterm newborns with the weight of below 1500 grams affiliated with respiratory distress syndrome: a randomised clinical trial. *Adv Biomed Res*. 2016;5:3.
116. Sai Sunil Kishore M, Dutta S, Kumar P. Early nasal intermittent positive pressure ventilation versus continuous positive airway pressure for respiratory distress syndrome. *Acta Paediatr*. 2009;98(9):1412–1415.
117. Salama GSA, Ayyash FF, Al-Rabadi AJ, Alquran ML, Shakkoury AG. Nasal -IMV versus Nasal-CPAP as an initial mode of respiratory support for premature infants with RD: a prospective randomized clinical trial. *Rawal Med J*. 2015;40(2):197–202.
118. Shi Y, Tang S, Zhao J, Shen J. A prospective, randomized, controlled study of NIPPV versus nCPAP in preterm and term infants with respiratory distress syndrome. *Pediatr Pulmonol*. 2014;49(7):673–678.
119. Zhou B, Zhai J, Jiang H, et al. Usefulness of DuoPAP in the treatment of very low birth weight preterm infants with neonatal respiratory distress syndrome. *Eur Rev Med Pharmacol Sci*. 2015;19(4):573–577.
120. Silveira CST, Leonardi KM, Melo APCF, Zaia JE, Brunherotti MAA. Response of preterm infants to 2 noninvasive ventilatory support systems: nasal CPAP and nasal intermittent positive-pressure ventilation. *Respir Care*. 2015;60(12):1772–1776.
121. Lemyre B, Laughon M, Bose C, Davis PG. Early nasal intermittent positive pressure ventilation (NIPPV) versus early nasal continuous positive airway pressure (NCPAP) for preterm infants. *Cochrane Database Syst Rev*. 2016; (12).
122. Wood F, Gupta S, Tin W, Sinha S. G170 randomised controlled trial of synchronised intermittent positive airway pressure (SiPAP™) versus continuous positive airway pressure (CPAP) as a primary mode of respiratory support in preterm infants with respiratory distress syndrome. *Arch Dis Child*. 2013;98(suppl 1). A78-A.
123. Friedlich P, Lecart C, Posen R, Ramicone E, Chan L, Ramanathan R. A randomized trial of nasopharyngeal-synchronized intermittent mandatory ventilation versus nasopharyngeal continuous positive airway pressure in very low birth weight infants after extubation. *J Perinatol*. 1999;19(6 Pt 1):413–418.

124. Barrington KJ, Bull D, Finer NN. Randomized trial of nasal synchronized intermittent mandatory ventilation compared with continuous positive airway pressure after extubation of very low birth weight infants. *Pediatrics.* 2001;107(4):638–641.
125. Khalaf MN, Brodsky N, Hurley J, Bhandari V. A prospective randomized, controlled trial comparing synchronized nasal intermittent positive pressure ventilation versus nasal continuous positive airway pressure as modes of extubation. *Pediatrics.* 2001;108(1):13–17.
126. Moretti C, Giannini L, Fassi C, Gizzi C, Papoff P, Colarizi P. Nasal flow-synchronized intermittent positive pressure ventilation to facilitate weaning in very low-birthweight infants: unmasked randomized controlled trial. *Pediatr Int.* 2008;50(1):85–91.
127. Khorana M, Paradeevisut H, Sangtawesin V, Kanjanapatanakul W, Chotigeat U, Ayutthaya J. A randomized trial of non-synchronized Nasopharyngeal Intermittent Mandatory Ventilation (nsNIMV) vs. Nasal Continuous Positive Airway Pressure (NCPAP) in the prevention of extubation failure in pre-term< 1,500 grams. *J Med Assoc Thailand.* 2008;91:S136–S142.
128. Gao W, Tan S, Chen Y, Zhang Y, Wang Y. Randomized trail of nasal synchronized intermittent mandatory ventilation compared with nasal continuous positive airway pressure in preterm infants with respiratory distress syndrome. *Zhongguo dang dai er ke za zhi.* 2010;12(7): 524–526.
129. O'Brien K, Campbell C, Brown L, Wenger L, Shah V. Infant flow biphasic nasal continuous positive airway pressure (BP-NCPAP) vs. infant flow NCPAP for the facilitation of extubation in infants'≤ 1,250 grams: a randomized controlled trial. *BMC Pediatrics.* 2012;12(1):43.
130. Kahramaner Z, Erdemir A, Turkoglu E, Cosar H, Sutcuoglu S, Ozer EA. Unsynchronized nasal intermittent positive pressure versus nasal continuous positive airway pressure in preterm infants after extubation. *J Matern Fetal Neonatal Med.* 2014;27(9):926–929.
131. Jasani B, Nanavati R, Kabra N, Rajdeo S, Bhandari V. Comparison of non-synchronized nasal intermittent positive pressure ventilation versus nasal continuous positive airway pressure as post-extubation respiratory support in preterm infants with respiratory distress syndrome: a randomized controlled trial. *J Matern Fetal Neonatal Med.* 2016;29(10):1546–1551.
132. Victor S, Roberts SA, Mitchell S, Aziz H, Lavender T. Biphasic positive airway pressure or continuous positive airway pressure: a randomized trial. *Pediatrics.* 2016; 138(2).
133. Ribeiro SNS, Fontes MJF, Bhandari V, Resende CB, Johnston C. Noninvasive ventilation in Newborns≤ 1,500 g after tracheal extubation: randomized clinical trial. *Am J Perinatol.* 2017;34(12):1190–1198.
134. Lemyre B, Davis PG, De Paoli AG, Kirpalani H. Nasal intermittent positive pressure ventilation (NIPPV) versus nasal continuous positive airway pressure (NCPAP) for preterm neonates after extubation. *Cochrane Database Syst Rev.* 2017;(2).
135. Roberts CT, Owen LS, Manley BJ, et al. Nasal high-flow therapy for primary respiratory support in preterm infants. *N Engl J Med.* 2016;375(12):1142–1151.
136. Yoder BA, Stoddard RA, Li M, King J, Dirnberger DR, Abbasi S. Heated, humidified high-flow nasal cannula versus nasal CPAP for respiratory support in neonates. *Pediatrics.* 2013;131(5):e1482–e1490.
137. Shin J, Park K, Lee EH, Choi BM. Humidified high flow nasal cannula versus nasal continuous positive airway pressure as an initial respiratory support in preterm infants with respiratory distress: a randomized, controlled non-inferiority trial. *J Korean Med Sci.* 2017;32(4): 650–655.
138. Murki S, Singh J, Khant C, et al. High-flow nasal cannula versus nasal continuous positive airway pressure for primary respiratory support in preterm infants with respiratory distress: a randomized controlled trial. *Neonatology.* 2018;113(3):235–241.
139. Ciuffini F, Pietrasanta C, Lavizzari A, et al. Comparison between two different modes of non-invasive ventilatory support in preterm newborn infants with respiratory distress syndrome mild to moderate: preliminary data. *La Pediatria Medica e Chirurgica.* 2014.
140. Lavizzari A, Colnaghi M, Ciuffini F, et al. Heated, humidified high-flow nasal cannula vs nasal continuous positive airway pressure for respiratory distress syndrome of prematurity: a randomized clinical noninferiority trial. *JAMA Pediatr.* 2016.
141. Wilkinson D, Andersen C, O'Donnell CP, De Paoli AG, Manley BJ. High flow nasal cannula for respiratory support in preterm infants. *Cochrane Database Syst Rev.* 2016;2. Cd006405.
142. Iranpour R, Sadeghnia A, Hesaraki M. 393 high-flow nasal cannula versus nasal continuous positive airway pressure in the management of respiratory distress syndrome. *Arch Dis Child.* 2012;97(Suppl 2): A115–A116.
143. Nair G, Karna P. Comparison of the effects of Vapotherm and nasal CPAP in respiratory distress in preterm infants. *E-PAS.* 2005;57:2054.
144. Soonsawad S, Swatesutipun B, Limrungsikul A, Nuntnarumit P. Heated humidified high-flow nasal cannula for prevention of extubation failure in preterm infants. *Indian J Pediatr.* 2017;84(4):262–266.
145. Manley BJ, Owen LS, Doyle LW, et al. High-flow nasal cannulae in very preterm infants after extubation. *N Engl J Med.* 2013;369(15):1425–1433.
146. Mostafa-Gharehbaghi M, Mojabi H. Comparing the effectiveness of nasal continuous positive airway pressure (NCPAP) and high flow nasal cannula (HFNC) in prevention of post extubation assisted ventilation. *Zahedan J. Res. Med. Sci.* 2015;17(6).
147. Campbell D, Shah P, Shah V, Kelly E. Nasal continuous positive airway pressure from high flow cannula versus infant flow for preterm infants. *J Perinatol.* 2006;26(9): 546.
148. Kadivar M, Mosayebi Z, Razi N, Nariman S, Sangsari R. High flow nasal cannulae versus nasal continuous

positive airway pressure in neonates with respiratory distress syndrome managed with Insure method: a randomized clinical trial. *Iran J Med Sci*. 2016;41(6):494.

149. Liu C. Efficacy and safety of heated humidified high-flow nasal cannula for prevention of extubation failure in neonates. *Zhonghua er ke za zhi*. 2014;52(4):271–276.
150. Collins CL, Holberton JR, Barfield C, Davis PG. A randomized controlled trial to compare heated humidified high-flow nasal cannulae with nasal continuous positive airway pressure postextubation in premature infants. *J Pediatr*. 2013;162(5):949–954.e1.
151. Kugelman A, Riskin A, Said W, Shoris I, Mor F, Bader D. A randomized pilot study comparing heated humidified high-flow nasal cannulae with NIPPV for RDS. *Pediatr Pulmonol*. 2015;50(6):576–583.
152. Zhu XW, Zhao JN, Tang SF, Yan J, Shi Y. Noninvasive high-frequency oscillatory ventilation versus nasal continuous positive airway pressure in preterm infants with moderate-severe respiratory distress syndrome: a preliminary report. *Pediatr Pulmonol*. 2017;52(8):1038–1042.
153. Malakian A, Bashirnezhadkhabaz S, Aramesh MR, Dehdashtian M. Noninvasive high-frequency oscillatory ventilation versus nasal continuous positive airway pressure in preterm infants with respiratory distress syndrome: a randomized controlled trial. *J Matern Fetal Neonatal Med*. 2018:1–151.
154. Mukerji A, Sarmiento K, Lee B, Hassall K, Shah V. Noninvasive high-frequency ventilation versus bi-phasic continuous positive airway pressure (BP-CPAP) following CPAP failure in infants< 1250 g: a pilot randomized controlled trial. *J Perinatol*. 2017;37(1):49.

CHAPTER 16

Pharmacological Therapies for the Prevention of Bronchopulmonary Dysplasia

ERIK A. JENSEN, MD, MSCE • BARBARA SCHMIDT, MD, MSC

INTRODUCTION

Bronchopulmonary dysplasia (BPD) is the most common and one of the most consequential morbidities in very preterm infants. BPD affects approximately half of all infants born with birth weights less than 1000g and is associated with long-term impairments of lung function, growth, and neurodevelopment.[1–7] Most data indicate that BPD rates have not improved in recent decades.[7–9] The lack of safe and effective means to provide the necessary respiratory support for very immature infants is one hindrance to reducing the high frequency of BPD. Despite the strong physiologic data implicating lung injury from positive airway pressure and supplemental oxygen in the development of BPD, use of "gentle" respiratory support strategies have produced only modest benefits.[10–13] As such, evidence-based drug therapy must be included in a comprehensive approach to the prevention of BPD. In this chapter, we review the evidence for pharmacological agents that have been shown in randomized controlled trials (RCTs), or meta-analyses of RCTs, to reduce the risks of BPD or the composite outcome of death or BPD in very preterm infants. In addition, we discuss several drug therapies that have been hypothesized to reduce the risk of BPD but lack robust evidence to support their current use for BPD prevention. BPD was defined throughout this chapter as the use of supplemental oxygen at a postmenstrual age (PMA) of 36 weeks.[14]

DATA PRESENTATION

We present all estimates of treatment effects using risk differences (RDs) and the numbers needed to treat (NNTs) or harm (NNH). For therapies evaluated in a single RCT only, the RD was calculated by subtracting the proportion of infants with the outcome of interest in the intervention group from that in the randomized comparison group.[15] For therapies evaluated in multiple RCTs, the pooled RD was calculated using a pooled relative risk.[15] All relative risks were derived from fixed effects meta-analyses unless a random effects model was utilized in the cited systematic review. All event rates were extracted from the cited references. The NNT or NNH is the inverse of the RD.

PHARMACOLOGICAL THERAPIES THAT REDUCE THE RISK OF BPD

Caffeine

Caffeine is a methylxanthine that stimulates breathing through competitive inhibition of adenosine, an endogenous downregulator of respiratory drive in the central nervous system.[16] In addition, caffeine reduces hypoxemic depression of breathing in premature infants, increases responsiveness to carbon dioxide, and improves pharyngeal tone and diaphragmatic contractility.[17,18] The Caffeine for Apnea of Prematurity (CAP) trial demonstrated that caffeine reduces the risk of BPD in infants with birth weights of 500–1250g (Fig. 16.1).[19] Follow-up data from the CAP trial that were collected through 11 years of age show that caffeine results in durable improvement in motor function.[20] Although the CAP trial did not report the composite outcome of death or BPD (Fig. 16.2), there is no suggestion in the trial data that caffeine affects the risk of mortality (Fig. 16.3).[19,21]

Caffeine is initiated with an intravenous or enteral loading dose of 20 mg/kg of caffeine citrate (10 mg/kg of caffeine base) followed by a once daily maintenance dose of 5–10 mg/kg beginning 24 hours later.[19] Unlike for other methylxanthines, routine measurement of serum drug levels is not necessary.[22] Observational

Updates on Neonatal Chronic Lung Disease. https://doi.org/10.1016/B978-0-323-68353-1.00016-6

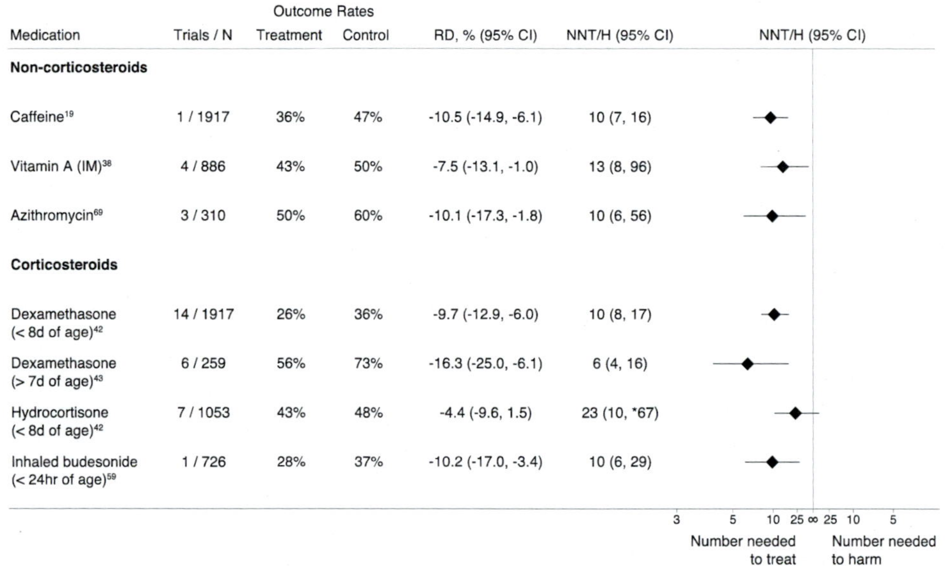

Medication	Trials / N	Outcome Rates: Treatment	Outcome Rates: Control	RD, % (95% CI)	NNT/H (95% CI)
Non-corticosteroids					
Caffeine[19]	1 / 1917	36%	47%	-10.5 (-14.9, -6.1)	10 (7, 16)
Vitamin A (IM)[38]	4 / 886	43%	50%	-7.5 (-13.1, -1.0)	13 (8, 96)
Azithromycin[69]	3 / 310	50%	60%	-10.1 (-17.3, -1.8)	10 (6, 56)
Corticosteroids					
Dexamethasone (< 8d of age)[42]	14 / 1917	26%	36%	-9.7 (-12.9, -6.0)	10 (8, 17)
Dexamethasone (> 7d of age)[43]	6 / 259	56%	73%	-16.3 (-25.0, -6.1)	6 (4, 16)
Hydrocortisone (< 8d of age)[42]	7 / 1053	43%	48%	-4.4 (-9.6, 1.5)	23 (10, *67)
Inhaled budesonide (< 24hr of age)[59]	1 / 726	28%	37%	-10.2 (-17.0, -3.4)	10 (6, 29)

FIG. 16.1 **Bronchopulmonary dysplasia (BPD) at 36 weeks postmenstrual age among surviving premature infants.** Therapies shown in a randomized trial and/or meta-analysis to reduce risk for BPD among survivors or the composite outcome of death or BPD. *indicates number needed to harm. *CI*, confidence interval; *IM*, intramuscular; *NNH*, number needed to harm; *NNT*, number needed to treat; *RD*, risk difference.

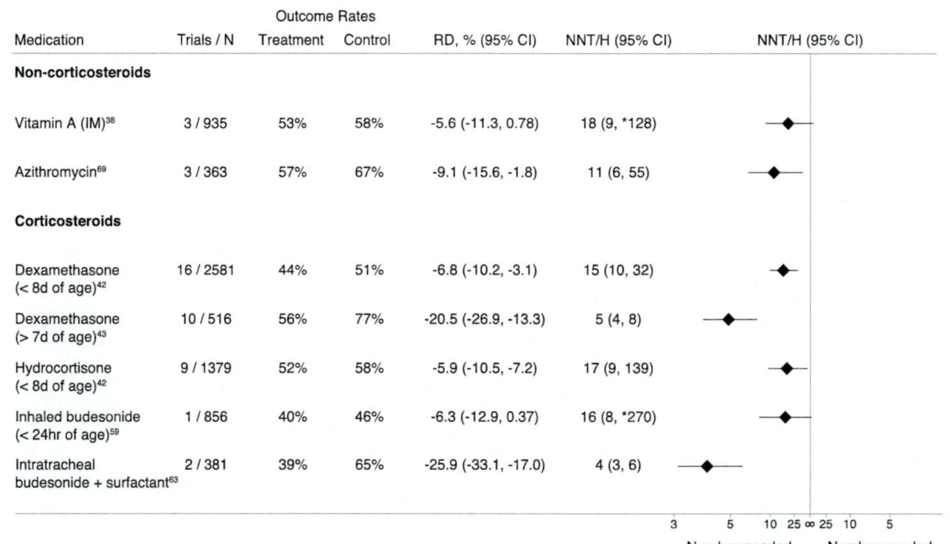

Medication	Trials / N	Outcome Rates: Treatment	Outcome Rates: Control	RD, % (95% CI)	NNT/H (95% CI)
Non-corticosteroids					
Vitamin A (IM)[38]	3 / 935	53%	58%	-5.6 (-11.3, 0.78)	18 (9, *128)
Azithromycin[69]	3 / 363	57%	67%	-9.1 (-15.6, -1.8)	11 (6, 55)
Corticosteroids					
Dexamethasone (< 8d of age)[42]	16 / 2581	44%	51%	-6.8 (-10.2, -3.1)	15 (10, 32)
Dexamethasone (> 7d of age)[43]	10 / 516	56%	77%	-20.5 (-26.9, -13.3)	5 (4, 8)
Hydrocortisone (< 8d of age)[42]	9 / 1379	52%	58%	-5.9 (-10.5, -7.2)	17 (9, 139)
Inhaled budesonide (< 24hr of age)[59]	1 / 856	40%	46%	-6.3 (-12.9, 0.37)	16 (8, *270)
Intratracheal budesonide + surfactant[63]	2 / 381	39%	65%	-25.9 (-33.1, -17.0)	4 (3, 6)

FIG. 16.2 **Death or bronchopulmonary dysplasia (BPD) at 36 weeks postmenstrual age.** Therapies shown in a randomized trial and/or meta-analysis to reduce risk for BPD among survivors or the composite outcome of death or BPD. *indicates number needed to harm. *CI*, confidence interval; *IM*, intramuscular; *NNH*, number needed to harm; *NNT*, number needed to treat; *RD*, risk difference.

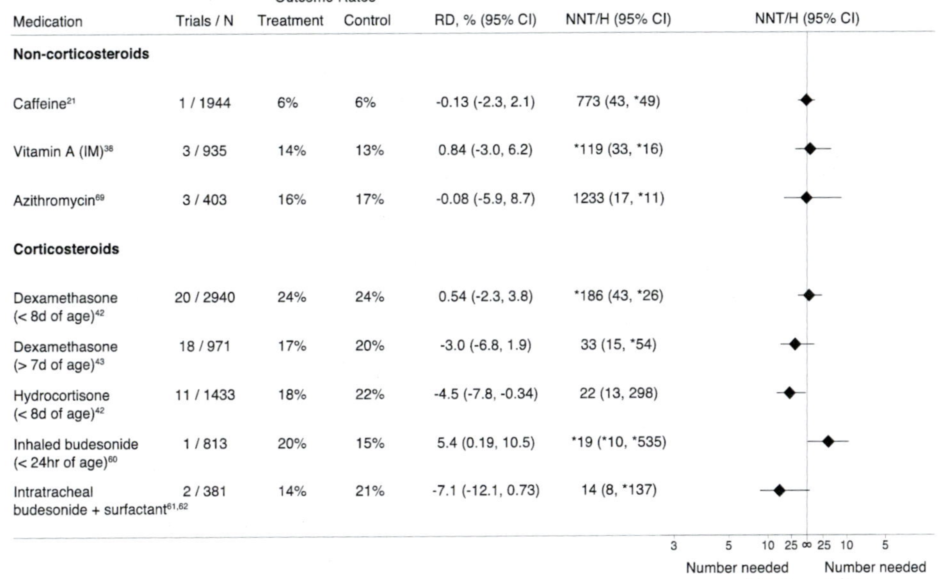

Medication	Trials / N	Outcome Rates Treatment	Control	RD, % (95% CI)	NNT/H (95% CI)
Non-corticosteroids					
Caffeine[21]	1 / 1944	6%	6%	-0.13 (-2.3, 2.1)	773 (43, *49)
Vitamin A (IM)[38]	3 / 935	14%	13%	0.84 (-3.0, 6.2)	*119 (33, *16)
Azithromycin[69]	3 / 403	16%	17%	-0.08 (-5.9, 8.7)	1233 (17, *11)
Corticosteroids					
Dexamethasone (< 8d of age)[42]	20 / 2940	24%	24%	0.54 (-2.3, 3.8)	*186 (43, *26)
Dexamethasone (> 7d of age)[43]	18 / 971	17%	20%	-3.0 (-6.8, 1.9)	33 (15, *54)
Hydrocortisone (< 8d of age)[42]	11 / 1433	18%	22%	-4.5 (-7.8, -0.34)	22 (13, 298)
Inhaled budesonide (< 24hr of age)[60]	1 / 813	20%	15%	5.4 (0.19, 10.5)	*19 (*10, *535)
Intratracheal budesonide + surfactant[61,62]	2 / 381	14%	21%	-7.1 (-12.1, 0.73)	14 (8, *137)

FIG. 16.3 **Death at last study follow-up.** Therapies shown in a randomized trial and/or meta-analysis to reduce risk for bronchopulmonary dysplasia (BPD) among survivors or the composite outcome of death or BPD. *indicates number needed to harm. *CI*, confidence interval; *IM*, intramuscular; *NNH*, number needed to harm; *NNT*, number needed to treat; *RD*, risk difference.

studies suggest that beginning caffeine therapy within the first 72 hours of age may produce the largest reduction in the risk of BPD.[23–27] It is uncertain whether these findings indicate a true benefit of earlier drug use or greater illness severity among infants in whom caffeine was started at later ages. Nevertheless, initiation of caffeine soon after birth is recommended for all very preterm infants who are at high risk of apnea, and who are either weaned from mechanical ventilation or maintained on noninvasive respiratory support.[28–30]

The optimal time to discontinue caffeine is not established. The CAP trial investigators recommended continued use of study drug until infants tolerated at least 5 consecutive days without positive airway pressure.[19] More recent data suggest that extending caffeine until term corrected age may reduce intermittent hypoxemia among infants receiving minimal respiratory support.[31] Further RCTs are needed to establish the safety and efficacy of prolonged caffeine therapy.

Vitamin A

Vitamin A is a group of nutritionally derived organic compounds that are essential for normal growth and maturation of the respiratory epithelium.[32,33] Early studies in preterm infants found lower plasma vitamin A levels among those who developed BPD compared to those who did not.[34–36] These data raised the hypothesis that relative vitamin A deficiency may play a role in the pathophysiology of BPD. Twenty years ago, a multicenter RCT showed that intramuscular (IM) injections of vitamin A (5000 IU 3 times per week) during the first 4 weeks of age reduced the rates of death or BPD and BPD among extremely low birth weight infants.[37] A 2016 meta-analysis of all trial data confirmed that IM vitamin A reduced the risk of BPD (Fig. 16.1) but not the risk of the composite outcome of death or BPD (Fig. 16.2).[38]

Several observational studies have called into question the effectiveness of IM vitamin A supplementation in the current era. One large study showed similar rates of BPD among infants who received vitamin A and untreated controls.[39] Another found that the prevalence of BPD did not increase during a period of limited IM vitamin A availability in the United States, despite a substantial drop in its use.[40] However, these observational findings provide lower quality of evidence and cannot supersede the data from RCTs. Ideally, a new trial of vitamin A would resolve this controversy.

Corticosteroids

Inflammation within the lung has been proposed to contribute to the pathophysiology of BPD.[41] This hypothesis is supported by the results of RCTs showing that corticosteroids reduce the risk of BPD in very preterm infants.[42,43] However, there is well-founded concern for long-term harm with indiscriminate corticosteroid use in this population.[42,43] Moreover, different corticosteroid medications, dosing routes, and dosing schedules as well as the variable quality of the published RCTs complicate the interpretation of the available evidence and hence the safe use of these drugs. Broadly, corticosteroids for BPD prevention can be divided into those that are administered systemically and those that are delivered directly into the lung. The meta-analyses of systemic corticosteroids by the Cochrane review group have been further divided by medication type and age of the infant at the initiation of drug therapy.

Systemic corticosteroids

Dexamethasone. Dexamethasone initiated within the first 8 days of age ("early use") reduces the risk of BPD in very preterm infants (Figs. 16.1 and 16.2).[42] However, this early use of dexamethasone increases the rates of gastrointestinal perforation, hypertrophic cardiomyopathy, cerebral palsy (CP), and major neurosensory disability.[42] This is why the use of dexamethasone therapy in the first week of life is not recommended in very preterm infants.[28,42,44]

The balance between risks and benefits is less certain if dexamethasone is initiated after the first week ("late use"). This use of dexamethasone lowers the risk of BPD (Fig. 16.1) and the composite outcome of death or BPD (Fig. 16.2), but short-term side effects include hyperglycemia, glycosuria, and hypertension.[43] It remains unclear if the late use of dexamethasone increases the risk of CP.[43] The statistical power of published RCTs is inadequate to evaluate long-term outcomes and the high rates of open label corticosteroid use in several trials may obscure actual treatment effects.[43,45]

When considering the safety of the late use of dexamethasone, clinicians must also weigh the risks of poor neurologic outcomes that are associated with BPD itself.[6,46–48] A meta-regression by Doyle et al. provides the best available means to balance these competing risks.[49,50] This analysis suggests that the size and direction of the effect of dexamethasone on the outcome of death or CP are both dependent on the rates of BPD in the trial control populations, akin to an infant's baseline risk of BPD.[50] According to this meta-regression, the adverse long-term neuromotor effects of dexamethasone likely outweigh the benefits in preterm infants with low to moderate risks of BPD.[50] Conversely, for ventilator-dependent infants with a greater than 60% risk of BPD the late use of dexamethasone may actually reduce the risk of death or CP.[50]

The optimal dose and treatment duration for late dexamethasone are unknown. General consensus favors low doses administered for 1–2 weeks.[44] The regimen utilized in the stopped early Dexamethasone: A Randomized Trial (DART) study (a total dose of 0.89 mg/kg administered over 10 days) is one such approach.[51] The DART investigators reported higher rates of successful extubation with dexamethasone and found no evidence of long-term neurologic harm.[51,52] However, enrollment for this RCT had to be abandoned after only 70 very preterm infants had been recruited.[51,52] Treatment with dexamethasone did not reduce the risk of BPD among this small number of trial participants.[51,52]

Hydrocortisone. Hydrocortisone has been hypothesized to produce similar respiratory benefits as dexamethasone but with less risk for adverse neurologic outcomes.[53,54] The largest trial to date of hydrocortisone for the prevention of BPD, the PREMILOC trial, compared a 10-day course of hydrocortisone, initiated within the first 24 hours of age, to placebo in infants born before 28 weeks of gestation.[55] Infants in the treatment arm received 1 mg/kg/day of hydrocortisone hemisuccinate divided into two daily doses for 7 days, followed by one dose of 0.5 mg/kg/day for 3 days.[55] BPD-free survival was more common among infants in the hydrocortisone group (NNT 12, 95% CI 6–200) although neurodevelopmental outcomes at 2 years of age were not improved.[55,56] In addition, a subgroup analysis found a nearly twofold increase in rate of late-onset sepsis among infants born at 24–25 weeks of gestation who were randomized to receive hydrocortisone (39.8% vs. 23.3%; NNH 6, 95% CI 3 to 36).[55] A 2017 Cochrane Review of all trials in which hydrocortisone was initiated during the first week after delivery showed a small reduction in the risks of mortality (Fig. 16.3) and the composite outcome of death or BPD (Fig. 16.2), but not BPD among survivors (Fig. 16.1).[42] Gastrointestinal perforation was more common in the hydrocortisone-treated infants.[42]

Intrapulmonary corticosteroids

Intrapulmonary corticosteroids offer the potential benefit of reducing inflammation within the lung while minimizing the adverse effects of systemically administered steroids. Inhalation has been most commonly used to deliver steroids directly into the lung. Four inhaled corticosteroids (budesonide, beclomethasone, fluticasone, flunisolide) have been studied in RCTs for the possible prevention of BPD.[57,58] A meta-analysis of all trials—irrespective of the drug used—found that infants treated with inhaled corticosteroids had lower risks of BPD and the composite of death or BPD.[57] The multicenter Neonatal European Study of Inhaled Steroids (NEUROSIS) contributed most of the weight to this analysis.[59] This RCT compared inhaled budesonide initiated within the first 24 hours after birth (400 μg every 12 hours for the first 14 days followed by 200 μg every 12 hours from day 15 until the infant was free of supplemental oxygen and respiratory support or reached 32 weeks PMA) to placebo among extremely premature infants receiving positive airway pressure.[59] Inhaled budesonide decreased the risk of BPD (Fig. 16.1), but significantly increased the risk of mortality at 18–22 months corrected age (Fig. 16.3).[59,60] Although no etiology for this adverse effect has been reported, this concerning finding outweighs the respiratory benefits of early inhaled budesonide.[60] Additional trials are needed to assess the safety and efficacy of inhaled corticosteroids initiated within the first few days of life. Use of inhaled corticosteroids after 7 days of age has not been shown to reduce the risk of BPD.[58]

A group of investigators in Taiwan used surfactant as a vehicle to administer budesonide into the lung.[61,62] They performed two RCTs to compare a mixture of intratracheal budesonide and surfactant to surfactant therapy alone in very low birth weight infants with severe respiratory distress syndrome (RDS).[61,62] A meta-analysis of these two trials indicated that the combination therapy reduced the risk of the composite outcome of death or BPD (Fig. 16.2); data for BPD alone were not reported.[63] While this finding is promising, the large effect size (NNT 4, 95% CI 3 to 6) that was obtained in a small numbers of trial participants raises the concern that this result may have arisen by chance.[63] Confirmation in larger trials is needed.

Azithromycin

Colonization of the respiratory tract with the mycoplasma species *Ureaplasma parvum and U. urealyticum* in very preterm infants is associated with the development of BPD.[64,65] Azithromycin, a macrolide antibiotic, achieves high concentration in lung fluid and has known activity against *Ureaplasma*.[66] Azithromycin also has anti-inflammatory properties.[67,68] Three small trials assessed the efficacy of azithromycin for preventing BPD.[69] Although none demonstrated benefit individually, the risks of BPD (Fig. 16.1) and the composite of death or BPD (Fig. 16.2) were reduced by azithromycin when data from all three trials were combined.[69] Importantly, the quality of evidence from these trials was low and enrollment was not restricted to infants with known *Ureaplasma* colonization.[28,69] Moreover, in 2013, the FDA issued a warning about the proarrhythmic potential of this drug in certain adults with cardiovascular risk factors. Larger trials are needed to establish the safety and efficacy of prophylactic azithromycin in very preterm infants before this therapy can be recommended for widespread use.[28]

PHARMACOLOGICAL THERAPIES WITH UNCERTAIN EFFECTS ON THE RISK OF BPD

Antenatal Corticosteroids

Over 30 RCTs have evaluated the effects of antenatal corticosteroids for pregnant women at risk of preterm delivery.[70] Antenatal corticosteroids reduce the risks of mortality, RDS, intraventricular hemorrhage, necrotizing enterocolitis (NEC), and early-onset sepsis in preterm infants.[70] However, none of the published trials, most of which were conducted over 20 years ago, reported the rates of supplemental oxygen use at a PMA of 36 weeks.[70] A meta-analysis of trials that used different definitions of BPD did not show any benefit of antenatal corticosteroids over control therapy on "chronic lung disease".[70] Lastly, no association between the exposure to antenatal corticosteroids and the risk of BPD was found in three more recent observational studies.[71–73]

Exogenous Surfactant

Meta-analyses of RCTs published in the 1980s and 1990s showed that animal-derived exogenous surfactant administered to preterm infants receiving invasive mechanical ventilation reduced the rates of mortality, pulmonary air leaks, and the use of supplemental oxygen at 28 days of age.[74–76] None of these older trials reported the rates of BPD at a PMA of 36 weeks.[74–76] Subsequent RCTs compared the early use of nasal continuous positive airway pressure (nCPAP) with prophylactic intubation and mechanical ventilation (without or without surfactant administration) and found a small reduction in the risk of death or BPD at 36 weeks PMA in favor of nCPAP (NNT: 25, 95% CI 14–147).[11] As a result, the early use of nCPAP rather than intubation and surfactant administration is now recommended for spontaneously breathing very preterm infants.[77] However, the majority of babies who are born before 29 weeks of gestation may still require mechanical ventilation during the first few days of life, despite attempts at noninvasive respiratory support.[78] It is unknown whether later administration of surfactant affects the risk of BPD in this subset of infants who cannot be maintained on noninvasive support.

The observation that avoiding endotracheal intubation and mechanical ventilation may lower the risk of BPD encouraged investigators to explore alternative means of surfactant administration. One such method is the INtubation, SURfactant administration during brief mechanical ventilation, followed by Extubation (INSURE) technique.[79] Although initial RCTs demonstrated reduced risk for oxygen therapy at 28 days of age, additional evidence from subsequent, larger trials suggests that the effects of INSURE on supplemental oxygen use at 36 weeks PMA are similar to those of nCPAP alone.[80,81] Efforts to administer surfactant without endotracheal intubation include "less invasive surfactant administration" (LISA) or "minimally invasive surfactant therapy" (MIST).[82,83] During LISA, surfactant is instilled into the trachea using a thin catheter (e.g., a feeding tube) while maintaining nCPAP therapy.[83] Four small trials in extremely preterm infants compared LISA to an alternative means of surfactant administration and 1 compared LISA to nCPAP therapy alone.[84–88] None of these trials demonstrated a reduction in the risk of BPD among infants treated with LISA versus control.[84–88] A meta-analysis combining all 5 studies showed that LISA reduced the risks of BPD and the composite of death or BPD.[83] An additional meta-analysis inclusive of one other trial enrolling moderately preterm infants found a similar result.[89,90]

Prevention or Treatment of a Patent Ductus Arteriosus

Observational data demonstrate an association between the presence of a patent ductus arteriosus (PDA) in very preterm infants and the subsequent development of BPD.[91,92] Despite this relationship, there are no robust data indicating that pharmacological closure of the PDA reduces the risk of BPD.[93–97] Prophylactic administration of ibuprofen or indomethacin to preterm infants reduces the rates of a subsequent symptomatic PDA, but does not prevent BPD (Fig. 16.4) or the composite of death or BPD (Fig. 16.5).[98,99] Similarly, selective treatment of a moderate to large PDA confirmed by echocardiography during the first week after delivery has not been shown to reduce the risks of either outcome (Figs. 16.4 and 16.5).[100–103] Moreover, neither prophylactic nor early therapy of a confirmed PDA reduce the risk of mortality (Fig. 16.6).[98–101] While some very preterm infants may benefit from pharmacological closure of the PDA, there are no evidence-based strategies to reliably identify these infants.[97]

Inhaled Nitric Oxide

Inhaled nitric oxide (iNO) is a potent pulmonary vasodilator and an evidence-based therapy for the treatment of persistent pulmonary hypertension in late preterm and full-term newborns.[104] In contrast, data from 16

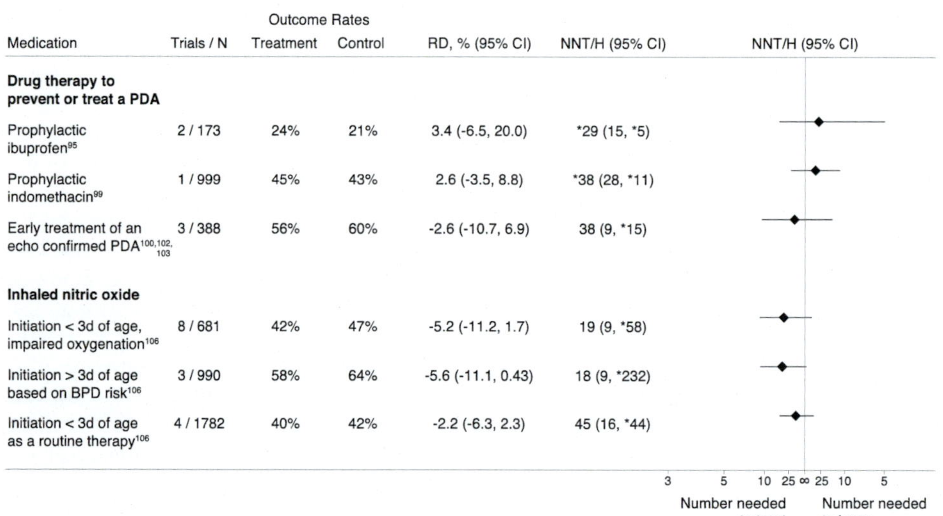

Medication	Trials / N	Outcome Rates Treatment	Outcome Rates Control	RD, % (95% CI)	NNT/H (95% CI)
Drug therapy to prevent or treat a PDA					
Prophylactic ibuprofen[95]	2 / 173	24%	21%	3.4 (-6.5, 20.0)	*29 (15, *5)
Prophylactic indomethacin[99]	1 / 999	45%	43%	2.6 (-3.5, 8.8)	*38 (28, *11)
Early treatment of an echo confirmed PDA[100,102,103]	3 / 388	56%	60%	-2.6 (-10.7, 6.9)	38 (9, *15)
Inhaled nitric oxide					
Initiation < 3d of age, impaired oxygenation[106]	8 / 681	42%	47%	-5.2 (-11.2, 1.7)	19 (9, *58)
Initiation > 3d of age based on BPD risk[106]	3 / 990	58%	64%	-5.6 (-11.1, 0.43)	18 (9, *232)
Initiation < 3d of age as a routine therapy[106]	4 / 1782	40%	42%	-2.2 (-6.3, 2.3)	45 (16, *44)

FIG. 16.4 **Bronchopulmonary dysplasia (BPD) at 36 weeks postmenstrual age among surviving premature infants.** Select therapies that have not been shown in a randomized trial and/or meta-analysis to reduce risk for BPD among survivors or the composite outcome of death or BPD. *indicates number needed to harm. *CI*, confidence interval; *echo*, echocardiogram, *IM*, intramuscular; *NNH*, number needed to harm; *NNT*, number needed to treat; *RD*, risk difference.

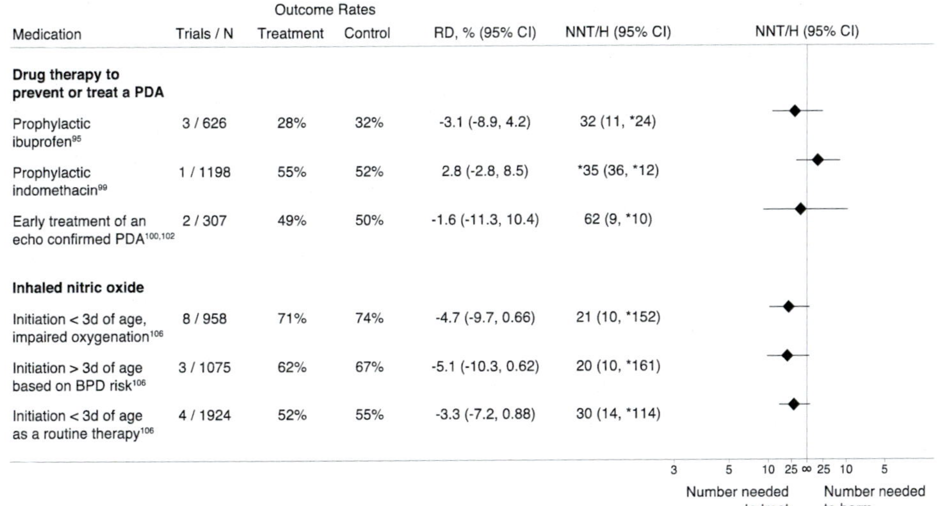

Medication	Trials / N	Outcome Rates: Treatment	Outcome Rates: Control	RD, % (95% CI)	NNT/H (95% CI)
Drug therapy to prevent or treat a PDA					
Prophylactic ibuprofen[95]	3 / 626	28%	32%	-3.1 (-8.9, 4.2)	32 (11, *24)
Prophylactic indomethacin[99]	1 / 1198	55%	52%	2.8 (-2.8, 8.5)	*35 (36, *12)
Early treatment of an echo confirmed PDA[100,102]	2 / 307	49%	50%	-1.6 (-11.3, 10.4)	62 (9, *10)
Inhaled nitric oxide					
Initiation < 3d of age, impaired oxygenation[106]	8 / 958	71%	74%	-4.7 (-9.7, 0.66)	21 (10, *152)
Initiation > 3d of age based on BPD risk[106]	3 / 1075	62%	67%	-5.1 (-10.3, 0.62)	20 (10, *161)
Initiation < 3d of age as a routine therapy[106]	4 / 1924	52%	55%	-3.3 (-7.2, 0.88)	30 (14, *114)

FIG. 16.5 **Death or bronchopulmonary dysplasia (BPD) at 36 weeks postmenstrual age.** Select therapies that have not been shown in a randomized trial and/or meta-analysis to reduce risk for BPD among survivors or the composite outcome of death or BPD. *indicates number needed to harm. *CI*, confidence interval; *echo*, echocardiogram, *IM*, intramuscular; *NNH*, number needed to harm; *NNT*, number needed to treat; *RD*, risk difference.

Medication	Trials / N	Outcome Rates: Treatment	Outcome Rates: Control	RD, % (95% CI)	NNT/H (95% CI)
Drug therapy to prevent or treat a PDA					
Prophylactic ibuprofen[95]	4 / 700	13%	14%	-1.5 (-5.4, 4.2)	68 (19, *24)
Prophylactic indomethacin[94]	18 / 2769	17%	18%	-0.75 (-3.3, 2.2)	133 (31, *46)
Early treatment of an echo confirmed PDA[100,101]	7 / 644	13%	12%	1.1 (-3.2, 7.6)	*89 (32, *13)
Inhaled nitric oxide					
Initiation < 3d of age, impaired oxygenation[106]	10 / 1066	41%	39%	0.90 (-4.4, 7.0)	*111 (23, *14)
Initiation > 3d of age based on BPD risk[106]	3 / 1075	10%	8%	1.5 (-1.6, 5.8)	*69 (64, *17)
Initiation < 3d of age as a routine therapy[106]	4 / 1924	16%	17%	-1.6 (-4.4, 1.8)	61 (23, *56)

NNT/H (95% CI)
3 5 10 25 ∞ 25 10 5
Number needed to treat
Number needed to harm

FIG. 16.6 **Death at last study follow-up.** Common therapies that have not been shown in a randomized trial and/or meta-analysis to reduce risk for bronchopulmonary dysplasia (BPD) among survivors or the composite outcome of death or BPD. *indicates number needed to harm. *CI*, confidence interval; *echo*, echocardiogram, *IM*, intramuscular; *NNH*, number needed to harm; *NNT*, number needed to treat; *RD*, risk difference.

RCTs that included over 3000 preterm infants have failed to show conclusively that iNO prevents BPD or the composite outcome of death or BPD, whether used as an early routine strategy or selectively in very preterm infants with an increased risk of BPD (Figs. 16.4 and 16.5).[105,106]

Diuretics

Diuretics are among the most common classes of medications administered in the neonatal intensive care unit.[107] Despite this regular use, there is little evidence from RCTs that administration of diuretics has any sustained clinical benefits in very preterm infants at high risk of BPD.[108–111] These medications may reduce pulmonary edema and provide short-term improvement in respiratory mechanics.[112] However, no published RCT has evaluated whether diuretics reduce the risk of BPD.[113] A large, multicenter observational study suggested an association between greater furosemide exposure and lower risk of BPD.[114] These findings require confirmation in an appropriately designed trial that includes an evaluation of the potential metabolic and renal adverse effects of chronic diuretic use in preterm babies.[115]

CONCLUSION

Caffeine and vitamin A are the only medications with high-quality evidence to support routine use for the prevention of BPD in most very preterm infants. Dexamethasone reduces the risk of developing BPD, but for many very preterm infants the risk of adverse long-term neurologic effects outweighs the benefits. For those at high risk of developing BPD, dexamethasone initiated after 7 days of age may be appropriate. Treatment with systemic hydrocortisone beginning in the first week after delivery has been shown in meta-analyses to reduce the risk of death or BPD. However, current evidence does not consistently show that early hydrocortisone reduces BPD risk among surviving very preterm infants and suggests it may not produce long-term improvement in neurodevelopment despite any potential respiratory benefits.

REFERENCES

1. Berkelhamer SK, Mestan KK, Steinhorn RH. Pulmonary hypertension in bronchopulmonary dysplasia. *Semin Perinatol*. 2013;37(2):124–131.
2. Bott L, Béghin L, Devos P, Pierrat V, Matran R, Gottrand F. Nutritional status at 2 years in former infants with bronchopulmonary dysplasia influences nutrition and pulmonary outcomes during childhood. *Pediatr Res*. 2006; 60(3):340–344.
3. Carraro S, Filippone M, Da Dalt L, et al. Bronchopulmonary dysplasia: the earliest and perhaps the longest lasting obstructive lung disease in humans. *Early Hum Dev*. 2013;89(S3):S3–S5.
4. Cristea AI, Carroll AE, Davis SD, Swigonski NL, Ackerman VL. Outcomes of children with severe bronchopulmonary dysplasia who were ventilator dependent at home. *Pediatrics*. 2013;132(3):e727–e734.
5. Doyle LW, Faber B, Callanan C, Freezer N, Ford GW, Davis NM. Bronchopulmonary dysplasia in very low birth weight subjects and lung function in late adolescence. *Pediatrics*. 2006;118(1):108–113.
6. Ehrenkranz RA, Walsh MC, Vohr BR, et al. Validation of the national institutes of health consensus definition of bronchopulmonary dysplasia. *Pediatrics*. 2005;116(6): 1353–1360.
7. Stoll BJ, Hansen NI, Bell EF, et al. Trends in care practices, morbidity, and mortality of extremely preterm neonates, 1993–2012. *JAMA*. 2015;314(10):1039–1051.
8. Botet F, Figueras-Aloy J, Miracle-Echegoyen X, R-M JM, Salvia-Roiges MD, Carbonell-Estrany X. Trends in survival among extremely-low-birth-weight infants (less than 1000g) without significant bronchopulmonary dysplasia. *BMC Pediatr*. 2012;12(1):63–70.
9. Horbar JD, Carpenter JH, Badger GJ, et al. Mortality and neonatal morbidity among infants 501 to 1500 grams from 2000 to 2009. *Pediatrics*. 2012;129(6): 1019–1026.
10. Fischer HS, Bührer C. Avoiding endotracheal ventilation to prevent bronchopulmonary dysplasia: a meta-analysis. *Pediatrics*. 2013;132(5):e1351–1360.
11. Schmölzer GM, Kumar M, Pichler G, Aziz K, O'Reilly M, Cheung P-Y. Non-invasive versus invasive respiratory support in preterm infants at birth: systematic review and meta-analysis. *BMJ*. 2013;347:f5980.
12. Subramaniam P, Ho JJ, Davis PG. Prophylactic nasal continuous positive airway pressure for preventing morbidity and mortality in very preterm infants. *Cochrane Database Syst Rev*. 2016;6:CD001243.
13. Doyle L, Carse E, Adams A, et al. Ventilation in extremely preterm infants and respiratory function at 8 years. *N Engl J Med*. 2017;377(4):329–337.
14. Shennan AT, Dunn MS, Ohlsson A, Lennox K, Hoskins EM. Abnormal pulmonary outcomes in premature infants: Prediction from oxygen requirement in the neonatal period. *Pediatrics*. 1988;82(4):527–532.
15. Mendes D, Alves C, Batel-Marques F. Number needed to treat (NNT) in clinical literature: an appraisal. *BMC Med*. 2017;15(1):112.
16. Daly J, Bruns R, Snyder S. Adenosine receptors in the central nervous system: relationship to the central actions of methylxanthines. *Life Sci*. 1981;28(19):2083–2097.
17. Julien C, Joseph V, Bairam A. Caffeine reduces apnea frequency and enhances ventilatory long-term facilitation in rat pups raised in chronic intermittent hypoxia. *Pediatr Res*. 2010;68:105–111.
18. Kassim Z, Greenough A, Rafferty G. Effect of caffeine on respiratory muscle strength and lung function in prematurely born, ventilated infants. *Eur J Pediatr*. 2009;168: 1491–1495.
19. Schmidt B, Roberts RS, Davis P, et al. Caffeine therapy for apnea of prematurity. *N Engl J Med*. 2006;354(20): 2112–2121.
20. Schmidt B, Roberts R, Anderson P, et al. Academic performance, motor function, and behavior 11 years after neonatal caffeine citrate therapy for apnea of

prematurity: an 11-year follow-up of the cap randomized clinical trial. *JAMA Pediatr.* 2017;171(6):564–572.
21. Schmidt B, Roberts RS, Davis P, et al. Long-term effects of caffeine therapy for apnea of prematurity. *N Engl J Med.* 2007;357(19):1893–1902.
22. Natarajan G, Botica M, Thomas R, Aranda J. Therapeutic drug monitoring for caffeine in preterm neonates: an unnecessary exercise? *Pediatrics.* 2007;119(5):936–940.
23. Lodha A, Seshia M, McMillan DD, et al. Association of early caffeine administration and neonatal outcomes in very preterm neonates. *JAMA Pediatr.* 2015;169(1):33–38.
24. Patel R, Leong T, Carlton D, Vyas-Read S. Early caffeine therapy and clinical outcomes in extremely preterm infants. *J Perinatol.* 2013;33(2):134–140.
25. Taha D, Kirkby S, Nawab U, et al. Early caffeine therapy for prevention of bronchopulmonary dysplasia in preterm infants. *J Matern Fetal Neonatal Med.* 2014;27(16):1698–1702.
26. Davis PG, Schmidt B, Roberts RS, et al. Caffeine for apnea of prematurity trial: benefits may vary in subgroups. *J Pediatr.* 2010;156(3):382–387.
27. Dobson NR, Patel RM, Smith PB, et al. Trends in caffeine use and association between clinical outcomes and timing of therapy in very low birth weight infants. *J Pediatr.* 2014;164(5), 992-998 e993.
28. Jensen EA, Foglia EE, Schmidt B. Evidence-based pharmacologic therapies for prevention of bronchopulmonary dysplasia: application of the grading of recommendations assessment, development, and evaluation methodology. *Clin Perinatol.* 2015;42(4):755–779.
29. Eichenwald EC. AAP committee on fetus and newborn: apnea of prematurity. *Pediatrics.* 2016;137(1):e20153757.
30. Sweet DG, Carnielli V, Greisen G, et al. European consensus guidelines on the management of respiratory distress syndrome - 2016 update. *Neonatology.* 2017;111(2):107–125.
31. Rhein L, Dobson N, Darnall R, et al. Effects of caffeine on intermittent hypoxia in infants born prematurely: a randomized clinical trial. *JAMA Pediatr.* 2014;168(3):250–257.
32. Niederreither K, Dolle P. Retinoic acid in development: towards an integrated view. *Nat Rev Genet.* 2008;9:541–553.
33. Biesalski H, Nohr I. Importance of vitamin A for lung function and development. *Mold Aspects Med.* 2003;24:431–440.
34. Shenai J, Chytil F, Stahlman M. Vitamin A status of neonates with bronchopulmonary dysplasia. *Pediatr Res.* 1985;19:185–188.
35. Hustead V, Gutcher G, Anderson S, Zachman R. Relationship of vitamin A (retinol) status to lung disease in the preterm infant. *J Pediatr.* 1984;104:610–615.
36. Chytil F. The lungs and vitamin A. *Am J Physiol.* 1992;262:L517–L527.
37. Tyson JE, Wright LL, Oh W, et al. Vitamin A supplementation for extremely-low-birth-weight infants. National institute of child health and human development neonatal research network. *N Engl J Med.* 1999;340(25):1962–1968.
38. Darlow B, Graham P, Rojas-Reyes M. Vitamin A supplementation to prevent mortality and short- and long-term morbidity in very low birth weight infants. *Cochrane Database Syst Rev.* 2016;8:CD000501.
39. Gadhia MM, Cutter GR, Abman SH, Kinsella JP. Effects of early inhaled nitric oxide therapy and vitamin A supplementation on the risk for bronchopulmonary dysplasia in premature newborns with respiratory failure. *J Pediatr.* 2014;164(4):744–748.
40. Tolia VN, Murthy K, McKinley PS, Bennett MM, Clark RH. The effect of the national shortage of vitamin A on death or chronic lung disease in extremely low-birth-weight infants. *JAMA Pediatr.* 2014;168(11):1039–1044.
41. Speer C. Pulmonary inflammation and bronchopulmonary dysplasia. *J Perinatol.* 2006;26(Suppl 1):S57–S62.
42. Doyle LW, Cheong J, Ehrenkranz RA, Halliday HL. Early (< 8 days) systemic postnatal corticosteroids for prevention of bronchopulmonary dysplasia in preterm infants. *Cochrane Database Syst Rev.* 2017;10:CD001146.
43. Doyle LW, Cheong J, Ehrenkranz RA, Halliday HL. Late (> 7 days) systemic postnatal corticosteroids for prevention of bronchopulmonary dysplasia. *Cochrane Database Syst Rev.* 2017;10:CD001145.
44. Watterberg KL, AAP Committee on Fetus and Newborn. Policy statement–postnatal corticosteroids to prevent or treat bronchopulmonary dysplasia. *Pediatrics.* 2010;126(4):800–808.
45. Onland W, van Kaam A, De Jaegere A, Offringa M. Open-label glucocorticoids modulate dexamethasone trial results in preterm infants. *Pediatrics.* 2010;2010(126):e954–964.
46. Linsell L, Malouf R, Morris J, Kurinczuk J, Marlow N. Prognostic factors for poor cognitive development in children born very preterm or with very low birth weight: a systematic review. *JAMA Pediatr.* 2015;169(12):1162–1172.
47. Linsell L, Malouf R, Morris J, Kurinczuk J, Marlow N. Prognostic factors for cerebral palsy and motor impairment in children born very preterm or very low birthweight: a systematic review. *Dev Med Child Neurol.* 2016;58(6):554–569.
48. Singer L, Yamashita T, Lilien L, Collin M, Baley J. A longitudinal study of developmental outcome of infants with bronchopulmonary dysplasia and very low birth weight. *Pediatrics.* 1997;100(6):987–993.
49. Doyle LW, Halliday HL, Ehrenkranz RA, Davis PG, Sinclair JC. Impact of postnatal systemic corticosteroids on mortality and cerebral palsy in preterm infants: effect modification by risk for chronic lung disease. *Pediatrics.* 2005;115(3):655–661.
50. Doyle LW, Halliday HL, Ehrenkranz RA, Davis PG, Sinclair JC. An update on the impact of postnatal systemic corticosteroids on mortality and cerebral palsy in preterm infants: effect modification by risk of bronchopulmonary dysplasia. *J Pediatr.* 2014;165(6):1258–1260.

51. Doyle L, Davis P, Morley C, McPhee A, Carlin J, DART Study Investigators. Low-dose dexamethasone facilitates extubation among chronically ventilator-dependent infants: a multicenter, international, randomized, controlled trial. *Pediatrics*. 2006;117(1):75–83.
52. Doyle L, Davis P, Morley C, McPhee A, Carlin J, DART Study Investigators. Outcome at 2 years of age of infants from the dart study: a multicenter, international, randomized, controlled trial of low-dose dexamethasone. *Pediatrics*. 2007;119(4):716–721.
53. Rademaker K, Uiterwaal C, Groenendaal F, et al. Neonatal hydrocortisone treatment: neurodevelopmental outcome and mri at school age in preterm-born children. *J Pediatr*. 2007;150(4):351–357.
54. van der Heide-Jalving M, Kamphuis P, van der Laan M, et al. Short- and long-term effects of neonatal glucocorticoid therapy: is hydrocortisone an alternative to dexamethasone? *Acta Paediatr*. 2003;92(7):827–835.
55. Baud O, Maury L, Lebail F, et al. Effect of early low-dose hydrocortisone on survival without bronchopulmonary dysplasia in extremely preterm infants (premiloc): a double-blind, placebo-controlled, multicentre, randomised trial. *Lancet*. 2016;387(10030):1827–1836.
56. Baud O, Trousson C, Biran V, et al. Association between early low-dose hydrocortisone therapy in extremely preterm neonates and neurodevelopmental outcomes at 2 years of age. *JAMA*. 2017;317(13):1329–1337.
57. Shinwell E, Portnov I, Meerpohl J, Karen T, Bassler D. Inhaled corticosteroids for bronchopulmonary dysplasia: a meta-analysis. *Pediatrics*. 2016;138(6):e20162511.
58. Onland W, Offringa M, van Kaam A. Late (≥ 7 days) inhalation corticosteroids to reduce bronchopulmonary dysplasia in preterm infants. *Cochrane Database Syst Rev*. 2017;8:CD002311.
59. Bassler D, Plavka R, Shinwell E, et al. Early inhaled budesonide for the prevention of bronchopulmonary dysplasia. *N Engl J Med*. 2015;373(16):1497–1506.
60. Bassler D, Shinwell E, Hallman M, et al. Long-term effects of inhaled budesonide for bronchopulmonary dysplasia. *N Engl J Med*. 2018;378(2):148–157.
61. Yeh TF, Chen CM, Wu SY, et al. Intratracheal administration of budesonide/surfactant to prevent bronchopulmonary dysplasia. *Am J Respir Crit Care Med*. 2016;193(1): 86–95.
62. Yeh TF, Lin HC, Chang CH, et al. Early intratracheal instillation of budesonide using surfactant as a vehicle to prevent chronic lung disease in preterm infants: a pilot study. *Pediatrics*. 2008;121(5):e1310–1318.
63. Venkataraman R, Kamaluddeen M, Hasan S, Robertson H, Lodha A. Intratracheal administration of budesonide-surfactant in prevention of bronchopulmonary dysplasia in very low birth weight infants: a systematic review and meta-analysis. *Pediatr Pulmonol*. 2017; 52(7):968–975.
64. Wang E, Ohlsson A, Kellner J. Association of ureaplasma urealyticum colonization with chronic lung disease of prematurity: results of a metaanalysis. *J Pediatr*. 1995; 127(4):640–644.
65. Schelonka R, Katz B, Waites K, Benjamin D. Critical appraisal of the role of ureaplasma in the development of bronchopulmonary dysplasia with metaanalytic techniques. *Pediatr Infect Dis J*. 2005;24(12): 1033–1039.
66. Matlow A, Th'ng C, Kovach D, Quinn P, Dunn M, Wang E. Susceptibilities of neonatal respiratory isolates of ureaplasma urealyticum to antimicrobial agents. *Antimicrob Agents Chemother*. 1998;42(5):1290–1292.
67. Jaffe A, Bush A. Anti-inflammatory effects of macrolides in lung disease. *Pediatr Pulmonol*. 2001;31(6):464–473.
68. Aghai Z, Kode A, Saslow J, et al. Azithromycin suppresses activation of nuclear factor-kappa b and synthesis of pro-inflammatory cytokines in tracheal aspirate cells from premature infants. *Pediatr Res*. 2007;62(4):483–488.
69. Nair V, Loganathan P, Soraisham AS. Azithromycin and other macrolides for prevention of bronchopulmonary dysplasia: a systematic review and meta-analysis. *Neonatology*. 2014;106(4):337–347.
70. Roberts D, Brown J, Medley N, Dalziel S. Antenatal corticosteroids for accelerating fetal lung maturation for women at risk of preterm birth. *Cochrane Database Syst Rev*. 2017;3:CD004454.
71. Carlo W, McDonald S, Fanaroff A, et al. Association of antenatal corticosteroids with mortality and neurodevelopmental outcomes among infants born at 22 to 25 weeks' gestation. *JAMA*. 2011;306(21):2348–2358.
72. Travers CP, Carlo WA, McDonald SA, et al. Mortality and pulmonary outcomes of extremely preterm infants exposed to antenatal corticosteroids. *Am J Obstet Gynecol*. 2018;218(1), 130.e131-130.e113.
73. Travers CP, Clark RH, Spitzer AR, Das A, Garite TJ, Carlo WA. Exposure to any antenatal corticosteroids and outcomes in preterm infants by gestational age: prospective cohort study. *BMJ*. 2017;356:j1039.
74. Soll RF. Prophylactic natural surfactant extract for preventing morbidity and mortality in preterm infants. *Cochrane Database Syst Rev*. 2000;2:CD000511.
75. Soll RF. Prophylactic synthetic surfactant for preventing morbidity and mortality in preterm infants. *Cochrane Database Syst Rev*. 2000;2:CD001079.
76. Soll RF. Synthetic surfactant for respiratory distress syndrome in preterm infants. *Cochrane Database Syst Rev*. 2000;2:CD001149.
77. Committee on Fetus and Newborn; American Academy of Pediatrics. Respiratory support in preterm infants at birth. *Pediatrics*. 2014;133(1):171–174.
78. Morley C, Davis P, Doyle L, et al. Nasal cpap or intubation at birth for very preterm infants. *N Engl J Med*. 2008;358(7):700–708.
79. Victorin LH, Deverajan LV, Curstedt T, Robertson B. Surfactant replacement in spontaneously breathing babies with hyaline membrane disease – a pilot study. *Biol Neonate*. 1990;58(3):121–126.
80. Stevens TP, Harrington EW, Blennow M, Soll RF. Early surfactant administration with brief ventilation vs. Selective surfactant and continued mechanical ventilation for preterm infants with or at risk for respiratory distress

syndrome. *Cochrane Database Syst Rev.* 2007;4: CD003063.
81. Isayama T, Chai-Adisaksopha C, McDonald SD. Noninvasive ventilation with vs without early surfactant to prevent chronic lung disease in preterm infants: a systematic review and meta-analysis. *JAMA Pediatr.* 2015;**169**(8): 731–739.
82. More K, Sakhuja P, Shah PS. Minimally invasive surfactant administration in preterm infants: a meta-narrative review. *JAMA Pediatr.* 2014;168(10):901–908.
83. Foglia E, Jensen E, Kirpalani H. Delivery room interventions to prevent bronchopulmonary dysplasia in extremely preterm infants. *J Perinatol.* 2017;37(11):1171–1179.
84. Bao Y, Zhang G, Wu M, Ma L, Zhu J. A pilot study of less invasive surfactant administration in very preterm infants in a Chinese tertiary center. *BMC Pediatr.* 2015;15(1): 342.
85. Kanmaz HG, Erdeve O, Canpolat FE, Mutlu B, Dilmen U. Surfactant administration via thin catheter during spontaneous breathing: randomized controlled trial. *Pediatrics.* 2013;131(2):e502–509.
86. Kribs A, Roll C, Göpel W, et al. Nonintubated surfactant application vs conventional therapy in extremely preterm infants: a randomized clinical trial. *JAMA Pediatr.* 2015; 169(8), 723-30.
87. Mirnia K, Heidarzadeh M, Hosseini MB, Sadeghnia A, Balila M, Ghojazadeh M. Comparison outcome of surfactant administration via tracheal catheterization during spontaneous breathing with insure. *Med J Islamic World Acad Sci.* 2013;21(4):143–148.
88. Göpel W, Kribs A, Ziegler A, et al. Avoidance of mechanical ventilation by surfactant treatment of spontaneously breathing preterm infants (AMV): an open-label, randomised, controlled trial. *Lancet.* 2011;378(9803): 1627–1634.
89. Aldana-Aguirre JC, Pinto M, Featherstone RM, Kumar M. Less invasive surfactant administration versus intubation for surfactant delivery in preterm infants with respiratory distress syndrome: a systematic review and meta-analysis. *Arch Dis Child Fetal Neonatal Ed.* 2017;102(1):F17–F23.
90. Mohammadizadeh M, Ardestani A, Sadeghnia A. Early administration of surfactant via a thin intratracheal catheter in preterm infants with respiratory distress syndrome: feasibility and outcome. *J Res Pharm Pract.* 2015;4(1):31–36.
91. Palta M, Gabbert D, Weinstein MR, Peters ME. Multivariate assessment of traditional risk factors for chronic lung disease in very low birth weight neonates. The newborn lung project. *J Pediatr.* 1991;119(2):285–292.
92. Oh W, Poindexter B, Perritt R, et al. Association between fluid intake and weight loss during the first ten days of life and risk of bronchopulmonary dysplasia in extremely low birth weight infants. *J Pediatr.* 2005;147(6):786–790.
93. Benitz WE. Patent ductus arteriosus: to treat or not to treat? *Arch Dis Child Fetal Neonatal Ed.* 2012;97(2): F80–F82.
94. Fowlie PW, Davis PG, McGuire W. Prophylactic intravenous indomethacin for preventing mortality and morbidity in preterm infants. *Cochrane Database Syst Rev.* 2010;(7):CD000174.
95. Ohlsson A, Walia R, Shah S. Ibuprofen for the treatment of patent ductus arteriosus in preterm or low birth weight (or both) infants. *Cochrane Database Syst Rev.* 2015;2: CD003481.
96. Ohlsson A, Shah P. Paracetamol (acetaminophen) for patent ductus arteriosus in preterm or low birth weight infants. *Cochrane Database Syst Rev.* 2018;4:CD010061.
97. Benitz W, AAP Committee on Fetus and Newborn. Patent ductus arteriosus in preterm infants. *Pediatrics.* 2016; 137(1):e20153730.
98. Ohlsson A, Shah SS. Ibuprofen for the prevention of patent ductus arteriosus in preterm and/or low birth weight infants. *Cochrane Database Syst Rev.* 2011;(7): CD004213.
99. Schmidt B, Davis P, Moddemann D, et al. Long-term effects of indomethacin prophylaxis in extremely-low-birth-weight infants. *N Engl J Med.* 2001;344(26): 1966–1972.
100. Clyman RI, Liebowitz M, Kaempf J, et al. PDA-TOLERATE Trial: an exploratory randomized controlled trial of treatment of moderate-to-large patent ductus arteriosus at 1 week of age. *J Pediatr.* 2018;205, 41-48.e6.
101. Farooqui MA, Elsayed Y, Jeyaraman MM, et al. Pre-symptomatic targeted treatment of patent ductus arteriosus in preterm newborns: a systematic review and meta-analysis. *J Neonatal Perinat Med.* 2019;12(1):1–7.
102. Sosenko I, Fajardo M, Claure N, Bancalari E. Timing of patent ductus arteriosus treatment and respiratory outcome in premature infants: a double-blind randomized controlled trial. *J Pediatr.* 2012;160(6), 929-935.e921.
103. Aranda J, Clyman R, Cox B, et al. A randomized, double-blind, placebo-controlled trial on intravenous ibuprofen L-lysine for the early closure of nonsymptomatic patent ductus arteriosus within 72 hours of birth in extremely low-birth-weight infants. *Am J Perinatol.* 2009;26(3): 235–245.
104. Barrington K, Finer N, Pennaforte T, Altit G. Nitric oxide for respiratory failure in infants born at or near term. *Cochrane Database Syst Rev.* 2017;1:CD000399.
105. Askie L, Ballard R, Cutter G, et al. Inhaled nitric oxide in preterm infants: an individual-patient data meta-analysis of randomized trials. *Pediatrics.* 2011;128(4):729–739.
106. Barrington K, Finer N, Pennaforte T. Inhaled nitric oxide for respiratory failure in preterm infants. *Cochrane Database Syst Rev.* 2017;1:CD000509.
107. Hsieh EM, Hornik CP, Clark RH, et al. Medication use in the neonatal intensive care unit. *Am J Perinatol.* 2014; 31(9):811–821.
108. Kassab M, Khriesat WM, Anabrees J. Diuretics for transient tachypnoea of the newborn. *Cochrane Database Syst Rev.* 2015;11:CD003064.
109. Stewart A, Brion LP. Intravenous or enteral loop diuretics for preterm infants with (or developing) chronic lung disease. *Cochrane Database Syst Rev.* 2011;(9): CD001453.

110. Stewart A, Brion LP, Ambrosio-Perez I. Diuretics acting on the distal renal tubule for preterm infants with (or developing) chronic lung disease. *Cochrane Database Syst Rev.* 2011;(9):CD001817.
111. Stewart A, Brion LP, Soll R. Diuretics for respiratory distress syndrome in preterm infants. *Cochrane Database Syst Rev.* 2011;12:CD001454.
112. Iyengar A, Davis J. Drug therapy for the prevention and treatment of bronchopulmonary dysplasia. *Front Pharmacol.* 2015;6:12.
113. Beam KS, Aliaga S, Ahlfeld SK, Cohen-Wolkowiez M, Smith PB, Laughon MM. A systematic review of randomized controlled trials for the prevention of bronchopulmonary dysplasia in infants. *J Perinatol.* 2014; 34(9):705–710.
114. Greenberg RG, Gayam S, Savage D, et al. Furosemide exposure and prevention of bronchopulmonary dysplasia in premature infants. *J Pediatr.* 2019;208: 134–140. e2.
115. Segar JL. Neonatal diuretic therapy: furosemide, thiazides, and spironolactone. *Clin Perinatol.* 2012;39(1): 209–220.

CHAPTER 17

Ventilation Strategies in Bronchopulmonary Dysplasia: Where We Are and Where We Should Be Going?

MARTIN KESZLER, MD • ROBIN MCKINNEY, MD

INTRODUCTION

Research regarding mechanical ventilation in preterm infants has almost exclusively focused on the early stages of lung disease. Very appropriately, the dominant theme has been the prevention of lung injury and mitigation of the risk of chronic lung disease. Much less high-quality research is available to guide the care of infants with evolving and established bronchopulmonary dysplasia (BPD). However, despite improvement in neonatal care, the incidence of BPD has not decreased appreciably over the past few decades, in part because of the increasing survival of extremely immature infants.[1] An arrest of normal alveolarization is probably inevitable when a second trimester fetus that is at the early saccular stage of lung development and lacks adequate antioxidant defenses is suddenly exposed to extrauterine levels of oxygen and therefore it is unlikely that BPD will disappear from our intensive care units in the foreseeable future. Thus clinicians continue to be faced with the need to provide long-term respiratory support to a substantial number of former extremely low gestational age newborns (ELGANs) with various degrees of respiratory insufficiency without a substantial body of evidence to support strong clinical recommendations. In this relative vacuum, there is a great degree of practice style variation and many neonatologists continue to treat chronically ventilator-dependent infants with strategies similar to those typically used in the acute stage of respiratory distress syndrome (RDS), despite important differences in the pathophysiologic manifestations of the lung disease. Additionally, there is often a lack of appreciation that the goals of support need to shift from an emphasis on extubation at the earliest opportunity to the recognition that once chronic lung disease has developed, adequate long-term support is essential for lung growth and eventual recovery.

In this chapter, we will review the important differences in the nature of the lung pathology between acute RDS and established chronic lung disease, examine available evidence for appropriate mechanical ventilation strategies, and provide recommendations for long-term ventilation of these infants.

WHEN DOES RESPIRATORY DISTRESS SYNDROME BECOME BRONCHOPULMONARY DYSPLASIA?

It should be self-evident that this transition occurs gradually and at variable rates in individual patients. There is no abrupt change in the pathophysiology and therefore there should not be a sudden change in ventilation strategy in ELGANs who remain ventilator-dependent beyond the first 2 or 3 weeks of life. Rather, there should be a periodic reassessment of the clinical condition, gas exchange, and lung mechanics as evidenced by pulmonary graphics displayed on the ventilator screen. Infants who ultimately develop long-term ventilator dependence may follow one of the following paths[2]: (1) severe RDS/respiratory insufficiency with a poor response to surfactant requiring moderately high ventilator settings—these infants' condition never substantially improves and progresses to worsening chronic lung disease; (2) mild-to-moderate RDS with initial improvement, sometimes successful extubation, followed by deteriorating respiratory status, requiring reintubation or increasing ventilator support, eventually

Updates on Neonatal Chronic Lung Disease. https://doi.org/10.1016/B978-0-323-68353-1.00017-8

leading to chronic ventilator dependence; and (3) minimal evidence of early lung disease with low ventilator settings or only noninvasive support and low oxygen requirement, followed by gradually worsening respiratory status with diffuse haziness of lung fields and early bubbly appearance of the lungs, ultimately leading to intubation and progressively increasing level of support. The infants in the first group may have an element of congenital pneumonia or pulmonary hypoplasia and their condition may be complicated by pulmonary hypertension. The second pathway appears to be the most common and probably represents the consequence of exposure to relative hyperoxia (by fetal standards) and ventilator-associated lung injury (VALI) of lungs at early stages of development.[3] The third path suggests accelerated lung maturation due to exposure to intrauterine inflammation, followed by increased susceptibility to VALI.[4]

The full-blown pathophysiology of BPD may not become manifested until the second month of life, but progressive increase in airway resistance begins as early as the first week of life,[5,6] with increasing heterogeneity of lung aeration, increased secretions leading to wandering atelectasis, and the tendency to hyperinflation by the second to third week of life.[7] Increasing tidal volume requirements despite permissive hypercapnia has been documented by 3 weeks of age in former ELGANs still requiring mechanical ventilation.[8]

PATHOPHYSIOLOGIC BASIS OF VENTILATOR SUPPORT IN BRONCHOPULMONARY DYSPLASIA

The term "bronchopulmonary dysplasia" accurately captures the fact that the condition affects both the airways and the lung parenchyma. In most infants, the airway obstructive component predominates, but the phenotype is quite variable and the proportion of parenchymal versus airway component varies from patient to patient and even within the lungs of a single infant. Both large and small airways are often affected and each leads to different manifestations. The large airways may be affected by mucosal/submucosal damage from prolonged intubation ultimately leading to subglottic stenosis, local obstruction from an airway granuloma at the opening of a bronchus, or vocal cord dysfunction. A common cause of large airway obstruction is tracheobronchomalacia that appears to be the result of prolonged cyclic stretch of immature airway structures. Tracheobronchomalacia may lead to dynamic obstruction during expiration, manifested by expiratory stridor and strikingly abnormal flow-volume loops on pulmonary graphics in ventilated infants[9] or by inspiratory stridor due to collapse of the extrathoracic trachea in infants breathing spontaneously. Small airway obstruction results from a combination of mucosal edema, smooth muscle hypertrophy, and increased secretions and is universally present at least to some degree and is commonly unresponsive to bronchodilators. An important contribution to small airway obstruction is airway closure at low lung volume caused by the paucity of alveolar attachment of the small airways due to the simplified lung of "new BPD," as discussed later.

The hallmark of BPD is substantial heterogeneity of parenchymal and airway involvement, resulting in marked regional variability in time constants. This variability leads to multicompartmental lung physiology, making it difficult to ventilate these lungs optimally. Areas with relatively low airway resistance, referred to as "fast compartments," are able to fill and empty relatively rapidly, whereas the regions with high airway resistance, the "slow compartments," require a longer period to inflate and even longer to deflate. Ventilation at relatively rapid rates with short inspiratory and expiratory times, such as is typically used in newborn infants with RDS, would preferentially direct gas flow to the fast compartments, resulting in increased dead space ventilation, poor ventilation/perfusion matching, and lung injury from overexpansion of that relatively healthy portion of the lungs. In addition, the limited volume of gas that did enter the slow compartments is likely to be trapped there, owing to the prolonged expiratory time constant, with small airway collapse at lower lung volumes. Emptying of the multicompartmental lung depends almost entirely on emptying of the slow compartments, which is impaired if expiratory time is inadequate, leading to air trapping (Fig. 17.1). Consequently, much slower respiratory rates and longer inspiratory and expiratory times are essential to optimize ventilation in infants with established BPD (Fig. 17.2).

Baraldi et al.[10] reported that the time constant of infants with BPD and on prolonged mechanical ventilation increased from 0.14 ± 0.01 s at 10–20 days of life to 0.33 ± 0.02 s at 6 months and 0.48 ± 0.03 s at 1 year. Three time constants are needed to exhale 95% of the tidal volume and, a complete exhalation requires five time constants. Using the reported value of approximately 0.3 s at 6 months of age, an expiratory time of 1.5 s is needed for complete exhalation ($5 \times 0.3\ s = 1.5\ s$). Inspiratory time constants are shorter than expiratory ones,[11] but inspiratory time should be at a minimum of 0.5 s. Consequently, the

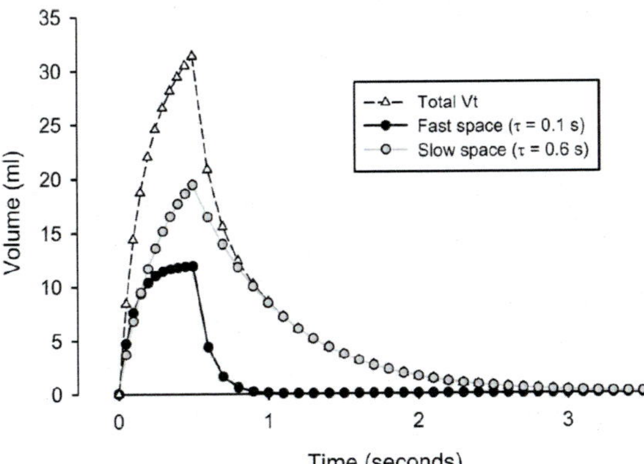

FIG. 17.1 Volume-time curves for one ventilator cycle in a patient with very severe BPD showing the filling and emptying of the fast and slow compartments. In this extreme example, the inspiratory time is 0.5 s and the ventilator rate is 17 cycles per minute. The fast compartment (*black circles*) has a compliance of 0.5 mL/cmH_2O, resistance of 0.2 cmH_2O/(mL/s), and time constant of 0.1 s. The slow compartment (*open circles*) has a compliance of 0.8 mL/cmH_2O, resistance of 0.75 cmH_2O/(mL/s), and a time constant of 0.6 s. The open triangles are the total tidal volume, which is the sum of the volumes in the two compartments. In this example the total tidal volume is 31.4 mL, the tidal volume of the fast space is 11.9 mL, and the tidal volume of the slow space is 19.5 mL. As can be seen, exhalation depends entirely on the slow space, as the fast compartment has completely emptied by 1 s, whereas the slow compartment has only completely emptied by 3.5 s, the total time for one ventilator cycle. (Reproduced with permission from Shepherd EG Durkin LS, Malleske DT, Nelin LD. Mechanical ventilation of the infant with severe bronchopulmonary dysplasia. In: Aly H, ed. *Respiratory Management of Newborns*: IntechOpen; 2016.)

respiratory rate in a 6-month-old infant with established type 2 severe BPD should be no more than 30/minute (60 s divided by 2 s per cycle [0.5 + 1.5 s] = 30/minute). Older infants with very severe BPD may need a rate as slow as 20/minute (60 s divided by 3 s per cycle [0.5 + 2.5 s] = 20/minute).

The second important difference is the need for a substantially higher tidal volume (V_T). Several factors contribute to the need for these unusually large (from the neonatal perspective) tidal volumes. First, there is increased alveolar dead space resulting from heterogeneous lung inflation and air trapping. Second, there is increased anatomic dead space caused by "acquired tracheomegaly" described by Bhutani et al.[12] more than 30 years ago. Its occurrence should not come as a surprise when one considers that a ventilator rate of 50 inflations/minute typical for acute RDS, which stretches the immature airway tissues 72,000 times in 24 hours and more than 1 million times in 2 weeks! Finally, the slow ventilator rate necessitated by the long time constants must be coupled with a higher V_T in order to maintain adequate minute ventilation (MV). If we assume an adequate MV is 250–300 mL/kg/min and the rate is limited to 20/minute, the tidal volume would need to be 12.5–15 mL/kg (12.5–15 mL/kg × 20 inflations/min = 250–300 mL/kg/min). The actual MV needed to achieve adequate CO_2 clearance in an individual patient would depend on the physiologic dead space (sum of alveolar and anatomic dead space); the amount of alveolar simplification that reduces the surface area available for gas exchange; the degree of permissive hypercapnia, which facilitates CO_2 removal by increasing the gradient for CO_2 diffusion; and the degree to which spontaneous breathing between the mechanical inflations augments total MV.

The third major difference in the approach to ventilation of infants with established BPD, compared with acute RDS, is the need for substantially higher levels of positive end-expiratory pressure (PEEP). Poorly supported small airways that lack intrinsic rigidity tend to collapse as the lungs empty, resulting in the characteristic expiratory flow limitation at low lung volume (Fig. 17.3).[13] Large airway collapse due to tracheobronchomalacia may result in a similar pattern of flow limitation and responds similarly to high applied PEEP. The use of higher PEEP in the face of air trapping seems counterintuitive but works by effectively splinting the airways open during the later stages of expiration and allows more complete emptying, especially of the slow compartment. High PEEP is also needed to prevent large airway collapse during strong inspiratory efforts of the infant with tracheomalacia that would result in collapse of the extrathoracic trachea. Failure to recognize this phenomenon often leads to inappropriate lowering of PEEP in the erroneous belief that the air trapping seen radiographically is a reflection of excessive set PEEP. In fact, the air trapping is typically the result of dynamic (also called intrinsic) PEEP, which results from inadequate expiratory time and/or airway closure at low lung volumes. With inadequate PEEP, the lungs remain overexpanded (ventilation is occurring on the flat upper portion of the pressure-volume relationship; Fig. 17.4), leading to poor lung compliance, increased work of breathing, increased pulmonary vascular resistance, tachypnea, and poor gas exchange. When the diaphragm is already depressed because of air trapping, the infant is unable to generate a high tidal volume and can only attempt to maintain MV by increasing the respiratory

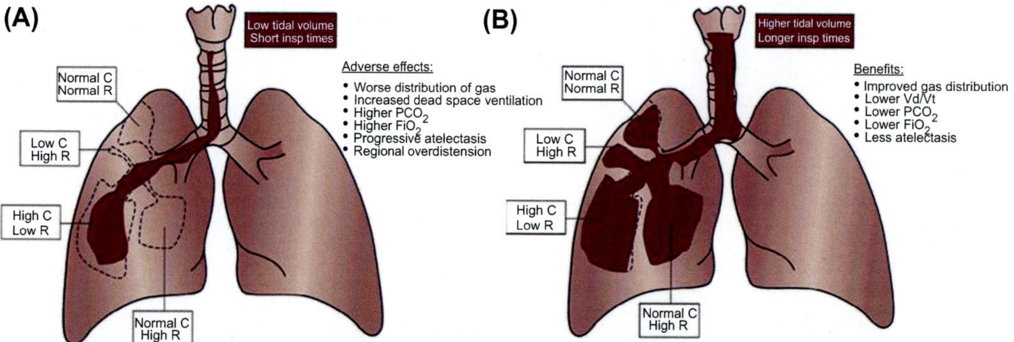

FIG. 17.2 The two-compartment lung pathophysiology. (A) The effect of ventilating with rapid rates, short inspiratory times, and low tidal volumes, which results in underventilation, increase in relative dead space, atelectasis, and increased ventilation/perfusion mismatch because the gas preferentially enters the fast lung compartments that have low airway resistance. (B) When slower rates and longer inspiratory rates are used, more even gas distribution is achieved with less atelectasis, improved ventilation, and lower oxygen requirement. C, compliance; R, resistance; Vd/Vt, dead space ventilation/total ventilation. (Reproduced with permission from Nelin LD, Abman SH, Panitch HB. A physiology-based approach to the respiratory care of children with severe bronchopulmonary dysplasia. In: Bancalari E, ed. *The Newborn Lung*: Elsevier; 2019.)

rate, which, as previously noted, leads to maldistribution of tidal volume, increased dead space ventilation, and ventilation/perfusion mismatch. Additionally, high intrinsic PEEP makes it more difficult for the infant to trigger the ventilator, which may lead to inconsistent pressure support (PS) with air hunger and agitation.

GENERAL APPROACH TO RESPIRATORY SUPPORT IN INFANTS WITH SEVERE BRONCHOPULMONARY DYSPLASIA

Although many infants with established BPD respond well to noninvasive distending airway pressure to promote airway patency, distending pressure alone may

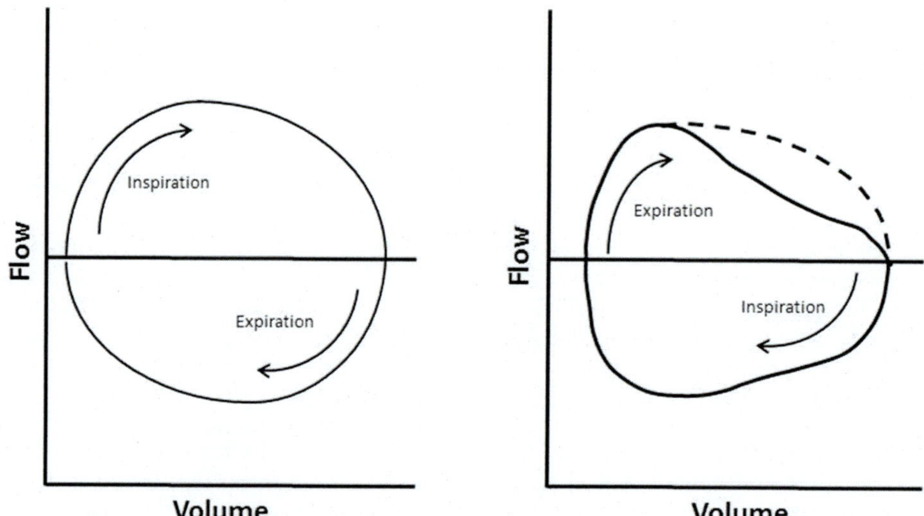

FIG. 17.3 Normal flow-volume curve in (A) illustrates the unconstrained inspiratory and expiratory flow throughout the respiratory cycle and in (B) demonstrates the characteristic drop in expiratory flow as the lung empties during expiration. This phenomenon is known as expiratory flow limitation at low lung volumes, which results from closure of the small airways that are inadequately supported by alveolar attachments of the simplified lung and lack intrinsic rigidity. The dashed line in (B) shows the response to increased positive end-expiratory pressure that now effectively maintains airway patency during expiration.

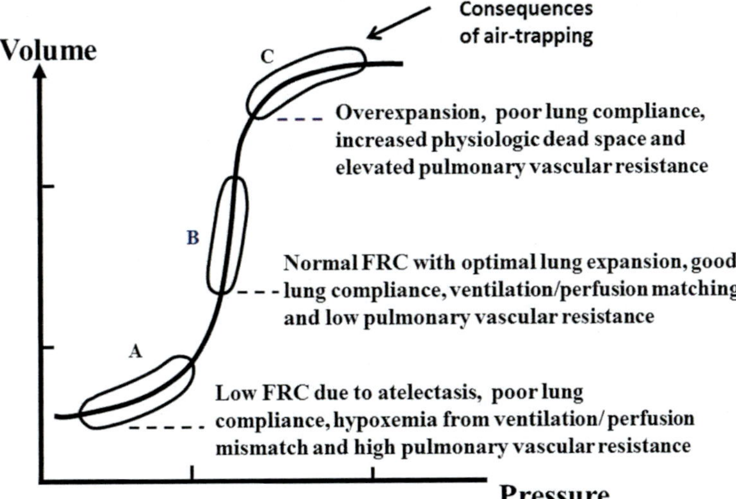

FIG. 17.4 Lung volume has an important effect on lung compliance as well as ventilation/perfusion matching, alveolar dead space, and pulmonary vascular resistance. The top right-hand portion of the S-shaped pressure-volume curve represents the situation that results from positive end-expiratory pressure with air trapping, such as commonly occurs in ventilated infants with bronchopulmonary dysplasia. *FRC*, functional residual capacity.

not provide sufficient support. Avoidance of invasive ventilation is an evidence-based strategy for prevention of BPD, but once severe BPD is established, the need for adequate support to facilitate somatic and pulmonary growth takes precedence over avoidance of intubation. The management of infants with established severe BPD requires a chronic care model and different treatment goals compared with the acute care model that neonatologists are accustomed to in the neonatal intensive care unot.[14] This model recognizes that BPD is a chronic condition that does not improve in days or even weeks. Optimal long-term respiratory and nutritional support facilitate a progrowth state, enable the patient to participate in developmentally appropriate activities, and promote lung recovery over a period of months, paving the way to eventual good outcome. The signs of the need for initiation or continuation of mechanical ventilation include high oxygen requirement, persistent respiratory distress, head-bobbing, retractions, tachypnea, frequent desaturation events, excessive CO_2 retention, intolerance of handling, and poor growth. The diagnosis of pulmonary hypertension is also considered by most clinicians an indication for mechanical ventilation. These signs may be present despite adequate gas exchange documented by blood gas measurement; it is essential to understand that an acceptable blood gas does not necessarily indicate adequate support.

In the absence of clinical trial evidence to recommend one mode of synchronized mechanical ventilation over another, the choice of modalities is driven by the pathophysiologic principles outlined earlier and the consensus of seasoned clinicians with experience in treating these infants.[15–17] Synchronized intermittent mandatory ventilation (SIMV) with or without PS appears to be the most widely used modality in this population. This choice is based on the need for longer inspiratory and expiratory times and the desire to control the rate of mechanical inflations. Assist control or PS ventilation as a primary mode has also been used successfully in these infants, but these modalities allow the infant to drive the ventilator rate, which can result in excessively rapid cycling and insufficient expiratory time, leading to air trapping. Volume-controlled or volume-targeted modes, such as volume-guarantee or pressure-regulated volume control, may be advantageous in terms of maintaining more stable MV in the face of changing lung mechanics, but because these infants typically require much higher tidal volumes than those to which neonatologists are accustomed to, clinicians seldom choose sufficiently high tidal volumes to provide adequate support.

It must be recognized that there is no single way that will optimally support all infants with severe established BPD because of the heterogeneity of the BPD phenotype. Consequently, an individualized approach is optimal with modes of support and specific settings chosen based on the best assessment of the individual infant's respiratory status using chest radiographs, lung mechanics, and other imaging modalities, if available. An important element in this process is the reassessment of the selected modalities and settings based on the patient's response and the information available by observing the waveforms on the ventilator display. Blood gas measurement has a limited role here because the values are not necessarily representative of the infant's overall status and may be distorted by the infant's response to the painful stimulus of obtaining the blood. The degree of metabolic compensation reflected by the bicarbonate level on serum electrolyte measurement may be a better reflection of the steady-state ventilatory status. End-tidal CO_2 measurement adds significant dead space and is unreliable in small infants in general[18] and even more so in the presence of increased dead space and multicompartmental lung[19] and thus should not be routinely relied on. Oxygenation status is best monitored by pulse oximetry. Persistence of tachypnea, retractions, and agitation with intermittent desaturations suggests suboptimal settings. A well-supported infant is calm, comfortable, and able to interact with the environment without the routine need for sedation/analgesia.

SPECIFIC RECOMMENDATIONS FOR MECHANICAL VENTILATION OF INFANTS WITH ESTABLISHED SEVERE BRONCHOPULMONARY DYSPLASIA

In infants with evidence of high airway resistance who require slow ventilation rates, SIMV is the preferred mode. PS of the spontaneous breaths is usually appropriate, but caution should be exercised to avoid a rapid rate with air trapping. The use of SIMV with PS may be uniquely suited to the multicompartmental lung of the infant with severe BPD. It appears that in many infants, the spontaneous breaths (with PS) ventilate the fast compartments with relatively faster respiratory rate and lower tidal volume, whereas the slow rate, high V_T mechanical inflations chiefly ventilate the slow compartments. If the pressure-control mode is used (PC-SIMV), peak inflation pressure (PIP) needs to be adjusted to achieve a V_T of 8–10 mL/kg for the mechanical inflations initially (measured at the airway opening) and adjusted as needed based on the infant's response. For infants with less severe BPD, 6–8 mL/kg may be sufficient. However, if the infant remains tachypneic with persistent high work of breathing, higher PIP and V_T is probably needed, sometimes as high as 12–15 mL/kg when a slow ventilator rate is used. This may result in PIP settings that are beyond the comfort level of many neonatologists, but appear to be both needed and well tolerated by older infants with established BPD. If using PS for spontaneous breaths, the PS level should be initially set at 10–12 cmH_2O and adjusted to achieve V_T of spontaneous breaths of 4–6 mL/kg and/or resolution of tachypnea. If volume-controlled SIMV (VC-SIMV) is used, the challenge is to determine the correct setting of V_T that will deliver an adequate V_T to the patient who often has an uncuffed endotracheal/tracheostomy tube and whose lung volume/lung compliance is relatively low to the ventilator circuit and humidifier, resulting in substantial and variable loss of V_T to compression of gas in the circuit and leak around the endotracheal tube, necessitating a V_T setting that is much higher than the actual delivered V_T (Fig. 17.5).[20] The option is to judge the adequacy of delivered V_T clinically (by chest rise and breath sounds, both of which are subjective) or to measure the exhaled V_T at the airway opening using a separate flow sensor.

If a volume-targeted mode that measures V_T at the airway opening is used (i.e., volume guarantee), the target V_T should initially be set at 6–8 mL/kg (8–10 mL/kg for older infants with more severe disease) and the PIP limit set sufficiently high to allow that target to be reliably reached without excessive alarms. If a volume-targeted mode that uses V_T measurement at the ventilator end of the patient circuit is used (i.e., pressure-regulated volume control of the Servo-i), the same issues as described earlier for volume-controlled ventilation are operative and substantially higher V_T settings will be needed because the circuit compliance feature available on that ventilator is ineffective when there is a leak around an uncuffed endotracheal tube. The newest version of PRVC now regulates V_T based on the measurement performed at the airway opening and this should eliminate this problem. Regardless of the initial settings, if evidence of insufficient support is noted, higher V_T target and PIP will be needed. This is especially likely when there is evidence of large physiologic dead space, which can be estimated by capnography using the equation $Paco_2 - EtCO_2/Paco_2$. A normal dead space fraction is less than 0.3.

Initial PEEP should be in the range of 8–10 cmH_2O to splint large and small airways open throughout the respiratory cycle. Ventilator rate should be set at 20–25 inflations/minute with an inspiratory time of 0.5–0.7 s. Flow waveform on the ventilator display should always be inspected for evidence of dynamic PEEP, demonstrated by failure of expiratory flow to return to zero before the onset of the next inflation (Fig. 17.6). If this phenomenon is observed, the expiratory time should be increased until the problem

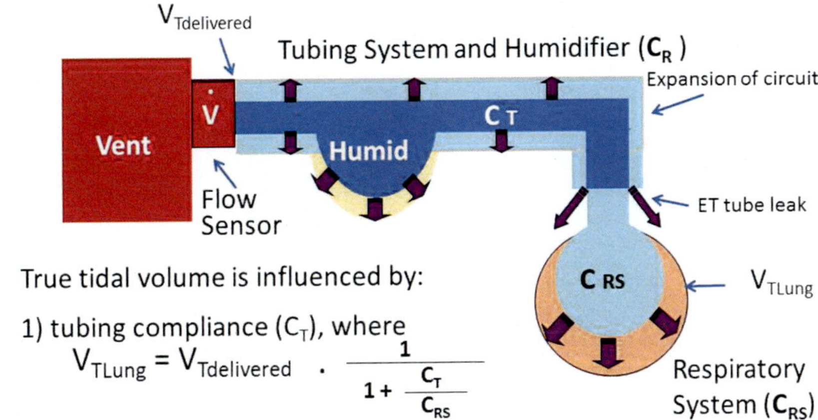

FIG. 17.5 Functional limitation of volume-controlled ventilation in newborn infants. Volume-controlled ventilation regulates the volume of gas delivered into the proximal end of the ventilator circuit ($V_{Tdelivered}$). The volume of gas entering the lungs (V_{TLung}) is affected by four factors: (1) tubing compliance (C_T), (2) compressible volume of the circuit and humidifier, (3) magnitude of the leak around an uncuffed endotracheal (ET) tube, and (4) baby's respiratory effort. In newborn infants the volume of the lungs is only a fraction of the circuit/humidifier volume and often poorly compliant. Thus the loss of volume to compression of gas in the circuit and to stretching of the compliant circuit is very substantial. Variable leak around ET tubes makes compensation very challenging.

resolves; this may result in ventilator rate as low as 15 inflations/minute in extreme cases. Evidence of high airway resistance is readily seen in the scalar flow waveform routinely displayed by modern ventilators. Flow-volume loops are useful in recognizing expiratory flow limitation at low lung volumes, and this suggests the need for higher end-expiratory pressure (Fig. 17.3). An alternate approach to determine an optimal PEEP is to vary the PEEP level systematically and determine the value that results in the best compliance and lowest resistance, so-called "best PEEP." However, the PEEP level that is needed to maintain airway patency may be higher than the level that results in best lung compliance in a given patient, so a subjective judgment still needs to be made as to the true optimal PEEP. Additionally, the compliance measurement does not account for the patient's contribution to transpulmonary pressure, and therefore compliance measurement in actively breathing infants is unreliable.

WEANING FROM MECHANICAL VENTILATION

There is little objective information regarding the optimal timing or method of weaning from mechanical ventilation in infants with established severe BPD. As previously mentioned, a long-term view is indicated and therefore lowering and eventually discontinuing mechanical ventilatory support should only be considered after a substantial period of stability, consistent adequate weight gain, and ability to interact with caregivers. In some infants, airway problems preclude weaning of support even when these conditions are met.

In general, if the fraction of inspired oxygen (FiO_2) has consistently remained below 0.40 without severe desaturation episodes and there is no evidence of pulmonary hypertension, it is reasonable to begin to reduce the respiratory support. There is no evidence base to suggest the best approach to reduce the support; gradual reduction of inflation pressure or V_T target is the usual approach, with changes made only one to two times per week. The infant's response to the attempt needs to be assessed each time, and if there is a substantial increase in FiO_2 or work of breathing, the change may need to be reversed and further weaning attempts deferred. If the weaning is tolerated without significant setback, gradual weaning can continue, being mindful of the chronicity of the condition and the possible contribution of airway disease to ventilator dependence. Gradually lowering PEEP may be alternated

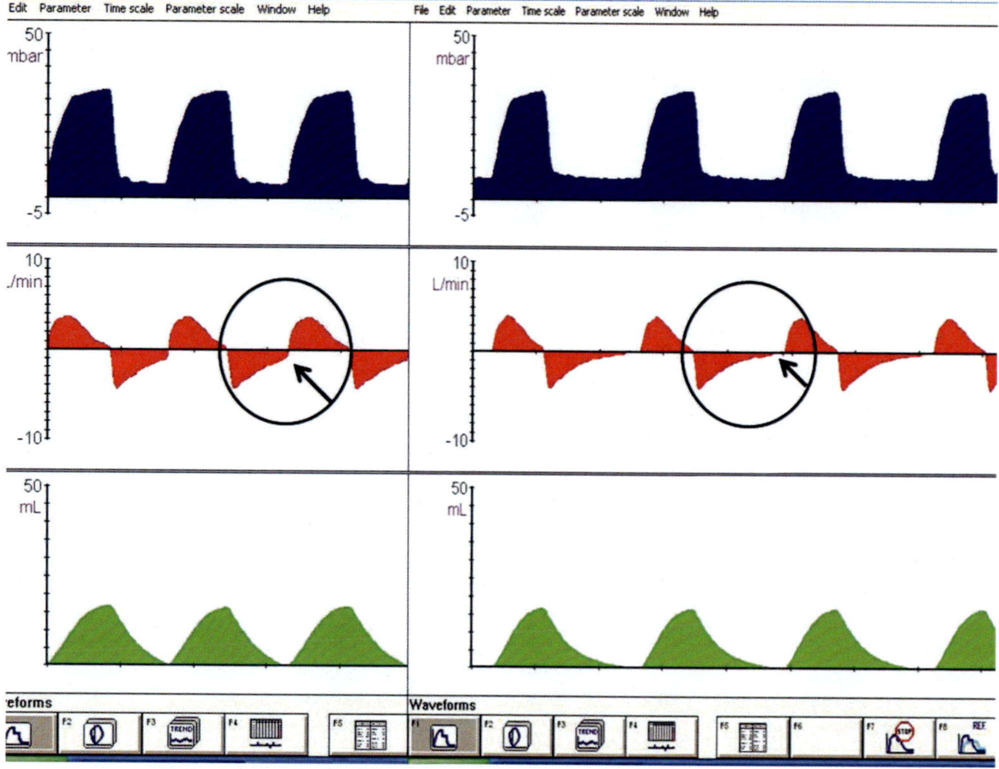

FIG. 17.6 A typical ventilator display showing (A) airway pressure, (B) flow, and (C) volume. The left panel illustrates dynamic positive end-expiratory pressure (PEEP) due to insufficient expiratory time in a patient with high airway resistance. This is recognized by the fact that there is still expiratory flow occurring when the next inflation begins. Flow can only occur if there is a pressure gradient between the trachea and the ventilator circuit, thus the pressure in the trachea must be higher than the set PEEP. The right panel demonstrates that with prolongation of the expiratory time (i.e., slower ventilator rate), the expiratory flow returns to baseline before the onset of the next inflation. The arrow indicates the difference between expiratory flow when inspiratory is insufficient in the left panel and when it is adequate in the right panel.

with reductions in PIP/V_T. There is no consensus regarding "extubatable" settings in infants with established BPD, but in general, they can be extubated from substantially higher PIP, V_T, and PEEP than small preterm infants, thus care should be taken to avoid reducing support too much. Some clinicians gauge readiness for extubation by allowing the infant progressively longer trials of PS without large SIMV inflations. Some form of noninvasive support is typically needed and we have become accustomed to extubating these infants to continuous positive airway pressure at pressures that match the mean airway pressure before extubation, typically 10–15 cmH_2O, which appear to be needed and well tolerated in these infants.

ALTERNATE VENTILATION MODES

High-Frequency Ventilation

High-frequency ventilation (HFV) has been studied extensively in infants with various causes of acute respiratory failure, but there is a paucity of literature on the use of HFV in infants with BPD. The physics of HFV would suggest that it is best suited to treat disorders characterized by short time constants. However, because hypercapnia is often a problem in infants with BPD and because they often require PIP and V_T that are beyond the comfort level of neonatal practitioners, the demonstrated ability of HFV to effectively ventilate with lower V_T entices clinicians to use it in this unproven manner. Some indirect evidence suggests that gas distribution with HFV may be less affected by regional time constants and that accelerated gas diffusion may contribute to improved gas exchange with low V_T. There is insufficient evidence to recommend the use of HFV, but anecdotally, both high-frequency oscillatory ventilation (HFOV) and high-frequency jet ventilation (HFJV) have been used in this setting. If used at all, both HFOV and HFJV need to be used with lower ventilator frequency/rate to account for the longer time constants and with high mean airway pressure to improve airway patency. The concern with HFOV is the potential of the active exhalation phase to collapse the poorly supported small airways as well as the segments of large airways affected by malacia. From a theoretic standpoint, HFJV, which relies on passive exhalation, may be more effective, but only two small case series are available to support this concept.[21,22]

Neurally Adjusted Ventilatory Assist

Neurally adjusted ventilatory assist (NAVA) is an emerging alternative to conventional flow-triggered ventilation that may be uniquely suitable to provide support to infants with severe established BPD, who are quite difficult to ventilate optimally with the conventional synchronized ventilation modes. During NAVA, the ventilator responds to the electric activity of the diaphragm (Edi) measured by an array of electrodes embedded in a special feeding tube and provides inflation pressure in synchrony and in proportion to the infant's inspiratory effort. This allows the patient to control not only the onset of inspiration but also the magnitude and duration of each inflation. In essence, the baby drives the ventilator and, at least in theory, receives the exact amount of support needed without depending on the bedside provider to select the appropriate inflation pressure or volume, inflation time, and ventilator rate. Several short-term crossover studies in preterm infants with RDS demonstrated that infants switched to NAVA have lower PIP, but no important clinical outcomes were assessed.[23] Only one randomized study in this population is available and it failed to demonstrate significant differences in outcome.[24] Lee et al.[25] showed that infants switched to NAVA after having been chronically ventilated had lower sedation requirements suggesting better patient ventilator synchrony. Jung et al. demonstrated lower peak and mean airway pressures, lower work of breathing, and improved gas exchange when preterm infants who had been ventilated for at least 4 weeks were switched from SIMV to NAVA.[26] No systematic data are available to evaluate the potential benefits of NAVA in infants with established severe BPD, but unpublished data from the BPD Collaborative indicate that it is being used with some frequency in this unique population.

Considerations for Tracheostomy

There is no consensus on the timing of tracheostomy in infants with established BPD. Traditionally, the need for tracheostomy signaled recognition that prolonged ventilation will be needed and was seen as a failure, thus approached with reluctance by both providers and parents. There are both risks and important benefits in tracheostomy in infants requiring prolonged mechanical ventilation (Box 17.1). The decision may be influenced by practical considerations, such as patient size and stability (or lack of thereof) but needs to be made sufficiently in advance of planned discharge to allow for discussion with the family who may need some time to come to terms with the situation and for the thorough teaching that is needed to allow for safe discharge home. In general, if an infant with established BPD reaches a postmenstrual age of 36 weeks and still requires invasive mechanical ventilation (i.e., type 2 severe BPD),[14] serious consideration should be given to moving forward with initiating the discussion regarding tracheostomy. Available evidence indicates that the timing of tracheostomy is highly variable among centers.[27] Our approach is to portray tracheostomy as a positive step that will enable the child to finally come home after months of hospitalization. Once healed, tracheostomy provides a stable airway to facilitate more effective ventilation with less discomfort and greater respiratory stability, which in turn improves the tolerance of handling by staff and family members, allowing better tolerance of developmentally appropriate activities, the acquisition of oral motor skills, greater family interaction with their child, and ultimately better neurodevelopmental outcomes. Data from a large

BOX 17.1
Risks and Benefits of Tracheostomy

Risks	Benefits
Surgical risk	Facilitates D/C
Postop critical period	Removal of ETT
Long-term commitment	Less discomfort/sedation
Infection	Safer airway
Impact on vocalization	Oral motor skills/PO feeding
Skin irritation	Better neurodevelopment
Tracheal erosion	Better growth

institution with extensive experience in the management of severe BPD indicate that, when compared to a period before performing tracheostomy, infants showed better linear growth, needed fewer calories, received less sedatives/analgesics, and were better able to participate in developmental therapy sessions.[28] An earlier study utilizing data from the *Eunice Kennedy Shriver* National Institute of Child Health and Human Development Neonatal Research Network found that babies undergoing tracheostomy earlier (<120 days of age) were less likely to die or have neurodevelopmental impairment than those who underwent tracheostomy later (odds ratio, 0.5; confidence interval, 0.3–0.9).[29] A multidisciplinary team needs to carefully evaluate the risks and benefits of tracheostomy in each patient and present a clear and consistent recommendation to the family.

FUTURE DIRECTIONS

With the increasing survival of extremely preterm infants at the borderline of viability, there will continue to be a population of former preterm infants who require long-term respiratory support and thus there is an urgent need for high-quality research to address the many knowledge gaps that currently challenge the care of this relatively orphan population. The attitude of neonatologists needs to shift from one of despair over a failure to prevent the development of BPD to one that embraces the reality that these patients continue to need the best possible care that we can offer and that, despite many challenges, they can ultimately have a good outcome. Although lung disease is the most critical problem in these infants, many comorbidities, such as pulmonary hypertension, aerodigestive problems, feeding difficulties, and neurodevelopmental delays, affect their progress, making a multidisciplinary approach mandatory.

Because of the heterogeneity of the disease, better phenotyping of BPD is needed in order to better understand how to optimize respiratory management. Currently, respiratory function monitoring is confined to infants who are mechanically ventilated and limited by the omission of the infant's spontaneous respiratory effort. Noninvasive methods of measuring airway resistance would be highly desirable to monitor disease progression and response to medication. Systematic data collection to define the population characteristics, respiratory support modalities, and level of support is needed as a starting point, followed by adequately powered clinical trials to evaluate the comparative effectiveness of different approaches to mechanical ventilation. Currently, there is still uncertainty regarding basic questions such as appropriate oxygen saturation and partial pressure of carbon dioxide (P_{CO_2}) targets, or indeed if P_{CO_2} matters at all, as long as pH is adequate.

A systematic evaluation of the optimal timing of tracheostomy is needed to provide the necessary evidence base for this critical decision. Promising novel modalities, such as NAVA, need to be evaluated systematically and compared to existing approaches. The challenge in designing such studies is the reality that there is substantial heterogeneity in this population and that the specific protocols for comparing different ventilation modes need to allow for individualized patient care. Important clinical outcomes, such as duration of hospitalization, growth, and neurodevelopmental outcomes, need to be evaluated, in addition to mortality, morbidity, and the need for sedation/analgesia.

Because these infants constitute a relatively small proportion of patients, multicenter collaboration is needed to reach an adequate sample size. The recognition that a collaboration of multiple institutions dedicated to study severe BPD is essential to move the field forward has led to the formation of the BPD Collaborative in 2012.[14] The Collaborative has grown from the initial 8 centers to the current 18 and is actively collecting descriptive data in a common database that will inform the design of prospective studies currently in the planning stages.

REFERENCES

1. Stoll BJ, Hansen NI, Bell EF, et al. Trends in care practices, morbidity, and mortality of extremely preterm neonates, 1993–2012. *JAMA*. 2015;314(10):1039–1051.
2. Charafeddine L, D'Angio CT, Phelps DL. Atypical chronic lung disease patterns in neonates. *Pediatrics*. 1999;103(4 Pt 1):759–765.
3. Keszler M, Sant'Anna G. Mechanical ventilation and bronchopulmonary dysplasia. *Clin Perinatol*. 2015;42(4):781–796.
4. Jobe AH. Effects of chorioamnionitis on the fetal lung. *Clin Perinatol*. 2012;39(3):441–457.
5. Goldman SL, Gerhardt T, Sonni R, et al. Early prediction of chronic lung disease by pulmonary function testing. *J Pediatr*. 1983;102(4):613–617.
6. Lui K, Lloyd J, Ang E, Rynn M, Gupta JM. Early changes in respiratory compliance and resistance during the development of bronchopulmonary dysplasia in the era of surfactant therapy. *Pediatr Pulmonol*. 2000;30(4):282–290.
7. Jarriel WS, Richardson P, Knapp RD, Hansen TN. A nonlinear regression analysis of nonlinear, passive-deflation flow-volume plots. *Pediatr Pulmonol*. 1993;15(3):175–182.
8. Keszler M, Nassabeh-Montazami S, Abubakar K. Evolution of tidal volume requirement during the first 3 weeks of life

in infants <800 g ventilated with volume guarantee. *Arch Dis Child Fetal Neonatal Ed.* 2009;94(4):F279–F282.
9. Reiterer F, Eber E, Zach MS, Muller W. Management of severe congenital tracheobronchomalacia by continuous positive airway pressure and tidal breathing flow-volume loop analysis. *Pediatr Pulmonol.* 1994;17(6):401–403.
10. Baraldi E, Filippone M, Trevisanuto D, Zanardo V, Zacchello F. Pulmonary function until two years of life in infants with bronchopulmonary dysplasia. *Am J Respir Crit Care Med.* 1997;155(1):149–155.
11. Wolfson MR, Bhutani VK, Shaffer TH, Bowen Jr FW. Mechanics and energetics of breathing helium in infants with bronchopulmonary dysplasia. *J Pediatr.* 1984; 104(5):752–757.
12. Bhutani VK, Ritchie WG, Shaffer TH. Acquired tracheomegaly in very preterm neonates. *Am J Dis Child.* 1986; 140(5):449–452.
13. Tepper RS, Morgan WJ, Cota K, Taussig LM. Expiratory flow limitation in infants with bronchopulmonary dysplasia. *J Pediatr.* 1986;109(6):1040–1046.
14. Abman SH, Collaco JM, Shepherd EG, et al. Interdisciplinary care of children with severe bronchopulmonary dysplasia. *J Pediatr.* 2017;181(12–28):e11.
15. Castile RG, Nelin LD. Lung function, structure and the physiologic basis for mechanical ventilation of infants with established BPD. In: Abman SH, ed. *Bronchopulmonary Dysplasia.* New York: Informa Healthcare USA; 2009: 328–346.
16. Shepherd EG, Durkin LS, Malleske DT, Nelin LD. Mechanical ventilation of the infant with severe bronchopulmonary dysplasia. In: Aly H, ed. *Respiratory Management of Newborns.* IntechOpen; 2016.
17. Nelin LD, Abman SH, Panitch HB. A physiology-based approach to the respiratory care of children with severe bronchopulmonary dysplasia. In: Bancalari E, ed. *The Newborn Lung.* Elsevier; 2019.
18. Schmalisch G. Current methodological and technical limitations of time and volumetric capnography in newborns. *Biomed Eng Online.* 2016;15(1):104.
19. Singh BS, Gilbert U, Singh S, Govindaswami B. Sidestream microstream end tidal carbon dioxide measurements and blood gas correlations in neonatal intensive care unit. *Pediatr Pulmonol.* 2013;48(3):250–256.
20. Keszler M. Volume-targeted ventilation: one size does not fit all. Evidence-based recommendations for successful use. *Arch Dis Child Fetal Neonatal Ed.* 2019 Jan;104(1): F108–F112.
21. Friedlich P, Subramanian N, Sebald M, Noori S, Seri I. Use of high-frequency jet ventilation in neonates with hypoxemia refractory to high-frequency oscillatory ventilation. *J Matern Fetal Neonatal Med.* 2003;13(6):398–402.
22. Plavka R, Dokoupilova M, Pazderova L, et al. High-frequency jet ventilation improves gas exchange in extremely immature infants with evolving chronic lung disease. *Am J Perinatol.* 2006;23(8):467–472.
23. Firestone KS, Beck J, Stein H. Neurally adjusted ventilatory assist for noninvasive support in neonates. *Clin Perinatol.* 2016;43(4):707–724.
24. Rossor TE, Hunt KA, Shetty S, Greenough A. Neurally adjusted ventilatory assist compared to other forms of triggered ventilation for neonatal respiratory support. *Cochrane Database Syst Rev.* 2017;10:CD012251.
25. Lee J, Kim HS, Jung YH, Choi CW, Jun YH. Neurally adjusted ventilatory assist for infants under prolonged ventilation. *Pediatr Int.* 2017;59(5):540–544.
26. Jung YH, Kim HS, Lee J, Shin SH, Kim EK, Choi JH. Neurally adjusted ventilatory assist in preterm infants with established or evolving bronchopulmonary dysplasia on high-intensity mechanical ventilatory support: a single-center experience. *Pediatr Crit Care Med.* 2016;17(12): 1142–1146.
27. Murthy K, Porta NFM, Lagatta JM, et al. Inter-center variation in death or tracheostomy placement in infants with severe bronchopulmonary dysplasia. *J Perinatol.* 2017; 37(6):723–727.
28. Luo J, Shepard S, Nilan K, et al. Improved growth and developmental activity post tracheostomy in preterm infants with severe BPD. *Pediatr Pulmonol.* 2018;53(9): 1237–1244.
29. DeMauro SB, D'Agostino JA, Bann C, et al. Developmental outcomes of very preterm infants with tracheostomies. *J Pediatr.* 2014;164(6), 1303-1310 e1302.

CHAPTER 18

Management of Severe BPD Requiring Chronic Medical Support

EDWARD G. SHEPHERD, MD • DANIEL T. MALLESKE, MD • SUSAN K. LYNCH, MD • LEIF D. NELIN, MD

INTRODUCTION

Bronchopulmonary dysplasia (BPD), first described in 1967 by Northway et al.,[1] is the most common complication of extreme prematurity, and its incidence is inversely proportional to gestational age (GA) at birth.[2,3] Severe BPD is defined currently as a need for ≥30% oxygen and/or respiratory support at 36 weeks postmenstrual age (PMA) in preterm infants born before 32 weeks GA.[4] Advances in neonatal care have led to improved survival in extremely low birthweight (ELBW) infants; however, rates of BPD, and severe BPD in particular, do not seem to be decreasing.[3,4] Numerous care practices, including avoidance of mechanical ventilation, implementation of "gentle ventilation" techniques, aggressive use of nasal continuous positive airway pressure (nCPAP), administration of caffeine, use of surfactant, etc., reduce the incidence of BPD in specific studies; however, these results have not translated into a reduced incidence of BPD, or severe BPD, nationally or internationally.[5] Indeed, despite proven implementation of multiple care practices that "should" prevent BPD, the rates of BPD seem to be increasing.[6,7]

Infants with BPD are at high risk for numerous complications above and beyond those associated with preterm birth, and the number and severity of which are strongly correlated with the severity of their BPD.[8–11] Indeed, infants with severe BPD suffer cerebral palsy at rates 50% higher than those with moderate BPD, have a 40%–50% chance of cognitive and/or motor delays on Bayley Scale assessments, have higher rates of deafness, are more likely to have growth impairments, and overall have a greater than 60% chance of experiencing some form of neurodevelopmental delay, if they survive to discharge.[8] It is not clear, however, why severe BPD is associated with neurodevelopmental delays. Multiple mechanisms, including hypoxic spells, exposure to systemic inflammation, the use of systemic steroids, and so forth, have been proposed as causal; however, these do not explain the wide variability in outcome.[4,11–13] For example, while some infants with severe BPD are negatively affected by hypoxic spells, systemic inflammation, exposure to systemic steroids, etc., others with the same exposures are not affected. Some infants with severe BPD receive tracheostomy placement while others with similar degrees of illness do not.[11] In addition, other childhood lung diseases, including cystic fibrosis and asthma, do not seem to be associated with neurodevelopmental delays. Why, then, do infants with severe BPD have such disproportionately high rates of complications?

We argue that the association between severe BPD and long-term neurodevelopmental impairment is not an intrinsic result of the disease process itself, but instead that the care practices employed to treat infants with established severe BPD contribute to neurodevelopmental impairment.[14] This notion is supported by recent publications demonstrating that there is extremely wide variability between centers in outcomes for infants with severe BPD and that neurodevelopmental outcomes can be influenced by care practices.[11,14,15] Specifically, infants with established severe BPD are beyond the period in which BPD can be prevented, but we continue to treat them using an acute-care, prevention-focused model.[4,16] This acute-care model assumes that there is a rapidly changing physiology that demands frequent changes in care, frequent laboratory assessments, and multiple noxious stimuli. Unfortunately, the literature is quite clear that the sum of noxious stimuli a preterm infant undergoes during their hospitalization is strongly correlated with worse neurodevelopmental outcomes.[17–20] In addition, there is substantial evidence that exposure to medications that are commonly used in the acute care of sick neonates,

Updates on Neonatal Chronic Lung Disease. https://doi.org/10.1016/B978-0-323-68353-1.00018-X

including systemic steroids, sedatives, and narcotics, may impair development as well.[21–23]

It is critical to understand and acknowledge that established severe BPD is much better conceptualized as a chronic disease as opposed to the acute respiratory diseases that neonatologists and intensive care physicians are more familiar treating. Indeed, unlike respiratory diseases in the first few days of life in preterm infants wherein physiology is rapidly changing and rapid responses to these changes are necessary, severe BPD has a relatively static physiology that is unlikely to improve rapidly and cannot be improved by rapidly weaning support.[4,15,16] Thus, a chronic approach to the patient with established severe BPD is needed to maximize not only pulmonary outcomes but neurodevelopmental outcomes. Furthermore, the natural history of severe BPD strongly suggests that weaning respiratory support rapidly or aggressive pharmacological interventions have negative effects on long-term outcomes. It is becoming clear that growth, particularly linear growth, over a relatively long time period, likely measured in months (not days or weeks), is the most important therapy for the patient with severe BPD. Therefore, it is imperative to employ a chronic-care model focused on maintaining comfort, avoiding neuroactive medications, avoiding noxious stimuli, and maximizing positive stimuli while providing excellent nutrition so that infants can progress through the phases of severe BPD.[4,15] In other words, care for infants with severe BPD must be laser-focused on maximizing positive neurodevelopmental interactions while minimizing negative ones. Critically, this care model must acknowledge that changes in care can only occur slowly, as the disease itself only progresses slowly.

The natural history of severe BPD from birth through discharge can be conceptualized as a progression through four predictable and sequential phases of illness which correlates with key clinical markers (Table 18.1). Critically, severe BPD itself represents a wide spectrum of disease,[4] and the pace of progress through these phases is inversely correlated with the degree of BPD severity. Infants with relatively "mild" severe BPD may conclude all phases within months, but infants with the most severe forms of BPD can require years. The clinician must accept, however, that nothing can be done to accelerate the process beyond the pace at

TABLE 18.1
Phases of Severe BPD.

Phase I (Unstable) *Ventilator management based on physiology*	**Phase II (Transitional)** *Adjust ventilator support for increased activity*	**Phase III (Pro-growth)** *Wean ventilator support while maintaining activity*	**Phase IV (Convalescence)** *Transition to home or referring center*
Characteristics: • High FiO2 requirements • Frequent desaturations • Air-trapping • IV sedation/paralysis • High systemic steroids • Pulmonary hypertension (PH)	**Characteristics:** • FiO2 <0.50 • Off of IV sedation/paralysis • Weaning enteric sedatives • PH stable or decreasing • Tolerates cares • Steroids <1 mg/kg/day	**Characteristics:** • FiO2 <0.40 • CPAP/PS trials or wean PIP • Maintains developmental activities • Tolerates postural activity • Good linear growth • Steroids <0.2 mg/kg/day	**Characteristics:** • Nasal cannula, nCPAP, or home ventilator • Happy child • Consistent interactions • Weaning bronchodilators and diuretics
Physiology: • Unstable; characterized by obstruction with long time constants • V/Q mismatch • Frequent bronchospasm	**Physiology:** • Obstruction with lability • Episodic bronchospasm	**Physiology:** • Continues with obstruction but stable • Bronchospasm rare • Extubation attempts feasible	**Physiology:** • Stable except for exacerbations • Tolerating weaning
Transition to Phase II: • Improvement in oxygenation • Systemic steroids able to be weaned even minimally • Central lines out • PH improved	**Transition to Phase III:** • No desaturations • Work of breathing improved • Systemic steroids ≤0.2 mg/kg	**Transition to Phase IV:** • Stable oxygenation • Comfortable breathing • Developmental progress • Good growth velocity	**Transition to discharge:** • No systemic steroids • Excellent growth • Parental teaching • Disposition

which healing and growth can occur, and efforts to circumvent the natural progression of the disease may paradoxically lengthen its time course.

Phase I is a period of physiologic instability that, in rare and extreme cases, may begin soon after birth but usually starts later during the first and second months of life. Phase I usually lasts 1 to 6 months. Patients in Phase I typically require significant ventilator support and high concentrations of oxygen to survive and maintain oxygenation and they have frequent desaturations that are not preventable with standard ventilator manipulations. Their physical examination is notable for increased work of breathing and poor neuroregulation. Some of these infants will require intermittent or continuous sedation and in extreme cases pharmacologic paralysis. They may have emerging evidence of pulmonary hypertension (PH), which can be an ominous complication. In some cases, they will require systemic steroid administration to achieve acceptable stability. With good growth, however, these patients gradually stabilize as they evolve into Phase II, the transitional stage.

Babies in Phase II are clinically more stable, but still may require significant respiratory support, including high ventilator settings that are aimed at assuring adequate and consistent ventilation-perfusion matching. Their oxygenation is much more stable with fewer spells, and the fraction of inspired oxygen (FiO_2) typically can be weaned to 0.6 or less while maintaining adequate oxygen saturations. Physical examination is typically notable for improved work of breathing, regular periods of quiet alertness, and improving tolerance of low-level activities. If present, PH is stable or improving, and weaning of narcotics and sedatives is usually possible. At the same time, babies in Phase II are often very active as they are rapidly growing, developing, and increasing muscle mass, and nonpharmacological comfort measures are critical. The primary goals of the care team during Phase II are to provide adequate respiratory support to ensure that patients can maintain appropriate developmental interactions, while continuing to provide outstanding nutrition to ensure optimal linear growth. Most often, Phase II is the period in which tracheostomies are placed if needed. Phase II typically lasts between 3 and 12 months, but progress may be excruciatingly slow in the most severe cases of BPD. By the end of Phase II, infants will typically be stable on an FiO_2 less than 0.5.

Phase III is the period of steady clinical improvement and can perhaps be best characterized as a "pro-growth" state. Infants in this phase have stable oxygenation and tolerate careful weaning of respiratory support without developmental compromise. On physical examination, these infants will have extended periods of calm interaction and substantial respiratory reserve even when challenged. Linear growth typically accelerates during Phase III, and weight/length ratios should normalize. During Phase III, it should be possible to wean systemic steroids either to physiologic replacement doses for those with adrenal insufficiency, or discontinue them completely. While improvement is usually steady, the pace remains relatively slow, and Phase III may last between 3 and 12 months.

The final or "convalescent" phase is notable for substantially improved respiratory reserve with consistent and robust interactions with the environment, steady motor development, and adequate clinical stability consistent with hospital discharge. Infants in Phase IV are continuously stable on respiratory support that is feasible at home. Typically, such infants will require supplemental oxygen via nasal cannula or tracheostomy collar; however, infants with the most severe forms of BPD may require home ventilation via tracheostomy. These infants should require an FiO_2 less than 0.4 and PH should be resolved or well controlled. Stable feeds must be ensured either with oral feeds or with gastrostomy tubes for those unable to achieve full PO feeds. Medications should be weaned to twice daily, if possible, to improve parental adherence, and all families and caregivers must be fully trained in all aspects of care.

FUNDAMENTALS OF BPD CARE

The keys to successfully navigating the four phases of severe BPD are the basic principles of chronic care which emphasize incremental change and continuous care. Care should be provided by a dedicated transdisciplinary team that maintains expertise in severe BPD.[4,15] This team must provide continuous and reliable feedback to the practitioners to ensure that patients are responding appropriately to changes in care and that progress remains steady. And finally, each team must also develop mechanisms to ensure continuity of care over the course of prolonged hospitalizations. Once these teams and mechanisms are in place, care can be focused on the fundamentals of outstanding BPD care, which are outlined in the following section.

There are five core principles that are fundamental to outstanding severe BPD care.[15] The first two principles are focused on avoiding the most common causes of death for infants with established severe BPD, while the last three are focused on maximizing the infant's ability to heal, grow, and develop. These principles are:

1. Avoid infections
2. Avoid pulmonary hypertensive crises
3. Optimize growth
4. Provide intensive developmental care
5. Provide minimal impact respiratory support

While these principles seem intuitive and simple, in practice they are difficult to achieve in a typical intensive care setting. Underlying all of these principles is a commitment to basic chronic care fundamentals, including mechanisms to ensure outstanding continuity of care, team empowerment, robust feedback mechanisms, and a strong commitment to parent-centered care. In the Nationwide Children's Hospital Comprehensive Center for BPD (CCBPD), we have concluded that infants with severe BPD care are best served in a separate unit for such infants; however, we believe it is entirely possible to apply these principles to individual patients within typical neonatal intensive care units. The following is a description of the critical aspects of applying the fundamentals of BPD.

Avoid infection

Infections are one of the leading causes of death for infants with severe BPD. Thus, meticulous hand hygiene is an absolute necessity in the routine care of patients with severe BPD. Furthermore, aggressive infection control programs must be utilized to prevent infections in these patients. For example, infants with severe BPD are particularly vulnerable to viral infections before and after discharge. Thus, units must achieve superior hand hygiene and restrict exposure to any person with symptoms of viral infection or recent exposures, including staff. Moreover, these babies and their families must receive timely immunizations, including influenza vaccination and pertussis boosters if indicated.

The most common fatal infections are central line–associated blood stream infections (CLABSIs). Therefore, the most important infection control practice for infants with severe BPD is to remove any central lines as soon as possible. This can be challenging since infants with severe BPD are often extremely ill and clinically unstable and thus practitioners are hesitant to remove central access. In addition, these babies usually require positive pressure at 36 weeks PMA and may be perceived as irritable, and this perception can lead to an escalation in the use of sedative, anxiolytic, and/or hypnotic medications given intravenously, thereby prolonging central line use. When caregivers are able to provide superb and continuous nonpharmacological pain and stress relief, the need for these intravenous medications is significantly decreased facilitating central line discontinuation.

Finally, it is critical to limit exposure to broad-spectrum antibiotics in this population, as each day of exposure increases the risk of death.[24] Given that these patients are by definition unstable and often suffer frequent spells, teams caring for infants with severe BPD should have judicious antibiotic stewardship practices in place, and must be comfortable with the use of serial clinical examinations to determine risk of infection.

Avoid Pulmonary Hypertensive Crises

PH is the most common morbidity in patients with severe BPD[25] and is discussed in detail in Chapter 8. Interestingly the incidence of PH in BPD is variable among centers; in one study the point prevalence of PH in patients with severe BPD ranged from 17% to 36%.[26] Although it is not clear what leads to this intercenter variability in BPD associated PH, we wonder if some of this intercenter variation may be attributable to differences in oxygenation targets. Lower oxygenation targets could potentially lead to areas of hypoxemia and pulmonary vasoconstriction in the lung that might exacerbate PH. Gold standard evidence is lacking on optimal oxygenation targets. However, a higher target for oxygen saturations in patients with established severe BPD than are routinely used in earlier neonatal pulmonary diseases may be beneficial, given that the diagnosis of severe BPD is made at 36 weeks PMA after concerns for the development of retinopathy of prematurity. We routinely target oxygen saturations 94%–98%, while the recently published AHA/ATS guidelines suggest targeting oxygen saturations between 92% and 95%.[27] It is also imperative to maintain optimal ventilation-perfusion matching using a ventilation strategy that adequately ventilates all compartments of the lung and maintains well-inflated lungs.[4,15,28] Finally, meticulous fluid management should be employed to avoid fluid overload in patients at risk for right heart failure.

Optimize Growth

Nutrition in patients with severe BPD is challenging and is discussed in detail in Chapter 12, but nutrition must be the leading priority as it is growth, particularly linear growth, that will lead to improvements in clinical status and progression through the phases of disease.[4,15] The dietician should be an integral part of the multidisciplinary team and should provide a regular assessment of nutritional status on rounds. Fenton growth charts are maintained, and the length and weight-for-length charts are the primary charts used in this population to assess adequacy of growth and nutrition.[4] It is imperative in this population to use a recumbent length board to get the most reliable measure of length.[15] Given the complex fluid status and need to maintain optimal cardiopulmonary status, these infants are usually fluid restricted. We aim for 120–140 kcal/kg/day to achieve growth and repair, and to achieve this often requires calorically dense feedings. Considering the importance of avoiding infection, the use of total parenteral nutrition to enhance caloric intake is highly discouraged.

Provide Intensive Developmental Care

Patients need to receive developmental therapies frequently while hospitalized to maximize neurodevelopmental outcomes. Treatments focus on creating an age-appropriate sensory and social environment, including promotion of normal sleep–wake cycles.[15] During the more acute phase of illness therapies may be limited to minimally stimulating activities such as parental instruction related to their child's stress and self-regulatory behaviors, encouragement of kangaroo care, and facilitated tucking. However, as the patient transitions into the transitional phase (Table 18.1), therapists begin to assess respiratory tolerance to position changes, provide tactile, proprioceptive and vestibular input, facilitate state organization, and provide visual and auditory stimuli. A formalized neurodevelopmental assessment should be carried out at about 40 weeks PMA so that subsequent therapies can be directed at improving identified areas of delay.

It cannot be overemphasized that neurodevelopmental care does not only involve the various therapies discussed earlier, but needs to be considered in every aspect of the patient's medical care. In general terms this includes avoidance of noxious stimuli such as arterial and heel sticks (when possible), elimination of neuroactive substances such as opioids/sedatives, and elimination or minimization of exposure to systemic corticosteroids.[4,15] Stated a little differently, positive experiences need to be maximized while negative experiences/stimuli need to be minimized or even eliminated. Blood draws must be limited to those that are absolutely necessary for monitoring, for example weekly to monthly electrolytes depending on phase of illness (Table 18.1). In the CCBPD we never monitor arterial or heel stick blood gases as they are a noxious painful stimulus, not necessarily reflective of a steady state, and seem to provide relatively little additional actionable information in this population.[15,29,30] Peripheral lines are discouraged as they too represent a noxious stimulus and in active infants must be frequently replaced. On the other hand, parental interaction with the patient is highly encouraged through all phases of disease (Table 18.1). Indeed, actively involved parents provide the best feedback on the patient's status and progression. Developmentally optimal care is care that allows attainment of appropriate developmental milestones despite severe illness and in the context of a "ticking clock". That is to say, we cannot afford to delay developmentally appropriate care until an infant has fully recovered since the window of opportunity for attaining a certain milestone may be lost.

Provide Minimal Impact Respiratory Support

Ventilator strategies in BPD are discussed in detail in Chapter 17. In the context of management, it is important to consider that the goals and strategies used in acute neonatal lung diseases are not physiologically appropriate in patients with severe BPD. In the newborn infant with respiratory distress in the first days of life the aim of respiratory support is to maintain adequate oxygenation to allow for self-limited lung diseases to run their course. In the patient with established severe BPD the aim of respiratory support is to maximize oxygenation to allow for good growth and development in a disease that is *not* self-limited. Clinical status in these patients may take weeks or months to improve. Thus, there is little expectation that rapid extubation or rapid weaning from respiratory support can be successfully accomplished in these patients, or for that matter that they are even desirable goals in this population.

Minimal impact respiratory support is not a lung protection strategy; the lungs are injured when the diagnosis of severe BPD is made at 36 weeks PMA. Therefore, minimal impact respiratory support does *not* focus on minimizing the tidal volumes delivered but rather focuses on adequate exhalation. By allowing adequate time for lung-emptying, areas of overinflation are reduced or prevented, thereby maximizing ventilation-perfusion matching. The vast majority of patients with severe BPD have a significant component of obstruction and most patients with severe BPD have normal or elevated lung compliance.[31] The time taken for air to get into or out of the alveoli can be conceptualized using the time constants for inhalation and exhalation, respectively.[28] The time constants are defined as the product of the resistance (R_L) and compliance (C_L) of the lung (time constant (τ) = R_L x C_L). Given the exponential nature of volume filling and emptying of the lung, it takes five inspiratory time constants for the lung to completely fill and five expiratory time

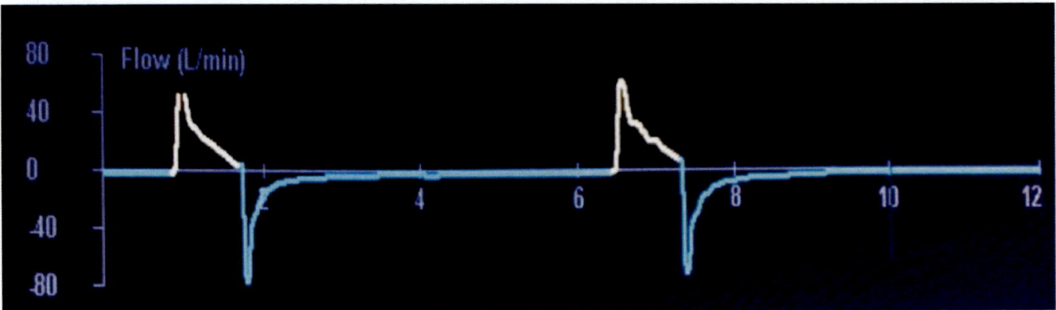

FIG. 18.1 Flow time curve in a patient with prolonged exhalation time. Please note that the time to achieve zero flow on exhalation is greater than 2 seconds, necessitating a slow IMV rate in order to achieve adequate emptying.

constants for the lung to completely empty. The high R_L seen in nearly all patients with severe BPD coupled with the normal or elevated C_L results in exceedingly long time constants. This means that the patient with severe BPD needs both relatively long inspiratory times and especially long expiratory times to adequately fill and empty the lung.[28] An inspiratory time between 0.5 and 1.0seconds is typically required in these patients. The relatively long expiratory times mandate slow rates, with set rates on the ventilator no more than 8 to 16 per minute in the vast majority of these patients. Inspection of the flow-time curves from the ventilator can provide information on the adequacy of filling and emptying of the lung. For example, in the flow-time tracing shown in Fig. 18.1 the time for the expiratory flow to return to zero is a little more than 2seconds. If the next ventilator breath starts before the expiratory flow has returned to zero then the expiratory time is not long enough to allow complete emptying of the lung and the rate should be further decreased.

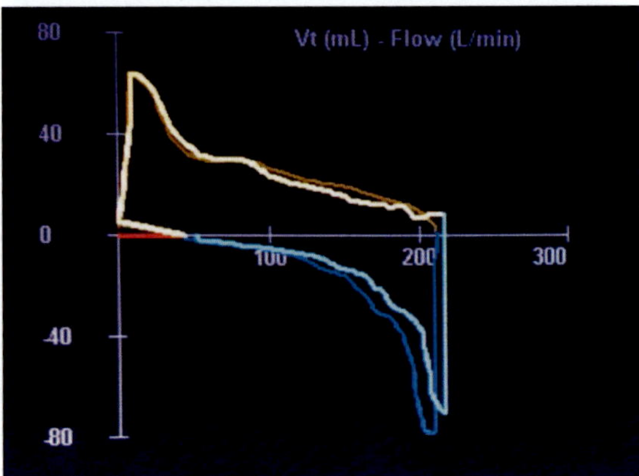

FIG. 18.2 Flow volume loop in a patient with prolonged exhalation time (yellow lines represents positive pressure inhalation; blue lines represents passive exhalation). It is of interest to note that both inhalation and exhalation curves are concave, suggesting heterogeneous lung filling and emptying. Please note that the exhalation flow in blue reaches zero flow prior to inhalation.

Similarly, as shown in the flow-volume loop from the ventilator in Fig. 18.2, expiratory flow has returned to 0 before the next inspiration begins. It is worthwhile noting that in both the flow-time and flow-volume loops exhalation is concave inward suggesting heterogeneity of lung emptying.

The lung is heterogeneous in terms of injury so there will be areas of the lung that are relatively normal in terms of R_L and C_L; however, the relatively normal parts of the lung account for only a small percentage of the total ventilation of the lung.[4,30] Therefore, to adequately ventilate the entirety of the lung in severe BPD, one needs to use not only longer inspiratory and expiratory times but also higher tidal volumes. In acute neonatal lung diseases a tidal volume of 4–6 mL/kg is usually targeted; however, in established severe BPD tidal volumes starting at 10–12 mL/kg and then increased as needed to get good chest rise and to make the patient comfortable.[29,31] We use pressure-limited ventilation to achieve the tidal volumes required to maximize ventilation-perfusion matching; however, whether any particular mode of ventilation is superior to any other mode has not been studied in established severe BPD. In the setting of severe BPD the set positive end-expiratory pressure (PEEP) should be relatively high (8–12 cmH_2O) to optimize gas exchange.[28] Patients with severe BPD may have evidence of expiratory flow limitation at lower PEEP settings due to expiratory collapse of small airways. Although these patients often have hyperinflation on chest X-ray, the use of long expiratory times combined with higher PEEP levels actually promotes emptying and alleviates hyperinflation in infants with established severe BPD.[4,30,31]

Weaning from mechanical ventilation in these patients is a slow process. Extubation should only be considered when the patient has entered Phase III of their disease and is in a progrowth state. The time needed to reach Phase III in this patient population is highly variable, and thus a "personalized" approach is needed. When the patient is stable in <40% oxygen, demonstrating good growth, and able to tolerate therapies and activities extubation can be considered. We generally extubate patients with severe BPD to nasal CPAP (nCPAP). The use of nCPAP in this population requires meticulous attention to the details of delivery of nCPAP for this mode of respiratory support to be successful in these older and larger patients. Often judicious use of anxiolytic medications such as diazepam or lorazepam are needed for 24–72 hours postextubation as the patient adjusts to the new mode of respiratory support. Consider switching nCPAP to nasal cannula when the patient is stable in <30% oxygen; the vast majority of our patients are discharged on supplemental oxygen via nasal cannula.

Obviously, there will be patients who do not move into Phase III of their disease in a time-frame that is compatible with continued endotracheal intubation and therefore tracheostomy placement needs to be considered. The decision to commit an infant with severe BPD to tracheostomy is complex and often difficult.[4,15] There is no evidence for the optimal timing of a tracheostomy in these infants to guide these considerations. It has been reported that ~13% of infants with severe BPD have a tracheostomy placed.[11,26,32] Underscoring the lack of evidence regarding optimal tracheostomy timing, Murthy et al.[11] using the Children's Hospitals Neonatal Consortium (CHNC) database found that there was significant intercenter variation (range 2%–37%) in the proportion of infants with severe BPD undergoing tracheostomy. The median age at tracheostomy in the CHNC cohort was 46 weeks PMA with an IQR of 43–52 weeks.[11] Thus, in the absence of evidence to guide the decision for tracheostomy placement, each patient must be considered individually and the decision has to involve extensive ongoing frank discussions between providers and family.

There are a relatively few infants with severe BPD who fail to respond to minimal impact respiratory support. In the rare nonresponding patient potential "hidden" phenotypes that may need to be addressed should be considered. In severe BPD patients unresponsive to this approach, structure-function studies should be obtained, which may include pulmonary function testing (PFT), lung CT, lung MRI, echocardiogram, and/or bronchoscopy. These tests are performed to rule out severe tracheobronchomalacia or other airway abnormalities, pulmonary vascular disease, as well as to determine if the patient has purely restrictive lung disease as potential causes of nonresponse to minimal impact ventilation.[31] An important "hidden" phenotype that can cause nonresponsiveness to usual management is pulmonary vascular disease, including PH, pulmonary venous stenosis, and/or the presence of systemic-to-pulmonary collaterals. To optimize ventilation-perfusion matching there will be some patients with severe BPD that require therapies (such as pulmonary vasodilators) to promote appropriate pulmonary blood flow as discussed in Chapter 8. We recently published a study of PFT results from a group of patients with the most severe forms of BPD that demonstrated, as expected, that 51% had purely obstructive disease (as defined as a forced expiratory volume at 0.5seconds (FEV0.5) <80% of predicted and total lung capacity (TLC) ≥90% of predicted). Somewhat surprising was the finding that ~9% of the published cohort had purely restrictive disease, defined as a total lung capacity (TLC) < 90% of predicted and a FEV0.5 divided by forced vital capacity (FEV0.5/FVC) ≥ 90% of predicted. The remaining 40% had a mixed picture defined as TLC <90% of predicted and FEV0.5/FVC <90% of predicted. In the setting of nonresponse to the usual obstructive lung disease approach outlined it is important to rule out restrictive lung disease since a very different approach to respiratory support is needed for the patient to move through the phases of severe BPD, and these patients usually respond very well to relative quickly stopping intermittent positive pressure ventilation and moving to nCPAP or nasal cannula. Given the difficulty in obtaining iPFTs in intubated neonates this diagnosis can be entertained when the other causes of nonresponsiveness to minimal impact ventilation are ruled out. It should be kept in mind that the occurrence of purely restrictive lung disease in sBPD is likely to be relatively rare, thus the diagnosis should only be entertained once all other potential causes of nonresponsiveness to minimal impact ventilation are ruled out.

Thus, the patient with severe BPD needs an approach to care that is focused on the chronic nature of the disease and maximizes the patient's ability to heal, grow, and develop. Using these principles, mortality and neurodevelopment can likely be improved for this very high-risk population. While evidence is limited, recent data suggest that centers that employ such methods have lower rates of the combined outcome of tracheostomy and/or death[11] and higher rates of typical neurodevelopment as defined by Bayley Scales.[15] Key to this approach is minimizing noxious stimuli, as the number and intensity of such stimuli is strongly associated with worse long-term outcomes. The most noxious stimuli that chronically ill babies typically suffer are repeated heel sticks for lab obtainment and thus all unnecessary lab draws should be eliminated. In our own center, for instance, we have eliminated entirely the use of capillary blood gases, as they are a painful procedure and may be unreliable indicators of steady-state respiratory status.[33] Instead, we use once weekly or once every other week ascertainment of serum bicarbonate to confirm that steady-state respiratory status is adequate.[34] A culture of multidisciplinary chronic care and moving away from the NICU culture of acute care is imperative for improving the outcomes of these patients. Utilizing the entire multidisciplinary team for feedback on patient status and progress helps to ensure that weaning proceeds at the appropriate pace and in the correct setting to optimize development. It is imperative to provide adequate support to enable development and to not wean support until all of the feedback and parameters suggest that it will be well tolerated. Finally, it is important to remember that infants with severe BPD will likely have long-term alterations in lung function due to their disease and are at greater risk for chronic lung dysfunction as adults.[35,36] Therefore as discussed in the next chapter, ongoing multidisciplinary follow-up is crucial for all patients with severe BPD following discharge from the neonatal intensive care unit.[4,37,38]

REFERENCES

1. Northway WJ, Rosan RC, Porter DY. Pulmonary disease following respirator therapy of hyaline-membrane disease. Bronchopulmonary dysplasia. *N Engl J Med.* 1967;276: 357–368.
2. Jensen EA, Schmidt B. Epidemiology of bronchopulmonary dysplasia. *Birth Defects Res A Clin Mol Teratol.* 2014; 100:145–157.
3. Stoll BJ, Hansen NI, Bell EF, et al. Trends in care practices, morbidity, and mortality of extremely preterm neonates, 1993–2012. *JAMA.* 2015;314:1039–1051.
4. Abman S, Collaco JM, shepherd EG, et al. Interdisciplinary care of children with severe bronchopulmonary dysplasia. *J Pediatr.* 2017;181:12–28.
5. McEvoy CT, Jain L, Schmidt B, et al. Bronchopulmonary dysplasia: NHLBI workshop on the primary prevention of chronic lung diseases. *Ann Am Thorac Soc.* 2014; 11(Suppl 3):S146–S153.
6. Doyle LW, Carse E, Adams AM, et al. Ventilation in extremely preterm infants and respiratory function at 8 years. *N Engl J Med.* 2017;377:329–337.
7. DeMauro SB. The impact of bronchopulmonary dysplasia on childhood outcomes. *Clin Perinatol.* 2018;45:439–452.
8. Ehrenkranz RA, Walsh MC, Vohr BR, et al. Validation of the National Institutes of Health consensus definition of bronchopulmonary dysplasia. *Pediatrics.* 2005;116: 1353–1360.
9. Walsh MC, Morris BH, Wrage LA, et al. Extremely low birthweight neonates with protracted ventilation: mortality and 18-month neurodevelopmental outcomes. *J Pediatr.* 2005;146:798–804.
10. Padula MA, Grover TR, Brozanski B, et al. Therapeutic interventions and short-term outcomes for infants with severe bronchopulmonary dysplasia born at <32 weeks' gestation. *J Perinatol.* 2013;33:877–881.
11. Murthy K, Porta NFM, Lagatta JM, et al. Inter-center variation in death or tracheostomy placement in infants with severe bronchopulmonary dysplasia. *J Perinatol.* 2017;37: 723–727.
12. Leroy S, Caumette E, Waddington C, et al. A time-based analysis of inflammation in infants at risk of bronchopulmonary dysplasia. *J Pediatr.* 2018;192, 60-65 e61.
13. Balena-Borneman J, Ambalavanan N, Tiwari HK, et al. Biomarkers associated with bronchopulmonary dysplasia/ mortality in premature infants. *Pediatr Res.* 2017;81: 519–525.
14. Logan JW, Burdo-Hartman W, Lynch SK. Optimizing neurodevelopment in severe bronchopulmonary dysplasia. *NeoReviews.* 2017;18:e598–e605.
15. Shepherd EG, Knupp AM, Welty SE, et al. An interdisciplinary bronchopulmonary dysplasia program is associated with improved neurodevelopmental outcomes and fewer rehospitalizations. *J Perinatol.* 2012;32:33–38.
16. Moore PE, Poston JT, Boyer D, et al. ATS core curriculum 2017: Part II. Pediatric pulmonary medicine. *Ann Am Thorac Soc.* 2017;14:S165–S181.
17. Brummelte S, Grunau RE, Chau V, et al. Procedural pain and brain development in premature newborns. *Ann Neurol.* 2012;71:385–396.
18. Valeri BO, Ranger M, Chau CM, et al. Neonatal invasive procedures predict pain intensity at school age in children born very preterm. *Clin J Pain.* 2016;32:1086–1093.
19. Maitre NL, Key AP, Chorna OD, et al. The dual nature of early-life experience on somatosensory processing in the human infant brain. *Curr Biol.* 2017;27:1048–1054.
20. Grunau RE, Whitfield MF, Petrie-Thomas J, et al. Neonatal pain, parenting stress and interaction, in relation to cognitive and motor development at 8 and 18 months in preterm infants. *Pain.* 2009;143:138–146.
21. Zwicker JG, Miller SP, Grunau RE, et al. Smaller cerebellar growth and poorer neurodevelopmental outcomes in very preterm infants exposed to neonatal morphine. *J Pediatr.* 2016;172:81–87 e82.
22. Kocek M, Wilcox R, Crank C, Patra K. Evaluation of the relationship between opioid exposure in extremely low birth weight infants in the neonatal intensive care unit

and neurodevelopmental outcome at 2 years. *Early Hum Dev*. 2016;92:29–32.
23. McPherson C. Morphine exposure in preterm infants correlates with impaired cerebellar growth and poorer neurodevelopmental outcome. *Evid Based Med*. 2016;21:234.
24. Ting JY, Synnes A, Roberts A, et al. Association between antibiotic use and neonatal mortality and morbidities in very low-birth-weight infants without culture-proven sepsis or necrotizing enterocolitis. *JAMA Pediatr*. 2016; 170:1181–1187.
25. Mourani PM, Abman SH. Pulmonary hypertension and vascular abnormalities in bronchopulmonary dysplasia. *Clin Perinatol*. 2015;42:839–855.
26. Guaman MC, Gien J, Baker CD, et al. Point prevalence, clinical characteristics, and treatment variation for infants with severe bronchopulmonary dysplasia. *Am J Perinatol*. 2015;32:960–967.
27. Abman SH, Hansmann G, Archer SL, et al. Pediatric pulmonary hypertension: guidelines from the American heart association and American thoracic society. *Circulation*. 2015;132:2037–2099.
28. Nelin LD, Abman SH, Panitch HB. A physiology-based approach to the respiratory care of children with severe bronchopulmonary dysplasia. In: Bancalari E, ed. *The Newborn Lung: Neonatology Questions and Controversies*. Elsevier; 2019:363–385.
29. Shepherd EG, Nelin LD. Physical examination. In: Goldsmith JP, et al., eds. *Assisted Ventilation of the Neonate, an Evidence-Based Approach to Newborn Respiratory Care*. Philadelphia, PA: Elsevier Saunders; 2017, 61-66.e61.
30. Shepherd EG, Lynch SK, Malleske DT, Nelin LD. Mechanical ventilation of the infant with severe bronchopulmonary dysplasia. In: Aly H, Abdel-Hady H, eds. *Respiratory Management of Newborns*. Crotia: Intech Rijeka; 2016:83–94.
31. Shepherd EG, Clouse BJ, Hasenstab KA, et al. Infant pulmonary function testing and phenotypes in severe bronchopulmonary dysplasia. *Pediatrics*. 2018;141:e20173350.
32. Mandy G, Malkar M, Welty SE, et al. Tracheostomy placement in infants with bronchopulmonary dysplasia: safety and outcomes. *Pediatr Pulmonol*. 2013;48:245–249.
33. Courtney SE, Weber KR, Breakie LA, et al. Capillary blood gases in the neonate. A reassessment and review of the literature. *Am J Dis Child*. 1990;144:168–172.
34. Bruno CM, Valenti M. Acid-base disorders in patients with chronic obstructive pulmonary disease: a pathophysiological review. *J Biomed Biotechnol*. 2012;915150:2012.
35. Cheong JLY, Doyle LW. An update on pulmonary and neurodevelopmental outcomes of bronchopulmonary dysplasia. *Semin Perinatol*. 2018;42:478–484.
36. Davidson LM, Berkelhamer SK. Bronchopulmonary dysplasia: chronic lung disease of infancy and long-term pulmonary outcomes. *J Clin Med*. 2017;6(4).
37. Collaco JM, McGrath-Morrow S. Respiratory phenotypes for preterm infants, children, and adults: bronchopulmonary dysplasia and more. *Ann Am Thorac Soc*. 2018;15: 530–538.
38. Katz SL, Luu TM, Nuyt AM, et al. Long-term follow-up of cardiorespiratory outcomes in children born extremely preterm: recommendations from a Canadian consensus workshop. *Paediatr Child Health*. 2017;22:75–79.

CHAPTER 19

Post–Neonatal Intensive Care Unit Management of Bronchopulmonary Dysplasia

JOSEPH M. COLLACO, MD, PHD • SHARON A. MCGRATH-MORROW, MD, MBA

INTRODUCTION

Advancements in neonatal care have led to large numbers of extremely low-birth-weight infants surviving to discharge from the hospital. This in turn has led to an increasing number of infants and children with respiratory disease related to prematurity, requiring outpatient care. Symptoms may range from mild respiratory symptoms that resolve within weeks of discharge from the neonatal intensive care unit (NICU) to those requiring home mechanical ventilation for years. In this chapter, we describe the post-NICU management of bronchopulmonary dysplasia (BPD), including medications, respiratory support, and preventing/treating common respiratory complications.

MEDICATIONS

There are several different types of medications commonly encountered in outpatient clinical settings for former preterm infants, including inhaled β-agonists, inhaled and systemic corticosteroids, diuretics, and antipulmonary hypertensive agents. The efficacy of these medications in infants and children with BPD has not been rigorously studied, despite their common usage in this population. With the exception of antipulmonary hypertensive agents, there has been minimal change in the outpatient management of BPD in the past several decades.[1] Most typically, administration of these medications is initiated during an infant's initial NICU admission and is carried over into the outpatient setting upon discharge. Given the paucity of evidence for these medications' use in both the inpatient and outpatient settings, it is likely that local inpatient practices dictate outpatient use leading to a significant variation. A snapshot study conducted in 2015 among eight tertiary care NICUs in the United States found significant variation in use for diuretics, inhaled corticosteroids, and inhaled β-agonists among infants diagnosed with severe BPD.[2]

INHALED β-AGONISTS

Obstructive airway disease is a common manifestation of BPD and can present with signs and symptoms similar to asthma. Both airway inflammation and structural changes may play a role in the obstructive lung disease related to BPD. Compared with asthma, structural changes to the BPD airways may play a larger role in the pathogenesis of the disease.[3,4] This dual physiology may give a picture of asthma partially responsive to standard asthma therapies based on the degree of airway inflammation versus structural changes present. The risk of childhood asthma may be 1.7–3.9 times higher in children with a history of BPD depending on gestational age at birth.[5] However, the burden of the disease may be decreasing over time as a 2014 meta-analysis of cross-sectional data demonstrated that obstruction as measured by spirometry (forced expiratory volume in the first second of expiration [FEV_1]) is becoming milder among preterm birth cohorts over the past several decades.[6]

Inhaled short-acting β-agonists (albuterol or levalbuterol) can be used as needed and/or as scheduled, ranging from daily to every 4 hours in an outpatient setting. Commonly, inhaled β-agonists are given as needed for acute respiratory symptoms such as wheezing, coughing, or unexplained tachypnea or work of breathing above baseline. Frequent use of or minimal responsiveness to short-acting β-agonists for chronic respiratory symptoms can occur with poorly controlled airway inflammation, bronchomalacia,

Updates on Neonatal Chronic Lung Disease. https://doi.org/10.1016/B978-0-323-68353-1.00019-1

and/or recurrent aspiration. Airway inflammation may respond to controller medications, such as inhaled steroids; however in the absence of improvement, further diagnostic testing should be considered to rule out other causes of chronic respiratory symptoms such as anatomic or functional airway abnormalities and/or aspiration. Frequent use of short-acting β-agonists for acute symptoms, such as those that accompany a viral upper respiratory tract infection, should prompt evaluation by a medical provider and consideration for initiating a short course of systemic steroids. Scheduled inhaled β-agonists can be given for preventing the aforementioned symptoms in infants or children with severe symptoms or for airway clearance. In the case of the former, the goal would be to wean β-agonist use to an as-needed basis as soon as the patient will tolerate it. In terms of airway clearance, in addition to relaxing smooth airway muscles, β-agonists can increase ciliary beat frequency thus aiding in mucociliary clearance.[7]

Inhaled albuterol and levalbuterol are the most commonly used short-acting β-agonists in the United States; enteral preparations may be associated with significant cardiac side effects.[8] Pediatric studies suggest that there is no difference in the degree of tachycardia resulting from albuterol use versus levalbuterol use,[9,10] but there are no studies in preterm infants who have higher resting heart rates at baseline. There are also no published studies for the use of long-acting β-agonists in preterm infants.

INHALED AND SYSTEMIC CORTICOSTEROIDS

There is a role for the use of corticosteroids in the management of BPD as airway inflammation is associated with the development of BPD.[11,12] Typically, inhaled corticosteroids are used as prophylactic medication to decrease chronic symptom burden and prevent acute exacerbations, whereas systemic steroids are more commonly used for treating acute exacerbations of respiratory symptoms that may be associated with respiratory infections, anesthesia, etc. Although there are a number of studies assessing the use of corticosteroids within the NICU, particularly for the prevention of BPD, there are fewer studies focused on outpatient outcomes in preterm infants. Several studies of inhaled corticosteroid use in the NICU have found no differences in neurodevelopmental disabilities at 1.5–3 years of age.[13–15] Although one long-term study found an increase in mortality (relative risk, 1.37) primarily in the NICU setting among preterm infants receiving inhaled corticosteroids,[13] other studies have not necessarily observed this.[14] A randomized controlled trial of inhaled corticosteroids in preterm infants with moderate-severe BPD reported in 2017, observed a trend toward reduced rehospitalizations and systemic steroid use over the 3 months following initial discharge.[16] However, another randomized controlled trial of 30 infants with chronic lung disease reported in 2002 did not see a difference in respiratory symptoms, systemic steroid courses, or hospital readmissions over a 1-year follow-up period.[17] There exists some evidence that adrenal suppression may occur in some children who are on inhaled corticosteroids,[18] but this is not consistently seen.[19] Given these mixed results, there is considerable variation in practice for the use of inhaled corticosteroids, ranging from 0% to 87% for infants with severe BPD among eight tertiary care centers in one snapshot study.[2]

Given the potential effects on both somatic growth and neurocognitive development,[20] the use of systemic steroids is limited in the NICU, but systemic steroids may be helpful for acute management of respiratory exacerbations or for failure of weaning respiratory support (e.g., to aid with extubation) after NICU discharge. There may be a small subset of infants with severe BPD and chronic respiratory failure who are dependent on systemic corticosteroids to maintain stability, and these are the rare patients who may be discharged from the NICU setting on a daily or every other day systemic steroid dosing.

In the outpatient setting, initiating inhaled corticosteroid use should be considered for chronic coughing/wheezing or frequent acute episodes of coughing/wheezing that result in multiple systemic steroid courses, emergency department visits, or hospital readmissions. There may also be a lower threshold to consider these medications if a susceptible patient is likely to be exposed to multiple viruses (e.g., in daycare) or has a dysfunctional swallow associated with intermittent aspiration.

The goal of management with steroids, inhaled or systemic, should always be to wean to the lowest possible dose while maintaining respiratory stability. The exact timing of weaning is dependent on a patient's chronic symptoms and ability to handle acute exacerbations, as wheezing or asthmalike symptoms may continue to be present over the lifespan of a preterm individual[21] or may improve within months to a few years after NICU discharge.[22] Many patients will require a gradual step-down of therapies, particularly if adrenal suppression is present. The use of spirometry for children over 4 years of age may be helpful to follow obstructive lung disease and titrate the inhaled steroid dosing[23] (see Table 19.1 for a list of useful diagnostic tests).

DIURETICS

Among preterm infants with BPD, diuretics are frequently used to manage interstitial pulmonary edema secondary to increased capillary permeability.[1] Within the NICU setting, there is limited published data demonstrating improvement of pulmonary mechanics with diuretics acting on the distal renal tubule,[24] but data to support the sustained use of loop diuretics for management of BPD are not present.[25] Although furosemide is commonly used in the NICU setting for time-limited courses,[26] it is less commonly used for long-term use owing to its potential adverse events such as electrolyte disturbances and nephrocalcinosis. More commonly used for long-term management are the thiazide diuretics (chlorothiazide and hydrochlorothiazide) often in combination with spironolactone.[1,26] They are associated with less electrolyte disturbances than furosemide and have been shown to improve respiratory mechanics and oxygen requirement in one randomized control trial of infants with BPD.[1,27]

As mentioned previously, there is significant variation in inpatient use of diuretics,[2] which likely translates into variation in which outpatients are receiving diuretic therapy. There are no guidelines for when and how to wean diuretics in outpatients with BPD. A survey of pediatric pulmonologists found that approximately half of respondents would wean oxygen before diuretic use, and vice versa for the other half.[28] In general, patients on home supplemental oxygen may wean from diuretic therapy at a later age than those not on supplemental oxygen.[29] When weaning off diuretic therapy at

TABLE 19.1
Outpatient Diagnostic Testing for Preterm Lung Disease.

	Intervention[a]	Comments
Follow-up studies to be considered	• Spirometry	• Only for patients aged ≥4 years. A reduction in FEV_1 may indicate the presence of small airway disease; a reduction in FVC may suggest exercise limitations.
	• Overnight polysomnography	• Useful for screening for obstructive sleep apnea or titrating respiratory support.
	• Chest computed tomography (±contrast)	• May be useful in assessing for parenchymal disease/cystic disease, but it does involve radiation exposure.
	• Echocardiography (±cardiac catheterization)	• Echocardiograms Can be used for screening for pulmonary hypertension or titration of therapies. Outpatient catheterization is typically reserved for procedural interventions or assessing pharmacotherapy failure.
	• Airway endoscopy	• May be useful in assessing for upper airway lesions and/or tracheobronchomalacia. In combination with observed feeding (FEES), it may be helpful in assessing dysphagia.
	• Exercise studies	• For older patients, they may be useful in assessing pulmonary reserve. Individual laboratories may have specific age/height criteria for completing studies.

FEES, fiberoptic endoscopic evaluation of swallowing; *FEV_1*, forced expiratory volume in the first second of expiration; *FVC*, forced vital capacity.
[a] The options presented in this table are not meant to be carried out for all patients, but are options that may or may not be pursued, given the individual patient presentations.

home, families should be advised to monitor for oxygen desaturations if on home pulse oximetry, changes in respiration, and facial/peripheral edema.

ANTIPULMONARY HYPERTENSIVE MEDICATIONS

Supportive therapies should be considered as the first-line management of pulmonary hypertension associated with BPD, particularly if the pulmonary hypertension is mild or moderate. These may include the use of supplemental oxygen for pulmonary vasodilation, optimal nutrition to maximize lung growth, avoidance of aspiration and infection, and treatment of hemodynamically significant shunts/airway obstruction.[30–32]

Ideally, the decision to initiate antipulmonary hypertensive pharmacotherapy for a moderate to severe disease that does not respond to supportive therapies should be done in consultation with a multidisciplinary team with expertise in pulmonary hypertension.[32] Although performing cardiac catheterization before initiating long-term pharmacotherapy has been recommended,[33] in practice, many infants with BPD and pulmonary hypertension are at high risk for adverse outcomes with anesthesia and/or this procedure.[30,34] It should be recognized that certain causes of pulmonary hypertension seen within the preterm infant population can be worsened with the initiation of antipulmonary hypertension therapy, including pulmonary vein stenosis, left ventricular dysfunction, certain intracardiac shunts, and/or collateral vessels.[35]

The most commonly used class of agents to treat pulmonary hypertension in patients with BPD is the selective phosphodiesterase type 5 (PDE5) inhibitors (most often, sildenafil). The evidence supporting its use is largely limited to retrospective single center studies.[36–39] Potential adverse effects that may limit its use include transient hypotension, ventilation-perfusion mismatch leading to desaturations, and priapism.[36] Concerns have been raised regarding 3-year mortality with sildenafil in one randomized controlled trial of pediatric patients with pulmonary hypertension,[40] but this has not been observed in other studies.[41] Tadalafil has seen limited use at some centers, but there are no published data concerning its use in preterm infants.

Two other classes of chronic antipulmonary hypertensive agents used with patients with severe pulmonary hypertension and BPD are endothelin receptor antagonists (bosentan) and prostacyclins (epoprostenol, iloprost, and treprostinil).[35] Bosentan is administered orally and requires periodic transaminase assessment owing to the risk of liver toxicity. The short half-life of prostacyclins makes effective delivery challenging; they are also associated with a risk of systemic hypotension.[35] In preterm infants, epoprostenol and treprostinil have been administered via continuous intravenous infusion via central line, although treprostinil has also been administered via pump subcutaneously. Iloprost can be delivered via inhalation. Lastly, inhaled nitric oxide may be used in an inpatient setting for the treatment of acute pulmonary hypertensive crises.[31,32]

RESPIRATORY SUPPORT

Oxygen

Hypoxemia is a common manifestation of BPD. Owing to its sometimes slow resolution, many infants with BPD are discharged from NICUs on home supplemental oxygen typically delivered via nasal cannula. Flows may range from 1/32 L per minute (LPM) to 2 LPM and use may be continuous or intermittent (e.g., with feeding and/or sleeping only). Patients with moderate or severe BPD are more likely to be discharged on supplemental oxygen; a 2005 validation study of the NICHD BPD criteria in 4866 infants reported that 64.4% of patients with moderate or severe BPD were discharged to home on supplemental oxygen compared with 2.8% of their peers with no or mild BPD.[42]

In general, home supplemental oxygen can be discontinued for most infants with BPD before 12 months of age.[43–47] The severity of BPD may be predictive of how long supplemental oxygen requirements will persist, as in the same study, infants with severe BPD were weaned from oxygen at a mean age of 9.7 months compared with their peers with milder disease who were weaned between 7 and 8 months of age on average.[42] Age of being weaned off of oxygen has also been shown to be associated with the flow of oxygen prescribed at discharge with patients on higher flows requiring supplemental oxygen until a later age.[43]

There are no published guidelines or protocols for how and when to wean supplemental oxygen in the outpatient setting.[28] Typically, pulse oximetry measurements are used to guide decision-making, although there is variation in the type of monitoring, ranging from single determinations in an outpatient clinic to providing a pulse oximeter in the home setting to the use of overnight polysomnography.[43] It is important to recognize that daytime pulse oximetry alone may be misleading because saturations may be lower with sleep overnight, and even short pauses in breathing lasting a few seconds may lead to desaturations owing to decreased pulmonary reserve.[48] There is no specific consensus regarding minimum acceptable oxygen saturation percentage, although a study of surveyed pulmonologists reported a range of values between 90% and 95%.[28] Although nocturnal saturations are the primary data used for weaning decisions by most pulmonologists, other factors to be considered include somatic growth, other vital signs, recent hospitalizations, and echocardiographic data.[28] There may also be a substantial fraction of parents (32.1%) who may undertake oxygen weaning without medical supervision, and in one study, unsupervised weaning was associated with pulmonary hypertension and public insurance.[43]

Tracheostomies and Home Mechanical Ventilation

Patients with the most severe forms of BPD may require long-term ventilation for optimal growth and development. Estimates vary as to how many children with BPD are chronically ventilated, but the incidence may be 200 infants annually with as many as 2000 preterm infants and children with severe BPD in the United States requiring home ventilation at any one time.[31,49,50] These patients typically have prolonged initial hospitalizations for months after birth for stabilization of respiratory status, managing other comorbidities, and coordinating care for discharge.[51,52]

Training of caregivers of patients with tracheostomies and ventilators is critical. Despite the use of monitoring devices, the risk of death is high, with a mortality rate of 18.6% among patients with BPD in one study.[50] In one retrospective study of 228 children on home mechanical ventilation, the mortality rate was 21%, including 19% of deaths related to tracheostomy complications that were likely preventable.[53] Factors that may contribute to these preventable deaths may include inadequate training of family and professional caregivers.[49]

The American Thoracic Society guidelines for pediatric patients on home mechanical ventilation recommend that they should be comanaged by a generalist and a respiratory subspecialist, have an alert and attentive caregiver at all times (in practice, this requires the use of home nurses for periods of time), and have two or more family members who are trained in all aspects of respiratory care.[54] The guidelines outline the use of standardized discharge criteria and specific pieces of critical equipment.

Currently, there are no published protocols for outpatient ventilator management of severe BPD, and ventilatory strategies may need to be personalized based on presenting needs. In contrast to the multiple modalities of ventilator support utilized in the NICU during various stages of evolving lung disease, most infants with BPD on home ventilators are on (1) synchronized intermittent mandatory ventilation (SIMV) mode with pressure control/pressure support, (2) continuous positive airway pressure (CPAP) mode with pressure support, or (3) CPAP only. Modes of ventilation incorporating volume control are less commonly used but may need to be considered for the most difficult-to-ventilate infants. For patients with established lung disease, lower rates and longer inspiratory times may promote more homogenous inflation of lung units with heterogeneous time constants due to cystic disease. For patients with significant tracheo- or bronchomalacia, a higher positive end-expiratory pressure (PEEP) may be required to maintain a patent airway. In such cases, direct visualization under flexible bronchoscopy can be useful in titrating ventilator pressures. While there are no published guidelines on the maximum acceptable fraction of inspired oxygen (FiO_2) for discharge, maintaining FiO_2 above 40% in the home setting is challenging owing to the amount of oxygen required. It is recommended to stabilize ventilator settings and oxygen requirements in an inpatient setting before the initial discharge.

Compared with chronic respiratory failure requiring long-term ventilation, BPD has a more favorable prognosis, with many children able to wean off ventilator support as they age. Limited data suggest that the median age for weaning from ventilatory support is 2 years.[50,55] Typically, ventilator weaning is conducted in an inpatient setting but may be considered with a more gradual approach in an outpatient setting with close monitoring. Essential elements for weaning ventilatory support include pulse oximetry, end-tidal CO_2 monitoring, and frequent clinical assessments. In general, it is advisable to wean daytime support before weaning overnight support. Overnight polysomnography can be helpful in determining the safety of reduced ventilator support or whether adequate ventilation/oxygenation occurs off of ventilator support. Even in patients who are unable to wean from ventilator support, repeat polysomnography should be considered every 12–36 months to reassess whether changes in settings are required. Caution is advised when weaning ventilator support for patients with BPD and pulmonary hypertension because the pulmonary hypertension may worsen or pulmonary hypertensive crises may occur with changes in gas exchange.[30]

Following weaning from mechanical ventilation, decannulation can be considered under supervision of a pediatric otolaryngologist, as preterm infants may also have airway anomalies (e.g., subglottic stenosis, granulomas) that require additional surgical management or preclude decannulation.[55,56] The approach to decannulation varies among centers.[55–57] Preparation and assessment for decannulation may include monitoring tolerance of downsized and/or capped tracheostomies. Typically, tolerance of capping is assessed overnight in an inpatient setting or with overnight polysomnography.[55–57] Increased respiratory symptoms or events (e.g., increased work of breathing, desaturations, hypercarbia) or higher apnea/hypopnea indexes during polysomnography when the tracheostomy is capped are associated with a higher rate of unsuccessful decannulation.[58,59] Decannulation should be planned during seasons when respiratory viruses are less frequent in the community; overnight inpatient observation should be strongly considered after decannulation as well.[58]

COMMON COMPLICATIONS AND THEIR MANAGEMENT (SEE TABLE 19.2)

Respiratory Infections

Perhaps one of the greatest sources of morbidity and mortality in preterm infants with BPD are respiratory infections, mostly viral. Up to half of infants and children are readmitted before 2 years of age after initial hospital discharge owing to respiratory illnesses.[60,61]

TABLE 19.2
Prevention of Common Complications.

Intervention	Comments
• Preventing lung injury	• Avoidance of active smoking, secondhand smoke, air pollution • Prevention of (or mitigation of) aspiration
• Preventing infection	• Hand hygiene • Avoidance of sick contact • Influenza and pneumococcal vaccinations • Palivizumab prophylaxis
• Preventing pulmonary hypertensive crises	• Reducing the risk of respiratory infections • Preoperative anesthesia consults for pulmonary hypertension

While patients may present with typical symptoms associated with respiratory viral infections, such as cough and nasal congestion, among infants and children with BPD, wheezing and increased work of breathing are common. In more severe presentations, acute respiratory failure may occur. Some viruses are certainly associated with more severe presentations and mortality, such as respiratory syncytial virus,[62] but it should be recognized that other common respiratory viruses, such as rhinovirus, can be associated with increased morbidities among patients with BPD.[63] Patients with BPD may have longer recovery times from respiratory infections than their peers without BPD, and emerging evidence suggests that severe respiratory infections in infancy and early childhood may lead to altered lung function in childhood and adulthood.[64–66]

Management of respiratory infections typically involves close observation and supportive care. Escalation of respiratory support is common, including the use of supplemental oxygen, high-flow nasal cannulas, noninvasive/invasive ventilation, or positive pressure ventilation with intubation, depending on patient needs. Scheduled β-agonist therapies may aid with both small airway disease and mucociliary clearance. Courses of systemic corticosteroids should be considered to aid with the airway inflammation that is commonly present; patients may require tapering courses depending on recovery from symptoms and whether underlying adrenal insufficiency is present. Antibiotics are appropriate when bacterial disease is suspected or diagnosed. Pulmonary hypertensive crises may occur in infants/children with a history of pulmonary hypertension (see the section Pulmonary Hypertension for additional description).

Preventing respiratory infections or mitigating their severity is an essential part of BPD outpatient management. Avoidance of sick contacts should be encouraged when possible. Families should be aware that daycare attendance may result in higher risk of emergency department visits, systemic corticosteroid use, antibiotic use for respiratory illnesses, and days with difficulty breathing, likely secondary to an increased risk of acquiring respiratory viral infections in day care.[67] Immunoprophylaxis (with palivizumab) for respiratory syncytial virus infection should be considered for high-risk infants.[68] Some centers also recommend the 23-valent pneumococcal vaccination for children with BPD over 2 years of age, but there is no published data to support this practice. Lastly, exposure to secondhand smoke may increase the risk of acquiring respiratory infections in general[69] and may be linked to an increased risk of hospital admission and activity limitations in infants and children with BPD.[70]

Pulmonary Hypertension

Pulmonary hypertension is a complication of BPD, and although more commonly seen with more severe BPD, it can be observed with any severity of BPD.[30,32] Few infants undergo the gold standard for the diagnosis of pulmonary hypertension (i.e., cardiac catheterization) owing to the risks of the procedure. In practice, echocardiography is used to diagnose the presence and severity of pulmonary hypertension, with severe pulmonary hypertension being associated with estimated pulmonary pressures >2/3 systemic pressures with severe ventricular septal flattening.[32] Appropriate follow-up for preterm infants and children with pulmonary hypertension cannot be understated, as given the identical severity of BPD, pulmonary hypertension is associated with higher rates of morbidity and mortality.[30,71–73]

In the outpatient settings, echocardiography also serves as the primary means of serial assessment of pulmonary hypertension. The frequency of follow-up echocardiography is dependent on the stability of the patient and the weaning of respiratory support and antipulmonary hypertensive agents (every 1–4 months).[32] Careful coordination between subspecialists weaning support and medications is essential to prevent pulmonary hypertensive crises. Limited prospective data demonstrates improvement of pulmonary hypertension over the first year of life.[71] Long-term data from school-aged children with a history of BPD suggest that pulmonary hypertension does not persist even under pulmonary vasoconstrictive settings (i.e., hypoxia).[74,75] Another study of 7-year-old children with a history of pulmonary hypertension found evidence of subclinical right ventricular dysfunction, but the significance of this is unclear.[76]

Pulmonary hypertensive crises represent an acute increase in pulmonary vascular pressures often accompanied by right-sided heart failure. Biomarkers of pulmonary hypertension may also demonstrate an acute increase from baseline (e.g., serum brain natriuretic peptide levels). These crises often occur in the setting of altered gas exchange such as surgery/anesthesia or respiratory infections[30,34] or other scenarios where cardiac output does not meet metabolic demands, such as fever or hypovolemia. These crises may resolve with management of the offending event, but in some cases, they may require more aggressive management of pulmonary hypertension, including increasing doses of chronic therapy or the acute use of inhaled nitric oxide.[32] Consultation with a team with expertise in pulmonary hypertension is essential, as crises may be fatal.[31,32] More insidiously, ongoing aspiration may increase pulmonary hypertension severity over time. Therefore the presence of dysphagia and/or gastroesophageal reflux may require more aggressive medical or surgical management if pulmonary hypertension is present.[30]

Aspiration

Aspiration of foreign materials into the upper and lower airways can have long-term consequences for the developing respiratory tract. For example, infants and toddlers who have a history of pneumonia confirmed by chest radiography have been observed to have worse lung function than those without pneumonia.[65] Infants with BPD may be more at risk for aspiration, as they frequently have respiratory rates exceeding 60 breaths per minute, which may result in insufficient pharyngeal transit time for safe swallowing.[77] Vocal cord paresis or paralysis may also be a risk for aspiration.[78] Infants with BPD and severe intraventricular hemorrhages may also be at increased risk for dysphagia and aspiration, with one study reporting that infants with BPD and ventricular shunts were more likely to have gastric tubes placed.[79] Common aspiration sources include aspiration during oral ingestion of liquids and/or solids, aspiration of oral and nasal secretions, and/or aspiration of gastric contents secondary to gastroesophageal reflux.

Signs and symptoms of aspiration can vary between patients.[80] Acute signs of aspiration may include choking, gagging, and coughing. Although oxygen desaturations can occur with aspiration while feeding, they may also be a sign of respiratory insufficiency with the exertion of feeding.[81–83] Aspiration pneumonia or bronchitis may ensue within 24–72 h of a significant aspiration event. Chronic aspiration may present more insidiously than acute aspiration events, as symptoms do not always occur at the time of feeding. Although chronic symptoms may be similar to acute symptoms, their lack of temporal correlation to feeding can make them nonspecific. There is also a subset of infants with BPD that do not necessarily manifest any acute symptoms with aspiration, frequently referred to as "silent aspiration."[84,85] For these patients, chronic symptoms, worsening radiologic chronic findings, worsening pulmonary hypertension, or increased hypercarbia on serial blood gases may suggest that aspiration is occurring.

Diagnosing aspiration frequently requires a tailored approach, including a careful history of respiratory and gastrointestinal symptoms, physical examination, observation of feeding within a clinical setting, and possible imaging or endoscopy. Standard imaging modalities such as chest radiography or computed tomography may demonstrate the sequelae of aspiration, although infiltrates secondary to acute aspiration may take up to 24 hours to be seen on radiography. Videofluoroscopic swallow studies can be used to diagnose aspiration secondary to oropharyngeal dysphagia, but they may overestimate the disease severity if a patient is not at his/her baseline respiratory status. Other imaging modalities to consider include upper gastrointestinal series and/or gastroesophageal scintigraphy ("milk scans"), which may or may not be diagnostic for aspiration secondary to gastroesophageal reflux.[86]

There are several types of endoscopy that may be helpful in diagnosing the cause and severity of aspiration in the respiratory and gastrointestinal tract. Flexible laryngoscopy and/or direct (rigid) laryngology/bronchoscopy of the upper airway performed by otolaryngologists can be used not only to diagnose upper airway anomalies (e.g., laryngeal clefts, vocal cord paresis) but also to characterize any upper airway inflammation secondary to gastroesophageal reflux. A specialized form of endoscopy during swallowing (fiberoptic endoscopic examination of swallowing) can be useful in characterizing the interactions between respiration and swallowing under direct visualization, but it does require trained providers.[87,88] Flexible bronchoscopy of the lower airways, performed by pulmonologists, can assess for inflammatory changes secondary to aspiration (e.g., lower airway malacia) and perform bronchoalveolar lavage. Bronchoalveolar fluid can be submitted for both microbiologic studies to rule out infection and some specialized tests for aspiration such as histologic examination for lipid-laden macrophages. The lack of sensitivity and specificity regarding the relationship between lipid-laden macrophages and chronic aspiration however has questioned the utility of this test.[89] Esophagogastroduodenoscopy performed by gastroenterologists can also assess for changes secondary to reflux and anatomic variants predisposing to reflux (e.g., hiatal hernia).

The amount of aspiration that can be tolerated without an increase in acute illness or worsening of chronic disease is unclear[90]; however, infants and children with BPD may have more limited tolerance of aspiration, given their already reduced respiratory reserve. There are a number of interventions that should be considered for preventing aspiration. For aspiration secondary to oropharyngeal dysphagia, therapeutic options may include modifying feeding positions/bottles/utensils or holding oral feeding altogether. In cases where NPO (nothing by mouth) status is warranted, use of nasogastric tubes or gastrostomy tubes should be considered. The use of a nasogastric tube in the home setting for a patient with BPD is not advocated by some providers owing to the risk associated with a malpositioned tube in an infant who would poorly tolerate any aspiration.[91] For aspiration secondary to gastroesophageal reflux, therapeutic options include restricting feeding volumes, using medications (i.e., histamine-2 blockers, motility agents, and/or proton pump inhibitors), and in the case of severe reflux considering the use of either postpyloric feeding tubes (i.e., nasoduodenal or nasojejunal feeding tubes, or jejunostomy) or surgical fundoplication. For aspiration of oral secretions, the mainstay of therapeutic options include decreasing secretions through pharmaceutical agents such as glycopyrrolate, scopolamine, inhaled ipratropium, and/or botulinum toxin injections.[92–94] It should be noted that decreasing secretions may also result in increasing their viscosity leading to plugging of airways (or tracheostomies) with mucus. For decreasing existing inflammation from aspiration, inhaled corticosteroids can be considered, but there are no published data to support their use.

Obstructive Sleep Apnea

Pediatric patients with a history of prematurity are at a higher risk of developing obstructive sleep apnea (OSA) than their full-term counterparts, including anatomic obstruction (e.g., relatively larger tongues, changes in palatal anatomy), acquired lesions (e.g., vocal cord paresis, subglottic narrowing), airway muscle hypotonia, and/or increased chest wall compliance.[95–99] Even the common childhood cause for OSA, adenotonsillar hypertrophy, is observed more frequently among school-aged children with a history of prematurity.[100] Regardless of the cause, OSA is more prevalent among patients with a history of prematurity, likely throughout their lifetimes, as it is more common on polysomnography in preterm infants[101–104] and school-aged children.[100] Additionally, young adults with a history of prematurity are more likely to chronically snore.[105]

It is important to diagnose and treat OSA, as untreated OSA may result in impaired somatic growth,[106,107] may worsen neurocognitive outcomes,[108,109] and may constitute a risk factor for pulmonary hypertension.[110] Overnight polysomnography is considered the gold standard for the diagnosis of OSA, but it should be noted that not all sleep laboratories can accommodate infants or young children and that normative pediatric data for polysomnography is lacking; infants with BPD may be overdiagnosed with obstructive or central eventsowing to desaturations that may be due in part to poor pulmonary reserve.[48] Although outcomes with commonly used therapies for OSA such as tonsillectomy/adenoidectomy or noninvasive positive pressure ventilation (i.e., CPAP or bilevel positive airway pressure [BiPAP]) have not been studied in pediatric patients with BPD, referral to an otolaryngologist or other respiratory specialists for the child diagnosed with OSA is recommended to determine treatment options.

CONCLUSIONS

Respiratory disease in infancy can have consequences extending through the life span of the individual. Preterm infants with a history of BPD are at risk for asthma-like obstructive lung disease, OSA, exercise intolerance, and potential cardiovascular diseases associated with a history of pulmonary hypertension when compared with individuals born full term.[111] Optimization of lung function and growth can be achieved through early diagnosis, or ideally, prevention, of complications. However, owing to the variable nature of preterm lung disease, a personalized approach to patients undertaken by providers familiar with BPD and its sequelae may be required.[111]

REFERENCES

1. Bhandari A, Panitch H. An update on the post-NICU discharge management of bronchopulmonary dysplasia. *Semin Perinatol.* 2018;42(7):471–477.
2. Guaman MC, Gien J, Baker CD, Zhang H, Austin ED, Collaco JM. Point prevalence, clinical characteristics, and treatment variation for infants with severe bronchopulmonary dysplasia. *Am J Perinatol.* 2015;32(10): 960–967.
3. Vom Hove M, Prenzel F, Uhlig HH, Robel-Tillig E. Pulmonary outcome in former preterm, very low birth weight children with bronchopulmonary dysplasia: a case-control follow-up at school age. *J Pediatr.* 2014; 164(1), 40-45 e44.
4. Baraldi E, Bonetto G, Zacchello F, Filippone M. Low exhaled nitric oxide in school-age children with bronchopulmonary dysplasia and airflow limitation. *Am J Respir Crit Care Med.* 2005;171(1):68–72.
5. Harju M, Keski-Nisula L, Georgiadis L, Raisanen S, Gissler M, Heinonen S. The burden of childhood asthma and late preterm and early term births. *J Pediatr.* 2014; 164(2), 295-299 e291.
6. Kotecha SJ, Edwards MO, Watkins WJ, et al. Effect of preterm birth on later FEV1: a systematic review and meta-analysis. *Thorax.* 2013;68(8):760–766.
7. Wong LB, Miller IF, Yeates DB. Stimulation of ciliary beat frequency by autonomic agonists: in vivo. *J Appl Physiol.* 1988;65(2):971–981.
8. Glatstein MM, Rimon A, Koren L, Marom R, Danino D, Scolnik D. Unintentional oral beta agonist overdose: case report and review of the literature. *Am J Therapeut.* 2013;20(3):311–314.
9. Kelly A, Kennedy A, John BM, Duane B, Lemanowicz J, Little J. A comparison of heart rate changes associated with levalbuterol and racemic albuterol in pediatric cardiology patients. *Ann Pharmacother.* 2013;47(5): 644–650.
10. Bio LL, Willey VJ, Poon CY. Comparison of levalbuterol and racemic albuterol based on cardiac adverse effects in children. *J Pediatr Pharmacol Ther.* 2011;16(3): 191–198.
11. Martinez FD. Early-life origins of chronic obstructive pulmonary disease. *N Engl J Med.* 2016;375(9):871–878.
12. Yeh TF, Chen CM, Wu SY, et al. Intratracheal administration of budesonide/surfactant to prevent bronchopulmonary dysplasia. *Am J Respir Crit Care Med.* 2016;193(1): 86–95.
13. Bassler D, Shinwell ES, Hallman M, et al. Long-term effects of inhaled budesonide for bronchopulmonary dysplasia. *N Engl J Med.* 2018;378(2):148–157.
14. Nakamura T, Yonemoto N, Nakayama M, et al. Early inhaled steroid use in extremely low birthweight infants: a randomised controlled trial. *Arch Dis Child Fetal Neonatal Ed.* 2016 Nov;101(6):F552–F556.
15. Jangaard KA, Stinson DA, Allen AC, Vincer MJ. Early prophylactic inhaled beclomethasone in infants less than 1250 g for the prevention of chronic lung disease. *Paediatr Child Health.* 2002;7(1):13–19.
16. Kugelman A, Peniakov M, Zangen S, et al. Inhaled hydrofluoalkane-beclomethasone dipropionate in bronchopulmonary dysplasia. A double-blind, randomized, controlled pilot study. *J Perinatol.* 2017;37(2):197–202.
17. Beresford MW, Primhak R, Subhedar NV, Shaw NJ. Randomised double blind placebo controlled trial of inhaled fluticasone propionate in infants with chronic lung disease. *Arch Dis Child Fetal Neonatal Ed.* 2002;87(1): F62–F63.
18. Leung JS, Johnson DW, Sperou AJ, et al. A systematic review of adverse drug events associated with administration of common asthma medications in children. *PLoS One.* 2017;12(8):e0182738.
19. Cole CH, Shah B, Abbasi S, et al. Adrenal function in premature infants during inhaled beclomethasone therapy. *J Pediatr.* 1999;135(1):65–70.
20. O'Shea TM, Shah B, Allred EN, et al. Inflammation-initiating illnesses, inflammation-related proteins, and cognitive impairment in extremely preterm infants. *Brain Behav Immun.* 2013;29:104–112.
21. Been JV, Lugtenberg MJ, Smets E, et al. Preterm birth and childhood wheezing disorders: a systematic review and meta-analysis. *PLoS Med.* 2014;11(1):e1001596.
22. Jaakkola JJ, Ahmed P, Ieromnimon A, et al. Preterm delivery and asthma: a systematic review and meta-analysis. *J Allergy Clin Immunol.* 2006;118(4):823–830.
23. Rosenfeld M, Allen J, Arets BH, et al. An official American Thoracic Society workshop report: optimal lung function

tests for monitoring cystic fibrosis, bronchopulmonary dysplasia, and recurrent wheezing in children less than 6 years of age. *Ann Am Thorac Soc*. 2013;10(2):S1–S11.
24. Stewart A, Brion LP, Ambrosio-Perez I. Diuretics acting on the distal renal tubule for preterm infants with (or developing) chronic lung disease. *Cochrane Database Syst Rev*. 2011;(9):CD001817.
25. Stewart A, Brion LP. Intravenous or enteral loop diuretics for preterm infants with (or developing) chronic lung disease. *Cochrane Database Syst Rev*. 2011;(9):CD001453.
26. Slaughter JL, Stenger MR, Reagan PB. Variation in the use of diuretic therapy for infants with bronchopulmonary dysplasia. *Pediatrics*. 2013;131(4):716–723.
27. Kao LC, Durand DJ, McCrea RC, Birch M, Powers RJ, Nickerson BG. Randomized trial of long-term diuretic therapy for infants with oxygen-dependent bronchopulmonary dysplasia. *J Pediatr*. 1994;124(5 Pt 1): 772–781.
28. Palm K, Simoneau T, Sawicki G, Rhein L. Assessment of current strategies for weaning premature infants from supplemental oxygen in the outpatient setting. *Adv Neonatal Care*. 2011;11(5):349–356.
29. Bhandari A, Chow U, Hagadorn JI. Variability in duration of outpatient diuretic therapy in bronchopulmonary dysplasia: a clinical experience. *Am J Perinatol*. 2010; 27(7):529–535.
30. Collaco JM, Romer LH, Stuart BD, et al. Frontiers in pulmonary hypertension in infants and children with bronchopulmonary dysplasia. *Pediatr Pulmonol*. 2012;47(11): 1042–1053.
31. Abman SH, Collaco JM, Shepherd EG, et al. Interdisciplinary care of children with severe bronchopulmonary dysplasia. *J Pediatr*. 2017;181:12–28 e11.
32. Krishnan U, Feinstein JA, Adatia I, et al. Evaluation and management of pulmonary hypertension in children with bronchopulmonary dysplasia. *J Pediatr*. 2017;188: 24–34 e21.
33. Abman SH, Hansmann G, Archer SL, et al. Pediatric pulmonary hypertension: guidelines from the American heart association and American thoracic society. *Circulation*. 2015;132(21):2037–2099.
34. Bernier ML, Jacob AI, Collaco JM, McGrath-Morrow SA, Romer LH, Unegbu CC. Perioperative events in children with pulmonary hypertension undergoing non-cardiac procedures. *Pulm Circ*. 2018;8(1), 2045893217738143.
35. Baker CD, Abman SH, Mourani PM. Pulmonary hypertension in preterm infants with bronchopulmonary dysplasia. *Pediatr Allergy, Immunol Pulmonol*. 2014;27(1): 8–16.
36. Mourani PM, Sontag MK, Ivy DD, Abman SH. Effects of long-term sildenafil treatment for pulmonary hypertension in infants with chronic lung disease. *J Pediatr*. 2009;154(3), 379-384, 384 e371-372.
37. Trottier-Boucher MN, Lapointe A, Malo J, et al. Sildenafil for the treatment of pulmonary arterial hypertension in infants with bronchopulmonary dysplasia. *Pediatr Cardiol*. 2015;36(6):1255–1260.
38. Tan K, Krishnamurthy MB, O'Heney JL, Paul E, Sehgal A. Sildenafil therapy in bronchopulmonary dysplasia-associated pulmonary hypertension: a retrospective study of efficacy and safety. *Eur J Pediatr*. 2015;174(8): 1109–1115.
39. Kadmon G, Schiller O, Dagan T, Bruckheimer E, Birk E, Schonfeld T. Pulmonary hypertension specific treatment in infants with bronchopulmonary dysplasia. *Pediatr Pulmonol*. 2017;52(1):77–83.
40. Barst RJ, Beghetti M, Pulido T, et al. STARTS-2: long-term survival with oral sildenafil monotherapy in treatment-naive pediatric pulmonary arterial hypertension. *Circulation*. 2014;129(19):1914–1923.
41. Unegbu C, Noje C, Coulson JD, Segal JB, Romer L. Pulmonary hypertension therapy and a systematic review of efficacy and safety of PDE-5 inhibitors. *Pediatrics*. 2017;139(3).
42. Ehrenkranz RA, Walsh MC, Vohr BR, et al. Validation of the National Institutes of Health consensus definition of bronchopulmonary dysplasia. *Pediatrics*. 2005; 116(6):1353–1360.
43. Yeh J, McGrath-Morrow SA, Collaco JM. Oxygen weaning after hospital discharge in children with bronchopulmonary dysplasia. *Pediatr Pulmonol*. 2016;51(11): 1206–1211.
44. Silva DT, Hagan R, Sly PD. Home oxygen management of neonatal chronic lung disease in Western Australia. *J Paediatr Child Health*. 1995;31(3):185–188.
45. Bertrand P, Alvarez C, Fabres J, Simonetti M, Sanchez I. Home oxygen therapy in children with chronic respiratory failure. *Rev Med Chile*. 1998;126(3):284–292.
46. Saletti A, Stick S, Doherty D, Simmer K. Home oxygen therapy after preterm birth in Western Australia. *J Paediatr Child Health*. 2004;40(9–10):519–523.
47. Norzila MZ, Azizi BH, Norrashidah AW, Yeoh NM, Deng CT. Home oxygen therapy for children with chronic lung diseases. *Med J Malays*. 2001;56(2):151–157.
48. McGrath-Morrow SA, Ryan T, McGinley BM, Okelo SO, Sterni LM, Collaco JM. Polysomnography in preterm infants and children with chronic lung disease. *Pediatr Pulmonol*. 2012;47(2):172–179.
49. Boroughs D, Dougherty JA. Decreasing accidental mortality of ventilator-dependent children at home: a call to action. *Home Healthcare Nurse*. 2012;30(2):103–111. quiz 112-103.
50. Cristea AI, Carroll AE, Davis SD, Swigonski NL, Ackerman VL. Outcomes of children with severe bronchopulmonary dysplasia who were ventilator dependent at home. *Pediatrics*. 2013;132(3):e727–734.
51. Baker CD, Martin S, Thrasher J, et al. A standardized discharge process decreases length of stay for ventilator-dependent children. *Pediatrics*. 2016;137(4).
52. Gien J, Kinsella J, Thrasher J, Grenolds A, Abman SH, Baker CD. Retrospective analysis of an interdisciplinary ventilator care program intervention on survival of infants with ventilator-dependent bronchopulmonary dysplasia. *Am J Perinatol*. 2017;34(2):155–163.

53. Edwards JD, Kun SS, Keens TG. Outcomes and causes of death in children on home mechanical ventilation via tracheostomy: an institutional and literature review. *J Pediatr*. 2010;157(6), 955-959 e952.
54. Sterni LM, Collaco JM, Baker CD, et al. An official American thoracic society clinical practice guideline: pediatric chronic home invasive ventilation. *Am J Respir Crit Care Med*. 2016;193(8):e16–35.
55. Henningfeld JK, Maletta K, Ren B, Richards KL, Wegner C, D'Andrea LA. Liberation from home mechanical ventilation and decannulation in children. *Pediatr Pulmonol*. 2016;51(8):838–849.
56. Cristea AI, Jalou HE, Givan DC, Davis SD, Slaven JE, Ackerman VL. Use of polysomnography to assess safe decannulation in children. *Pediatr Pulmonol*. 2016; 51(8):796–802.
57. Liptzin DR, Connell EA, Marable J, Marks J, Thrasher J, Baker CD. Weaning nocturnal ventilation and decannulation in a pediatric ventilator care program. *Pediatr Pulmonol*. 2016;51(8):825–829.
58. Prickett KK, Sobol SE. Inpatient observation for elective decannulation of pediatric patients with tracheostomy. *JAMA Otolaryngol Head Neck Surg*. 2015;141(2):120–125.
59. Robison JG, Thottam PJ, Greenberg LL, Maguire RC, Simons JP, Mehta DK. Role of polysomnography in the development of an algorithm for planning tracheostomy decannulation. *Otolaryngol Head Neck Surg*. 2015;152(1): 180–184.
60. Doyle LW, Ford G, Davis N. Health and hospitalisations after discharge in extremely low birth weight infants. *Semin Neonatol*. 2003;8(2):137–145.
61. Bhandari A, Panitch HB. Pulmonary outcomes in bronchopulmonary dysplasia. *Semin Perinatol*. 2006;30(4): 219–226.
62. Deshpande SA, Northern V. The clinical and health economic burden of respiratory syncytial virus disease among children under 2 years of age in a defined geographical area. *Arch Dis Child*. 2003;88(12): 1065–1069.
63. Chidekel AS, Rosen CL, Bazzy AR. Rhinovirus infection associated with serious lower respiratory illness in patients with bronchopulmonary dysplasia. *Pediatr Infect Dis J*. 1997;16(1):43–47.
64. Greenough A, Alexander J, Boit P, et al. School age outcome of hospitalisation with respiratory syncytial virus infection of prematurely born infants. *Thorax*. 2009; 64(6):490–495.
65. Chan JY, Stern DA, Guerra S, Wright AL, Morgan WJ, Martinez FD. Pneumonia in childhood and impaired lung function in adults: a longitudinal study. *Pediatrics*. 2015;135(4):607–616.
66. Edmond K, Scott S, Korczak V, et al. Long term sequelae from childhood pneumonia; systematic review and meta-analysis. *PLoS One*. 2012;7(2):e31239.
67. McGrath-Morrow SA, Lee G, Stewart BH, et al. Day care increases the risk of respiratory morbidity in chronic lung disease of prematurity. *Pediatrics*. 2010;126(4): 632–637.
68. American Academy of Pediatrics Committee on Infectious Diseases, American Academy of Pediatrics Bronchiolitis Guidelines Committee. Updated guidance for palivizumab prophylaxis among infants and young children at increased risk of hospitalization for respiratory syncytial virus infection. *Pediatrics*. 2014;134(2):e620–638.
69. Moritsugu KP. The 2006 Report of the Surgeon General: the health consequences of involuntary exposure to tobacco smoke. *Am J Prev Med*. 2007;32(6):542–543.
70. Collaco JM, Aherrera AD, Breysse PN, Winickoff JP, Klein JD, McGrath-Morrow SA. Hair nicotine levels in children with bronchopulmonary dysplasia. *Pediatrics*. 2015;135(3):e678–686.
71. Bhat R, Salas AA, Foster C, Carlo WA, Ambalavanan N. Prospective analysis of pulmonary hypertension in extremely low birth weight infants. *Pediatrics*. 2012; 129(3):e682–689.
72. An HS, Bae EJ, Kim GB, et al. Pulmonary hypertension in preterm infants with bronchopulmonary dysplasia. *Korean Circ J*. 2010;40(3):131–136.
73. Stuart BD, Sekar P, Coulson JD, Choi SE, McGrath-Morrow SA, Collaco JM. Health-care utilization and respiratory morbidities in preterm infants with pulmonary hypertension. *J Perinatol*. 2013;33(7):543–547.
74. Joshi S, Wilson DG, Kotecha S, Pickerd N, Fraser AG, Kotecha S. Cardiovascular function in children who had chronic lung disease of prematurity. *Arch Dis Child Fetal Neonatal Ed*. 2014;99(5):F373–F379.
75. Korhonen P, Hyodynmaa E, Lautamatti V, Iivainen T, Tammela O. Cardiovascular findings in very low birth-weight schoolchildren with and without bronchopulmonary dysplasia. *Early Human Development*. 2005;81(6): 497–505.
76. Kwon HW, Kim HS, An HS, et al. Long-term outcomes of pulmonary hypertension in preterm infants with bronchopulmonary dysplasia. *Neonatology*. 2016;110(3): 181–189.
77. Newman LA, Cleveland RH, Blickman JG, Hillman RE, Jaramillo D. Videofluoroscopic analysis of the infant swallow. *Investig Radiol*. 1991;26(10):870–873.
78. de Jong AL, Kuppersmith RB, Sulek M, Friedman EM. Vocal cord paralysis in infants and children. *Otolaryngol Clin N Am*. 2000;33(1):131–149.
79. McGrath-Morrow SA, Ahn ES, Collaco JM. Respiratory outcomes after initial hospital discharge in children with ventricular shunts and bronchopulmonary dysplasia. *Pediatr Pulmonol*. 2017;52(10):1323–1328.
80. Arvedson JC, Lefton-Greif MA. *Pediatric Videofluoroscopic Swallow Studies*. San Antonio, TX: The Psychological Corporation; 1998.
81. Lee JH, Chang YS, Yoo HS, et al. Swallowing dysfunction in very low birth weight infants with oral feeding desaturation. *World J Pediatr*. 2011;7(4):337–343.
82. Colodny N. Comparison of dysphagics and nondysphagics on pulse oximetry during oral feeding. *Dysphagia*. 2000;15(2):68–73.
83. Singer L, Martin RJ, Hawkins SW, Benson-Szekely LJ, Yamashita TS, Carlo WA. Oxygen desaturation

complicates feeding in infants with bronchopulmonary dysplasia after discharge. *Pediatrics.* 1992;90(3): 380–384.

84. Davis NL, Liu A, Rhein L. Feeding immaturity in preterm neonates: risk factors for oropharyngeal aspiration and timing of maturation. *J Pediatr Gastroenterol Nutr.* 2013; 57(6):735–740.
85. Newman LA, Keckley C, Petersen MC, Hamner A. Swallowing function and medical diagnoses in infants suspected of Dysphagia. *Pediatrics.* 2001;108(6):E106.
86. Boesch RP, Daines C, Willging JP, et al. Advances in the diagnosis and management of chronic pulmonary aspiration in children. *Eur Respir J.* 2006;28(4):847–861.
87. Hartnick CJ, Hartley BE, Miller C, Willging JP. Pediatric fiberoptic endoscopic evaluation of swallowing. *Ann Otol Rhinol Laryngol.* 2000;109(11):996–999.
88. Leder SB, Karas DE. Fiberoptic endoscopic evaluation of swallowing in the pediatric population. *Laryngoscope.* 2000;110(7):1132–1136.
89. Lahiri T. The utility of the lipid-laden macrophage index for the evaluation of aspiration in children. *Cancer Cytopathol.* 2014;122(3):161–162.
90. Lefton-Greif MA, Arvedson JC. Pediatric feeding/swallowing: yesterday, today, and tomorrow. *Semin Speech Lang.* 2016;37(4):298–309.
91. Sorokin R, Gottlieb JE. Enhancing patient safety during feeding-tube insertion: a review of more than 2,000 insertions. *J Parenter Enter Nutr.* 2006;30(5):440–445.
92. Zeller RS, Davidson J, Lee HM, Cavanaugh PF. Safety and efficacy of glycopyrrolate oral solution for management of pathologic drooling in pediatric patients with cerebral palsy and other neurologic conditions. *Ther Clin Risk Manag.* 2012;8:25–32.
93. Eiland LS. Glycopyrrolate for chronic drooling in children. *Clin Ther.* 2012;34(4):735–742.
94. Faria J, Harb J, Hilton A, Yacobucci D, Pizzuto M. Salivary botulinum toxin injection may reduce aspiration pneumonia in neurologically impaired children. *Int J Pediatr Otorhinolaryngol.* 2015;79(12):2124–2128.
95. Katz ES, Mitchell RB, D'Ambrosio CM. Obstructive sleep apnea in infants. *Am J Respir Crit Care Med.* 2012;185(8): 805–816.
96. Macey-Dare LV, Moles DR, Evans RD, Nixon F. Long-term effect of neonatal endotracheal intubation on palatal form and symmetry in 8-11-year-old children. *Eur J Orthod.* 1999;21(6):703–710.
97. Don GW, Kirjavainen T, Broome C, Seton C, Waters KA. Site and mechanics of spontaneous, sleep-associated obstructive apnea in infants. *J Appl Physiol.* 2000;89(6): 2453–2462.
98. Tonkin SL, McIntosh C, Gunn AJ. Does tongue size contribute to risk of airway narrowing in preterm infants sitting in a car safety seat? *Am J Perinatol.* 2014;31(9): 741–744.
99. Arens R, Marcus CL. Pathophysiology of upper airway obstruction: a developmental perspective. *Sleep.* 2004; 27(5):997–1019.
100. Rosen CL, Larkin EK, Kirchner HL, et al. Prevalence and risk factors for sleep-disordered breathing in 8- to 11-year-old children: association with race and prematurity. *J Pediatr.* 2003;142(4):383–389.
101. Dransfield DA, Spitzer AR, Fox WW. Episodic airway obstruction in premature infants. *Am J Dis Child.* 1983; 137(5):441–443.
102. Huang YS, Paiva T, Hsu JF, Kuo MC, Guilleminault C. Sleep and breathing in premature infants at 6 months post-natal age. *BMC Pediatrics.* 2014;14:303.
103. Qubty WF, Mrelashvili A, Kotagal S, Lloyd RM. Comorbidities in infants with obstructive sleep apnea. *J Clin Sleep Med.* 2014;10(11):1213–1216.
104. Ortiz LE, McGrath-Morrow SA, Sterni LM, Collaco JM. Sleep disordered breathing in bronchopulmonary dysplasia. *Pediatr Pulmonol.* 2017;52(12):1583–1591.
105. Paavonen EJ, Strang-Karlsson S, Raikkonen K, et al. Very low birth weight increases risk for sleep-disordered breathing in young adulthood: the Helsinki Study of Very Low Birth Weight Adults. *Pediatrics.* 2007;120(4): 778–784.
106. Stone RS, Spiegel JH. Prevalence of obstructive sleep disturbance in children with failure to thrive. *J Otolaryngol Head Neck Surg.* 2009;38(5):573–579.
107. Bonuck K, Parikh S, Bassila M. Growth failure and sleep disordered breathing: a review of the literature. *Int J Pediatr Otorhinolaryngol.* 2006;70(5):769–778.
108. Hunter SJ, Gozal D, Smith DL, Philby MF, Kaylegian J, Kheirandish-Gozal L. Effect of sleep-disordered breathing severity on cognitive performance measures in a large community cohort of young school-aged children. *Am J Respir Crit Care Med.* 2016;194(6):739–747.
109. Emancipator JL, Storfer-Isser A, Taylor HG, et al. Variation of cognition and achievement with sleep-disordered breathing in full-term and preterm children. *Arch Pediatr Adolesc Med.* 2006;160(2):203–210.
110. Ingram DG, Singh AV, Ehsan Z, Birnbaum BF. Obstructive sleep apnea and pulmonary hypertension in children. *Paediatr Respir Rev.* 2017 Jun;23:33–39.
111. Collaco JM, McGrath-Morrow SA. Respiratory phenotypes for preterm infants, children, and adults: bronchopulmonary dysplasia and more. *Ann Am Thorac Soc.* 2018;15(5):530–538.

CHAPTER 20

Short- and Long-Term Outcomes After Bronchopulmonary Dysplasia

ELIZABETH K. BAKER, MBBS(HONS) • JEANIE L.Y. CHEONG, MD • LEX W. DOYLE, MD

INTRODUCTION

Bronchopulmonary dysplasia (BPD), also referred to as "chronic lung disease", is an important morbidity following preterm birth. It is associated with adverse respiratory outcomes in childhood, adolescence, and adulthood.[1–3] BPD is also a risk factor for poorer neurodevelopment in preterm infants. As neonatal intensive care has evolved, survival of the smallest and most immature infants has increased[4–6] but at the cost of increasing rates of BPD.[7–9]

This review will discuss the short- and long-term respiratory and neurodevelopmental outcomes of BPD survivors compared with preterm infants without BPD and with infants born at term or of normal birth weight (NBW, >2499 g).

PATHOGENESIS OF BRONCHOPULMONARY DYSPLASIA

The diagnosis and classification of BPD on the basis of respiratory support and oxygen requirement at 36 weeks' postmenstrual age[10,11] correlates with longer term pulmonary outcomes. Infants born preterm who do not fulfill the diagnostic criteria for BPD still demonstrate adverse pulmonary outcomes in childhood[12] and adolescence.[13] Rather than considering a categoric diagnosis of BPD at 36 weeks, it is preferable to conceptualize the pulmonary sequelae of preterm birth as a spectrum of illness. Certainly, infants diagnosed with BPD represent the more severe end of that spectrum; however, the absence of a diagnosis of BPD does not preclude longer term respiratory sequelae. This will become increasingly important as survivors born in the current era of "new BPD" reach adulthood and trends develop toward alternate modes of respiratory support as infants convalesce, such as high-flow oxygen therapy, challenging our current definitions of BPD.

BPD, first described by Northway and colleagues in 1967,[14] was associated with the use of mechanical ventilation and high oxygen concentrations to treat hyaline membrane disease. Histologically, Northway's BPD was characterized by areas of hyperinflation, interspersed with atelectasis, smooth muscle hypertrophy, and inflammatory infiltrates, with increased elastin and collagen deposition.[14] The mean gestation of survivors in Northway's original cohort, born in 1962–65, was 34 weeks. Today, infants at greatest risk of BPD are born more preterm, i.e., in the canalicular phase of lung development before alveolar and distal capillary development has commenced. Thus the pathogenesis of BPD has changed. "New" BPD is characterized predominantly by arrested alveolar development with fewer, simplified alveoli and abnormal angiogenesis.[15,16]

PULMONARY CONSEQUENCES OF VERY AND EXTREMELY PRETERM BIRTH, AND THE IMPACT OF BRONCHOPULMONARY DYSPLASIA

Mortality

As the survival of our smallest and most immature infants increases, mortality due to pulmonary causes is also decreasing.[17] For infants born at ≤28 weeks' gestation in centers across the National Institute of Child Health and Human Development (NICHD) Neonatal Research Network, mortality decreased from 83 per 1000 live births (95% confidence interval [CI], 77, 90) in 2004–07 and 84 per 1000 live births (95% CI, 78, 90) in 2000–03 to 68 per 1000 live births (95% CI, 63, 74) in 2008–11.[17] For infants who survived beyond 12 hours, deaths occurring in the first 14 days and in the first month of life were most commonly (49.5% and 42.8%, respectively) attributed to the

Updates on Neonatal Chronic Lung Disease. https://doi.org/10.1016/B978-0-323-68353-1.00020-8

respiratory distress syndrome (20). Deaths beyond 60 days of life, however, were mostly due to BPD.[17]

Oxygen Dependency

By virtue of the diagnosis, infants with BPD are more likely than those without BPD to be dependent on oxygen therapy both for a longer duration and at the time of discharge. In the EPICure 2006 cohort of births at <27 weeks' gestation in the United Kingdom, around one-third (36%) of infants with moderate BPD and two-thirds (62%) of those with severe BPD were discharged home with supplemental oxygen.[6] When compared with the first EPICure cohort (1995), the subgroup of infants born between 22 and 25 weeks' gestation in the 2006 cohort had an overall rate of discharge home with supplemental oxygen of 41%, which was an increase by 7% (95% CI, −0.2%, 14%).[6] For those treated with oxygen at home, the median duration of oxygen therapy post discharge in the EPICure 2006 cohort was 2.5 months (75th percentile 8.5 months).[6]

In survivors born at <28 weeks' gestation in the state of Victoria, Australia, the rate of oxygen dependence at 36 weeks' postmenstrual age was 46% for those born in 1991–92 and 43% for those born in 1997, but rose to 56% for those born in 2005.[9] After adjustment for other perinatal variables, infants born in 2005 required more than 3 weeks of additional oxygen therapy than those born in 1997.[9]

Hospital Readmission

Preterm infants are rehospitalized at higher rates over the first 2 years of life than term-born controls.[12,18] Readmission rates are higher in preterm infants with BPD than in preterm infants without BPD.[12,19] BPD survivors experience more respiratory illness during the first 2 years of life than preterm infants without BPD[12,19,20] and infants born at term.[12,21]

In a cohort of 133 infants born at less than 32 weeks who survived to discharge in New York State between 1985 and 1986, Cunningham et al.[12] reported a 36% readmission rate during the first 2 years of life for respiratory illness, compared with 2.5% in term controls ($P < .001$). BPD was a risk factor for rehospitalization; 45% of infants with BPD compared with 25% of infants without BPD were readmitted ($P < .05$).[12]

As survival rates for the smallest and least mature infants have increased, the rate of readmission in the first 2 years of life has also increased.[18] The UK Millennium Cohort Study[22] reported an adjusted odds ratio (OR) of 13.7 (95% CI, 6.5, 29.2) for three or more readmissions by 9 months of age for infants born at <32 weeks when compared with babies born between 39 and 41 weeks. Doyle et al.[18] reported that extremely low-birth-weight (ELBW) infants were 2–3 times more likely to be readmitted in the first 2 years of life than NBW term infants. The hospital readmission rates for ELBW infants ranged from 52% to 66%, compared with 18%–23% in the controls.[18]

Respiratory morbidity during the first 2 years of life for three cohorts of preterm infants born in the Netherlands in 1996–97, 2003–04, and 2008–09, at 25–29 completed weeks of gestation, was reported.[20] Readmission rates for infants with BPD (73% in 1996–97, 60% in 2003–04, and 78% in 2008–09) did not differ much between the three cohorts studied. However, the rate of rehospitalization was increased for infants with BPD (78%) compared with infants without BPD (48%) in the 2008–09 cohort ($P = .05$). Over the time spanned by the three cohorts, the proportion of hospitalizations for respiratory illness increased in infants with BPD. In the 2008–09 cohort, 78% of hospitalizations for infants with BPD were for respiratory illness compared with 50% and 66% for the 1996–97 and 2003–04 cohorts, respectively. Importantly, the relatively small sample studied, 380 in total, limited its statistical power to detect differences over time and between infants with and without BPD. Despite the lack of statistical power, the burden of rehospitalization and respiratory morbidity for preterm infants was evident.

Kuint et al.[19] reported that 62% (3956/6385) of very low-birth-weight (VLBW) infants born in Israel from 1995 to 2012 and followed up to a median age of 10.7 years (interquartile range, 6.2, 15.7) were rehospitalized at least once, with rehospitalization rates of 16.2 per 100 patient-years (100 PY). BPD, surgically treated necrotising enterocolitis, severe intraventricular hemorrhage, periventricular leukomalacia, and severe retinopathy of prematurity were risk factors for rehospitalization. Infants with BPD had higher rates of hospital readmission (33.6 per 100 PY) than infants without BPD (14.4 per 100 PY) with an adjusted relative risk (aRR) of rehospitalization of 1.94 (95% CI, 1.72, 2.17). The influence of BPD on the risk of readmission was substantial in the first decade after initial hospital discharge, with the highest aRR, 2.01 (95% CI, 1.60, 2.54) reported in the fifth to sixth year post discharge. However, by the 11th to 14th years and the 15th to 18th years post initial hospital discharge the difference in risk of readmission between infants with and those without BPD was diminished (aRR, 1.15 [95% CI, 0.75, 1.75] and 1.26 [95% CI, 0.67, 2.39], respectively).

The EPICure study group reported the respiratory morbidity of 236 infants born at ≤25 weeks' completed gestation in 1995 in the United Kingdom and Ireland.[23] Importantly this cohort of infants was born in an era of widespread antenatal corticosteroid and surfactant use, both of which alter the pathogenesis of neonatal lung disease. By 30 months of age, 64% of the preterm infants had been readmitted to hospital. Respiratory morbidity was the most common reason for readmission. Survivors of BPD were no more likely to require multiple (three or more) readmissions than preterm children without BPD; however, those discharged home with oxygen were at increased risk of multiple readmissions (OR, 2.7; 95% CI, 1.39, 5.27) compared with those not discharged home on oxygen.

Although the incidence of hospital readmission decreases with increasing age, increased readmission rates for VLBW infants compared with NBW infants are still evident in late childhood.[21] McCormick et al.[21] found VLBW infants were three to four times more likely to be admitted to hospital compared with NBW infants both since birth (54.7% vs. 22%) and in the year before interview at 8–10 years of age (6.9% vs. 1.8%; OR, 2.98; 95% CI, 2.00, 4.45). Respiratory illness was the predominant reason for readmission. However, the risk of hospitalization in the year before interview did not differ between VLBW infants with and those without BPD (6.2% vs. 7.1%, $P = .85$).[21]

By adolescence the increased incidence of respiratory ill health and hospital readmission observed in children who were born prematurely was less evident.[24] In the year before assessment, the clinical respiratory health of 14-year-old children born with birth weight ≤1500 g (n = 180) was comparable to term-born controls (n = 42) with only infrequent reports of hospitalization for pneumonia (n = 1) and asthma (n = 1).[24] In this cohort, the readmission rate for respiratory illness was 5% in those children who had BPD in the newborn period compared with 0% in those without BPD.[24]

Asthma and Wheeze

Preterm survivors experience more symptoms of respiratory ill health than term infants,[22,25,26] and the rates are increased for preterm infants with BPD compared with those without BPD.

In a cohort of 257 infants born with birth weight ≤1500 g in 1988–91, radiographic evidence of BPD at days 25–35 was strongly associated with bronchodilator use up to 2 years of age (OR, 10.1; 95% CI, 4.07, 25.2) and with asthma between 2 and 5 years of age (OR, 4.83; 95% CI, 2.18, 10.7).[27] Reports of increased wheeze, asthma, and chronic cough in preterm survivors compared with term-born controls continue into later childhood[26] and adolescence.[25] When assessed at 8 years of age a cohort of VLBW infants born in Scotland in 1984 were twice as likely as age-matched classroom controls to experience wheeze, either alone or associated with a viral respiratory illness or exercise.[26] Preterm survivors born in 1980–81 experienced cough, wheeze, and asthma at 5 years of age two to three times more than age- and sex-matched controls.[25]

The aforementioned studies describe infants born before the widespread use of surfactant and antenatal corticosteroids. However, similar respiratory symptoms are still observed in preterm survivors in the modern era. In a Norwegian cohort of 372 infants born at <28 weeks' gestation or with birth weight <1000 g during 1999–2000, BPD was associated with wheeze in the first year of life and asthma medications from 2 to 5 years of age.[28] The UK Millennium Cohort Study[22] reported an adjusted OR of 2.6 (95% CI, 1.7, 4.0) at 3 years and 2.9 (95% CI, 1.9, 4.6) at 5 years for wheezing in children born at <32 weeks' gestation compared with term-born controls (39–41 weeks). Infants diagnosed with BPD in the 1995 EPICure cohort received more treatment for "chest problems" by 30 months, and at 6 years of age, they experienced more wheeze and associated symptoms and were more likely to have used bronchodilators or corticosteroids in the previous 12 months than those without BPD.[23] This trend continued at 11 years of age when more extremely preterm (EP) infants with BPD experienced wheeze in the previous 12 months compared with EP infants without BPD (mean difference, 13%; 95% CI, 2, 25).[29]

Reports of asthma and wheezing in preterm survivors are more variable during the early adult years. Gough et al.[30] reported that adult survivors of BPD were twice as likely to report wheeze and three times as likely to use asthma medication compared with term-born controls. Caskey et al.[13] reported that preterm survivors with BPD when asked at 24 years of age were 10 times more likely to report being woken by cough and four times more likely to report experiencing breathlessness when wheezing than term-born controls. However, Gibson et al.[31] reported no difference in the rates of asthma or symptoms such as dry cough or wheeze with exercise at a mean age of 25.7 years between survivors born with birth weight <1501 g from 1977 to 1982 and NBW controls born in 1980–82.

Airway Growth and Lung Function

The airways grow throughout childhood, peaking in the early 20s, after which there is a gradual decline with age[32] (Fig. 20.1). In most people, the decline with age is not a problem because other causes of death will intervene before airway function is so reduced with age that they would become symptomatic; tobacco smokers are an obvious exception. As the lungs of preterm infants require exposure to much higher concentrations of oxygen than they would be exposed to if they remained in the uterus, and many very preterm (VP) infants require assisted ventilation and exposure to even higher concentrations of oxygen than the concentration available in air, it is vital to study airway growth in preterm survivors, particularly in those who had BPD, compared with those born at term.

Spirometric lung function measurements provide an objective assessment of airway growth. However, lung function tests are not without limitations—spirometry requires cooperation on behalf of the subject and as such is of limited value early in childhood. Furthermore, it may present additional challenges to those with physical and cognitive impairments. Often individuals most at risk of respiratory impairment are those who may find compliance with testing most challenging and are excluded from follow-up, thus adding to the bias of reporting in research studies. Despite these limitations, lung function tests provide a valuable means to assess the pulmonary sequelae of preterm birth and BPD.

The lung function of preterm survivors from the presurfactant era has been documented into early adulthood, whereas outcomes of infants born in the postsurfactant era have been documented in childhood and adolescence, with reports of lung function into early adulthood only just emerging. What remains unknown is the trajectory of lung function of survivors

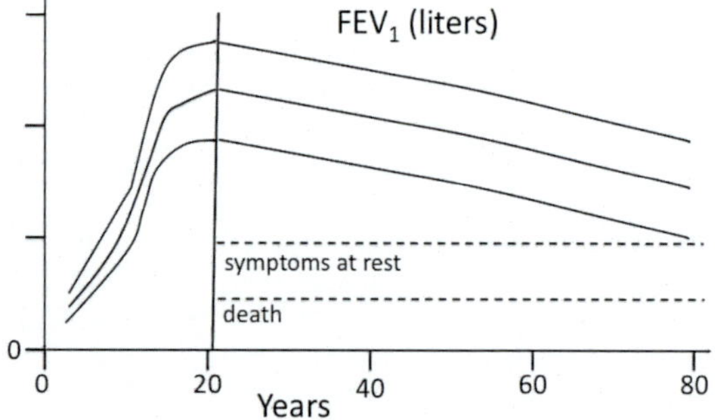

FIG. 20.1 Changes in forced expiratory volume in the first second of expiration (FEV_1) with age: mean and 95% confidence interval shown. Vertical line at age when peak of airway growth occurs. Dashed horizontal lines represent values where symptoms may appear at rest and when death from chronic obstructive lung disease ensues.

of extreme prematurity, particularly those who had BPD, into middle and late adulthood of both eras.

Lung Function in Childhood

Reports of lung function in childhood can be considered in two eras: pre-1990 when respiratory distress syndrome was managed expectantly with mechanical ventilation and oxygen therapy and after the early 1990s when the widespread use of endogenous surfactant and antenatal corticosteroids significantly altered the course of neonatal respiratory distress syndrome. The major findings from the studies are summarized in Table 20.1.

Before the widespread use of surfactant and antenatal corticosteroids: pre-1990

Survivors born before the widespread use of surfactant and antenatal corticosteroids demonstrate more abnormalities of lung function in childhood than their term-born counterparts,[26] and these abnormalities are more marked in children who had BPD.[26,33–36]

McLeod and colleagues[26] reported that VLBW children born in Scotland in 1984 had, after adjustment for height, reduced forced vital capacity (FVC) (1.81 L; 95% CI, 1.76, 1.85) compared with term-born controls (1.91 L; 95% CI, 1.89, 1.95) at 8–9 years of age. More VLBW infants had poor expiratory flows (defined as forced expiratory volume in 1 second to FVC [FEV_1/FVC] ratio of <70%) suggestive of obstructive lung pathology compared with term born controls. In this cohort, poorer expiratory function was associated with respiratory distress syndrome, duration of ventilation, and prolonged need for supplemental oxygen >40% in the neonatal period.

Chan et al.[33] compared the lung function at 7 years of age of 130 low-birth-weight (LBW) infants born in 1979–80 with 120 age-matched controls. LBW (<2500 g birth weight) infants had lower forced expiratory volume in 0.75 seconds to FVC ($FEV_{0.75}$/FVC) ratio compared with the control group (mean [standard deviation {SD}]: 0.86 (0.10) vs. 0.89 (0.07); $P < .001$), suggestive of airway obstruction.[33] In this cohort of children, LBW infants who received treatment for neonatal respiratory disease (oxygen therapy or mechanical ventilation) had poorer lung function than those who did not.

In a cohort of VLBW infants born in Melbourne, Australia,[34] in the late 1970s to early 1980s, those with BPD (n = 44) had significantly poorer lung function at 8 years of age than those without BPD (n = 126). Infants with BPD had reduced mean FVC and FEV_1 and higher mean residual volume (RV) and

TABLE 20.1
Lung Function in Childhood.

Author, Year Published	Year of Birth	Participants	Controls	Age	Major Findings (Compared With Controls)
BEFORE THE WIDESPREAD USE OF SURFACTANT AND ANTENATAL CORTICOSTEROIDS: PRE-1990S					
McLeod[26] 1996	1984	BW < 1500 g, n = 292	Classroom controls matched for age and sex, n = 574	8–9 years	Reduced FVC More preterm infants with FEV_1/FVC <70% Poorer respiratory function associated with RDS, duration of ventilation, and prolonged oxygen >40%
Chan[33] 1989	1979–80	BW < 2000 g, n = 130	Age matched BW > 2000 g, n = 123	7 years	Lower $FEV_{0.75}$/FVC Oxygen therapy and mechanical ventilation associated with poorer lung function
Kitchen[34] 1992	1977–82	BW ≤ 1500 g, n = 188	BW > 2500 g, n = 15	8 years	Obstructive pattern of lung disease, worse in subjects with BPD Decreased FVC and FEV_1 Increased RV, RV/TLC (BPD vs. NBW)
Kennedy[35] 2000	1981–82	BW ≤ 1500 g, n = 102	Classmates BW > 2000 g, except one, n = 82	11 years	Reduced expiratory flow Decreased FVC Increased RV/TLC Lowest expiratory flow in subjects with BPD Duration of O_2 therapy associated with lower FEV_1
Siltanen[36] 2004	1987–88	BW < 1500 g, n = 72	School children from same grade BW > 2500 g, n = 65	10 years	Reduced expiratory flow, BPD worse Decreased FEV_1, FVC, FEV_1/FVC, FEF_{50}, and $FEF_{25\%-75\%}$
AFTER WIDESPREAD USE OF SURFACTANT AND ANTENATAL CORTICOSTEROIDS, BEYOND EARLY 1990S					
Doyle[37] 2006	1991–92	<28 weeks' GA BW < 1000 g, n = 240	BW > 2499 g, n = 208	8–9 years	Reduced airflow, BPD worse BPD more likely to have FEV_1<75% of predicted Increased RV and RV/TLC
Fawke[29] 2010	1995	≤25 weeks' GA n = 182	Classmates matched for age, sex, and ethnicity, n = 161	11 years	Reduced expiratory flow FEV_1, $FEF_{25-75\%}$ reduced by 1.5 *z*-scores More infants with BPD had clinically significant airflow reduction

Continued

TABLE 20.1
Lung Function in Childhood.—cont'd

Author, Year Published	Year of Birth	Participants	Controls	Age	Major Findings (Compared With Controls)
Fortuna[38] 2016	1999–2002	<28 weeks' GA BW < 1000 g, n = 48	Age- and sex-matched term-born infants, n = 27	8 and 12 years	Reduced expiratory flow Infants with BPD had lower FEV_1, FVC, FEV_1/FVC, and $FEF_{25\%-75\%}$ BPD FEV_1 *z*-score decreased over time
MacLean[39] 2016	1997–2004	≤28 weeks' GA, n = 103	Term-born infants, n = 64	8 and 12 years	Airflow limitation Decreased FEV_1, FEV_1/FVC, $FEF_{25\%-75\%}$ *z*-scores Increased RV, RV/TLC in moderate/severe BPD
Doyle[9] 2017	1991/92 1997 2005	<28 weeks' GA 1991/92, n = 183 1997, n = 112 2005, n = 123		8 years	Reduced expiratory flow 2005 versus 1997 lower FEV_1 *z*-score 2005 versus 1997 and 1991/92 lower FEV_1/FVC *z*-score
Simpson[40] 2017	1997–2003	≤32 weeks' GA, n = 163	Term-born infants, n = 58	9–11 years	Airflow limitations Reduced FEV_1, $FEF_{25\%-75\%}$, FEV_1/FVC Worse in BPD More BPD had abnormally low FEV_1, $FEF_{25\%-75\%}$, and FEV_1/FVC

BPD, bronchopulmonary dysplasia; *BW*, birth weight; *$FEF_{25\%-75\%}$*, forced expiratory flow during 25%–75% of FVC; *FEV_1*, forced expiratory volume in the first second of expiration; *FVC*, forced vital capacity; *GA*, gestational age; *NBW*, normal birth weight; *RDS*, respiratory distress syndrome; *RV*, residual volume; *TLC*, total lung capacity.

RV to total lung capacity (RV/TLC) ratio compared with those without BPD.

A cohort of VLBW infants born in Adelaide, Australia, between 1981 and 1982[35] showed reduced expiratory flows, reduced FVC, and increased RV/TLC compared with controls (birth weight >2000 g). Among this cohort, infants with BPD (defined as oxygen supplementation 1 month postnatally associated with respiratory distress and chest radiographic changes consistent with the diagnosis) had the lowest expiratory flows.[35] Supplemental oxygen duration of 20 days or less had little effect on FEV_1; however, FEV_1 was reduced by 3% for each week of oxygen therapy beyond 20 days.[35]

When tested at 10 years of age, VLBW infants born in the late 1980s in Helsinki,[36] compared with NBW controls, had lower values for FVC, FEV_1, FEV_1/FVC, FEF after 50% of vital capacity (VC) has been exhaled ($FEF_{50\%}$), and forced expiratory flow at 25%–75% of VC ($FEF_{25\%-75\%}$). BPD and oxygen supplementation at 36 weeks' postmenstrual age were associated with lower FEV_1, FEV_1/FVC, $FEF_{50\%}$, and $FEF_{25\%-75\%}$, suggestive of airway obstruction.[36]

After widespread use of surfactant and antenatal corticosteroids, beyond early 1990s

The introduction of antenatal corticosteroids and endogenous surfactant in the early 1990s heralded a changed neonatal practice. Classic respiratory distress syndrome could be managed beyond supportive care alone, and less mature infants survived. However, long-term pulmonary sequelae remained. The possible benefits of antenatal corticosteroids and endogenous surfactant on long-term lung function may have been offset by the survival of smaller and less mature infants.

Variables reflecting airflow were reduced in a cohort of ELBW/EP infants with BPD born in 1991–92 in Victoria, Australia, compared with those without BPD.[37] During this era, surfactant was reserved for rescue therapy and was administered to just under 40% of the cohort of preterm infants.[37] At 8 years of age, preterm children had reduced FEV_1 *z*-scores compared with controls (mean difference [95% CI], −1.02 [−1.21 to −0.82]; $P < .001$). Furthermore, preterm children with BPD had reduced FEV_1 *z*-scores compared with preterm children without BPD (mean difference [95% CI], −0.47 [−0.75 to −0.20]; $P = .001$). However, Fig. 20.2 illustrates the variability in FEV_1 *z*-scores within each group, highlighting the challenge of predicting individual respiratory outcomes.

In the same Victorian cohort, infants with BPD were more likely to have an FEV_1 <75% of predicted at 8 years of age compared with infants without BPD (27.3% [24/88] vs. 15.2% [23/151], $\chi^2 = 5.1$, $P = .024$).[37] Those with BPD also had evidence of gas trapping with increased RV and RV/TLC compared with infants without BPD.[37]

Baseline spirometry was reduced by up to 1.5 SD for both FEV_1 and $FEF_{25\%-75\%}$ in the 1995 EPICure cohort of EP infants when lung function was studied at 11 years of age.[29] The changes were more marked in EP infants with BPD (n = 129) than in those without BPD (n = 53). More children with BPD had baseline lung function in the clinically significant range (*z*-scores ≤1.96) (66%; 85/129) compared with both EP children without BPD (32%, 17/53) and classmate controls (9%, 14/161).[29]

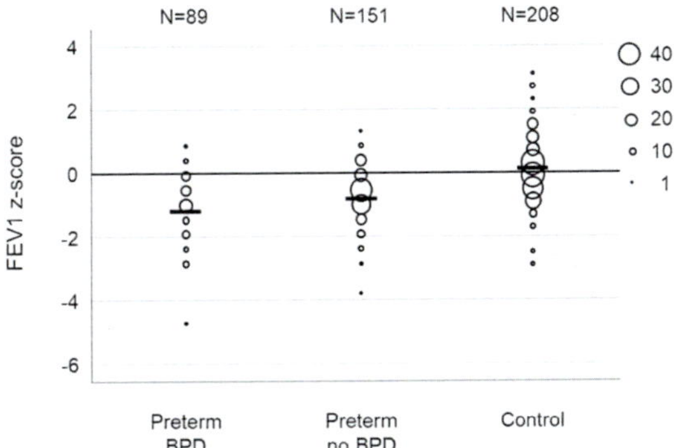

FIG. 20.2 Distribution of *z*-scores for forced expiratory volume in the first second of expiration (FEV_1) at 8 years of age contrasted between preterm children with bronchopulmonary dysplasia (BPD), preterm children without BPD, and controls, born in Victoria, Australia, in 1991–92. The size of circles is proportional to the sample size. Solid lines indicate means for each group.

Fortuna et al.[38] reported the lung function at 8 and 12 years of children born <28 weeks and <1000 g in 1999–2002 in Veneto, Italy. At both ages children with BPD had significantly lower *z*-scores for FEV_1, FVC, FEV_1/FVC, and $FEF_{25\%-75\%}$ than term controls. Children with BPD had significantly lower FEV_1 *z*-scores (mean [SD], −1.27 [1.07] vs. −0.47 [0.82]; $P = .007$) and FVC *z*-scores (−1.03 [1.08] vs. −0.28 [0.73]; $P = .004$) than children without BPD at 8 years of age.[38] The findings were similar at 12 years of age; those with BPD demonstrated greater airflow limitations than those without BPD. Children with BPD showed a decrease in FEV_1 *z*-score from −1.27 (1.07) at 8 years to −1.67 (1.1) at 12 years.

Lung function at 8–12 years in a cohort of children born at ≤28 weeks between 1997 and 2004 in Western Canada was compared with term-born controls.[39] The preterm cohort was subdivided into two categories: moderate/severe BPD and no/mild BPD. Both preterm groups had airflow limitation, with decreased FEV_1 *z*-scores, FEV_1/FVC *z*-scores, and $FEF_{25\%-75\%}$ *z*-scores compared with term infants. The difference between the moderate/severe BPD group and the mild/no BPD group was not significant. However, other parameters such as the RV and RV/TLC were increased in the moderate/severe BPD group compared with term controls, reflecting gas trapping.

Comparison of lung function among the 1991–92, 1997, and 2005 Victorian Infant Collaborative Study (VICS) cohorts (infants born at <28 weeks and/or with birth weight <1000 g in Victoria, Australia) demonstrated that, despite increased use of noninvasive respiratory support, the incidence of BPD increased and expiratory airflow values at 8 years of age declined in the most recent cohort compared with earlier cohorts.[9]

Preterm children born at ≤32 weeks' gestation during 1997–2003 in Perth, Australia, had lower spirometry values at 9–11 years of age (FEV_1, $FEF_{25\%-75\%}$, FEV_1/FVC) than the control children, which decreased further in preterm children with BPD.[40] More children with BPD had abnormally low values for FEV_1, $FEF_{25\%-75\%}$, and/or FEV_1/FVC (defined as <−1.96 *z*-score) compared with preterm children without BPD and term controls (46.8% vs. 13.5% vs. 0%, respectively).[40] About 92% of preterm children had changes on computed tomography (CT) of the chest; increased subpleural opacities, bronchial wall thickening, and areas of hypoattenuation were associated with obstructive patterns of lung disease on spirometry.[40] Assessment at three time points between the ages of 4 and 12 years showed FEV_1, $FEF_{25\%-75\%}$, and FEV_1/FVC values all declined by at least 0.1 *z*-score per year in children with BPD when compared with controls.[41] Additionally, respiratory mechanics (reactance at 8 Hz) decreased by -0.05 *z*-score per year (95% CI, -0.08, -0.01) and gas exchange (diffusing capacity of carbon monoxide) decreased by -0.03 *z*-score per year (95% CI, -0.06, -0.61) for infants with BPD relative to controls.

Lung Function in Adolescence and Beyond

Before the widespread use of surfactant and antenatal corticosteroids: pre-1990

Several studies have reported the lung function during adolescence and early adulthood of preterm infants born in the presurfactant era (Table 20.2). Preterm infants with BPD surviving into late adolescence and adulthood show obstructive patterns of lung disease,[1,2,42,43] reduced peak lung function, and a more rapid decline in lung function[42] compared with preterm infants without BPD and healthy term-born infants.

Pulmonary outcomes in late adolescence and early adulthood of preterm survivors were first reported by Northway et al. in 1990.[2] The respiratory function at 18 years of age of 26 survivors born between 1964 and 1973, with a mean gestation of 33.2 weeks (SD, 3.8) and diagnosed with BPD, were compared with a control group of preterm infants without BPD and healthy term-born controls. Those infants with BPD had evidence of obstructive airway disease with significantly lower peak expiratory flow rates, FVC, FEV_1, $FEF_{25\%-75\%}$, and $FEF_{50\%}$ than matched cohort controls and term-born controls. Although neonatal intensive care has evolved since these infants were born, similar lung function abnormalities are reported in survivors of BPD in more recent eras.

Halvorsen et al.[1] reported the lung function of 46 adolescents born at ≤28 weeks' gestation or with birth weight ≤1000 g in Norway from 1982 to 85 compared with term-born controls at a mean age of 17.7 years. Adolescents born preterm had significantly lower peak expiratory flow rates and FEV_1 than controls; the more severe the BPD, the larger the discrepancy in these parameters compared with control participants. Although $FEF_{50\%}$ and flow with 75% of VC exhaled ($FEF_{75\%}$) were also reduced significantly in those born preterm, the severity of BPD was not associated with a worsening of these measures.

Doyle et al.[42] reported that VLBW adolescents with BPD born between 1977 and 82 and studied at 18 years of age had evidence of more obstructive airway disease than VLBW adolescents without BPD. FEV_1, FEV_1/FVC, and $FEF_{25\%-75\%}$ expressed as a percentage of predicted were significantly lower in infants with BPD than in those without BPD. Importantly, more VLBW adolescents with BPD than those without BPD had values in the clinically important ranges. Moreover, lung function declined more rapidly (greater reduction in FEV_1/FVC) between 8 and 18 years in those with BPD than those without BPD.

Vrijlandt et al.[43] reported the lung function of 42 preterm adolescents, with a mean of 30 weeks' gestation and mean birth weight of 1246 g, at 19 years of age compared with 44 healthy term controls. Those born preterm showed more airway obstruction, as demonstrated by lower FVC, FEV_1, FEV_1/FVC, peak expiratory flow, flow with 25% of VC exhaled ($FEF_{25\%}$), $FEF_{50\%}$, $FEF_{75\%}$, and specific airway conductance (corrected for lung volume) compared with healthy term controls. However, the lung function parameters measured, with the exception of $FEF_{25\%}$, $FEF_{50\%}$, and $FEF_{75\%}$ were within the normal range. In this cohort of preterm infants, the lung function abnormalities observed did not differ between those infants with BPD ($n = 8$) and those without ($n = 12$) BPD, although it must be noted that the sample size was small and may not have had adequate power to detect a difference between the groups.

Gough et al.[30] compared 72 adult survivors of BPD born between 1978 and 93 in Belfast to preterm survivors without BPD and term-born controls. Adult survivors of BPD had significantly lower than predicted lung function measures (FEV_1, FVC, FEV_1/FVC, and $FEF_{25\%-75\%}$) than term-born controls. Additionally, significantly more BPD survivors had evidence of airflow limitation in the abnormally low range compared with non-BPD preterm survivors and term controls.

Gibson et al.[31] reported the lung function of three groups of adults: BW < 1000 g, BW = 1000−1500 g, and normal weight controls at a mean age of 25.7 years (SD, 1.0) born between 1977 and 1982. Both groups with birth weight <1501 g had lower *z*-scores for FEV_1, FEV_1/FVC, and $FEV_{25\%-75\%}$ than controls, but the mean values were within the expected range. Those with birth weight <1501 g diagnosed with BPD had lower lung function variables than those without BPD; however, this only reached statistical significance for *z*-score of FEV_1. There were no differences in lung function variables between those born with birth weight <1000 g compared with those born with birth weight 1000−1500 g.

Vollsaeter and colleagues[44] reported significantly lower *z*-scores for FEV_1, $FEF_{25\%-75\%}$, FEV_1/FVC, and higher airway resistance in adults born with birth weight ≤1000 g or at ≤28 weeks' gestation between 1982 and 1985 than adult term-born controls when studied at 25 years of age. In this cohort, RV/TLC increased with severity of BPD.

TABLE 20.2
Lung Function in Adolescence and Beyond: Presurfactant Era.

Author, Year Published	Year of Birth	Participants	Controls	Age	Major Findings
Northway[2] 1990	1964–1973	BPD survivors, mean GA 33.2 weeks, n = 26	Preterm survivors without BPD, mean GA 34.5 weeks, n = 26 Age-matched normal subjects, n = 53	18 years	Compared to preterm and age-matched controls, BPD survivors had lower FVC, FEV_1, $FEF_{25\%-75\%}$, $FEF_{50\%}$
Halvorsen[1] 2004	1982–85	≤28 weeks' gestation or BW ≤ 1000 g, n = 46	Term-born infants, sex-matched, BW = 3000–4000 g, n = 35	17.7 years	Lower PEF and FEV Worse in BPD
Doyle[43] 2006	1977–1982	BW = 500–999 g, n = 63 (born in 1977–80) BW = 1000–1500 g, n = 86 (born in 1980–82)	BW > 2499 g, n = 37 (born in 1980–82)	18 years	More obstructive airways disease in BPD; lower FEV_1, FEV_1/FVC, $FEF_{25\%-75\%}$ FEV_1/FVC declines more rapidly in subjects with BPD
Vrijlandt[44] 2006	1983	GA <32 weeks BW < 1500 g, n = 42	Healthy term-born infants, n = 44	19 years	Preterm versus term; lower FVC, FEV_1, FEV_1/FVC, PEF, $FEF_{25\%}$, $FEF_{50\%}$, $FEF_{75\%}$, and sGaw No difference between with BPD and without BPD
Gough[30] 2014	1978–93	BPD survivors, n = 72	Preterm survivors without BPD, n = 57 Sex- and age-matched term-born controls, n = 78	24–25 years	BPD survivors versus term; lower FEV_1, FVC, FEV_1/FVC, and $FEF_{25\%-75\%}$ BPD survivors versus term and non-BPD survivors; more clinically significant airflow limitation
Gibson[31] 2015	1977–82	BW < 1000 g, n = 86 BW = 1000–1500 g, n = 124	BW > 2499 g, n = 60 (born in 1980–82)	25.7 years	Preterm versus control; Lower *z*-scores for FEV_1, FEV_1/FVC, and $FEV_{25\%-75\%}$ BPD versus non-BPD; lower *z*-score for FEV_1
Vollsaeter[45] 2015	1982–85	BW ≤ 1000 g or GA ≤ 28 weeks, n = 45	Term born, age and sex matched, n = 39	25 years	Preterm versus control; lower *z*-scores for FEV_1, $FEF_{25\%-75\%}$, FEV_1/FVC, and higher airway resistance RV/TLC increased with BPD severity
Caskey[13] 2016	1977–93	<1500 g with BPD, n = 25	BW < 1500 g without BPD, n = 24 Term born, n = 25	Mean, 24–28 years	BPD versus term; lower FEV_1, FVC, and $FEF_{25\%-75\%}$

BPD, bronchopulmonary dysplasia; *BW*, birth weight; *$FEF_{25\%}$*, forced expiratory flow at 25% of FVC; *$FEF_{25-75\%}$*, forced expiratory flow during 25%–75% of FVC; *$FEF_{50\%}$*, forced expiratory flow at 50% of FVC; *$FEF_{75\%}$*, forced expiratory flow at 75% of FVC; *FEV_1*, forced expiratory volume in the first second of expiration; *FVC*, forced vital capacity; *GA*, gestational age; *PEF*, peak expiratory flow; *sGaw*, specific airway conductance corrected for lung volume.

Wong et al.[3] reported emphysematous lung changes on CT in 84% of a small cohort (n = 21) of survivors born in Western Australia in 1980–87 with a birth weight of <1500 g diagnosed with moderate-severe BPD. About 71% of participants reported persistent respiratory symptoms; FEV_1 (median 89.0% predicted; range, 22.6, 121.9) and $FEF_{25\%-75\%}$ (median 63.7% predicted; range, 6.1, 117.2) values were lower than those expected for age, height, and sex, consistent with other reports.

Caskey et al.[13] reported greater airway obstruction in preterm survivors both with (n = 25) and without BPD (n = 24) compared with term-born controls (n = 25). Preterm survivors with BPD had lower FEV_1, FVC, and $FEF_{25\%-75\%}$ values than term-born controls. Although this was also the case for preterm survivors without BPD, the difference did not reach statistical significance. Similar to Wong et al.,[3] Caskey et al.[13] reported abnormalities on high-resolution CT in all BPD survivors. Although the emphysematous changes observed were consistent with those reported by Wong et al.,[3] the most common finding was of subpleural opacities. It is important to note that participants studied by Caskey et al. were born over the 15 years from 1978 to 1993, during which neonatal care evolved, particularly with the introduction of antenatal corticosteroids and exogenous surfactant.

After widespread use of surfactant and antenatal corticosteroids, beyond early 1990s

Preterm infants born in the era of widespread surfactant use are reaching adulthood and reports of their long-term lung function are emerging. Doyle et al.[45] reported respiratory function of preterm survivors of the 1991–92 VICS cohort at 18 years compared with term-born controls. Preterm survivors had airflow limitation compared with term controls; mean difference in FEV_1 *z*-score was −0.92 (95% CI, −1.14, −0.71).[45] Moreover, among the preterm survivors, those who had BPD (n = 77) had even worse airflow limitation than those who did not have BPD (n = 132) (mean difference in FEV_1 *z*-score, −0.68 (95% CI, −0.98, −0.39).

In a recent individual participant data meta-analysis of 11 cohort studies, which includes those studies mentioned earlier, where expiratory flows were measured from at least 16 years of age (up to 33 years of age) in 935 survivors born either VP (<32 weeks' gestation) or with VLBW and 722 controls born either with NBW or at term, it was clear that VP/VLBW survivors are not reaching the normal peak of airway capacity in their early 20s.[46] The reductions in airflow capacity in VP/VLBW survivors in early adulthood (mean age, 21 years) were large (e.g., mean difference in *z*-score for FEV_1, −0.78, 95% CI, −0.96, −0.61). Moreover, at least four fold more had low values for expiratory flows in worrying clinical ranges compared with controls. VP/VLBW survivors who had BPD in the newborn period had even worse airflow capacity than those who did not have BPD, with reductions ranging between −0.5 and −1.0 SD in those with BPD compared with those without BPD, after adjustment for other potential confounders, such as sex and smoking.

Changes in Lung Function Over Time

The few cohort studies that have followed the trajectory of lung function with age report mixed results. Vollsaeter et al.[44] compared lung function at age 18 and 25 years of a preterm cohort (birth weight ≤1000 g or ≤28 weeks' gestation) with a term cohort born in 1982–85 in Norway. The trajectory of respiratory function variables of the preterm groups when subdivided on BPD severity was comparable with the term-born cohort. However, when the preterm groups were studied as a single cohort, changes in mean FEV_1 and FVC *z*-scores were increased in the preterm group compared with term controls (0.23 vs. 0.04, $P = .028$ and 0.58 vs. 0.26, $P = .017$, respectively). However, others suggest lung function may decline more rapidly in preterm survivors as they age.[41,42] In the VICS cohort of infants born at <28 weeks and/or with birth weight <1000 g in 1991–92, infants with BPD had airway obstruction that increased over time demonstrated by decreases in *z*-scores for FEV_1, FEV_1/FVC, $FEF_{25\%-75\%}$, and $FEF_{75\%}$ between 8 and 18 years.[45]

In the recent individual participant data meta-analysis mentioned earlier,[46] there were 117 VP/VLBW participants and 53 controls who had airflow measured on two occasions, i.e., at 18 and 25 years of age. *z*-Scores for FVC increased between 18 and 25 years in both groups, but less so in the VP/VLBW group; however, differences in rates of change among the VP/VLBW cohorts with and without BPD were not reported.

Exercise Capacity

Survivors born preterm have reduced exercise capacity compared with term-born survivors.[13,43,47] When compared using a standardized symptom limited maximal exercise protocol (modified Bruce protocol[48]) with term-born controls at a mean age of 24 years, preterm survivors, both with and without BPD, had significantly lower peak oxygen consumption (VO_2) and traveled less distance.[13] Smith et al.[47] reported reduced exercise capacity, measured by the 20–minute shuttle test, at a mean age of 10.1 years in 126 infants born with birth weight <1000 g and at <32 weeks' gestation in 1992–94, an era of widespread surfactant use, compared with term-born controls. This cohort of infants also had expiratory flows worse than those of term-born controls but still within the normal range, i.e., lower FEV_1 (85% vs. 95% of predicted) and $FEF_{25\%-75\%}$ (71.8% vs. 91.4% of predicted), as well as evidence of air trapping, with a higher RV (141% vs. 99%). Similarly, Vrijlandt et al.[43] described lower exercise capacity in preterm infants born at <32 weeks and/or with birth weight <1500 g when studied at 19 years of age compared with term-born controls. This finding remained significant following correction for smoking status. Interestingly, there was no difference reported in the exercise capacity or lung function of preterm infants with and without BPD, although the numbers of infants in these subgroups were small.

ASSOCIATIONS OF BRONCHOPULMONARY DYSPLASIA WITH NEURODEVELOPMENTAL OUTCOMES

BPD is an independent risk factor for adverse neurodevelopmental outcomes in preterm infants.[49–53] We will review outcomes in the domains of neurosensory, cognitive and academic performance, language, and visuomotor performance.

Neurosensory Outcomes

Preterm infants are at greater risk of developing cerebral palsy (CP) than term-born infants. BPD is a risk factor for CP.[49,50] Analysis of the Trial of Indomethacin for Prophylaxis in Preterms (TIPP)[49] reported that BPD was a risk factor for the combined outcome of death, CP, cognitive delay, hearing loss or bilateral blindness, independent of the other serious preterm morbidities of severe retinopathy of prematurity and ultrasonographic brain injury. The OR for death or major neurosensory impairment was 2.4 (95% CI, 1.8, 3.2) for those who had BPD. Similarly, BPD was a risk factor for death or neurosensory impairment at 2 years of age in a Swiss cohort of infants born at 24–27 weeks' gestation in 2000–08.[50] The OR for the combined outcomes of death, moderate or major neurosensory impairment was 1.92 (95% CI, 1.24, 2.99)[50] for those with BPD. Natarajan et al.[54] reported the NICHD Neonatal Research Network outcomes of infants born with birth weight <1000 g between 2006 and 2007. Infants with BPD, determined using a physiologic definition, were more frequently diagnosed with severe CP (7.0% vs. 2.1%), spastic diplegia (7.8% vs. 4.1%), and quadriplegia (3.9% vs. 0.9%) than infants without BPD.

Majnemar et al.[51] found 71% of infants born in 1982–88 with severe BPD, defined as requiring home oxygen for at least 1 month post discharge, had neurologic abnormalities compared with 19% of control preterm infants ($P < .005$). This high rate of abnormality reflects both the severity of lung disease in the cohort and the era, presurfactant and preantenatal corticosteroids, in which they were born. Although neurosensory outcomes have improved over time in some studies,[50,55] BPD continues to be a risk factor for neurodevelopmental impairment. Kobaly et al.[56] report infants born at <28 weeks' gestation in 2000–03 with BPD had lower rates of neurosensory abnormalities than infants with BPD born in the earlier period of 1996–99, 31% versus 16%. Neonatal practice changed between these two cohorts with increased use of antenatal corticosteroids, decreased use of postnatal corticosteroids, and increased use of surfactant and indomethacin. BPD was a risk factor for CP for infants born at <25 weeks' gestation during 1993–99, OR, 1.66 (95% CI, 1.01, 2.74), in an NICHD study.[52] Although the two epochs studied, 1993–96 and 1996–99, differed in their exposure to surfactant and antenatal corticosteroids (increased rate of exposure in the latter epoch), the rate of neurosensory impairment did not change over time. Importantly the rate of postnatal corticosteroid exposure did not differ and was high in both epochs (73% in the earlier epoch vs. 79% in the latter epoch, $P = .052$).[52]

BPD severity correlates with the risk of neurosensory impairment.[53] The ELGANS study[53] examined the severity of BPD (defined at 36 weeks' postmenstrual age as mechanical ventilation with supplemental oxygen, supplemental oxygen alone, or no requirement for supplemental oxygen) as a risk factor for neurosensory impairment. More severe BPD was associated with a nearly sixfold increase in quadriparesis and a fourfold increase in diparesis. The risk, compared with no BPD, was also increased for the group who required supplemental oxygen without mechanical ventilation, albeit to a lesser degree.

Non-CP motor impairments, such as developmental coordination disorder (DCD), are also common in preterm survivors.[57] A weak association was observed in a cohort of ELBW/VP survivors between BPD and DCD; the incidence of BPD in children with DCD was 50%, whereas 30.5% of infants without DCD had BPD ($P = .062$). However, the difference in postnatal corticosteroid exposure between those with and those without DCD was substantial (50.0% vs. 24.7%, $P = .031$). BPD, postnatal corticosteroid exposure, and neurosensory outcome are clearly interrelated; however, caution must be exercised while using postnatal corticosteroid exposure as a surrogate for BPD.

Cognitive Function and Academic Achievement

The lower cognitive function and poorer academic achievement of children and adolescents born EP compared with term-born controls has been widely reported.[58–62] A number of biological and social factors influence the risk of poorer cognitive function and academic achievement in the preterm population,[58] of which BPD is one.[54,60,61,63]

A group of preterm infants with BPD born in Cleveland, Ohio, between 1989 and 91, showed poorer cognitive and academic outcomes that persisted during childhood compared with VLBW infants without BPD and term-born controls.[64] The Bayley Scales of Infant and Toddler Development were used to assess infants at 8, 12, 24, and 36 months of age corrected for prematurity. At all ages, infants with BPD scored significantly lower on the Mental Development Index (MDI) and Psychomotor Development Index (PDI) compared with VLBW infants without BPD and term controls.[64] Moreover, at 3 years of age corrected for prematurity, more infants with BPD (20%) had an MDI <70 compared with VLBW infants without BPD (11%) and term controls (4%).[64] Similarly, 20% of infants with BPD had a PDI <70 at 3 years compared with 9% of VLBW infants without BPD and 1% of term controls.[64]

Poorer neurodevelopmental outcomes, demonstrated in terms of cognition and academic performance, persisted when the Cleveland group were assessed at 8 years of age.[61] Infants with BPD showed deficits compared with VLBW and term infants in intelligence, reading, and mathematics and required more special education services. Infants with BPD also had poorer attention when compared with term-born infants.[61] More children with BPD (20%) had full-scale IQ < 70 than VLBW infants without BPD (11%) and term-born infants (3%). More children with BPD (54%) used special education classes than VLBW infants without BPD (37%) and term-born infants (25%). After controlling for birth weight and neurologic abnormalities, BPD and severity of BPD predicted lower performance IQ, perceptual organization, full-scale IQ, and attentional skills, as well as more special education placement.[61] When compared with infants with moderate or mild BPD, infants with severe BPD, defined using NICHD consensus definitions,[65] had lower performance IQ (mean, 75 vs. 86), poorer perceptual organization (mean, 76 vs. 86), and increased special education needs (69% vs. 44%).[60]

Exposure to postnatal corticosteroids may, in part, contribute to the poorer neurodevelopmental outcomes observed in BPD survivors of the Cleveland cohort.[61] Infants with BPD exposed to postnatal corticosteroids compared with those who did not receive corticosteroids had significantly lower performance IQ (72.8 vs. 84.8), full-scale IQ (77 vs. 85.2), and perceptual organization (74.0 vs. 85.2).[61] In addition, those who received corticosteroids were more likely to participate in special education services (78% vs. 48%), occupational therapy (71% vs. 44%), and physical therapy (71% vs. 41%).[61] In a large cohort of infants born at <28 weeks' gestation or with birth weight <1000 g in Victoria, Australia, in 1991–92 and studied at 2, 5, 8, and 18 years of age, having BPD not treated with postnatal corticosteroids had little effect on cognitive and academic outcomes at any age. However, postnatal corticosteroid exposure was associated with lower cognitive scores at age 8 and 18 years and with worse academic performance at 8 years.[58]

Language

Natarajan[54] reported ELBW infants born between 2006 and 2007 with BPD had significantly higher rates of language delay at 18–22 months (language composite score <70 assessed on Bayley Scales of Infant and Toddler Development III, 24.2% vs. 12.3%, $P < .0001$) than ELBW infants without BPD.

Singer et al.[66] reported in a cohort of VLBW infants at 3 years of age that those with BPD had lower language competence scores assessed using the Communication Domain Subscale of the Battelle Developmental Inventory than those without BPD. The mean (SD) developmental quotient (DQ) was significantly lower for children with BPD than for those without BPD for both receptive (84.7 (17) vs. 91.5 (17)) and expressive language (92.8 (22) vs. 99.7 (17)).[66] Not only was the mean DQ lower but also more children with BPD had scores within the impaired range of functioning (DQ < 85) than children without BPD for both receptive (49% vs. 34%) and expressive language (44% vs. 25%).[66] After controlling for lower IQ, children with BPD demonstrated impairment only in the receptive language domain. The same cohort of infants was assessed at 8 years of age.[67] Deficits in receptive language skills persisted in those VLBW infants with BPD compared with those without BPD. Articulation, as measured by mean percentile score (SD) for the Goldman-Fristoe Test of Articulation Sound in Word Subtest, was poorer for those infants with BPD compared with those without BPD (56 (38) vs. 78 (30)).[67] The delays in language that children with

BPD experience were reflected in increased enrollment in speech pathology services (infants with BPD, 48% vs. infants without BPD, 21%).[67] In this cohort of children, the severity of BPD correlated with the degree of language deficit.[60]

Visuospatial Perception

Visuospatial and visuomotor performance, the ability to interpret visual stimuli in the environment and respond with action, is diminished in children with BPD compared with children without BPD.[51] When studied at a mean age of 9.9 years, children with severe BPD born between 1982 and 89 scored lower than matched preterm controls without BPD on the Developmental Test of Visual Motor Integration (VMI) (mean (SD), 93.7 (12.6) vs. 101.0 (16.8); $P = .03$). They also scored higher, indicating more difficulty, on the Quick Neurological Screening Test (21.0 (10.60) vs. 12.5 (11.1); $P = .039$).[51] Gray et al.[68] reported similar findings of reduced VMI score for infants with BPD compared with birth weight-matched controls at 8 years of age (difference in mean 4.4, 95% CI, 1.1, 7.8); however, after adjusting for confounding variables the difference was no longer significant. Regression analysis showed increasing duration of oxygen therapy to be a risk factor for poorer performance on tests of visuomotor skill in VLBW survivors at 16 years of age.[69]

Quality of Life

Reports of quality of life in BPD survivors compared with preterm survivors without BPD are mixed. In a study by Bozzetto et al.[70] of self-reported health-related quality of life, determined using the Short Form 36, BPD survivors did not differ compared with healthy term-born children, despite poorer lung function (lower FEV_1, FVC, FEV_1/FVC, $FEF_{25\%-75\%}$ values). This study selected adolescents followed up in the Pneumology and Allergy Unit of the Department of Women's and Children's Health, Padova, Italy, and excluded BPD survivors with neurologic complications of prematurity, a group at increased risk of poorer quality of life. On the other hand, a cohort of BPD survivors, including some with neurologic sequelae of prematurity, reported lower quality of life scores at using the EuroQol EQ-5D instrument than term-born controls in early adulthood.[13]

SUMMARY

Pulmonary and neurologic sequelae of preterm delivery in the era of modern neonatal intensive care and the subsequent neonatal diagnosis of BPD have been described to early adulthood, but trajectories into later adult life are unclear. As increasing numbers of infants survive extreme prematurity, and the nature of neonatal lung disease continues to evolve, it is imperative we continue to document lung function and respiratory health, as well as neurocognitive functioning, beyond the nursery. We need to know the effectiveness, or otherwise, of changes in clinical practice. The vulnerable group of survivors who had BPD should be afforded additional surveillance and early intervention in the event of late-onset respiratory and neurologic illnesses. Clearly the consequences of prematurity are not confined to the nursery, preschool, or even adolescent years but must rather be considered a lifelong risk factor for respiratory and neurologic sequelae.

REFERENCES

1. Halvorsen T, Skadberg BT, Eide GE, et al. Pulmonary outcome in adolescents of extreme preterm birth: a regional cohort study. *Acta Paediatr, Int J Paediatr*. 2004;93:1294–1300.
2. Northway WH, Moss RB, Carlisle KB, et al. Late pulmonary sequelae of bronchopulmonary dysplasia. *N Engl J Med*. 1990;323:1793–1799.
3. Wong PM, Lees AN, Louw J, et al. Emphysema in young adult survivors of moderate-to-severe bronchopulmonary dysplasia. *Eur Respir J*. 2008;32:321–328.
4. Field DJ, Dorling JS, Manktelow BN, et al. Survival of extremely premature babies in a geographically defined population: prospective cohort study of 1994-9 compared with 2000-5. *BMJ*. 2008;336:1221.
5. Saigal S, Doyle LW. An overview of mortality and sequelae of preterm birth from infancy to adulthood. *Lancet*. 2008;371:261–269.
6. Costeloe KL, Hennessy EM, Haider S, et al. Short term outcomes after extreme preterm birth in England: comparison of two birth cohorts in 1995 and 2006 (the EPICure studies). *BMJ*. 2012;345:e7976.
7. Lorch SA. A decade of improvement in neonatal intensive care: how do we continue the momentum? *JAMA Pediatr*. 2017;171:e164395.
8. Stoll BJ, Hansen NI, Bell EF, et al. Trends in care practices, morbidity, and mortality of extremely preterm neonates, 1993–2012. *JAMA*. 2015;314:1039–1051.
9. Doyle LW, Carse E, Adams AM, et al. Ventilation in extremely preterm infants and respiratory function at 8 years. *N Engl J Med*. 2017;377:329–337.
10. Jobe A, Bancalari E. Bronchopulmonary dysplasia. *Am J Respir Crit Care Med*. 2001;163:1723–1729.
11. Walsh MC, Wilson-Costello D, Zadell A, et al. Safety, reliability, and validity of a physiologic definition of bronchopulmonary dysplasia. *J Perinatol*. 2003;23:451–456.
12. Cunningham CK, McMillan JA, Gross SJ. Rehospitalization for respiratory illness in infants of less than 32 weeks' gestation. *Pediatrics*. 1991;88:527–532.

13. Caskey S, Gough A, Rowan S, et al. Structural and functional lung impairment in adult survivors of bronchopulmonary dysplasia. *Ann Am Thorac Soc.* 2016;13: 1262–1270.
14. Northway Jr WH, Rosan RC, Porter DY. Pulmonary disease following respirator therapy of hyaline-membrane disease. Bronchopulmonary dysplasia. *N Engl J Med.* 1967;276: 357–368.
15. Coalson JJ. Pathology of new bronchopulmonary dysplasia. *Semin Neonatol.* 2003;8:73–81.
16. Voynow JA. "New" bronchopulmonary dysplasia and chronic lung disease. *Paediatr Respir Rev.* 2017;24:17–18.
17. Patel RM, Kandefer S, Walsh MC, et al. Causes and timing of death in extremely premature infants from 2000 through 2011. *N Engl J Med.* 2015;372:331–340.
18. Doyle LW, Ford G, Davis N. Health and hospitalisations after discharge in extremely low birth weight infants. *Semin Neonatol.* 2003;8:137–145.
19. Kuint J, Lerner-Geva L, Chodick G, et al. Rehospitalization through childhood and adolescence: association with neonatal morbidities in infants of very low birth weight. *J Pediatr.* 2017;188:135–141 e132.
20. Mulder EEM, Rijken M, de Smet L, et al. Respiratory morbidity was an important consequence of prematurity in the first two years after discharge in three cohorts from 1996 to 2009. *Acta Paediatr.* 2018;107:68–72.
21. McCormick MC, Workman-Daniels K, Brooks-Gunn J, et al. Hospitalization of very low birth weight children at school age. *J Pediatr.* 1993;122:360–365.
22. Boyle EM, Poulsen G, Field DJ, et al. Effects of gestational age at birth on health outcomes at 3 and 5 years of age: population based cohort study. *BMJ.* 2012;344:e896.
23. Hennessy EM, Bracewell MA, Wood N, et al. Respiratory health in pre-school and school age children following extremely preterm birth. *Arch Dis Child.* 2008;93:1037.
24. Doyle LW, Cheung MMH, Ford GW, et al. Birth weight <1501 g and respiratory health at age 14. *Arch Dis Child.* 2001;84:40–44.
25. Anand D, Stevenson CJ, West CR, et al. Lung function and respiratory health in adolescents of very low birth weight. *Arch Dis Child.* 2003;88:135–138.
26. McLeod A, Ross P, Mitchell S, et al. Respiratory health in a total very low birthweight cohort and their classroom controls. *Arch Dis Child.* 1996;74:188–194.
27. Evans M, Palta M, Sadek M, et al. Associations between family history of asthma, bronchopulmonary dysplasia, and childhood asthma in very low birth weight children. *Am J Epidemiol.* 1998;148:460–466.
28. Skromme K, Leversen KT, Eide GE, et al. Respiratory illness contributed significantly to morbidity in children born extremely premature or with extremely low birthweights in 1999-2000. *Acta Paediatr.* 2015;104: 1189–1198.
29. Fawke J, Lum S, Kirkby J, et al. Lung function and respiratory symptoms at 11 years in children born extremely preterm: the EPICure study. *Am J Respir Crit Care Med.* 2010; 182:237–245.
30. Gough A, Linden M, Spence D, et al. Impaired lung function and health status in adult survivors of bronchopulmonary dysplasia. *Eur Respir J.* 2014;43:808–816.
31. Gibson AM, Reddington C, McBride L, et al. Lung function in adult survivors of very low birth weight, with and without bronchopulmonary dysplasia. *Pediatr Pulmonol.* 2015;50:987–994.
32. Stocks J, Hislop A, Sonnappa S. Early lung development: lifelong effect on respiratory health and disease. *Lancet Respir Med.* 2013;1:728–742.
33. Chan KN, Noble-Jamieson CM, Elliman A, et al. Lung function in children of low birth weight. *Arch Dis Child.* 1989;64:1284.
34. Kitchen WH, Olinsky A, Doyle LW, et al. Respiratory health and lung function in 8-year-old children of very low birth weight: a cohort study. *Pediatrics.* 1992;89: 1151–1158.
35. Kennedy JD, Edward LJ, Bates DJ, et al. Effects of birthweight and oxygen supplementation on lung function in late childhood in children of very low birth weight. *Pediatr Pulmonol.* 2000;30:32–40.
36. Siltanen M, Savilahti E, Pohjavuori M, et al. Respiratory symptoms and lung function in relation to Atopy in children born preterm. *Pediatr Pulmonol.* 2004;37:43–49.
37. Doyle LW. Respiratory function at age 8-9 years in extremely low birthweight/very preterm children born in Victoria in 1991–1992. *Pediatr Pulmonol.* 2006;41: 570–576.
38. Fortuna M, Carraro S, Temporin E, et al. Mid-childhood lung function in a cohort of children with "new bronchopulmonary dysplasia. *Pediatr Pulmonol.* 2016;51: 1057–1064.
39. MacLean JE, DeHaan K, Fuhr D, et al. Altered breathing mechanics and ventilatory response during exercise in children born extremely preterm. *Thorax.* 2016;71:1012–1019.
40. Simpson SJ, Logie KM, O'Dea CA, et al. Altered lung structure and function in mid-childhood survivors of very preterm birth. *Thorax.* 2017;72:702–711.
41. Simpson SJ, Turkovic L, Wilson AC, et al. Lung function trajectories throughout childhood in survivors of very preterm birth: a longitudinal cohort study. *Lancet Child Adolesc Health.* 2018;2:350–359.
42. Doyle LW, Faber B, Callanan C, et al. Bronchopulmonary dysplasia in very low birth weight subjects and lung function in late adolescence. *Pediatrics.* 2006;118:108–113.
43. Vrijlandt EJLE, Gerritsen J, Boezen HM, et al. Lung function and exercise capacity in young adults born prematurely. *Am J Respir Crit Care Med.* 2006;173:890–896.
44. Vollsaeter M, Clemm HH, Satrell E, et al. Adult respiratory outcomes of extreme preterm birth. A regional cohort study. *Ann Am Thorac Soc.* 2015;12:313–322.
45. Doyle LW, Adams AM, Robertson C, et al. Increasing airway obstruction from 8 to 18 years in extremely preterm/low-birthweight survivors born in the surfactant era. *Thorax.* 2017;72:712–719.
46. Doyle LW, Andersson S, Bush A, et al. Expiratory airflow in late adolescence/early adulthood in survivors born very preterm or very low birthweight compared with controls

– an individual participant data meta-analysis. *Lancet Respir Med*. 2019;7:677–686.
47. Smith LJ, Van Asperen PP, McKay KO, et al. Reduced exercise capacity in children born very preterm. *Pediatrics*. 2008;122:e287–e293.
48. Bruce RA. Exercise testing of patients with coronary heart disease. Principles and normal standards for evaluation. *Ann Clin Res*. 1971;3:323–332.
49. Schmidt B, Asztalos EV, Roberts RS, et al. Impact of bronchopulmonary dysplasia, brain injury, and severe retinopathy on the outcome of extremely low-birth-weight infants at 18 months: results from the trial of indomethacin prophylaxis in preterms. *JAMA*. 2003;289:1124–1129.
50. Schlapbach LJ, Adams M, Proietti E, et al. Outcome at two years of age in a Swiss national cohort of extremely preterm infants born between 2000 and 2008. *BMC Pediatr*. 2012;12:198.
51. Majnemer A, Riley P, Shevell M, et al. Severe bronchopulmonary dysplasia increases risk for later neurological and motor sequelae in preterm survivors. *Dev Med Child Neurol*. 2000;42:53–60.
52. Hintz SR, Kendrick DE, Vohr BR, et al. Changes in neurodevelopmental outcomes at 18 to 22 months' corrected age among infants of less than 25 weeks' gestational age born in 1993–1999. *Pediatrics*. 2005;115:1645–1651.
53. Van Marter LJ, Kuban KC, Allred E, et al. Does bronchopulmonary dysplasia contribute to the occurrence of cerebral palsy among infants born before 28 weeks of gestation? *Arch Dis Child Fetal Neonatal Ed*. 2011;96:F20–F29.
54. Natarajan G, Pappas A, Shankaran S, et al. Outcomes of extremely low birth weight infants with bronchopulmonary dysplasia: impact of the physiologic definition. *Early Hum Dev*. 2012;88:509–515.
55. Doyle LW, Roberts G, Anderson PJ, et al. Changing long-term outcomes for infants 500–999 g birth weight in Victoria, 1979–2005. *Arch Dis Child Fetal Neonatal Ed*. 2011; 96. F443-447.
56. Kobaly K, Schluchter M, Minich N, et al. Outcomes of extremely low birth weight (<1 kg) and extremely low gestational age (<28 weeks) infants with bronchopulmonary dysplasia: effects of practice changes in 2000 to 2003. *Pediatrics*. 2008;121:73–81.
57. Davis NM, Ford GW, Anderson PJ, et al. Developmental coordination disorder at 8 years of age in a regional cohort of extremely-low-birthweight or very preterm infants. *Dev Med Child Neurol*. 2007;49:325–330.
58. Doyle LW, Cheong JL, Burnett A, et al. Biological and social influences on outcomes of extreme-preterm/low-birth weight adolescents. *Pediatrics*. 2015;136: e1513–1520.
59. Saigal S, den Ouden L, Wolke D, et al. School-age outcomes in children who were extremely low birth weight from four international population-based cohorts. *Pediatrics*. 2003;112:943–950.
60. Short EJ, Kirchner HL, Asaad GR, et al. Developmental sequelae in preterm infants having a diagnosis of bronchopulmonary dysplasia: analysis using a severity-based classification system. *Arch Pediatr Adolesc Med*. 2007;161: 1082–1087.
61. Short EJ, Klein NK, Lewis BA, et al. Cognitive and academic consequences of bronchopulmonary dysplasia and very low birth weight: 8-year-old outcomes. *Pediatrics*. 2003; 112:e359.
62. Anderson P, Doyle LW, The Victorian Infant Collaborative Study Group. Neurobehavioral outcomes of school-age children born extremely low birth weight or very preterm in the 1990s. *JAMA*. 2003;289:3264–3272.
63. Robertson CM, Etches PC, Goldson E, et al. Eight-year school performance, neurodevelopmental, and growth outcome of neonates with bronchopulmonary dysplasia: a comparative study. *Pediatrics*. 1992;89:365–372.
64. Singer L, Yamashita T, Lilien L, et al. A longitudinal study of developmental outcome of infants with bronchopulmonary dysplasia and very low birth weight. *Pediatrics*. 1997;100:987–993.
65. Jobe AH, Bancalari E. Bronchopulmonary dysplasia. *Am J Respir Crit Care Med*. 2001;163:1723–1729.
66. Singer LT, Siegel AC, Lewis B, et al. Preschool language outcomes of children with history of bronchopulmonary dysplasia and very low birth weight. *J Dev Behav Pediatr*. 2001;22:19–26.
67. Lewis BA, Singer LT, Fulton S, et al. Speech and language outcomes of children with bronchopulmonary dysplasia. *J Commun Disord*. 2002;35:393–406.
68. Gray PH, O'Callaghan MJ, Rogers YM. Psychoeducational outcome at school age of preterm infants with bronchopulmonary dysplasia. *J Paediatr Child Health*. 2004;40: 114–120.
69. Taylor HG, Minich N, Bangert B, et al. Long-term neuropsychological outcomes of very low birth weight: associations with early risks for periventricular brain insults. *J Int Neuropsychol Soc*. 2004;10:987–1004.
70. Bozzetto S, Carraro S, Tomasi L, et al. Health-related quality of life in adolescent survivors of bronchopulmonary dysplasia. *Respirology*. 2016;21:1113–1117.

CHAPTER 21

Emerging Therapies in BPD: Stem Cells and Extracellular Vesicles

LANNAE STRUEBY, MSC, MD, FRCPC • BERNARD THÉBAUD, MD, PHD, FRCPC

Prematurity and its associated mortality and morbidity are among the most important health consequences facing infants and children worldwide. An estimated 14.8 million children are born preterm yearly.[1] The impact on individual quality of life, the family unit,[2] health spending, and the overall economy is undeniable.[3–5] Thankfully, improvements in neonatal and perinatal medicine have permitted significant strides in the survival of preterm infants. Continued progress to minimize common morbidities of prematurity has proven more challenging in recent years.[6] Bronchopulmonary dysplasia (BPD), the chronic lung disease of prematurity, remains one of the most frequent complications of extreme preterm birth.[7] Even before their earliest breaths extreme preterm infants are exposed to essential, yet potentially noxious, intra- and extrauterine stimuli that initiate processes of inflammation and injury in multiple organs, including the lung. The capacity of susceptible preterm infants to tamponade these processes and repair sustained injury may easily be overwhelmed, contributing to the development of multiple morbidities, including BPD.[8]

The scarcity of effective, safe therapies in combination with the recognized long-term implications of BPD continues to inspire researchers to investigate novel approaches to treat, and importantly prevent, the development of these lung sequelae in vulnerable neonates.[9] The multifactorial pathogenesis of BPD and potential for subtypes of this clinically defined disease make the identification of a single effective traditional therapy unlikely. Stem cells and stem cell–derived therapies are emerging as promising avenues of research to potentially identify suitable therapies for treating or preventing BPD in the neonatal population.[10]

STEM CELL AND SECRETOME ESSENTIALS

Stem cells possess exceptional properties in comparison to somatic cells. They exist in an undifferentiated state owning the ability to differentiate into numerous cell types, while maintaining the capacity for self-renewal. This is possible through two types of cell division: symmetric and asymmetric. Symmetric division generates two undifferentiated identical daughter cells while asymmetric division produces one undifferentiated cell together with a second cell programmed to differentiate.[11]

Traditionally, stem cells are either embryonic or adult in origin. Embryonic stem cells are solely acquired from the blastocyst or fertilized egg while stem cells from all other sources are adult in nature. Adult stem cells can be derived from a variety of sources (umbilical cord, bone marrow, brain, skin)[11] and are essential for repair and regeneration of injured tissues. Recent advances have created a new category of induced pluripotent stem cells (iPSCs).[12] iPSCs are fully differentiated somatic cells reprogrammed to become pluripotent stem cells with the ability to generate cells of all three germ layers.[12] Stem cells are classified by potency or differential potential, of which there are four subgroups: unipotent, multipotent, pluripotent, and totipotent (Table 21.1). Although unipotent stem cells only generate one defined cell type they are distinct from nonstem cells as they retain the ability to self-renew.[11,13]

The potential therapeutic applications of stem cell arise not only from their intrinsic regenerative capacity but also from their potential paracrine properties. Stem cells, like many cells, secrete bioactive molecules that comprise their individual secretome. The secretome refers to the collection of factors secreted by a cell into the extracellular space. Elements of the secretome include, but are not limited to, proteins, lipids, nucleic acids, and extracellular vesicles.[15] Secreted molecules are essential to intercellular communication locally via the interstitial space and distally by entering body fluids such as plasma and cerebrospinal fluid.[16] The cellular secretome varies in response to alterations in

Updates on Neonatal Chronic Lung Disease. https://doi.org/10.1016/B978-0-323-68353-1.00021-X

the cell niche or environment. The secretome of in vitro cultured cells is represented in the surrounding media and commonly referred to as conditioned media.[15]

Recently, extracellular vesicles have garnered significant research interest as potential biomedical applications are explored and their role as essential components of the secretome is confirmed. The exponential growth of this field prompted the formation of the International Society for Extracellular Vesicles (ISEV) in 2011. The collective term extracellular vesicles is endorsed by the ISEV and encompasses an assortment of vesicles, including exosomes, microparticles, ectosomes, and nanovesicles (Table 21.2).[20] Extracellular vesicles are phospholipid enclosed particles 30 nm to 1 μm in size containing lipids, proteins, RNA, and DNA.[20,21] These vesicles exist in all body fluids and are essential communicators capable of delivering their heterogeneous cargo to recipient cells, thereby affecting function and phenotype. Extracellular vesicles have potential roles in diagnosis, monitoring, and treatment of disease states.[20] The subclass of vesicles termed exosomes are smaller in diameter (30–150 nm) and are secreted thru fusion of multivesicular bodies with the plasma membrane, as opposed to the direct budding mechanism.[21] Evidence indicates that numerous beneficial properties attributed to stem cells, including mesenchymal stromal cells (MSCs), are conferred by secreted exosomes.[15]

TABLE 21.1
Stem Cells Classification by Differential Potential.[11,13,14]

Cell Potency	Differentiation Potential
Totipotent	Capacity to generate mesoderm, endoderm, ectoderm, germ cells, and extraembryonic tissues. For example, zygote
Pluripotent	Capacity to generate mesoderm, endoderm, ectoderm, and germ cells. For example, embryonic stem cells from inner blastocyst
Multipotent	Capacity to generate multiple related cell types. For example, mesenchymal stem cells
Unipotent	Capacity to generate only one defined cell type. For example, type II alveolar epithelial cells in the lung

MESENCHYMAL STROMAL CELLS

MSCs are highly proliferative multipotent adult stem cells.[22] They were originally identified by Friedenstein et al. as discrete colony-forming fibroblasts, isolated from the bone marrow, and capable of demonstrating in vitro osteogenesis.[23] These fibroblast-like cells were demonstrated to support hematopoiesis; current literature identifies MSCs as potent repair cells with anti-inflammatory, immunomodulatory, and angiogenic properties. Additionally, MSCs are now isolated from a variety of sources, including adipose, bone marrow, lung, placenta, and the umbilical cord.[15]

MSCs isolated from diverse sources by individual techniques and subsequently expanded in vitro by various culture conditions are not uniform in nature. Due to the heterogeneity of this cell population, the International Society for Cellular Therapy (ISCT) recommends the term MSC as opposed to mesenchymal stem cell. Authentic mesenchymal stem cells occur; however, for clarity and accuracy the ISCT reserves the designation "stem" for cells uniformly demonstrating stem cell properties (undifferentiated state, self-renewal, differentiation potential).[24] The variable nature of MSC isolation also led the ISCT to identify minimal criteria for defining a human multipotent MSC (Table 21.3).[22] These criteria require expansion to permit the identification of consistent pharmaceutical grade MSCs for clinical trial use.[25] In 2016 the ISCT proposed potency release

TABLE 21.2
Principal Categories of Extracellular Vesicles.[17–19]

Extracellular Vesicle	Size	Mechanism of Release	Characteristic Markers
Apoptotic bodies	50–5000 nm	Generated by disintegrating cells during apoptosis	DNA, histones
Microparticles or ectosomes	50 or 100–1000 nm	Direct budding of plasma membrane	Integrins, selectins
Exosomes	30–150 nm	Fusion of multivesicular body with plasma membrane	Tetraspanins, TSG101

criteria based on the consensus that, despite variances in MSC populations, the fundamental mechanisms of action underlying MSC anti-inflammatory and/or repair functions are shared. Although these criteria represent significant progress, validated and robust MSC potency assays that predict therapeutic efficacy and are acceptable to regulatory agencies remain a challenge,[26] as does the definition of MSCs.[27]

MSCs are the primary cell therapy currently under investigation as a therapeutic agent for BPD.[10] Multiple factors contribute to this phenomenon (Table 21.4). MSCs have already demonstrated safety as a therapeutic agent, primarily in adults, through investigational and clinical use spanning more than 2 decades.[28,32] MSC therapy is associated with limited adverse events with no confirmed human cases of tumorigenicity arising from administered cells.[33] In 2012 graft-versus-host disease became the first pathology to secure conditional approval (Canada and New Zealand) for pharmaceutical use of MSCs in children,[34] almost 10 years after it was successfully used for this indication in a 9-year-old boy.[35] Allogeneic cell therapy is typically accompanied by the potential risk of immune rejection in recipients. MSC transplantation is thought to involve a diminished immune rejection risk. The extent and origin of the immune-evasive MSC nature requires further clarity. Hypotheses include reduced expression of class I and/or II major histocompatibility complex (MHC) molecules or the limited engraftment/persistence of administered cells minimizes immune recognition.[34,36]

TABLE 21.3
Minimal Criteria to Define a Human Multipotent MSC.[22]

Criteria	MSC Attribute
In vitro differentiation	Osteoblasts, adipocytes, chondroblasts
Culture characteristic	Plastic-adherent
Positive markers	CD105, CD73, CD90
Negative markers	CD45, CD34, CD14 or CD11b, CD79α or CD19, HLA-DR

TABLE 21.4
Therapeutic Advantages of MSCs and Umbilical Cord–Derived MSCs.[10,28–31].

Advantages of MSCs
Established safety profile (adults)
Immune-evasive potential
Relative ease of isolation/culture
Anti-inflammatory profile
Immunomodulatory capacity
Proangiogenic properties
Advantages of Umbilical cordderived MSCs
Ethically acceptable source
Safe and painless retrieval
Greater proliferative potential
Potentially enhanced healing properties

Another distinct advantage of MSCs is that they can be painlessly derived from ethically acceptable sources such as the umbilical cord. Umbilical cord MSCs are of interest in treating neonatal diseases not only secondary to their convenient source but also due to the putative enhanced proliferation and healing properties associated with cells isolated from this source.[29–31,37] Despite the abovementioned safety and advantages, preterm neonates represent a particularly vulnerable population for which long-term safety needs to be demonstrated prior to therapeutic use outside the context of a clinical trial.

PRECLINICAL INVESTIGATION OF MSC POTENTIAL TO PREVENT BPD

The fetal lung possesses abundant MSCs[38] which are recognized as critical components of normal lung growth and maturation. Lung MSCs are precursors to mature mesenchymal cells (myofibroblasts, lipofibroblasts, and fibroblast) and engage as directors of complex cellular interactions integral to early lung development.[39] Preterm birth alters the natural fetal environment exposing the immature lung to deleterious stimuli, including higher oxygen concentrations (21% and greater), a critical risk factor in the development of BPD. These adverse exposures are thought to create perturbations in lung MSCs which subsequently contributes to the development of BPD.[38] This hypothesis is supported by early rodent studies demonstrating that hyperoxia-induced lung injury is associated with a significant reduction in both circulating and resident lung MSCs.[40] More recent research indicates that human fetal lung MSCs (16–18 weeks gestational age) exhibit impaired function on exposure in vitro to 21% or 60% oxygen. Exposure to extrauterine oxygen concentrations altered MSC surface marker profile, created excessive proliferation, reduced colony forming ability, and adversely modified the secretome profile. Conversely, human umbilical cord–derived MSCs retain a lung protective secretome profile despite exposure to hyperoxia in vitro.[38] Depletion and/or dysfunction of MSCs as a contributor to the development of BPD, and the potential to rescue this phenotype with "healthy" MSCs, have spurred extensive preclinical research.

The protective effects of exogenous MSC administration on the immature lung are most frequently examined in hyperoxia rodent models of BPD.[40] Rodents models are employed to mimic BPD as mice and rats possess structurally immature lungs at the time of birth, similar to extreme preterm infants.[41,42] Intratracheally or intravenously administered bone marrow–derived MSCs were shown to improve survival and prevent the inflammation, alveolar simplification, vascular rarefaction, and pulmonary hypertension demonstrated in untreated hyperoxia exposed mouse and rat pups.[40,43] Subsequently, umbilical cord–derived MSCs were reported to repair established lung injury in addition to prevent injury in the hyperoxia rodent model; beneficial effects persisted up to 6 months after treatment.[44] The quantity of preclinical evidence available permitted the first meta-analysis assess the effectiveness of MSCs as a therapy in animal models of BPD. All included studies utilized the hyperoxia rodent model of BPD totaling 483 animals. MSC administration significantly improved the primary outcome of alveolarization (standardized mean difference (SMD) −1.330, 95% confidence interval (CI) −1.724 to −0.94, I^2 69%) and secondary outcomes of pulmonary hypertension, lung inflammation, fibrosis and angiogenesis.[45]

Paracrine mechanisms are thought to be pivotal to the beneficial effects conveyed by MSC administration in animal models of BPD. Although significant benefits are documented, a very limited number of MSCs engraft in the recipient lung[40] and engrafted MSC survival is of limited duration.[46] Therefore, it is possible that the cell itself is not required for the therapeutic benefits.[47,48] This hypothesis is supported by a multitude of individual articles and the subsequent meta-analysis demonstrating cell-free MSC-conditioned media significantly improves alveolarization (SMD -2.04, 95% CI -2.74 to −1.33, I^2 69%), angiogenesis, and pulmonary artery remodeling.[45] The potential of cell-free therapies is particularly intriguing given the possibility they may be accompanied by fewer adverse effects[15,49] and are thought to represent a static product with reduced potential for adverse alterations following administration. Live cell therapies are complicated by cell death, before or after administration to a patient, creating dosing variabilities.[48] Cells are physically larger (MSCs typically 18 μm or greater)[50,51] limiting passage through small capillaries and increasing emboli risk.[50] Microvesicles, such as exosomes, circulate easily through capillaries[51] (Table 21.5). These findings, and others, lead investigators to delve further into examining the role of the MSC secretome in protecting the immature lung.

MSCS' POTENTIAL MECHANISMS OF ACTION

Cellular Interactions

MSCs' therapeutic benefits are not exclusively conveyed by paracrine factors. Preserving the cell, in stem cell therapy, creates direct interaction between exogenous MSCs and injured lung, permitting cellular sensing and response to the extracellular environment. This interaction may be critical to optimizing MSC therapy as it enables the production and delivery of intelligent and personalized mediators to the injured lung.39 Direct cell-to-cell interaction may also be essential for selected therapeutic effects as MSCs are known to engage in intercellular organelle transfer. MSCs delivered intratracheally, in an LPS mouse model of lung injury, generate microtubules to transfer mitochondria to the alveolar epithelium. Transferred mitochondria and the ensuing increased alveolar adenosine triphosphate levels are proposed as a mechanism by which lung injury is prevented in this model.[53]

TABLE 21.5
Theoretical Advantages/Disadvantages of Cell-Free MSC-Derived Therapies (Conditioned Media and Exosomes)[15,19,48,51,52].

Advantages of Cell Free Therapies
Reduced risk of the following:
- Immune reaction
- Tumorigenicity
- Emboli formation
- Transmission of Infections
More conventional and stable dosing regime
Reduced risk of diminishing potency during storage
Stable composition after collection
Increased potential for readily available products
Potentially reduced cost
Disadvantages of Cell-Free Therapies
Static therapy (unable to respond to recipient niche)
Possible challenges producing required quantities
Ensuring purity of product
No historically comparable therapy

Communicators of Paracrine Effects

Paracrine-mediated actions appear to be the predominant mechanism by which MSC convey therapeutic benefits in BPD models.[39] MSC-derived extracellular vesicles are proposed as critical paracrine mediators[54,55] with various bioactive molecules or mechanisms postulated.[56–58] Exosomes represent the smallest spectrum of extracellular vesicles known to contain protein, lipids, mRNA, and miRNA.[51,56] Physiologic effects are accomplished by delivery of exosome contents to recipient cells (membrane fusion, endocytosis, or phagocytosis) or via ligand receptor signaling pathways. In a hyperoxia rat model of BPD, intratracheally administered human umbilical cord–derived MSC extracellular vesicles reduced hyperoxia-induced damage and demonstrated improved alveolarization and lung vascularization parameters compared to traditional MSC therapy, supporting the hypothesis that extracellular vesicles, including exosomes, mediate the therapeutic efficacy of MSCs.[54]

Exosome contents are reflective of their cell of origin which is responsive to the extracellular microenvironment.[59] This permits preconditioning of MSCs to potentially tailor or enhance exosome contents and therapeutic capability.[60] This responsiveness also indicates that diverse mediators, and diverse biologic actions, may predominate depending on cell source, isolation technique, and culture conditions.[51,60] As crucial paracrine communicators MSC exosomes have the potential to exert favorable therapeutic effects via modulation of angiogenesis, inflammation, oxidative stress, and/or the immune response. Multiple investigators have sought to identify pivotal factors associated with these pathways to inform on MSC mechanism of action and potential therapeutic options.

Vascular endothelial growth factor (VEGF) is a potent angiogenic protein essential to pulmonary vascular development and consequently alveolarization.[61] VEGF is identified as a component of MSC-conditioned media[62] and specifically exosomes.[56] Improved survival and enhanced lung vascular development and alveolarization occur with VEGF gene therapy in hyperoxia rodent models of BPD.[63] Exosomes' proangiogenic properties appear, in part, mediated by VEGF protein. Daily intraperitoneal injection of bone marrow–derived MSC exosomes protect alveolarization and angiogenesis in a rat hyperoxia model of BPD, and anti-VEGF antibodies were able to disrupt the exosome-mediated angiogenic properties in vitro.[56] Tumor necrosis factor alpha-stimulated gene-6 (TSG-6) protein is an anti-inflammatory molecule similarly identified in MSC secretome[56,64] and exosomes. Umbilical cord–derived MSC exosomes reduced lung injury and pulmonary hypertension in the murine hyperoxia BPD model, and this study identified TSG-6 protein as a required exosomal factor for prevention of lung injury.[57] Although discrete molecules demonstrate favorable effects and integral roles in simplified experimental models, as individual therapies they typically are unable to capture the pleiotropic coordinated benefits attributed to MSC therapies.[65]

Macrophages are an essential cellular component of the lung immune response.[58] Diverse macrophage phenotypes exist on a spectrum, participating as both initiators and resolvers of inflammation. Traditionally, macrophages were thought to exist in either an M1 proinflammatory state or the M2 anti-inflammatory state; macrophage plasticity and function are now recognized as more complex.[66] Modulation of macrophage phenotype may represent an underlying mechanism by which MSCs and their products ameliorate lung injury. A single dose of either umbilical cord–derived or bone marrow–derived MSC exosomes equally prevented hyperoxia-induced alveolar simplification and attenuated lung inflammation, fibrosis, and vascular remodeling. Long-term functional outcomes, including hyperoxia-induced pulmonary hypertension and pulmonary function testing, also demonstrated significant improvement over a month after exosome injection. Mechanistic experiments suggest that MSC exosomes suppressed inflammation and lung injury via modulation of the macrophage phenotype from the M1 toward the M2 "healer" state.[58] Interestingly the anti-inflammatory actions of TSG-6 protein have also, in part, been attributed to inducing a shift in macrophages from the M1 to the M2 phenotype.[67]

CLINICAL EVIDENCE INVESTIGATING MSCS EFFECT ON BPD

The vast majority of research addressing MSCs therapeutic abilities pertaining to preterm neonates and BPD is in the preclinical arena.[45] However, the first cautious steps in translating MSC therapy from the lab to the NICU have occurred. In 2014, the first phase I dose escalation trial investigating allogenic cord blood–derived MSC therapy in neonates was published. Nine preterm infants born between 23 and 29 weeks gestation and requiring mechanical ventilation were enrolled at 5–14 days of age. A single intratracheal MSC transplantation occurred at a dose of 10^7 or 2×10^7 cells. The study concluded that the transplantation procedure was feasible and well tolerated with no serious adverse events reported. Effectiveness of MSCs as a therapy for BPD was unable to be commented on.[68] Follow-up at 2 years of age indicates no adverse growth, respiratory, or neurodevelopmental outcomes.[69] The same investigators have completed, but not yet published, a phase II double blind, multicenter, controlled, randomized trial using the low-dose MSC transplantation (NCT01828957). Five-year follow-up of the phase I participants is also completed (NCT02023788) and similar long-term follow-up is planned for the phase II participants (NCT01897987). The success of preclinical studies and apparent safety of the first trial in neonates has prompted additional trials. An American phase I/II clinical trial of similar design was recently completed and results are awaited (NCT02381366). A third Spanish phase I trial intends to enroll 14 day old mechanically ventilated infants born at less than 28 weeks gestation for treatment with three doses of intravenous umbilical cord–derived MSCs (NCT02443961).[70]

Outside the context of clinical trials, the sole other report of MSC therapy for neonatal BPD is a small case series outlining off-label intravenous use of allogenic bone marrow–derived MSCs. Two infants born in the 24th week of gestation with severe ventilatory-dependent BPD and severe pulmonary hypertension were treated with multiple doses of intravenous MSCs starting at 5 months and 85 days of life. No acute adverse reactions occurred during MSC administration. MSC therapy was not associated with evident respiratory improvement and both infants eventually succumbed to their respiratory illness. A reduction in mRNA levels of selected inflammatory cytokines and an endogenous VEGF antagonist were documented in peripheral blood cells after MSC administration. Lung autopsy findings were consistent with preclinical studies demonstrating no evidence of donor MSC engraftment. The authors conclude that repeated intravenous MSC administration is feasible, with no observed toxicity, and recommend treatment at earlier stages of BPD.[71]

The therapeutic possibilities perceived to exist within MSC therapy inspire excitement. The results of pending phase I and II trials are anxiously awaited as the MSC/BPD story continues to unravel through preclinical investigations.[72,73] Additional insight into the safety and potential of cell therapies in neonates may arise from investigation of alternate cell types. The first open-label phase I safety trial investigating the intravenous administration of allogenic human amnion epithelial cells (hAECs) to preterm infants with established BPD identified transient cardiorespiratory compromise, consistent with pulmonary microembolic event, during cell infusion to the first infant. The cell administration protocol was adjusted (inclusion of inline filter and reduced cell concentration and rate of infusion) for the subsequent five infants and tolerated well with no adverse events. There was no significant change in respiratory support requirements after hAECs therapy and the authors conclude that allogeneic hAECs can be safely administered to infants.[74] Although no proposed trials investigating MSC exosomes or conditioned media for treatment of BPD are registered in the clinical trials database (clinicaltrials.gov), phase I and phase II trials utilizing exosomes for alternate diseases, such as graft-versus-host disease and non–small-cell lung cancer, are underway.[75,76]

TRANSLATIONAL CHALLENGES

One of the foundations of medicine is basic science, yet promising therapies with preclinical evidence are rarely realized as licenced agents in clinical practice. Fewer than 1 in 10 promising technologies enter routine clinical use within 20 years.[77] Although early phase clinical trial are ongoing, many challenges remain to successfully translate MSC-derived therapies to clinical practice for BPD prevention (Table 21.6). Understandably, the majority of MSC preclinical research is conducted in rodent models of BPD, potentially limiting applicability to humans.[45] Mice have structurally immature lungs, but unlike preterm infants they are adequately equipped for gas exchange and have mature respiratory drive.[58]

TABLE 21.6
Potential Obstacles to Translation of MSCs Therapeutic Promise[10,34,45]

Preclinical Model Factors
Oversimplified animal models
Predominantly single species
Nonrigorous design or reporting
Preclinical MSC Factors
Higher dosing regimens frequently utilized
Often xenogeneic
Variable potency/purity of product
Clinical Trial Factors
Selection of patients most likely to benefit
Dose, route, timing, and frequency of therapy
Potency/purity of therapy
Long-term safety in immunocompromised preterm infants
Logistical Factors
Economic implications
Regulatory concerns (safety, efficacy)

The discrepancy between human and rodent physiology should not be underestimated.[45] Additionally, the common hyperoxia model of BPD oversimplifies the truly multifactorial pathogenesis of BPD and may result in diminished realization of benefits in true BPD. More complex models exist, including a mouse model of BPD combining supplemental oxygen and mechanical ventilation.[78] Investigation of MSC therapies in large animal, particularly nonhuman primate models, would arguably provide more definitive evidence of effectiveness.[79] Preclinical research must be conducted rigorously if results are anticipated to translate to human trials, the ARRIVE guidelines aim to improve reporting and thereby quality of animal research.[80]

Appropriate design and execution of clinical trials is essential to recognizing the potential of MSC therapies for BPD. Every variable in a clinical trial has the potential to alter or obscure the true outcome. Particular attention must be paid to the MSC product; acquiring and testing a pharmaceutical grade MSC therapy isolated from the preferred source with meticulous culture and expansion techniques is crucial. Further preclinical and early clinical investigation is required to adequately inform decisions regarding dose, route, timing and frequency of MSC therapy.[81] Logistical and regulatory concerns such as economic implications, potency testing, and safety, all require addressing for hope of successful translation. Currently MSC-based therapy holds significant promise for treating BPD but clinical application of this emerging therapy should remain restricted to clinical trial use.

SUMMARY

A decade following publication of the lung protective effects of exogenous MSC administration in rodent models of BPD, much remains to be elucidated. MSCs show extreme therapeutic potential, both for cell and cell-free therapies. It is possible that the challenge of BPD multifactorial pathogenesis will be met by an equally multifactorial therapy: MSCs. Earlier therapies, such as dexamethasone, have taught clinicians and researchers to be wary of unintended outcomes in preterm neonates. MSC-derived therapies are under investigation for various conditions and importantly have also demonstrated benefit in sepsis[82] and brain injury animal models,[57,83] recognized potential adverse effects and known comorbidities of prematurity. In order to minimize inadvertent outcomes, identification and possible clinical translation of single bioactive molecules is of interest; however, this reductionist approach is not always advantageous. The true potential of stem cell–derived therapies likely lies in the integration of potencies (anti-inflammatory, anti-apoptotic, antifibrotic, proangiogenic).

As with any new therapy, excitement and forward progress must be tempered by caution, to ensure continued safety of our vulnerable preterm neonates while opening opportunities for innovative therapies. It remains to be seen if MSC-derived therapies will fulfill their perceived therapeutic potential and address a long-standing need for effective BPD therapy.

REFERENCES

1. Chawanpaiboon S, Vogel JP, Moller AB, et al. Global, regional, and national estimates of levels of preterm birth in 2014: a systematic review and modelling analysis. *Lancet Glob Health*. 2019;7(1):e37–e46.
2. Amorim M, Alves E, Kelly-Irving M, et al. Quality of life of parents of very preterm infants 4 months after birth: a mixed methods study. *Health Qual Life Outcomes*. 2018;16(1):178.
3. Frey HA, Klebanoff MA. The epidemiology, etiology, and costs of preterm birth. *Semin Fetal Neonatal Med*. 2016; 21(2):68–73.
4. Johnston KM, Gooch K, Korol E, et al. The economic burden of prematurity in Canada. *BMC Pediatr*. 2014;14:93.
5. Canadian Neonatal Network, Canadian Neonatal Follow-Up Network Investigators, Shafey A, et al. Outcomes and resource usage of infants born at ≤ 25 weeks gestation in Canada. *Paediatr Child Health*. 2019.
6. Twilhaar ES, Wade RM, de Kieviet JF, et al. Cognitive outcomes of children born extremely or very preterm since the 1990s and associated risk factors: a meta-analysis and meta-regression. *JAMA Pediatr*. 2018;172(4):361–367.
7. Stoll BJ, Hansen NI, Bell EF, et al. Trends in care practices, morbidity, and mortality of extremely preterm neonates, 1993–2012. *JAMA*. 2015;314(10):1039–1051.
8. Patra A, Huang H, Bauer JA, et al. Neurological consequences of systemic inflammation in the premature neonate. *Neural Regen Res*. 2017;12(6):890–896.
9. Strueby L, Thebaud B. Advances in bronchopulmonary dysplasia. *Expert Rev Respir Med*. 2014;8(3):327–338.
10. Thebaud B. Stem cell-based therapies in neonatology: a new hope. *Arch Dis Child Fetal Neonatal Ed*. 2018;103(6): F583–f588.
11. Wagers AJ, Weissman IL. Plasticity of adult stem cells. *Cell*. 2004;116(5):639–648.
12. Kang M, Thebaud B. Stem cell biology and regenerative medicine for neonatal lung diseases. *Pediatr Res*. 2018; 83(1–2):291–297.
13. Lakshmipathy U, Verfaillie C. Stem cell plasticity. *Blood Rev*. 2005;19(1):29–38.
14. Strueby L, Thebaud B. Mesenchymal stromal cell-based therapies for chronic lung disease of prematurity. *Am J Perinatol*. 2016;33(11):1043–1049.
15. Vizoso FJ, Eiro N, Cid S, et al. Mesenchymal stem cell secretome: toward cell-free therapeutic strategies in regenerative medicine. *Int J Mol Sci*. 2017;18(9).
16. Skalnikova H, Motlik J, Gadher SJ, et al. Mapping of the secretome of primary isolates of mammalian cells, stem cells and derived cell lines. *Proteomics*. 2011;11(4):691–708.

17. Szatanek R, Baj-Krzyworzeka M, Zimoch J, et al. The methods of choice for extracellular vesicles (evs) characterization. *Int J Mol Sci*. 2017;18(6).
18. Colombo M, Raposo G, Thery C. Biogenesis, secretion, and intercellular interactions of exosomes and other extracellular vesicles. *Annu Rev Cell Dev Biol*. 2014;30:255–289.
19. Muraca M, Piccoli M, Franzin C, et al. Diverging concepts and novel perspectives in regenerative medicine. *Int J Mol Sci*. 2017;18(5).
20. Nieuwland R, Falcon-Perez JM, Soekmadji C, et al. Essentials of extracellular vesicles: posters on basic and clinical aspects of extracellular vesicles. *J Extracell Vesicles*. 2018; 7(1):1548234.
21. Vestad B, Llorente A, Neurauter A, et al. Size and concentration analyses of extracellular vesicles by nanoparticle tracking analysis: a variation study. *J Extracell Vesicles*. 2017;6(1):1344087.
22. Dominici M, Le Blanc K, Mueller I, et al. Minimal criteria for defining multipotent mesenchymal stromal cells. The international society for cellular therapy position statement. *Cytotherapy*. 2006;8(4):315–317.
23. Friedenstein AJ, Chailakhjan RK, Lalykina KS. The development of fibroblast colonies in monolayer cultures of Guinea-pig bone marrow and spleen cells. *Cell Tissue Kinet*. 1970;3(4):393–403.
24. Horwitz EM, Le Blanc K, Dominici M, et al. Clarification of the nomenclature for msc: the international society for cellular therapy position statement. *Cytotherapy*. 2005; 7(5):393–395.
25. Krampera M, Galipeau J, Shi Y, et al. Immunological characterization of multipotent mesenchymal stromal cells–the international society for cellular therapy (isct) working proposal. *Cytotherapy*. 2013;15(9):1054–1061.
26. Galipeau J, Krampera M, Barrett J, et al. International society for cellular therapy perspective on immune functional assays for mesenchymal stromal cells as potency release criterion for advanced phase clinical trials. *Cytotherapy*. 2016;18(2):151–159.
27. Sipp D, Robey PG, Turner L. Clear up this stem-cell mess. *Nature*. 2018;561(7724):455–457.
28. Herrmann RP, Sturm MJ. Adult human mesenchymal stromal cells and the treatment of graft versus host disease. *Stem Cells Cloning*. 2014;7:45–52.
29. Jin HJ, Bae YK, Kim M, et al. Comparative analysis of human mesenchymal stem cells from bone marrow, adipose tissue, and umbilical cord blood as sources of cell therapy. *Int J Mol Sci*. 2013;14(9):17986–18001.
30. Hsieh JY, Wang HW, Chang SJ, et al. Mesenchymal stem cells from human umbilical cord express preferentially secreted factors related to neuroprotection, neurogenesis, and angiogenesis. *PLoS One*. 2013;8(8):e72604.
31. Yannarelli G, Dayan V, Pacienza N, et al. Human umbilical cord perivascular cells exhibit enhanced cardiomyocyte reprogramming and cardiac function after experimental acute myocardial infarction. *Cell Transplant*. 2013;22(9): 1651–1666.
32. Lazarus HM, Haynesworth SE, Gerson SL, et al. Ex vivo expansion and subsequent infusion of human bone marrow-derived stromal progenitor cells (mesenchymal progenitor cells): implications for therapeutic use. *Bone Marrow Transplant*. 1995;16(4):557–564.
33. Lalu MM, McIntyre L, Pugliese C, et al. Safety of cell therapy with mesenchymal stromal cells (safecell): a systematic review and meta-analysis of clinical trials. *PLoS One*. 2012;7(10):e47559.
34. Galipeau J, Sensebe L. Mesenchymal stromal cells: clinical challenges and therapeutic opportunities. *Cell Stem Cell*. 2018;22(6):824–833.
35. Le Blanc K, Rasmusson I, Sundberg B, et al. Treatment of severe acute graft-versus-host disease with third party haploidentical mesenchymal stem cells. *Lancet*. 2004; 363(9419):1439–1441.
36. Ankrum JA, Ong JF, Karp JM. Mesenchymal stem cells: immune evasive, not immune privileged. *Nat Biotechnol*. 2014;32(3):252–260.
37. Amable PR, Teixeira MV, Carias RB, et al. Protein synthesis and secretion in human mesenchymal cells derived from bone marrow, adipose tissue and wharton's jelly. *Stem Cell Res Ther*. 2014;5(2):53.
38. Mobius MA, Freund D, Vadivel A, et al. Oxygen disrupts human fetal lung mesenchymal cells: implications for bronchopulmonary dysplasia. *Am J Respir Cell Mol Biol*. 2019 May;60(5):592–600. https://doi.org/10.1165/rcmb.2018-0358OC.
39. Mobius MA, Rudiger M. Mesenchymal stromal cells in the development and therapy of bronchopulmonary dysplasia. *Mol Cell Pediatr*. 2016;3(1):18.
40. van Haaften T, Byrne R, Bonnet S, et al. Airway delivery of mesenchymal stem cells prevents arrested alveolar growth in neonatal lung injury in rats. *Am J Respir Crit Care Med*. 2009;180(11):1131–1142.
41. Amy RW, Bowes D, Burri PH, et al. Postnatal growth of the mouse lung. *J Anat*. 1977;124(Pt 1):131–151.
42. Hansmann G, Fernandez-Gonzalez A, Aslam M, et al. Mesenchymal stem cell-mediated reversal of bronchopulmonary dysplasia and associated pulmonary hypertension. *Pulm Circ*. 2012;2(2):170–181.
43. Aslam M, Baveja R, Liang OD, et al. Bone marrow stromal cells attenuate lung injury in a murine model of neonatal chronic lung disease. *Am J Respir Crit Care Med*. 2009; 180(11):1122–1130.
44. Pierro M, Ionescu L, Montemurro T, et al. Short-term, long-term and paracrine effect of human umbilical cord-derived stem cells in lung injury prevention and repair in experimental bronchopulmonary dysplasia. *Thorax*. 2013; 68(5):475–484.
45. Augustine S, Avey MT, Harrison B, et al. Mesenchymal stromal cell therapy in bronchopulmonary dysplasia: systematic review and meta-analysis of preclinical studies. *Stem Cells Transl Med*. 2017;6(12):2079–2093.
46. Eggenhofer E, Benseler V, Kroemer A, et al. Mesenchymal stem cells are short-lived and do not migrate beyond the lungs after intravenous infusion. *Front Immunol*. 2012;3:297.
47. Fung ME, Thebaud B. Stem cell-based therapy for neonatal lung disease: it is in the juice. *Pediatr Res*. 2014;75(1–1): 2–7.

48. Maguire G. Stem cell therapy without the cells. *Commun Integr Biol.* 2013;6(6):e26631.
49. Xu S, Liu C, Ji HL. Concise review: therapeutic potential of the mesenchymal stem cell derived secretome and extracellular vesicles for radiation-induced lung injury: progress and hypotheses. *Stem Cells Transl Med.* 2019 Apr;8(4):344–354. https://doi.org/10.1002/sctm.18-0038. Epub 2019 Jan 7.
50. Boltze J, Arnold A, Walczak P, et al. The dark side of the force - constraints and complications of cell therapies for stroke. *Front Neurol.* 2015;6:155.
51. Phinney DG, Pittenger MF. Concise review: msc-derived exosomes for cell-free therapy. *Stem Cells.* 2017;35(4): 851–858.
52. Willis GR, Mitsialis SA, Kourembanas S. "Good things come in small packages": application of exosome-based therapeutics in neonatal lung injury. *Pediatr Res.* 2018; 83(1–2):298–307.
53. Islam MN, Das SR, Emin MT, et al. Mitochondrial transfer from bone-marrow-derived stromal cells to pulmonary alveoli protects against acute lung injury. *Nat Med.* 2012; 18(5):759–765.
54. Porzionato A, Zaramella P, Dedja A, et al. Intratracheal administration of clinical-grade mesenchymal stem cell-derived extracellular vesicles reduces lung injury in a rat model of bronchopulmonary dysplasia. *Am J Physiol Lung Cell Mol Physiol.* 2019;316(1):L6–l19.
55. Phinney DG, Di Giuseppe M, Njah J, et al. Mesenchymal stem cells use extracellular vesicles to outsource mitophagy and shuttle micrornas. *Nat Commun.* 2015;6:8472.
56. Braun RK, Chetty C, Balasubramaniam V, et al. Intraperitoneal injection of msc-derived exosomes prevent experimental bronchopulmonary dysplasia. *Biochem Biophys Res Commun.* 2018;503(4):2653–2658.
57. Chaubey S, Thueson S, Ponnalagu D, et al. Early gestational mesenchymal stem cell secretome attenuates experimental bronchopulmonary dysplasia in part via exosome-associated factor tsg-6. *Stem Cell Res Ther.* 2018;9(1):173.
58. Willis GR, Fernandez-Gonzalez A, Anastas J, et al. Mesenchymal stromal cell exosomes ameliorate experimental bronchopulmonary dysplasia and restore lung function through macrophage immunomodulation. *Am J Respir Crit Care Med.* 2018;197(1):104–116.
59. Monsel A, Zhu YG, Gudapati V, et al. Mesenchymal stem cell derived secretome and extracellular vesicles for acute lung injury and other inflammatory lung diseases. *Expert Opin Biol Ther.* 2016;16(7):859–871.
60. Ferreira JR, Teixeira GQ, Santos SG, et al. Mesenchymal stromal cell secretome: influencing therapeutic potential by cellular pre-conditioning. *Front Immunol.* 2018;9:2837.
61. Yun EJ, Lorizio W, Seedorf G, et al. Vegf and endothelium-derived retinoic acid regulate lung vascular and alveolar development. *Am J Physiol Lung Cell Mol Physiol.* 2016; 310(4):L287–L298.
62. Makridakis M, Roubelakis MG, Vlahou A. Stem cells: insights into the secretome. *Biochim Biophys Acta.* 2013; 1834(11):2380–2384.
63. Thebaud B, Ladha F, Michelakis ED, et al. Vascular endothelial growth factor gene therapy increases survival, promotes lung angiogenesis, and prevents alveolar damage in hyperoxia-induced lung injury: evidence that angiogenesis participates in alveolarization. *Circulation.* 2005; 112(16):2477–2486.
64. Choi H, Lee RH, Bazhanov N, et al. Anti-inflammatory protein tsg-6 secreted by activated mscs attenuates zymosan-induced mouse peritonitis by decreasing tlr2/ nf-kappab signaling in resident macrophages. *Blood.* 2011;118(2):330–338.
65. Ortiz LA, Dutreil M, Fattman C, et al. Interleukin 1 receptor antagonist mediates the antiinflammatory and antifibrotic effect of mesenchymal stem cells during lung injury. *Proc Natl Acad Sci USA.* 2007;104(26):11002–11007.
66. Willis GR, Fernandez-Gonzalez A, Reis M, et al. Macrophage immunomodulation: the gatekeeper for mesenchymal stem cell derived-exosomes in pulmonary arterial hypertension? *Int J Mol Sci.* 2018;19(9).
67. Mittal M, Tiruppathi C, Nepal S, et al. Tnfalpha-stimulated gene-6 (tsg6) activates macrophage phenotype transition to prevent inflammatory lung injury. *Proc Natl Acad Sci USA.* 2016;113(50):E8151–e8158.
68. Chang YS, Ahn SY, Yoo HS, et al. Mesenchymal stem cells for bronchopulmonary dysplasia: phase 1 dose-escalation clinical trial. *J Pediatr.* 2014;164(5), 966–972.e966.
69. Ahn SY, Chang YS, Kim JH, et al. Two-year follow-up outcomes of premature infants enrolled in the phase i trial of mesenchymal stem cells transplantation for bronchopulmonary dysplasia. *J Pediatr.* 2017;185, 49–54.e42.
70. Pierro M, Thebaud B, Soll R. Mesenchymal stem cells for the prevention and treatment of bronchopulmonary dysplasia in preterm infants. *Cochrane Database Syst Rev.* 2017;11:Cd011932.
71. Alvarez-Fuente M, Arruza L, Lopez-Ortego P, et al. Off-label mesenchymal stromal cell treatment in two infants with severe bronchopulmonary dysplasia: clinical course and biomarkers profile. *Cytotherapy.* 2018;20(11): 1337–1344.
72. Chen CM, Chou HC. Human mesenchymal stem cells attenuate hyperoxia-induced lung injury through inhibition of the renin-angiotensin system in newborn rats. *Am J Transl Res.* 2018;10(8):2628–2635.
73. Kim YE, Park WS, Ahn SY, et al. Intratracheal transplantation of mesenchymal stem cells attenuates hyperoxia-induced lung injury by down-regulating, but not direct inhibiting formyl peptide receptor 1 in the newborn mice. *PLoS One.* 2018;13(10):e0206311.
74. Lim R, Malhotra A, Tan J, et al. First-in-human administration of allogeneic amnion cells in premature infants with bronchopulmonary dysplasia: a safety study. *Stem Cells Transl Med.* 2018;7(9):628–635.
75. Chen J, Hu C, Pan P. Extracellular vesicle microrna transfer in lung diseases. *Front Physiol.* 2017;8:1028.
76. Cheng L, Zhang K, Wu S, et al. Focus on mesenchymal stem cell-derived exosomes: opportunities and challenges in cell-free therapy. *Stem Cell Int.* 2017;2017:6305295.
77. Contopoulos-Ioannidis DG, Ntzani E, Ioannidis JP. Translation of highly promising basic science research into clinical applications. *Am J Med.* 2003;114(6):477–484.

78. Alejandre Alcazar MA, Kaschwich M, Ertsey R, et al. Elafin treatment rescues egfr-klf4 signaling and lung cell survival in ventilated newborn mice. *Am J Respir Cell Mol Biol.* 2018; 59(5):623–634.
79. Yoder BA, Coalson JJ. Animal models of bronchopulmonary dysplasia. The preterm baboon models. *Am J Physiol Lung Cell Mol Physiol.* 2014;307(12):L970–L977.
80. Kilkenny C, Browne WJ, Cuthill IC, et al. Improving bioscience research reporting: the arrive guidelines for reporting animal research. *PLoS Biol.* 2010;8(6): e1000412.
81. Mueller M, Kramer BW. Stem cells and bronchopulmonary dysplasia - the five questions: which cells, when, in which dose, to which patients via which route? *Paediatr Respir Rev.* 2017;24:54–59.
82. Zhu Y, Xu L, Collins JJP, et al. Human umbilical cord mesenchymal stromal cells improve survival and bacterial clearance in neonatal sepsis in rats. *Stem Cells Dev.* 2017; 26(14):1054–1064.
83. Mitsialis SA, Kourembanas S. Stem cell-based therapies for the newborn lung and brain: possibilities and challenges. *Semin Perinatol.* 2016;40(3):138–151.

CHAPTER 22

Burden of Chronic Lung Disease on the Caregivers: Families, Nurses, and Physicians

MARIANNE C. CHIAFERY, DNP, PNP-C, MS • CARL T. D'ANGIO, MD

Bronchopulmonary dysplasia (BPD), the most common of the neonatal chronic lung diseases, begins as an acute process, encompassing the ethical concerns and stresses associated with acute, serious, and life-threatening illness. As the infant survives the initial acute physiologic hurdles, the disease becomes chronic in nature. A chronic illness can be defined as a health condition that, at the time of diagnosis, is predicted to last more than 3 months, results in functional impairment or medical needs greater than those of other children of similar age, and will lead to limitation of function, disfigurement, the need for medication, diet or technology dependency, and the increased need for services and special ongoing treatments.[1–3] The chronic illness phase brings its own challenges and stressors. For children with severe BPD, these challenges can last into adolescence and beyond. In this chapter, we will review the ethical challenges, stressors, and burdens faced by caregivers, including parents/guardians, nurses, physicians, and other vital personnel who make up the circle of support required to achieve best outcomes for optimal child development, and family growth, resiliency, and cohesiveness.

OUTCOMES OF BRONCHOPULMONARY DYSPLASIA

Although the sequelae of BPD are covered in detail in other chapters, it is useful to review briefly the health burdens faced by children with BPD and their parents. Some of the abnormalities in pulmonary function seen in BPD resolve in the first 2 years after birth, but airflow limitation persists into childhood, adolescence, and even adulthood.[4–8] Symptoms such as wheezing and dyspnea are similar to those of asthma, but are less likely to be responsive to bronchodilator therapy than asthma.[9–12] Preterm children, including those with BPD, have diminished exercise tolerance, and adults who had BPD as children report increased sedentary behavior and limitations in mobility that affect activities of daily living and result in a lower reported quality of life (QOL) than their peers.[4,13–16] BPD increases healthcare resource use, respiratory medications, doctor and emergency room visits, and hospitalizations throughout childhood and adolescence.[17–23] Sleep-disordered breathing is elevated among former premature children with BPD.[24] At age 5 years, survivors with BPD have over double the odds of death or severe disability than former preterm children without BPD.[25] The elevated risk persists through 10–15 years, when the increase is estimated at fivefold compared with peers,[26] although some studies[27] suggest that BPD may not be an independent risk factor. Preschool- and school-aged children with BPD have poorer academic, behavioral, motor, and cognitive outcomes than their preterm or full-term peers.[17,28–30] Although 11-year-old extremely preterm children showed no difference in physical activity habits or difficulty with activities of daily living, compared to matched classroom controls, their lung function tests and peak oxygen consumption demonstrated persistent impairments.[14] Twelve-year-old children with BPD have nearly five times the odds of abnormal overall health status, compared with full-term infants.[31] Parents of 10 to 15-year-old children with BPD have threefold elevated odds of reporting at least one significant physical, psychologic, or cognitive consequence of chronic diseases, when compared with preterm infants without BPD.[26] In addition to more asthmalike symptoms and reports of shortness of breath, adult survivors of BPD exhibit continued decrements in executive function.[4,32]

Updates on Neonatal Chronic Lung Disease. https://doi.org/10.1016/B978-0-323-68353-1.00022-1

Severe Bronchopulmonary Dysplasia

Survivors of severe BPD, especially those who still require mechanical ventilation at 36 weeks' postmenstrual age (type 2 severe BPD), face additional challenges.[33] Children with severe BPD are at risk for multiple pulmonary and nonpulmonary sequelae, including growth failure and neurodevelopmental impairment, and may be at risk for chronic obstructive pulmonary disease in later life.[33,34] Up to a quarter of patients with severe BPD have pulmonary hypertension, which carries a mortality of 12%–38%.[35,36] Children with BPD aged 11–14 years have higher pulmonary arterial pressures than both term controls and other preterm children.[37] Chronic lung disease accounts for nearly 40% of the children in the United States who receive home ventilation; the majority of these children have BPD.[38] Children on home ventilation for severe BPD have about a one in five chance of death, with about 20% of the deaths due to tracheostomy complications.[39,40] One-third of the surviving children discharged with a tracheostomy remain technology dependent at 5–10 years of age.[41] Discharge on home oxygen for BPD is associated with a slowing of the recovery in neurodevelopment seen in premature infants.[42]

THEORETIC FRAMEWORK

A child is not a lone entity. Myriad people and organizations at varying levels of proximity have an impact on the child's well-being. Recognition of the interplay between the many relationships and potential stressors can facilitate planning to achieve the best possible outcomes for the child and family. Bronfenbrenner's bioecological systems theory[43] provides a framework to identify and assess factors that affect the child's development. The theory views child development in the context of a system of relationships, with the child and his innate biology as the primary factor and central to the system (Fig. 22.1). The components of the theory include expanding rings of influence, with bidirectional interactions between each component. The *Microsystem* is in most direct contact to the *Individual* (the child) and likely most influential on the child. In the hospital setting the *Microsystem* consists primarily of the parents and healthcare providers. The child, parents, and healthcare providers are together in a relationship dance (the *Mesosystem*). The child's status affects parental action and behavior and the parents' beliefs and behaviors impact the child, and both affect the providers, who themselves exert reciprocal effects. Further components include the *Exosystem* (of supports and

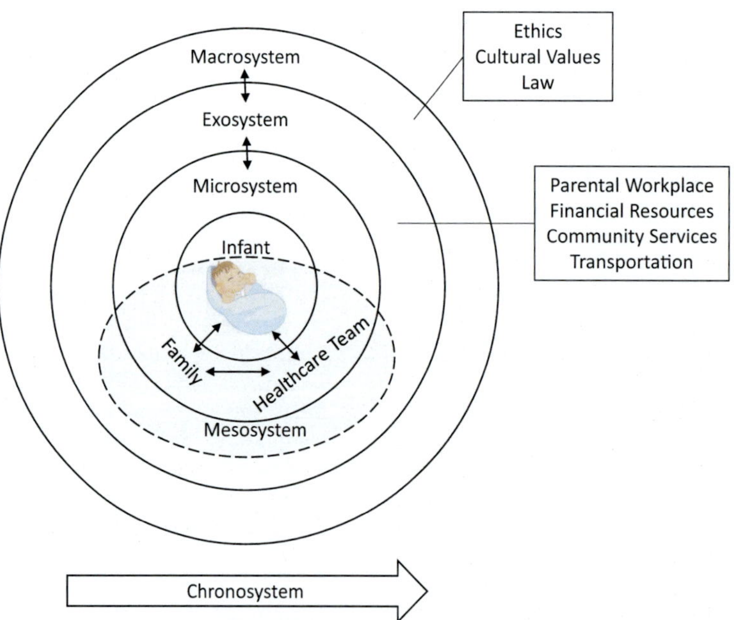

FIG. 22.1 **Bronfenbrenner's bioecological systems theory.** The theory views child development in the context of a system of relationships, including expanding rings of influence, all playing out over time.

community factors), the *Macrosystem* (of the societal environment), and the *Chronosystem* (of change over time). Environmental and supportive factors will change as the child transitions over time from acute to chronic level of care and from hospital to home.

BURDENS ON PARENTS

The story of BPD begins in the neonatal intensive care unit (NICU). The NICU environment is one that is foreign to most, and parents enter a land that they often did not prepare for or anticipate.[44] Parents note that stress is immediately elicited by the appearance and behavior of their ill infant, the challenges of parenting a sick infant, the unfamiliar routines of the NICU, and the stress of developing collaborative relationships with the multiple staff members caring for their baby (Fig. 22.2).[45–47] It is a roller-coaster ride of emotions, such as uncertainty, grief, sadness, fatigue, anxiety, happiness, confusion, anger, shame, and helplessness.[48,49] Loss of control over the environment and the ability to have contact with their infant adds to stress.[50] Parents also face the sudden and often unfamiliar responsibility of making healthcare decisions that may affect an infant's life or health. In the absence of evidence that parents are making decisions contrary to an infant's best interests, the authority for decision-making appropriately rests with the parents.[51] Healthcare providers can and should provide guidance and recommendations, but parents often feel the weight of responsibility heavily.

Parents suffer high levels of anxiety, fatigue, depression, and sleep disturbances. Poor sleep and the resultant chronic fatigue place mothers at increased risk for postpartum depression.[52] These physical and emotional stressors correlate with difficulties in parental role enactment, as well as poor self-perception of competence in the parental role.[53] Depression is not uncommon and may last for prolonged periods. About 13% of mothers are still depressed 2 years after the birth of their infant.[54] Fathers also suffer from stress and depression, with a study of 146 fathers of NICU infants showing incidences of minor and major depression of 41% and 16%, respectively.[55] Minor and major depression among fathers decreased at 4 months post hospital discharge to 10% and 2%, respectively. Mackley and colleagues[56] also found that one-third of fathers demonstrated symptoms of depression, which may last for months. Routine screening for symptoms of depression and anxiety among parents is indicated, but there are no consensus guidelines for how to approach this common problem.[57]

Posttraumatic stress disorder is present in up to 33% of fathers and 9% of mothers at 4 months after birth of their infants.[57,58] Mothers of premature infants in the NICU have higher stress levels than mothers of infants born at term.[59–61] Sources of stress include personal/family concerns, as well as situational and

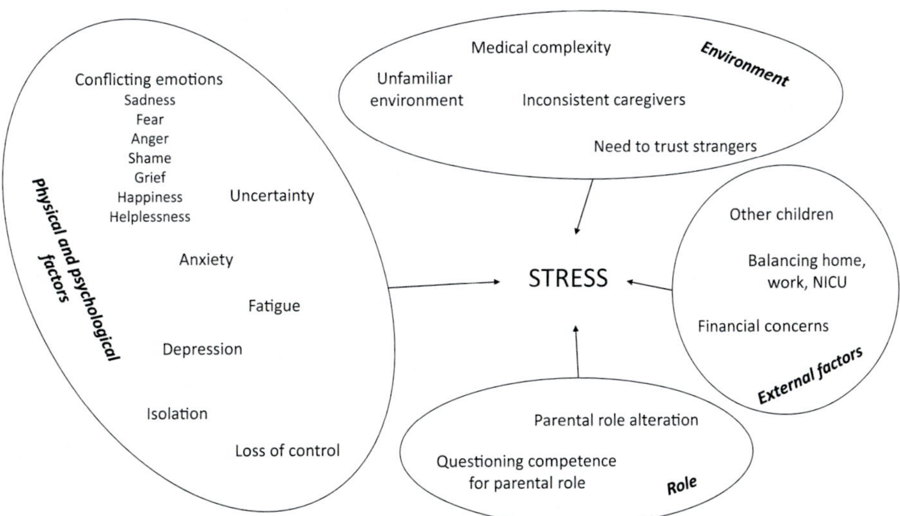

FIG. 22.2 Parental stressors. Parents experience stress from a variety of factors in the neonatal intensive care unit (NICU), including physical and psychologic stressors, alteration of role, the NICU environment, and external concerns.

environmental factors.[62] Loss of the maternal role is a major source of stress for mothers.[63,64] Akkoyun and Arslan[65] found particularly high stress levels among mothers whose infants were receiving ventilator support and parenteral feeds and among those who were in the lower- to middle-income category.

Effect on Fathers

Fathers report stressors that are similar to mothers, such as parental role alteration and concern for the baby's appearance.[66–70] Fathers also carry different stressors that are no less important and tend to tie in to traditional gender role expectations, such as financial burden and the stress of maintaining a job.[71,72] Protecting and supporting the mother and infant are high priorities for fathers, and often this means allowing the mother to do all the "firsts" such as first bath or first time to hold the infant.[73] Many fathers express a desire to "stay strong" for the mother and family unit.[73] Going to work is often a mixed blessing and concern: fathers often find work to be a time away from the stress of the NICU, but the pressure of maintaining an income to support the family is ever-present.[73]

The first moment of holding their infant is important for fathers to affirm the connection to their child and provides a solid feeling of truly being a father.[71,73,74] Even with that positive experience, many still fear that they will accidently harm their "frail" infant. Noergaard and colleagues[75] found that fathers who were purposely drawn into providing more care for their infants demonstrated higher levels of stress, perhaps due to the added expectation of yet-another role. Many fathers also provide emotional support for the infant's mother and assure the care of other children at home. Such changes in parental duties may contribute to stress for all family members.[50,76] Cultural factors and family dynamics should be considered before an expectation is made about the amount and type of paternal involvement that is comfortable. Fathers may need a different type of support than mothers, so individual assessment of parental stressors is warranted.

Supporting Parents

Janvier and colleagues,[77] in a manuscript authored by physicians whose family members underwent NICU hospitalization, note that from adversity come strength and the potential for positive outcomes for all stakeholders. This is best achieved when crucial supports are in place (Table 22.1). Parents may not be aware of available resources, so the healthcare team needs to provide guidance within the context of nonjudgmental regard as they help families cope with the crisis of an NICU admission. The healthcare team must be aware of the long-term impact of their interventions and actions with the family in order to help parents develop the strength needed for the current and future well-being of the individual parent, infant, and family unit.

The parent-child relationship is important for the infant's intellectual, social, and emotional development.[78,79] Parental involvement has been shown to decrease the length of hospital stay.[80] Parents who receive support to address stressors, develop coping strategies, and learn how to parent a sick child are more readily able to develop important parent-child bonds. Infants who spent more time during the NICU stay in skin-to-skin contact with their parents scored higher on the Bayley psychomotor developmental indexes at 6 months of age.[81] Family integrated care of NICU infants at risk for developing BPD has been shown to improve a number of NICU outcomes, including lowering the amount of time on respiratory support.[82]

Assessing and alleviating stressors

Nurses often have the most contact and opportunity to help relieve parental burden and stress and help parents gain confidence in parenting skills. Excellent communication skills and the ability to listen well are crucial to these tasks. Listening with the intent to understand the parents' perceptions is the fundamental basis to develop effective strategies to teach, guide, and relieve the stressors/burdens of parents and is cited as among the most common positive experiences by NICU parents.[83] Mothers desire a nurse who is sensitive to their needs, makes eye contact, takes time to sit to talk, treats their babies as normally as possible, and allows them to provide as much care for their babies as possible.[84,85] Trust is essential for a mother to be able to leave the hospital to see other children at home and to rest and refresh.[84]

Actions that diminish trust include frequent changes of the healthcare providers responsible for their infant and inconsistent communication.[73,85,86] As noted, an important parental role is one of protection of their vulnerable infant. This can be facilitated by keeping them informed of their infant's condition and providing ways to be actively involved in the baby's care. Taking time to provide factual information and clarify misunderstanding helps promote a trusting relationship.[87] As best as possible, communication should be balanced with good news, such as developmental and physical advances, as well as setbacks.[77] Parents who perceive they are only hearing bad news may be less likely to visit.

TABLE 22.1
Methods of Parental Support in the Neonatal Intensive Care Unit and Beyond[a].

Communication
Active listening
Transparent communication
Ascertaining values, concerns, and wishes
Understanding culture
Assessing and improving knowledge of the infant's condition
Nonjudgmental guidance
Reinforcing and validating parental role
Behavioral Support
Assessing affect and stress
Depression screening
Psychologic support
Attention to parental health and well-being
Supporting hope
Supporting resilience
Care Practices
Involving parents in care
Family-informed/centered care, including rooming-in
Skin-to-skin contact/kangaroo care
Developmental care and education
Providing privacy
Permission to leave/rest
Services
Social work and financial counseling support
Support groups
One-to-one peer support
Language and cultural interpreters
Spiritual care
In-home nursing care

[a] See text for references.

Attention must be paid to each parent as an individual. Members of the healthcare team must assess parental affect and ascertain values, concerns, wishes, culture, and knowledge of their infant's status and disease process.[88] Misunderstanding about the disease process and treatments should be addressed and clarified so that informed treatment and care decisions can be made.

Supporting the parental role

Mothers bemoan the lack of privacy in the NICU and the feeling of mothering in public, so efforts to provide privacy are welcome.[84] Breastfeeding can be difficult even in the best of situations, so nurses and breastfeeding educators should be available and sensitive to the needs of mothers who want to provide breast milk for their infants. Pumping breast milk to be delivered through a feeding tube can provide mothers with a tangible way to care for their infants.

Mothers report not feeling the baby is "hers" until they are discharged to home.[84] Nurses must find and define personal and professional boundaries to avoid acting like a surrogate and assuming what is best for the infant and parents. Allowing parents to experience the baby's "firsts" of milestones as frequently as possible helps to foster a feeling of parenthood.[84]

Fathers can easily feel like an outsider in the NICU, so measures to invite and include are critical. Skin-to-skin contact is a compelling moment for fathers and should be initiated as soon as possible. They need special encouragement that they are not too big or too clumsy and that the infant will be fine in their hands. Visitation should be encouraged, no matter the time of day, as fathers will likely have to plan visits around their work schedules.

Kangaroo care, a holding technique where the infant has skin-to-skin contact with the parent, has been shown to reduce parental stress, improve infants' physiologic parameters, and promote parent-infant bonding.[81,89,90] Additionally, the technique may prevent infection, reduce energy consumption to improve weight gain, and improve infant brain development.[91] Parental rooming-in has also been shown both to reduce the length of stay and to decrease the likelihood of moderate-to-severe BPD.[92]

Parents should be encouraged to find a balance between caring for the self and caring for their infant. Parents may be hesitant to leave their child and may need permission to take breaks from the bedside or even the NICU to recharge, refresh, or check on other family members. Parents may need to be reminded that it is necessary that they address their own basic needs for sleep, healthy diet, exercise, and social support. Parents may need help prioritizing the demands on their time.

Parents, especially mothers, may feel that they "caused" their infant's medical condition, resulting in lingering feelings of guilt. Sensitive listening for cues that this is a concern can alert the staff to provide reassurance that this situation is not their fault. Parents often need to be reminded of the ways they are being good parents.[77]

Parents balance hope with anxiety.[93] Hope is often the impetus that gives parents the energy to continue to visit and bond with their infant and be engaged with care. It is not unusual for staff and parents to predict different outcomes for an infant, with staff more likely to see risks and a poor QOL than parents. Parents also maintain optimism that their infant will have a good QOL. Even if the infant's prognosis is grave, there are positive steps that can be taken to provide hope and reassurance, such as emphasizing that the healthcare team will not abandon them or their infant or clarifying that their child will be kept as comfortable as possible.

Additional supports

A buddy system of pairing mothers of NICU infants with mothers who have previously undergone the experience may be helpful. Through shared experiences, the mother may feel less alone in the experience, find other resources, and realize that the current situation will not last forever. To address cultural needs in their diverse city, Preyde and Ardal[94] paired mothers of similar ethnicity and culture and found that mothers in the study group demonstrated less anxiety and less depression and perceived greater social support than the control group. Cultural interpreters to translate language as well as cultural mores and traditions, and to provide educational resources in the parents' primary language can be helpful.[95]

Father support groups may be helpful.[55,96] Offering fathers supportive counseling should be routine, yet in one study, only 27% of the nurses had made an attempt to discover if fathers were under stress and less than 20% offered assistance in seeking helpful resources.[97]

Multiple programs have been studied to determine how best to support parents. Generally, the programs include content on general neonatal physiology, infant development, parent interventions to promote development and bonding, and orientation to the NICU environment.[64,98,99] The Creating Opportunities for Parent Empowerment (COPE) program for parent education and behavioral interventions has been shown to diminish maternal stress and facilitate better cognitive growth among hospitalized infants than a control group.[80,100] Additionally, length of stay was shortened for infants in the experimental group.

Spiritual care can also facilitate coping, diminish parental stress, and help strengthen bonds with staff.[101,102] Regular visits by the families' spiritual leaders or hospital chaplaincy may be helpful. Other staff can provide spiritual support by exploring family beliefs in an open and compassionate way, sitting quietly, listening and praying with them, or simply honoring and making space for spiritual rituals.[103,104]

Parents come to the NICU with varying resources and support systems, so conversations about these topics is crucial. Social workers and other staff can help direct families to resources in the hospital or community to meet their particular needs and assist with applications for secondary insurance, or other financial resources.[68] Child Life specialists and occupational and physical therapists are also important because they teach parents how to be engaged with their baby, as well as skills and techniques to promote development and make adaptations to meet each infant's unique needs. Child Life specialists are also uniquely positioned to advise parents on how to provide information and support for siblings of the preterm or, later, chronically ill child.

BURDENS ON HOSPITAL STAFF

Vulnerable infants who are in distress and in harm's way tend to bring out emotional responses from those who care for them, and members of the healthcare team are not immune to such a reaction. A study of salivary cortisol levels from neonatal and pediatric intensive care physicians and nurses showed endocrinologic evidence of a stress response in 12.5% of samples.[105] Over 70% of the stress responses occurred without staff members having conscious awareness of stress. The ability to maintain professional distance can be challenging, as staff balance the obligation to honor the rights of parent to make decisions for their child and to develop a strong relationship with the parents, while maintaining a professional demeanor, often while caring for multiple patients at once. Knowledge of basic ethical reasoning, guiding ethical principles in neonatal care, the shared decision-making process, and the maintenance of professional boundaries is critical for the successful navigation of difficult situations in order to determine the best treatment plan for the infant.

Moral Distress

Moral dilemmas are not uncommon in the NICU, as parents, physicians, and nurses may disagree as to the best course of action. Moral distress is the "psychological response to morally challenging situations such as those of moral constraint, moral conflict, or both."[106] The cause of greatest moral distress for nurses is reported as being required to follow a family's wishes to continue life support when such action is viewed as not in the child's best interest or seems futile.[107] NICU patients undergo an average of 14 invasive procedures per day, and the close proximity to and involvement in causing pain may cause feelings of moral distress.[108,109] Poor communication and disagreements among team members, particularly around prognosis and perceived nonbeneficial treatment, are often cited as a significant cause of moral distress.[110–112]

Moral distress is felt by all professionals.[113] Solomon[114] reported that 38% of critical care physicians and 48% of nurses reported taking actions that went against their consciences. Work-related burnout and occupational stress take a toll on the staff that may manifest in physical and emotional responses such as anger, sleeplessness, guilt, early retirement, leaving medicine/nursing, or suicide.[115]

Hospital-wide moral distress consultation teams may decrease distress by providing an opportunity for interprofessional discussion about ethically challenging cases, enabling teams to find common ground and share and accept differing values, identifying recurring issues, and providing validation to staff members that their insights are valued.[116,117] Moral distress may also be decreased by unit-based discussions led by a clinical nurse ethicist.[118] Continued ethics education and case discussion in an interprofessional setting may promote team building, team trust, and understanding of the ethical obligations/beliefs held by individual team members.[119]

The overarching ethical climate of an organization is perhaps the most important factor to mitigate and prevent moral distress. An ethical climate is one where there is shared understanding of criteria that guide moral decision-making, that has leaders who are benevolent and acknowledge the contributions and concerns of each team member, and where the staff care for each other and make decisions that demonstrate primary concern for the patient and family.[120–122] Leaders can work to minimize barriers to open communication and flatten the power imbalances among staff, thus promoting intrateam trust.[123] de Boer and colleagues[124] implemented a five-step process to promote ethical decision-making to include all direct care professionals. The steps include (1) group exploration of medical facts and contextual factors, (2) determining the ethical dilemma and possible solutions, (3) analyzing the pros and cons and the likely effects of each option, (4) consensus decision-making, and (5) deriving an action plan to implement the decision. Participants reported better understanding about the ethical dilemma and that the observations and concerns of all participants in the infant's care were considered.

Supporting Nurses, Physicians, and Other Providers

Supporting nurses and staff

Nurses have a significant influence on the parental experience, and many parents remember forever the nurses who cared for their baby. However, many nurses do not feel adequately prepared to assess parental needs or support parents.[125] Staff are also at risk for adverse reactions due to chronic exposure to the stress of an NICU, which includes a fast-paced and noisy environment, frequent life/death situations with vulnerable infants, disagreements over treatment decisions, team/colleague work relationships, and the emotional stress of working with parents in crisis.[126] Staff who are not prepared for the environment, or do not have adequate coping methods, can suffer from burnout, defined as a state of physical, emotional, and mental exhaustion.[127] Staff who are depleted do not have the energy or internal resources to care for others and are at risk to emotionally distance themselves from patients and families.[126] It is crucial that appropriate and adequate support be in place for nursing staff and all who provide care for the infant and family.

Education of all staff who work with NICU families should start at orientation and continue on a regular basis, with the goal of developing staff who are able to provide psychosocial care to families as well as physical care to infants. Interdisciplinary education is recommended, as it supports effective team building via discussion and sharing of experiences.[126] Education topics should include parental experience and responses to the stressors of having a seriously ill infant in the NICU, common mood and anxiety disorders experienced by parents, family development, provision of culturally sensitive care, effective communication skills with parents and team members, end-of-life care, and education on self-care.[126]

Palliative care services can be very helpful, as the team members are comfortable with shared decision-making with families around burdens of care when the prognosis is uncertain. The benefits of palliative care in cases of BPD include parent and provider support, transparency in decision-making, and balancing medical status and best interests.[128] Observing palliative care teams at work can be educational for staff, as they can learn and emulate communication skills around difficult topics.

Additionally, local spiritual and community leaders can educate staff on beliefs, social norms, and ceremonies particular to religious and ethnic groups in the geographic referral area for the NICU. Such knowledge can help staff provide culturally sensitive care and prevent miscommunication and rifts with families who may have different beliefs than the staff.[129] Pastoral care providers can also bring important observations and insights to ethics case discussions.

Other support personnel include mental health professionals who can help recognize and counsel for signs of burnout and compassion fatigue and clinical ethicists who can help teams and individuals work through ethical dilemmas and identify and address moral distress.

Supporting physicians

Neonatologists are also at risk for burnout.[130] In a survey of US neonatologists, 16% reported experiencing compassion fatigue, while 21% reported signs of burnout.[131] Female gender, distress from specific clinical situations, emotional distress, lack of opportunity to discuss distress, personal health concerns, and interpersonal and work environment difficulties increased the likelihood of fatigue and burnout. Although the relationship between gender and burnout is inconsistent across studies of physicians, women physicians report high expectations, fulfilling multiple roles, and work environment factors, including workload, gender discrimination, and verbal and physical abuse, as factors contributing to stress and burnout.[132–134] Physicians are also likely to report moral distress in the course of their duties, with a majority experiencing such distress at least monthly.[116] Although the sources of stress for physicians differ from those of nurses (Table 22.2), physicians are more likely than nurses to report negative effects of work on their private lives.[135]

Potential opportunities to improve physicians' distress include a focus on increasing compassion satisfaction (fulfillment in helping others), an experience reported by 22% of US neonatologists and reported at 4.3 on a 6-point scale by Swiss neonatologists.[131,135] In studies of healthcare professionals and social workers, supervisor support, programs teaching self-care (self-compassion, mindfulness), practicing self-care, and dedicated caregiver support teams to provide real-time emotional assistance have all been reported to improve compassion satisfaction.[136–139] Even moral distress is perceived by physicians as a potentially valuable opportunity for robust discussion of medical decision-making, with only 8% of physicians wishing to eliminate it.[116] Signs of job dissatisfaction and burnout are ameliorated as physicians gain experience.[135] This correlates with endocrinologic evidence of decreased stress responses among intensive care staff with over 8 years of experience.[105]

TABLE 22.2
Sources of Distress Among Neonatal Intensive Care Unit Physicians and Nurses[a].

Communication
Lack of regular staff meetings[b]
Lack of routine discussion of difficult cases
Disagreements among caregivers
Poor information transmission
Decision-Making
Lack of ethics training
Dissatisfaction with decision-making process
End-of-life decision-making
Patient Characteristics
Caring for dying patients
Providing futile treatment
Others
Lack of psychologic support

[a] Items rated as occurring "often" or "sometimes" by >40% of providers.

[b] Items in italics reported more commonly by nurses than physicians.

Drawn from Klein, SD et al., Sources of distress for physicians and nurses working in Swiss neonatal intensive care units. *Swiss Med Wkly* 2017; 147:w14477.

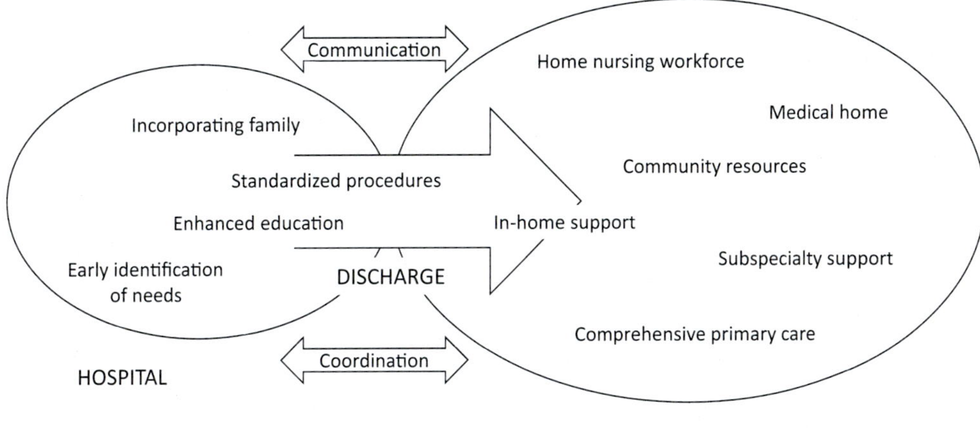

FIG. 22.3 Decreasing the stress of transition to home. Elements of a successful transition to home include early parental involvement and intensive education in the neonatal intensive care unit, in-home nursing support, robust community resources, and communication and collaboration between the inpatient and outpatient settings.

BURDENS OF BRONCHOPULMONARY DYSPLASIA BEYOND THE NURSERY

The challenges for parents caring for children at home with BPD begin even before discharge. A recent survey of Norwegian NICU parents found dissatisfaction with incorporating parents and siblings during the later phases of NICU hospitalization and with guidance and training to meet their child's needs.[83] Parents of children with BPD sent home on oxygen report increased anxiety at discharge.[140] This improves as infant respiratory status improves and further lessens when home oxygen is discontinued. Several studies have evaluated programs designed to ease the transition to home for premature infants, although few of these have focused specifically on infants expected to have complex needs.[80,141–148] Most programs included some form of enhanced education while the infant remained hospitalized and in-home support, by physical or virtual visits. The component most closely associated with program success (longer time on maternal breast milk, fewer emergency department visits, fewer and shorter rehospitalization, increased quality of mother-infant interactions, improved parental satisfaction) was the provision of in-home nursing support.[80,141,142,144,146] Hospital-based programs that provide comprehensive primary care to former very low-birth-weight infants have also been shown to decrease life-threatening illness and intensive care readmissions.[149] Successful transition to home for a medically complex infant requires a multifaceted approach involving close coordination between hospital and community resources (Fig. 22.3).[150] The Ohio Perinatal Quality Collaborative recently released a guide to improve mechanisms for the transition home that cites early identification of needs, strengthened community resources, improved hospital-community communication and collaboration, standardized procedures, and an adequate, trained home-nursing workforce.[151]

Caregiver Quality of Life

Mothers[i] of 1-year-old children with BPD being managed with home oxygen reported, on a semistructured questionnaire, multiple effects on their lives, including loss of career to become the primary caretaker for their infant, emotional distress, low self-esteem, self-blame, and unresolved grief.[152] In addition, many of the mothers reported isolation, in part from fear of infection.

Mothers of young children with BPD also report caregiver burden and stress above those experienced by parents of healthy children and similar to those experienced by other parents of children with chronic medical needs, such as home enteral nutrition and peanut allergy.[153] Families caring for 3-month-old infants

[i]The majority of research done on the effect of having a former premature infant with bronchopulmonary dysplasia at home has been performed with mothers, not fathers. Although data gathered from mothers may be generalizable to both parents, this section will refer to both parents only when the research supports this.

with BPD have higher scores for measures of impact on the family (which include financial, internal and external interactional, and primary caretaker burdens).[154] It is also common for children with severe BPD to have a combination of chronic health problems in addition to breathing issues, including failure to thrive, inability to eat by mouth, need to receive multiple medications throughout the day, oral aversion, neurologic irritability, abnormal muscle tone, and atypical responses to normal stimulation. Caring for a child with BPD is independently associated with poorer reported QOL among mothers of 3-year-old children.[155] Mothers of young children with BPD also report poor sleep, with an average sleep time of about 6 hours a night, and about a third reporting sleep quality as bad.[153] Poor sleep quality increases depressive symptoms and stress in the mothers and is the single largest predictor of decreased perceived QOL.[153] Increased infant respiratory morbidity also worsens parental QOL.[156] Factors that improve the perceived QOL among mothers of former preterm children include a stable marital union, higher family income, evangelical religious beliefs, and lower measures of depression.[155] As children grow, the physical, worry, and daily domains of parental QOL assessment also improve.[156] An evaluation of the QOL among parents of very preterm infants when their children were 27 years old showed no difference in reported QOL from parents of full-term infants.[157] Of note, however, QOL among all parents was affected by their children's mental health and peer relationships during childhood.

External Factors

Parents also face challenges from external factors that make it more difficult to care for their children with BPD. Among parents of very low-birth-weight infants, single parents and those with lower education attainment face additional challenges, with their children having poorer intellectual functioning at the age 3 years.[158] Concurrent BPD increases this risk. Parents of children with severe BPD are less likely to attend follow-up visits for their children, citing barriers including complex logistics, time commitment, negative perceptions, and emotional stress.[159] Even day care, which might provide some respite for parents of children with a chronic medical condition, increases respiratory morbidity among children under 3 years old with BPD by increasing emergency department visits, medication use, and the number of days with respiratory symptoms.[160]

Children's Quality of Life

Parents of 18- to 36-month-old infants with severe BPD rate the infants' health-related QOL as poorer than that of premature infants without BPD or full-term controls.[161] Additional neonatal morbidities further worsen parental impressions of QOL. This assessment also holds true at school age, with children with severe BPD scoring more poorly on tests of cognition, language, and executive and social function, as well as having lower scores on tests of health-related QOL.[162,163] A recently designed BPD-specific QOL measure for school-aged children shows good construct validity.[164] Further work will be needed to assess the value of this scale. Children with other congenital anomalies, such as diaphragmatic hernia, also have lower health-related QOL than healthy children; concomitant chronic and intermittently exacerbating lung disease enhances this effect.[165] Parental assessment of QOL among survivors with congenital diaphragmatic hernia was more optimistic than the children's. Conversely, adolescent survivors of extreme prematurity report a health-related QOL similar to that of their term-born peers and better than that of asthmatic teens.[166] Lung function was unrelated to the adolescents' assessment of QOL. In adulthood, some investigators find that survivors of BPD report increased respiratory impairment and poorer QOL than former preterm infants without BPD or full-term controls.[13] Others note no differences in reported QOL, despite increased respiratory symptoms, limitations in physical functioning, and poorer educational and employment opportunities.[167,168] Both the respiratory impairment and poorer health-related QOL persist over time among adults.[8,13]

Psychologic distress experienced during the first year of life may also cause mothers to perform fewer activities that foster cognitive development in their children with BPD.[169] Mothers of infants with BPD report fewer responsive, clear interactions with their infants than mothers of term infants; this dichotomy increases over the first year of life.[169] Caregivers of 5- to 10-year-old children with tracheostomy also report decreased responsiveness, activity, and interpersonal function among their children, particularly among children who are younger and/or those with maternal public insurance.[41]

It should be noted that standard QOL measures capture specific, quantifiable limitations of function. Some commentators have called for broader, more qualitative analysis of both challenges and strengths, noting that parents report both negative and positive themes in response to open-ended questions about their former premature infants.[170] There was no relationship between reporting positive themes by parents and the degree of neurodevelopmental impairment of the child. The potential lack of correlation between quantitative and qualitative measures may explain some of the discordant results of the QOL data reported.

Improving Outcomes

Programs that provide increased family involvement, enhanced education, support in the home and disease-specific follow-up improve some health measures during infancy, and have been discussed above.[147–149] Such programs may also help to improve parental stress and neurodevelopmental outcomes among children with BPD, but most are not tested beyond early childhood.[100] A Dutch proprietary behavioral intervention program aimed at very low-birth-weight infants showed promise in improving motor, mental, and behavioral function through 24 months of age among infants with BPD.[171,172] However, this effect waned by school age.[173]

Lessons From Other Chronic Diseases

The experiences of families of children with other chronic illnesses may inform our understanding of what is faced by families of children with BPD. Muscara and colleagues[174] identified three patterns of recovery among 159 parents whose children had experienced a serious childhood illness over the 18 months following the illness. "Resilient" parents (33% of the total) exhibited low levels of posttraumatic stress symptoms across the observation period. Parents in the "Recovery" group (52%) exhibited high initial distress, which abated over several months. Parents in the "Chronic" class (13%) had persistently elevated distress levels over the study period. Parent psychologic factors, including mood and anxiety, but not demographics or illness characteristics, were associated with the type of response.

Chronic illness impacts the family and can disrupt social relations within the family.[175] Higher degree of illness, greater levels of dependence, poor developmental function, siblings in the home, poor social support, lower parental income, and lower maternal education all increase the impact of chronic disease on the family structure.[154,175] In addition, poor levels of support from close relatives can negatively impact the relationship between the parents.[176] Parents of children with chronic illness, particularly those with lower health-related QOL and under the age of 7 years, are particularly likely to see their children as vulnerable.[177] Parents of school-aged children with serious chronic illness see themselves as major facilitators of positive social interactions for their children.[178] Parents of children with critical congenital heart defects identified significant psychologic impacts caring for their children and were supportive of providing mental health services as part of their family's care.[179] Limbers and Skipper[180] identified a risk for poorer health-related QOL among the siblings of children with chronic illness. The siblings rated their own QOL more poorly than did their parents. Exercise training of children with cystic fibrosis and asthma increases exercise capacity and QOL, but similar studies have not been performed among BPD survivors.[181] Adolescents with chronic illness and their parents identified gaps in transition to adult care, including inadequate education, emotional attachment to pediatric providers, and lack of adult specialists in their diseases, that led to an expected postponement of transfer to adult providers until about the age of 25 years.[182] However, a similar study among former very low-birth-weight infants during young adulthood found no similar concern about transition to adulthood.[168]

CONCLUSION

In summary, BPD evolves from an acute illness cared for in the hospital to a chronic illness cared for at home. Like many diseases experienced in the NICU, it places significant stress on both parents and healthcare providers, with the experiences of each group bound in a complex web with the infant at the center. Like many chronic diseases, it continues to exact an emotional and physical toll on parents as their children grow and mature and leaves lasting effects on the QOL of the children themselves as they reach adolescence and adulthood.

REFERENCES

1. Perrin EC, Newacheck P, Pless IB, et al. Issues involved in the definition and classification of chronic health conditions. *Pediatrics*. 1993;91:787–793.
2. McPherson M, Arango P, Fox H, et al. A new definition of children with special health care needs. *Pediatrics*. 1998; 102:137–140.
3. Stein RE, Bauman LJ, Westbrook LE, Coupey SM, Ireys HT. Framework for identifying children who have chronic conditions: the case for a new definition. *J Pediatr*. 1993;122:342–347.
4. Malleske DT, Chorna O, Maitre NL. Pulmonary sequelae and functional limitations in children and adults with bronchopulmonary dysplasia. *Paediatr Respir Rev*. 2018; 26:55–59.

5. Baraldi E, Filippone M, Trevisanuto D, Zanardo V, Zacchello F. Pulmonary function until two years of life in infants with bronchopulmonary dysplasia. *Am J Respir Crit Care Med.* 1997;155:149−155.
6. Caskey S, Gough A, Rowan S, et al. Structural and functional lung impairment in adult survivors of bronchopulmonary dysplasia. *Ann Am Thorac Soc.* 2016;13: 1262−1270.
7. MacLean JE, DeHaan K, Fuhr D, et al. Altered breathing mechanics and ventilatory response during exercise in children born extremely preterm. *Thorax.* 2016;71: 1012−1019.
8. Gough A, Spence D, Linden M, Halliday HL, McGarvey LPA. General and respiratory health outcomes in adult survivors of bronchopulmonary dysplasia: a systematic review. *Chest.* 2012;141:1554−1567.
9. Baraldi E, Bonetto G, Zacchello F, Filippone M. Low exhaled nitric oxide in school-age children with bronchopulmonary dysplasia and airflow limitation. *Am J Respir Crit Care Med.* 2005;171:68−72.
10. Brostrom EB, Thunqvist P, Adenfelt G, Borling E, Katz-Salamon M. Obstructive lung disease in children with mild to severe BPD. *Respir Med.* 2010;104:362−370.
11. Fawke J, Lum S, Kirkby J, et al. Lung function and respiratory symptoms at 11 years in children born extremely preterm: the EPICure study. *Am J Respir Crit Care Med.* 2010;182:237−245.
12. Filippone M, Bonetto G, Corradi M, Frigo AC, Baraldi E. Evidence of unexpected oxidative stress in airways of adolescents born very pre-term. *Eur Respir J.* 2012;40: 1253−1259.
13. Gough A, Linden M, Spence D, Patterson CC, Halliday HL, McGarvey LP. Impaired lung function and health status in adult survivors of bronchopulmonary dysplasia. *Eur Respir J.* 2014;43:808−816.
14. Welsh L, Kirkby J, Lum S, et al. The EPICure study: maximal exercise and physical activity in school children born extremely preterm. *Thorax.* 2010;65:165−172.
15. Landry JS, Tremblay GM, Li PZ, Wong C, Benedetti A, Taivassalo T. Lung function and bronchial hyperresponsiveness in adults born prematurely. A cohort study. *Ann Am Thorac Soc.* 2016;13:17−24.
16. Lovering AT, Elliott JE, Laurie SS, et al. Ventilatory and sensory responses in adult survivors of preterm birth and bronchopulmonary dysplasia with reduced exercise capacity. *Ann Am Thorac Soc.* 2014;11:1528−1537.
17. DeMauro SB. The impact of bronchopulmonary dysplasia on childhood outcomes. *Clin Perinatol.* 2018; 45:439−452.
18. Stevens TP, Finer NN, Carlo WA, et al. Respiratory outcomes of the surfactant positive pressure and oximetry randomized trial (SUPPORT). *J Pediatr.* 2014;165, 240-249 e4.
19. Smith VC, Zupancic JA, McCormick MC, et al. Rehospitalization in the first year of life among infants with bronchopulmonary dysplasia. *J Pediatr.* 2004;144:799−803.
20. Gross SJ, Iannuzzi DM, Kveselis DA, Anbar RD. Effect of preterm birth on pulmonary function at school age: a prospective controlled study. *J Pediatr.* 1998;133: 188−192.
21. Chye JK, Gray PH. Rehospitalization and growth of infants with bronchopulmonary dysplasia: a matched control study. *J Paediatr Child Health.* 1995;31:105−111.
22. Kuint J, Lerner-Geva L, Chodick G, et al. Rehospitalization through childhood and adolescence: association with neonatal morbidities in infants of very low birth weight. *J Pediatr.* 2017;188, 135-141 e2.
23. Walter EC, Koepsell TD, Chien JW. Low birth weight and respiratory hospitalizations in adolescence. *Pediatr Pulmonol.* 2011;46:473−482.
24. Ortiz LE, McGrath-Morrow SA, Sterni LM, Collaco JM. Sleep disordered breathing in bronchopulmonary dysplasia. *Pediatr Pulmonol.* 2017;52:1583−1591.
25. Schmidt B, Roberts RS, Davis PG, et al. Prediction of late death or disability at age 5 Years using a count of 3 neonatal morbidities in very low birth weight infants. *J Pediatr.* 2015;167, 982-986 e2.
26. Holsti A, Serenius F, Farooqi A. Impact of major neonatal morbidities on adolescents born at 23-25 weeks of gestation. *Acta Paediatr.* 2018;107:1893−1901.
27. Farooqi A, Hagglof B, Sedin G, Serenius F. Impact at age 11 years of major neonatal morbidities in children born extremely preterm. *Pediatrics.* 2011;127:e1247−e1257.
28. Gray PH, O'Callaghan MJ, Poulsen L. Behaviour and quality of life at school age of children who had bronchopulmonary dysplasia. *Early Hum Dev.* 2008;84:1−8.
29. Short EJ, Klein NK, Lewis BA, et al. Cognitive and academic consequences of bronchopulmonary dysplasia and very low birth weight: 8-year-old outcomes. *Pediatrics.* 2003;112:e359.
30. Singer L, Yamashita T, Lilien L, Collin M, Baley J. A longitudinal study of developmental outcome of infants with bronchopulmonary dysplasia and very low birth weight. *Pediatrics.* 1997;100:987−993.
31. Miller RJ, Sullivan MC, Hawes K, Marks AK. The effects of perinatal morbidity and environmental factors on health status of preterm children at age 12. *J Pediatr Nurs.* 2009; 24:101−114.
32. Gough A, Linden MA, Spence D, Halliday HL, Patterson CC, McGarvey L. Executive functioning deficits in young adult survivors of bronchopulmonary dysplasia. *Disabil Rehabil.* 2015;37:1940−1945.
33. Abman SH, Collaco JM, Shepherd EG, et al. Interdisciplinary care of children with severe bronchopulmonary dysplasia. *J Pediatr.* 2017;181, 12-28 e1.
34. Doyle LW, Faber B, Callanan C, Freezer N, Ford GW, Davis NM. Bronchopulmonary dysplasia in very low birth weight subjects and lung function in late adolescence. *Pediatrics.* 2006;118:108−113.
35. Collaco JM, Romer LH, Stuart BD, et al. Frontiers in pulmonary hypertension in infants and children with bronchopulmonary dysplasia. *Pediatr Pulmonol.* 2012;47: 1042−1053.
36. Slaughter JL, Stenger MR, Reagan PB, Jadcherla SR. Inhaled bronchodilator use for infants with bronchopulmonary dysplasia. *J Perinatol.* 2015;35:61−66.

37. Zivanovic S, Pushparajah K, Calvert S, et al. Pulmonary artery pressures in school-age children born prematurely. *J Pediatr*. 2017;191:42–49. e3.
38. Boroughs D, Dougherty JA. Decreasing accidental mortality of ventilator-dependent children at home: a call to action. *Home Healthc Nurse*. 2012;30:103–111.
39. Cristea AI, Carroll AE, Davis SD, Swigonski NL, Ackerman VL. Outcomes of children with severe bronchopulmonary dysplasia who were ventilator dependent at home. *Pediatrics*. 2013;132:e727–e734.
40. Edwards JD, Kun SS, Keens TG. Outcomes and causes of death in children on home mechanical ventilation via tracheostomy: an institutional and literature review. *J Pediatr*. 2010;157, 955-959 e2.
41. Rane S, Shankaran S, Natarajan G. Parental perception of functional status following tracheostomy in infancy: a single center study. *J Pediatr*. 2013;163:860–866.
42. Moon NM, Mohay HA, Gray PH. Developmental patterns from 1 to 4 years of extremely preterm infants who required home oxygen therapy. *Early Hum Dev*. 2007;83:209–216.
43. Bronfenbrenner U, Ceci SJ. Nature-nurture reconceptualized in developmental perspective: a bioecological model. *Psychol Rev*. 1994;101:568–586.
44. Hall EO. Being in an alien world: Danish parents' lived experiences when a newborn or small child is critically ill. *Scand J Caring Sci*. 2005;19:179–185.
45. Arnold L, Sawyer A, Rabe H, et al. Parents' first moments with their very preterm babies: a qualitative study. *BMJ Open*. 2013;3(4).
46. Russell G, Sawyer A, Rabe H, et al. Parents' views on care of their very premature babies in neonatal intensive care units: a qualitative study. *BMC Pediatr*. 2014;14:230.
47. Miles MS, Funk SG, Carlson J. Parental Stressor Scale: neonatal intensive care unit. *Nurs Res*. 1993;42:148–152.
48. Holditch-Davis D, Miles MS, Weaver MA, et al. Patterns of distress in African-American mothers of preterm infants. *J Dev Behav Pediatr*. 2009;30:193–205.
49. Heidari H, Hasanpour M, Fooladi M. The Iranian parents of premature infants in NICU experience stigma of shame. *Med Arh*. 2012;66:35–40.
50. Whittingham K, Boyd RN, Sanders MR, Colditz P. Parenting and prematurity: understanding parent experiences and preferences for support. *J Child Fam Stud*. 2014; 23:1050–1061.
51. D'Angio CT, Mercurio MR. Evidence-based ethics in the "gray zone" of neonatal viability: promises and limitations. *Pediatr Health*. 2008;2:777–786.
52. Dorheim SK, Bondevik GT, Eberhard-Gran M, Bjorvatn B. Sleep and depression in postpartum women: a population-based study. *Sleep*. 2009;32:847–855.
53. Busse M, Stromgren K, Thorngate L, Thomas KA. Parents' responses to stress in the neonatal intensive care unit. *Crit Care Nurse*. 2013;33:52–59.
54. Miles MS, Holditch-Davis D. Parenting the prematurely born child: pathways of influence. *Semin Perinatol*. 1997;21:254–266.
55. Cyr-Alves H, Macken L, Hyrkas K. Stress and symptoms of depression in fathers of infants admitted to the NICU. *J Obstet Gynecol Neonatal Nurs*. 2018;47:146–157.
56. Mackley AB, Locke RG, Spear ML, Joseph R. Forgotten parent: NICU paternal emotional response. *Adv Neonatal Care*. 2010;10:200–203.
57. Shaw RJ, Lilo EA, Storfer-Isser A, et al. Screening for symptoms of postpartum traumatic stress in a sample of mothers with preterm infants. *Issues Ment Health Nurs*. 2014;35:198–207.
58. Lefkowitz DS, Baxt C, Evans JR. Prevalence and correlates of posttraumatic stress and postpartum depression in parents of infants in the Neonatal Intensive Care Unit (NICU). *J Clin Psychol Med Settings*. 2010;17:230–237.
59. Doering LV, Moser DK, Dracup K. Correlates of anxiety, hostility, depression, and psychosocial adjustment in parents of NICU infants. *Neonatal Netw*. 2000;19:15–23.
60. Hummel P. Parenting the highrisk infant. *Nborn Infant Nurs Rev*. 2003;3:88–92.
61. Lubbe W, Bornman J. Early intervention care programme for parents of neonates. *Curationis*. 2005;28:73–82.
62. Miles MS, Brunssen SH. Psychometric properties of the parental stressor scale: infant hospitalization. *Adv Neonatal Care*. 2003;3:189–196.
63. Cleveland LM. Parenting in the neonatal intensive care unit. *J Obstet Gynecol Neonatal Nurs*. 2008;37:666–691.
64. Turan T, Basbakkal Z, Ozbek S. Effect of nursing interventions on stressors of parents of premature infants in neonatal intensive care unit. *J Clin Nurs*. 2008;17: 2856–2866.
65. Akkoyun S, Tas Arslan F. Investigation of stress and nursing support in mothers of preterm infants in neonatal intensive care units. *Scand J Caring Sci*. 2018; 32. Nov 14 [epub ahead of print].
66. Wormald F, Tapia JL, Torres G, et al. Stress in parents of very low birth weight preterm infants hospitalized in neonatal intensive care units. A multicenter study. *Arch Argent Pediatr*. 2015;113:303–309.
67. Baia I, Amorim M, Silva S, Kelly-Irving M, de Freitas C, Alves E. Parenting very preterm infants and stress in neonatal intensive care units. *Early Hum Dev*. 2016;101: 3–9.
68. Carter J, Dwyer N, Roselund J, et al. Systematic changes to help parents of medically complex infants manage medical expenses. *Adv Neonatal Care*. 2017;17:461–469.
69. Ichijima E, Kirk R, Hornblow A. Parental support in neonatal intensive care units: a cross-cultural comparison between New Zealand and Japan. *J Pediatr Nurs*. 2011;26: 206–215.
70. Joseph RA, Mackley AB, Davis CG, Spear ML, Locke RG. Stress in fathers of surgical neonatal intensive care unit babies. *Adv Neonatal Care*. 2007;7:321–325.
71. Deeney K, Lohan M, Parkes J, Spence D. Experiences of fathers of babies in intensive care. *Paediatr Nurs*. 2009; 21:45–47.
72. Dutta S, Mahajan R, Agrawal SK, Nehra R, Narang A. Stress in fathers of premature newborns admitted in a

neonatal intensive care unit. *Indian Pediatr.* 2016;53:311–313.
73. Logan RM, Dormire S. Finding my way: a phenomenology of fathering in the NICU. *Adv Neonatal Care.* 2018;18:154–162.
74. Martel MJ, Milette I, Bell L, Tribble DS, Payot A. Establishment of the relationship between fathers and premature infants in neonatal units. *Adv Neonatal Care.* 2016;16:390–398.
75. Noergaard B, Ammentorp J, Garne E, Fenger-Gron J, Kofoed PE. Fathers' stress in a neonatal intensive care unit. *Adv Neonatal Care.* 2018;18:413–422.
76. Swift MC, Scholten I. Not feeding, not coming home: parental experiences of infant feeding difficulties and family relationships in a neonatal unit. *J Clin Nurs.* 2010;19:249–258.
77. Janvier A, Lantos J, Aschner J, et al. Stronger and more vulnerable: a balanced view of the impacts of the NICU experience on parents. *Pediatrics.* 2016;138:e20160655.
78. Fegran L, Helseth S, Fagermoen MS. A comparison of mothers' and fathers' experiences of the attachment process in a neonatal intensive care unit. *J Clin Nurs.* 2008;17:810–816.
79. Sarkadi A, Kristiansson R, Oberklaid F, Bremberg S. Fathers' involvement and children's developmental outcomes: a systematic review of longitudinal studies. *Acta Paediatr.* 2008;97:153–158.
80. Melnyk BM, Feinstein NF, Alpert-Gillis L, et al. Reducing premature infants' length of stay and improving parents' mental health outcomes with the creating opportunities for parent empowerment (COPE) neonatal intensive care unit program: a randomized, controlled trial. *Pediatrics.* 2006;118:e1414–e1427.
81. Feldman R, Eidelman AI, Sirota L, Weller A. Comparison of skin-to-skin (kangaroo) and traditional care: parenting outcomes and preterm infant development. *Pediatrics.* 2002;110:16–26.
82. He SW, Xiong YE, Zhu LH, et al. Impact of family integrated care on infants' clinical outcomes in two children's hospitals in China: a pre-post intervention study. *Ital J Pediatr.* 2018;44:65.
83. Hagen IH, Iversen VC, Nesset E, Orner R, Svindseth MF. Parental satisfaction with neonatal intensive care units: a quantitative cross-sectional study. *BMC Health Serv Res.* 2019;19:37.
84. Hall EO, Brinchmann BS, Aagaard H. The challenge of integrating justice and care in neonatal nursing. *Nurs Ethics.* 2012;19:80–90.
85. Gallagher K, Shaw C, Aladangady N, Marlow N. Parental experience of interaction with healthcare professionals during their infant's stay in the neonatal intensive care unit. *Arch Dis Child Fetal Neonatal Ed.* 2018;103:F343–F348.
86. Enlow E, Faherty LJ, Wallace-Keeshen S, Martin AE, Shea JA, Lorch SA. Perspectives of low socioeconomic status mothers of premature infants. *Pediatrics.* 2017;139.
87. Al Maghaireh DF, Abdullah KL, Chan CM, Piaw CY, Al Kawafha MM. Systematic review of qualitative studies exploring parental experiences in the neonatal intensive care unit. *J Clin Nurs.* 2016;25:2745–2756.
88. Speziale H, Streubert H, Carpenter D. *Qualitative Research in Nursing: Advancing the Humanistic Imperative.* Philadelphia, PA: Wolters Kluwer; 2011.
89. Cho ES, Kim SJ, Kwon MS, et al. The effects of kangaroo care in the neonatal intensive care unit on the physiological functions of preterm infants, maternal-infant attachment, and maternal stress. *J Pediatr Nurs.* 2016;31:430–438.
90. Jones H, Santamaria N. Physiological benefits to parents from undertaking skin-to-skin contact with their neonate, in a neonatal intensive special care unit. *Scand J Caring Sci.* 2018;32:1012–1017.
91. Bera A, Ghosh J, Singh AK, Hazra A, Som T, Munian D. Effect of kangaroo mother care on vital physiological parameters of the low birth weight newborn. *Indian J Community Med.* 2014;39:245–249.
92. Ortenstrand A, Westrup B, Brostrom EB, et al. The stockholm neonatal family centered care study: effects on length of stay and infant morbidity. *Pediatrics.* 2010;125:e278–e285.
93. Aagaard H, Hall EO. Mothers' experiences of having a preterm infant in the neonatal care unit: a meta-synthesis. *J Pediatr Nurs.* 2008;23:e26–36.
94. Preyde M, Ardal F. Effectiveness of a parent "buddy" program for mothers of very preterm infants in a neonatal intensive care unit. *Can Med Assoc J.* 2003;168:969–973.
95. Bracht M, Kandankery A, Nodwell S, Stade B. Cultural differences and parental responses to the preterm infant at risk: strategies for supporting families. *Neonatal Netw.* 2002;21:31–38.
96. Prouhet PM, Gregory MR, Russell CL, Yaeger LH. Fathers' stress in the neonatal intensive care unit: a systematic review. *Adv Neonatal Care.* 2018;18:105–120.
97. Massoudi P, Wickberg B, Hwang CP. Fathers' involvement in Swedish child health care - the role of nurses' practices and attitudes. *Acta Paediatr.* 2011;100:396–401.
98. Meijssen DE, Wolf MJ, Koldewijn K, van Wassenaer AG, Kok JH, van Baar AL. Parenting stress in mothers after very preterm birth and the effect of the Infant Behavioural Assessment and Intervention Program. *Child Care Health Dev.* 2011;37:195–202.
99. Matricardi S, Agostino R, Fedeli C, Montirosso R. Mothers are not fathers: differences between parents in the reduction of stress levels after a parental intervention in a NICU. *Acta Paediatr.* 2013;102:8–14.
100. Melnyk BM, Alpert-Gillis L, Feinstein NF, et al. Improving cognitive development of low-birth-weight premature infants with the COPE program: a pilot study of the benefit of early NICU intervention with mothers. *Res Nurs Health.* 2001;24:373–389.
101. Modjarrad K. STUDENTJAMA. Medicine and spirituality. *JAMA.* 2004;291:2880.
102. Wilson SM, Miles MS. Spirituality in African-American mothers coping with a seriously ill infant. *J Soc Pediatr Nurses.* 2001;6:116–122.

103. Grant D. Spiritual interventions: how, when, and why nurses use them. *Holist Nurs Pract*. 2004;18:36–41.
104. Kucuk Alemdar D, Kardas Ozdemir F, Guducu Tufekci F. The effect of spiritual care on stress levels of mothers in NICU. *West J Nurs Res*. 2018;40:997–1011.
105. Fischer JE, Calame A, Dettling AC, Zeier H, Fanconi S. Experience and endocrine stress responses in neonatal and pediatric critical care nurses and physicians. *Crit Care Med*. 2000;28:3281–3288.
106. Fourie C. Moral distress and moral conflict in clinical ethics. *Bioethics*. 2015;29:91–97.
107. Trotochaud K, Coleman JR, Krawiecki N, McCracken C. Moral distress in pediatric healthcare providers. *J Pediatr Nurs*. 2015;30:908–914.
108. Barker DP, Rutter N. Exposure to invasive procedures in neonatal intensive care unit admissions. *Arch Dis Child Fetal Neonatal Ed*. 1995;72:F47–F48.
109. Hanna DR. The lived experience of moral distress: nurses who assisted with elective abortions. *Res Theory Nurs Pract*. 2005;19:95–124.
110. Baggs JG, Schmitt MH. Nurses' and resident physicians' perceptions of the process of collaboration in an MICU. *Res Nurs Health*. 1997;20:71–80.
111. Karanikola MN, Papathanassoglou ED, Kalafati M, Stathopoulou H. Exploration of the association between professional interactions and emotional distress of intensive care unit nursing personnel. *Dimens Crit Care Nurs*. 2012;31:37–45.
112. Bruce CR, Miller SM, Zimmerman JL. A qualitative study exploring moral distress in the ICU team: the importance of unit functionality and intrateam dynamics. *Crit Care Med*. 2015;43:823–831.
113. Whitehead PB, Herbertson RK, Hamric AB, Epstein EG, Fisher JM. Moral distress among healthcare professionals: report of an institution-wide survey. *J Nurs Scholarsh*. 2015;47:117–125.
114. Solomon MZ, Sellers DE, Heller KS, et al. New and lingering controversies in pediatric end-of-life care. *Pediatrics*. 2005;116:872–883.
115. Privitera MR, Rosenstein AH, Plessow F, LoCastro TM. Physician Burnout and Occupational Stress: an inconvenient truth with unintended consequences. *J Hosp Adm*. 2015;4:27–35.
116. Prentice T, Janvier A, Gillam L, Davis PG. Moral distress within neonatal and paediatric intensive care units: a systematic review. *Arch Dis Child*. 2016;101:701–708.
117. Hamric AB, Epstein EG. A health system-wide moral distress consultation service: development and evaluation. *HEC Forum*. 2017;29:127–143.
118. Chiafery MC, Hopkins P, Norton SA, Shaw MH. Nursing ethics huddles to decrease moral distress among nurses in the intensive care unit. *J Clin Ethics*. 2018;29:217–226.
119. Epstein S, Geniteau E, Christin P, et al. Role of a clinical nurse specialist within a paediatric multidisciplinary weight-management programme team. *J Clin Nurs*. 2010;19:2649–2651.
120. Victor B, Cullen J. The organizational bases of ethical work climates. *Adm Sci Q*. 1988;33:101–125.
121. Edmondson AC. Psychological safety, trust, and learning in organizations: a group-level lens. In: Kramer RM, Cook KS, eds. *Trust and Distrust in Organizations: Dilemmas and Approaches*. New York: Russell Sage; 2004:239–272.
122. Rathert C, Fleming DA. Hospital ethical climate and teamwork in acute care: the moderating role of leaders. *Health Care Manag Rev*. 2008;33:323–331.
123. Nembhard IM, Edmondson AC. Making it safe: the effects of leader inclusiveness and professional status on psychological safety and improvement efforts in health care teams. *J Organ Behav*. 2006;27:941–966.
124. de Boer JC, van Blijderveen G, van Dijk G, Duivenvoorden HJ, Williams M. Implementing structured, multiprofessional medical ethical decision-making in a neonatal intensive care unit. *J Med Ethics*. 2012;38:596–601.
125. Placencia FX, McCullough LB. Biopsychosocial risks of parental care for high-risk neonates: implications for evidence-based parental counseling. *J Perinatol*. 2012; 32:381–386.
126. Hall SL, Cross J, Selix NW, et al. Recommendations for enhancing psychosocial support of NICU parents through staff education and support. *J Perinatol*. 2015; 35(Suppl 1):S29–S36.
127. Pines A, Aronson E. *Career Burnout. Causes and Cures*. New York: The Free Press; 1988.
128. Porta NFM. Palliative care approaches to neonates with chronic respiratory failure. *Semin Perinatol*. 2017;41: 124–127.
129. Caldeira S, Hall J. Spiritual leadership and spiritual care in neonatology. *J Nurs Manag*. 2012;20:1069–1075.
130. Bellieni CV, Righetti P, Ciampa R, Iacoponi F, Coviello C, Buonocore G. Assessing burnout among neonatologists. *J Matern Fetal Neonatal Med*. 2012;25:2130–2134.
131. Weintraub AS, Geithner EM, Stroustrup A, Waldman ED. Compassion fatigue, burnout and compassion satisfaction in neonatologists in the US. *J Perinatol*. 2016;36: 1021–1026.
132. Stewart DE, Ahmad F, Cheung AM, Bergman B, Dell DL. Women physicians and stress. *J Women's Health Gend Based Med*. 2000;9:185–190.
133. Moore LR, Ziegler C, Hessler A, Singhal D, LaFaver K. Burnout and career satisfaction in women neurologists in the United States. *J Womens Health (Larchmt)*. 2019; 28(4), 515-52.
134. Rotenstein LS, Torre M, Ramos MA, et al. Prevalence of burnout among physicians: a systematic review. *JAMA*. 2018;320:1131–1150.
135. Klein SD, Bucher HU, Hendriks MJ, et al. Sources of distress for physicians and nurses working in Swiss neonatal intensive care units. *Swiss Med Wkly*. 2017; 147:w14477.
136. Hunsaker S, Chen HC, Maughan D, Heaston S. Factors that influence the development of compassion fatigue, burnout, and compassion satisfaction in emergency department nurses. *J Nurs Scholarsh*. 2015;47:186–194.
137. Cuartero ML, Campos-Vidal Jf PhD L. Self-care behaviours and their relationship with Satisfaction and

Compassion Fatigue levels among social workers. *Soc Work Health Care*. 2019;58:274–290.

138. Delaney MC. Caring for the caregivers: evaluation of the effect of an eight-week pilot mindful self-compassion (MSC) training program on nurses' compassion fatigue and resilience. *PLoS One*. 2018;13:e0207261.
139. Graham P, Zerbi G, Norcross W, Montross-Thomas L, Lobbestael L, Davidson J. Testing of A Caregiver support team. *Explore*. 2019;15:19–26.
140. Zanardo V, Freato F. Home oxygen therapy in infants with bronchopulmonary dysplasia: assessment of parental anxiety. *Early Hum Dev*. 2001;65:39–46.
141. Willis V. Parenting preemies: a unique program for family support and education after NICU discharge. *Adv Neonatal Care*. 2008;8:221–230.
142. Paul IM, Phillips TA, Widome MD, Hollenbeak CS. Cost-effectiveness of postnatal home nursing visits for prevention of hospital care for jaundice and dehydration. *Pediatrics*. 2004;114:1015–1022.
143. Lindberg B, Axelsson K, Ohrling K. Experience with videoconferencing between a neonatal unit and the families' home from the perspective of certified paediatric nurses. *J Telemed Telecare*. 2009;15:275–280.
144. Lasby K, Newton S, von Platen A. Neonatal transitional care. *Can Nurse*. 2004;100:18–23.
145. Glazebrook C, Marlow N, Israel C, et al. Randomised trial of a parenting intervention during neonatal intensive care. *Arch Dis Child Fetal Neonatal Ed*. 2007;92: F438–F443.
146. Broedsgaard A, Wagner L. How to facilitate parents and their premature infant for the transition home. *Int Nurs Rev*. 2005;52:196–203.
147. Vohr BR, Yatchmink YE, Burke RT, et al. Factors associated with rehospitalizations of very low birthweight infants: impact of a transition home support and education program. *Early Hum Dev*. 2012;88:455–460.
148. Lopez GL, Anderson KH, Feutchinger J. Transition of premature infants from hospital to home life. *Neonatal Netw*. 2012;31:207–214.
149. Broyles RS, Tyson JE, Heyne ET, et al. Comprehensive follow-up care and life-threatening illnesses among high-risk infants: a randomized controlled trial. *JAMA*. 2000;284:2070–2076.
150. Kuo DZ, Lyle RE, Casey PH, Stille CJ. Care system redesign for preterm children after discharge from the NICU. *Pediatrics*. 2017;139:e20162969.
151. Ohio Perinatal Quality Collaborative. *Improving Transition from NICU to Home for Infants Requiring Complex Care: NICU Graduates Change Package*. 2018.
152. Manns SV. Life after the NNU: the long term effects on mothers' lives, managing a child at home with broncho-pulmonary dysplasia and on home oxygen. *Neuroendocrinol Lett*. 2004;25(Suppl 1):127–132.
153. Feeley CA, Turner-Henson A, Christian BJ, et al. Sleep quality, stress, caregiver burden, and quality of life in maternal caregivers of young children with bronchopulmonary dysplasia. *J Pediatr Nurs*. 2014;29:29–38.
154. Balakrishnan A, Stephens BE, Burke RT, et al. Impact of very low birth weight infants on the family at 3 months corrected age. *Early Hum Dev*. 2011;87:31–35.
155. Moura MR, Araujo CG, Prado MM, et al. Factors associated with the quality of life of mothers of preterm infants with very low birth weight: a 3-year follow-up study. *Qual Life Res*. 2017;26:1349–1360.
156. McGrath-Morrow SA, Ryan T, Riekert K, Lefton-Greif MA, Eakin M, Collaco JM. The impact of bronchopulmonary dysplasia on caregiver health related quality of life during the first 2 years of life. *Pediatr Pulmonol*. 2013;48: 579–586.
157. Wolke D, Baumann N, Busch B, Bartmann P. Very preterm birth and parents' quality of life 27 Years later. *Pediatrics*. 2017;140.
158. Lodha A, Lakhani J, Ediger K, et al. Do preterm infants with a birth weight </=1250 g born to single-parent families have poorer neurodevelopmental outcomes at age 3 than those born to two-parent families? *J Perinatol*. 2018; 38:900–907.
159. Brady JM, Pouppirt N, Bernbaum J, et al. Why do children with severe bronchopulmonary dysplasia not attend neonatal follow-up care? Parental views of barriers. *Acta Paediatr*. 2018;107:996–1002.
160. McGrath-Morrow SA, Lee G, Stewart BH, et al. Day care increases the risk of respiratory morbidity in chronic lung disease of prematurity. *Pediatrics*. 2010;126:632–637.
161. Brady JM, Zhang H, Kirpalani H, DeMauro SB. Living with severe bronchopulmonary dysplasia-parental views of their child's quality of life. *J Pediatr*. 2018;207. Nov 5 [epub ahead of print].
162. Sriram S, Schreiber MD, Msall ME, et al. Cognitive development and quality of life associated with BPD in 10-year-olds born preterm. *Pediatrics*. 2018;141:e20172719.
163. Ronkainen E, Kaukola T, Marttila R, Hallman M, Dunder T. School-age children enjoyed good respiratory health and fewer allergies despite having lung disease after preterm birth. *Acta Paediatr*. 2016;105:1298–1304.
164. Meijer-Schaap L, Dubois AEJ, Kollen BJ, Tijmens-van der Hulst J, Flokstra-de Blok BMJ, Vrijlandt E. Development and construct validation of a parent-proxy quality of life instrument in children with bronchopulmonary dysplasia aged 4-8 years old. *Qual Life Res*. 2019;28: 523–533.
165. Bojanic K, Grizelj R, Vukovic J, et al. Health-related quality of life in children and adolescents with congenital diaphragmatic hernia: a cross-sectional study. *Health Qual Life Outcomes*. 2018;16:50.
166. Bozzetto S, Carraro S, Tomasi L, Berardi M, Zanconato S, Baraldi E. Health-related quality of life in adolescent survivors of bronchopulmonary dysplasia. *Respirology*. 2016; 21:1113–1117.
167. Beaudoin S, Tremblay GM, Croitoru D, Benedetti A, Landry JS. Healthcare utilization and health-related quality of life of adult survivors of preterm birth complicated by bronchopulmonary dysplasia. *Acta Paediatr*. 2013; 102:607–612.

168. Gaddlin PO, Finnstrom O, Sydsjo G, Leijon I. Most very low birth weight subjects do well as adults. *Acta Paediatr.* 2009;98:1513–1520.
169. Singer LT, Fulton S, Davillier M, Koshy D, Salvator A, Baley JE. Effects of infant risk status and maternal psychological distress on maternal-infant interactions during the first year of life. *J Dev Behav Pediatr.* 2003;24: 233–241.
170. Jaworski M, Janvier A, Lefebvre F, Luu TM. Parental perspectives regarding outcomes of very preterm infants: toward a balanced approach. *J Pediatr.* 2018;200, 58-63 e1.
171. Koldewijn K, Wolf MJ, van Wassenaer A, et al. The Infant Behavioral Assessment and Intervention Program for very low birth weight infants at 6 months corrected age. *J Pediatr.* 2009;154, 33-8 e2.
172. Koldewijn K, van Wassenaer A, Wolf MJ, et al. A neurobehavioral intervention and assessment program in very low birth weight infants: outcome at 24 months. *J Pediatr.* 2010;156:359–365.
173. Verkerk G, Jeukens-Visser M, Houtzager B, et al. The infant behavioral assessment and intervention program in very low birth weight infants; outcome on executive functioning, behaviour and cognition at preschool age. *Early Hum Dev.* 2012;88:699–705.
174. Muscara F, McCarthy MC, Hearps SJC, et al. Featured article: trajectories of posttraumatic stress symptoms in parents of children with a serious childhood illness or injury. *J Pediatr Psychol.* 2018;43:1072–1082.
175. Simsek IE, Erel S, Simsek TT, et al. Factors related to the impact of chronically disabled children on their families. *Pediatr Neurol.* 2014;50:255–261.
176. Laakkonen H, Taskinen S, Ronnholm K, Holmberg C, Sandberg S. Parent-child and spousal relationships in families with a young child with end-stage renal disease. *Pediatr Nephrol.* 2014;29:289–295.
177. Houtzager BA, Moller EL, Maurice-Stam H, Last BF, Grootenhuis MA. Parental perceptions of child vulnerability in a community-based sample: association with chronic illness and health-related quality of life. *J Child Health Care.* 2015;19:454–465.
178. Janin MMH, Ellis SJ, Lum A, Wakefield CE, Fardell JE. Parents' perspectives on their child's social experience in the context of childhood chronic illness: a qualitative study. *J Pediatr Nurs.* 2018;42:e10–e18.
179. Woolf-King SE, Arnold E, Weiss S, Teitel D. "There's no acknowledgement of what this does to people": a qualitative exploration of mental health among parents of children with critical congenital heart defects. *J Clin Nurs.* 2018;27:2785–2794.
180. Limbers CA, Skipper S. Health-related quality of life measurement in siblings of children with physical chronic illness: a systematic review. *Fam Syst Health.* 2014;32: 408–415.
181. Joschtel B, Gomersall SR, Tweedy S, Petsky H, Chang AB, Trost SG. Effects of exercise training on physical and psychosocial health in children with chronic respiratory disease: a systematic review and meta-analysis. *BMJ Open Sport Exerc Med.* 2018;4:e000409.
182. Fernandes SM, O'Sullivan-Oliveira J, Landzberg MJ, et al. Transition and transfer of adolescents and young adults with pediatric onset chronic disease: the patient and parent perspective. *J Pediatr Rehabil Med.* 2014;7:43–51.

Index

Note: Page numbers followed by "f" indicate figures, "t" indicates tables and "b" indicates boxes.